A PRACTICAL GUIDE TO GLOBAL HEALTH SERVICE

EDWARD O'NEIL, JR, MD

AMA
AMERICAN
MEDICAL
ASSOCIATION

American Medical Association
Vice President, Business Products: Anthony J. Frankos
Executive Director, Editorial and Operations: Mary Lou White
Director, Production and Manufacturing: Jean Roberts
Senior Acquisitions Editor: Suzanne Fraker
Developmental Editors: Katharine Dvorak and Carol Brockman
Director, Marketing: Pamela Palmersheim
Director, Sales: J.D. Kinney
Marketing Manager: Amy Burgess
Senior Production Coordinator: Boon Ai Tan
Senior Print Coordinator: Ronnie Summers

Cover photo credits: top left, photo courtesy of Father Bill Fryda, MD; top right, photo courtesy of James Eadie, MD; bottom left, © Dang Ngo/ZUMA Press; bottom right, © Ian Berry/Magnum Photos.

www.ama-assn.org

This book is for informational purposes only. It is not intended to constitute legal or other professional advice. If legal or other professional advice is required, the services of a competent professional should be sought. The views expressed in this book are the author's and do not necessarily reflect the views of the AMA. The names of organizations appearing in the book are for informational purposes only. Their incluson does not imply AMA endorsement.

Additional copies of this book may be ordered by calling 800 621-8335 or from the secure AMA Web site at www.amabookstore.com. Refer to product number OP420805.

Library of Congress Cataloging-in-Publication Data

O'Neil, Edward.
A practical guide to global health service / Edward O'Neil Jr.
p. ; cm.
Includes bibliographical references.
Summary: "A health providers guide to the practical aspects of serving internationally, including data on more then 300 organizations that send health providers overseas"—Provided by publisher.
ISBN 1-57947-673-2
1. Medical assistance, American. 2. Public health—International cooperation. 3. Voluntary health agencies—Directories. 4. Volunteer workers in medical care. 5. World health.
[DNLM: 1. World Health—Directory. 2. International Cooperation—Directory. 3. Organizations—Directory. 4. Voluntary Workers. WA 22.1 O58p 2006] I. American Medical Association. II. Title.

RA390.U5O54 2006
610.73'7—dc22 2005037136

ISBN 1-57947-673-2
BP08:05-P-044:04/06

Dedication

To my colleagues at Omni Med: Drs John O'Brien, James Eadie, Michael Morley, Katharine Morrow, John Varallo, and Peter and Nancy Mogielnicki. Where you have gone, may many more of our colleagues follow. To our many volunteers who have given so much through the years. And to Roger Sublett, Robert Sparks, Kathryn Johnson, Harry Barnes, Loretta Garcia Palacio, and Fran Wang for standing by me from the beginning and making this all possible.

To my colleagues in the medical profession: I stand in awe of your abilities to heal, to restore, and to improve life. I hope you will extend your reach to those who most need you and join in the struggle to heal our world.

And, finally, to the many people in developing countries—particularly Belize, Tanzania, Kenya, and Guyana—who have taught me so much. I hope this book will encourage more people to work *with* you to bring to fruition the dream of the ancient prophets—a just world order with health, longevity, and basic rights for all.

Contents

Acknowledgments

This book began as a concept in 1993 and evolved into a quest during the ensuing 13 years. Its roots go back further to my experiences as a medical student working in rural Tanzania in 1987. The wealth of information that has been generated from this quest has resulted in two books, this one and its companion text *Awakening Hippocrates: A Primer on Health, Poverty, and Global Service.* It took a great number of people many years to compile the data contained within this book. Similarly, many others have played important roles, whether as supporters, advisors, or sounding boards. I devoted an inordinate number of pages to the important task of thanking all of these people in *Awakening Hippocrates.* I will attempt to restrain my impulses here and ask readers to refer to the Acknowledgments of *Awakening Hippocrates* for a more complete listing. Some acknowledgments, however, bear repetition.

I will start with the group that has played the most important role: my family. I can never thank my wife Judy enough for her willingness to put aside her own careers to care for our kids at home while I pursued this quest. Judy has been a constant source of wisdom, support, and strength during this entire process. I avoid clichés whenever possible, but this one is unavoidable—without you, neither of these books would have happened. The writing of both books has spanned the births of our three children, James, Michaela, and Sean. There is no doubt that the writing has taken me away from them far more than we had hoped, either through missed vacations or years of late night and weekend writing sessions, but it is time I hope to make up. When my son James crept downstairs to visit late at night or my daughter insisted that I draw "fishies" all over an early manuscript, they gave me reprieves from the work and brought more clearly into focus the reasons to continue.

Both of my parents instilled a strong sense of justice, and the strong moral tone of both of these books very much reflects their influence on me. For years, both sacrificed to pay for college and help with medical school tuitions. They have always been there for me, and I hope this book in some small way repays their efforts. My three older sisters, too, have always been there for me, something of which I am ever mindful. My uncle Frank became a close friend and strong supporter of this work; I was fortunate to spend his last days with him, and I carry his love and support with me.

This book is inextricably linked to Omni Med, the nongovernmental organization (NGO) I founded in 1998. Belize became the site of the first Omni Med program and introduced me to an impressive group of people, including Loretta and

Vincent Palacio, Peter Allen, Austin Flores, Francis Smith, Bill Butcher, Fred Martinez, and many others. I have long admired the scores of physicians, nurses, and technicians throughout the hospitals in Belize who have allowed me to work among them and learn from their steadfast dedication. Many of the lessons I have learned about global health, I have learned in Belize and from these people. My heartfelt thanks to all of them. Similarly, Father Bill Fryda in Kenya has been a long-time teacher and friend. I hope many more people learn about St Mary's Hospital in Nairobi through these books, and I thank Bill for his visionary leadership and his influence.

I came to Belize only because of an extraordinary group of individuals that came together under the banner of Rotary International. From the time I first met Richard Bridges, Sheldon Daly, Harold Lincoln, and Jim Roberts from the Hingham Rotary Club, I knew this group was special. Richard Bridges became a good friend and a model of ethical and servant leadership, while a host of other club members impressed me with their dedication to service. In Belize, a small group of people that comprised the Orange Walk Rotary Club joined up with the Hingham Rotarians to turn a small idea into a multi-million dollar service effort. I have the good fortune to count its many members among my teachers and friends in Belize.

This book also owes an enormous debt to the people who make up Omni Med. All of the author's royalties will go to Omni Med and directly into our programs, one of which is the maintenance of the database information featured within this book. To those who question why someone would work gratis for nearly 10 years at an NGO, I can only advise them to look at our results. I am proud of those who have come into the Omni Med family and done such extraordinary things with so little funding. Dr John O'Brien has become a close friend and an indispensable part of our NGO's work in Belize and Guyana. Drs Michael Morley and Katharine Morrow joined our little effort in Belize and founded a successful program in Thailand that continues to expand. Dr James Eadie evolved from a promising student at Harvard Medical School into a seasoned physician who founded and now directs our program in Guyana. Dr John Varallo joined Omni Med and has turned a novel idea into a cervical cancer-screening program that is becoming a national model in Guyana. Peter and Nancy Mogielnicki have participated in almost all of our programs and introduced several other Dartmouth-Hitchcock physicians to Omni Med. For that and your ongoing support and involvement, thanks. None of these physicians is compensated for their time or effort; all cover their own travel expenses, and all of us share an ideal that we should be doing this. I can never thank each of you enough for your time, your sacrifice, and your extraordinary dedication to this cause. To the scores of health providers that have served through our various programs, I offer a heartfelt thanks.

Behind any effort like that of Omni Med's exists a group that supports and sustains it. I could not have a better board of directors than the one we have, all with Kellogg Foundation roots. Roger Sublett has supported my efforts from the beginning. He became the first board member, the first donor, and encouraged me from the outset to turn these ideas into a book and a functioning, living organization.

Omni Med, and most likely this book, would not exist if not for the support, encouragement, friendship, and wise counsel of Dr Sublett. My study of ethical leadership offered no better example than the man who became an important mentor. Roger, thanks.

Our other board members have helped guide Omni Med and me through some turbulent times, many brought on by our dire finances. Robert Sparks has always been there for me, always with the right take on any complicated situation that arises. Likewise, Kathryn Johnson has always been there personally and professionally and has lent her great vision and strategic thinking to help plot our future course. Harry Barnes has been a great friend and asset and adds the seasoned experience that only a former US ambassador can add. Other supporters of Omni Med who warrant thanks include my good friends Mal Visser and Darin Samaraweera. Drs Rick Foster and Thomas Bruce have also backed our efforts and have earned our eternal thanks.

During the roughly 12 years of data collection and several years of writing, a number of people have contributed to this book within the context of Omni Med. Ted Kordis designed the original Omni Med database, getting this all started back in 1994. I thank him for his brilliant design and lifelong friendship. Fran Wang updated and greatly expanded the database, making it into the user-friendly version it is now. Fran has been Omni Med's longest running, part-time employee and has rescued our database from spontaneous combustion time and again. We wouldn't have such a comprehensive work without her input. Many other people worked on the database throughout the years. This finished product is as much a testimony to their dedication and skill as anything else. Among them: Dr Doreen Ho, Dr Jamie McCabe, Phillip Choi, Ian McClure, Maggie Zraly, Leila Strachan, David Monteiro, Ethan Merlin, Jane Humphries, Edward Chan, and Yioula Sigounas. Many others also warrant thanks. The Lahey Clinic's Patty Newton offered her help and that of her staff during the early years of this text's development. Anne Lauriat came at just the right time and helped move some crucial things along. Peter Cuomo lent his considerable legal skills to developing a glossary, editing hundreds of sources in the bibliography, and putting the final touches on the Omni Med database. Peter will no doubt make important contributions at whatever legal firm is fortunate enough to land him.

Dr John Ross, my colleague at St Elizabeth's Hospital, read two chapters and offered key insights and encouragement; I thank him for both. A number of other people were kind enough to share their international experiences with me; I thank them for sharing so freely their life stories with me. They include Dr Chris Hudson, Dr Joseph Bowlds, Dr Ed Wyman, Dr James Meyer, Dr Duane Dowell, Mr Austin Flores, Dr Edmund Browne, and Dr Stephen and Kayleen Merry. As of this writing, Kayleen's health has deteriorated sharply. I thank her for her candor and wish her and her family strength through such a difficult period as this. I hope many more follow the example, depicted herein, that she has shared with us all.

Suzanne Fraker, the senior acquisition editor at the American Medical Association (AMA), believed in this concept from the beginning and pushed hard for more than two years to make it a reality. I owe her an enormous debt of gratitude for her perseverance, her strong will, her political acumen, and, most importantly, her basic humanity in seeing this through. I also thank the AMA for going out on a limb with this entire project. Both of these books express ideas that are far from the mainstream and I am grateful that I had the editorial freedom to say things that I think need to be said, even if some disagree. My editors, Katherine Dvorak and Carol Brockman, were patient and meticulous in their edits, and this final manuscript reflects their professional touch. Thanks also to Amy Burgess for her persistence in getting these books out to a wider audience.

Every book has a contract making it legal, and I am indebted to all of those attorneys from Kirkland and Ellis who worked for several months pro bono on behalf of Omni Med and me to see this through. Thanks to Dr Doreen and Derek Ho for making the connection and to Monica Tay for starting the ball rolling so many years ago. Rebecca Hazard and Kevin Rothman were models of patience and sage counsel, while Kate Dubin, Cristin Bolsinger, and Bradley Silver all contributed at key times. Micah Burch also gave generously of his time and modeled a professionalism and competency that I greatly admire and appreciate. All of these legal experts helped to steer this and the accompanying text to becoming Omni Med enterprises. It is right and fitting that all royalties will go to Omni Med. I'd also like to thank Bill Mahony for his considerable pro bono work in making Omni Med a legal entity back in 1998.

Any effort of this magnitude also owes a considerable amount to those who have so greatly influenced this work. Their voices course through this text. The scores of doctors, nurses, and other allied health personnel who have been brave enough to stake their lives firmly to a belief that the world order is imperfect and warrants fixing have influenced my writing. Furthermore, the oft-muted voices of those who find themselves at the bottom of economic orders in societies throughout the world have greatly influenced the tone of what follows herein.

This text and its companion took shape during the formative years of my Kellogg fellowship in 1994 through 1997. In fact, one might view these books as the end products of my fellowship experience. Thanks to the W.K. Kellogg Foundation for making this all possible. In addition to the previous people mentioned from the Kellogg Foundation, I would like to thank Linda Chamberlain for her advice in the early stages of compiling the data. She helped to design our first questionnaire—one that worked out very well. Thanks also to Roger Casey, Jim Kim, and Ellen Kahler for sharing their thoughts on culture.

I divide my time between Omni Med and the emergency department at St Elizabeth's Medical Center in Boston. Before that, I worked at Lahey Clinic NorthShore; I'd like to thank the nursing staff there for their support during the early years of this writing. At St Elizabeth's, I'd like to thank the nursing staff in the Emergency Department for your support during the past six years. Your encouragement has provided me with an important source of strength during the more difficult times of this work. It has always been a pleasure and a privilege to work with you. A special thanks to Kathy Dawley for your interest and support; it has meant a lot. Three physicians, Drs Sush Prusty, Howard Tarko, and Gian Corrado, took an active interest and offered plenty of encouragement; for that and your friendship, thanks. I am fortunate to work with such an incredible collection of doctors, nurses, and support staff at St Elizabeth's, where most of my family and I receive our health care.

Finally, I'd like to thank our friends and family for their patience during the writing of this book. John and Joan Stilla, Nancy, Corky, DJ, Rob and Jan, Ed D., Ed U., Joe, George, Rich, Ted, Mal, and several other close friends, thanks for putting up with my frequent absences during these past several years. I hope the time can be made up.

Preface

Wednesday June 9, 2004, was another steamy day in the emergency department at the Georgetown Public Hospital in Guyana. A couple of standing fans blew the hot, heavy air around and virtually everyone was drenched in sweat, a daily ritual for those who work in the tropics. A crush of people idled the time away in the waiting area, and the staff shuttled one patient after another through the congested treatment rooms. I had spent much of the morning seeing patients with the local staff as part of our nongovernmental organization (NGO) Omni Med's education program in Guyana. As had been the case in many other locales, I learned as much from these dedicated providers as I had taught to them.

Toward the end of the morning, one of the nurses asked me to look at a young boy who didn't look "right." He was two-years-old and "may have gotten into something," according to his worried mother. He was hopelessly thin, lying on a gurney near the hallway, and breathing faintly, not moving. I could elicit no response from him despite several attempts, and we quickly moved him to the treatment area with the best-stocked equipment. We dispatched an uncle to go and find out what he might have ingested, while the boy's breathing rate rapidly declined. Soon a crowd of nurses, students, and physicians gathered around in frantic attempts to revive him. We were able to place the "breathing tube" and soon, through two quickly placed IV lines, we poured in fluids and medications. Chest compressions soon followed, but it very quickly became clear that we were up against an unbeatable adversary. His breathless uncle came in to tell us that the child had ingested "rat poison," though not coumadin, the blood-thinning type used in rodent poisons in the United States. The type used in Guyana is far more lethal, and impossible to reverse. We continued our attempts to revive him for another half hour. Yet his cardiac tracing eventually showed a "flat-line" rhythm and we stopped.

I have worked in emergency medicine since 1992, and internationally since 1987, and have been present for scores of deaths. However, there is no amount of experience that can ever prepare one sufficiently for the task of informing a young mother that her two-year-old son has just died. I walked outside the immediate treatment area and told this frantic woman that we had done all we could, but we had been unable to save her young son. She screamed and cried, and for a minute, I thought she was going to hit me—I would not have blamed her if she had. But family members surrounded and consoled her, and soon she embraced me in a dying sob, crying uncontrollably for what seemed the longest time. As always happens in such cases, I felt awful, responsible, and retraced every step of our care. No, there really was nothing more that we could have done, though that didn't stop the second-guessing that continued to haunt me for a long time afterward.

This young boy comprised yet one more hard-luck story of life in a developing country, this time in Guyana. Poisonings happen everywhere, including the United States and Europe, and perhaps no amount of public health warnings about the dangers of poison in the house would have prevented his death. However, young, innocent lives are so frequently and needlessly lost in the developing world, that the event itself, though tragic, is commonplace. There may well be no more heart-wrenching occurrence in life than the loss of a child. Yet, poor mothers throughout the developing world play and replay scenes of grief and loss like this thousands of times every day. We in the "developed" world seem to have grown a protective covering over our collective consciences so that such images don't overly trouble us. Yet trouble us they should, given the frequency with which such deaths occur.

According to the United Nations, over 28,000 children under age five die every single day of treatable illnesses, mostly diarrhea, respiratory infections, malaria, and AIDS. That translates into roughly 1200 deaths every hour, or one death every three seconds (United Nations Development Programme 2005, 1). After the horrific tsunamis on December 26, 2004, roughly 300,000 people died. The event shocked the world, prompting one of the largest public outpourings of pledges for aid relief ever recorded. Yet for the unfortunate kids who inhabit the poorest areas of our world, their death rates are the equivalent of those tsunamis hitting three times per month, every month. If only the rich world would respond to these dying kids with the same urgency that it responded to the Asian tsunamis, perhaps fewer kids would have to die so young.

Yet these deaths are a mere part of a much larger, and far more troubling picture, comprised of two interrelated but quite disparate worlds—one rich and one poor. The larger picture is sometimes hard for those of us in the rich world to grasp. But ours is a world in which 1.1 billion people live on less than $1 per day and 2.6 billion people live on less than $2 per day (Sachs 2005, 18). Nearly one third of the people in the least developed countries, mostly in sub-Saharan Africa, will die before reaching age 40 (UNDP 1997, 5), while the life expectancy gap between those in the wealthiest and poorest countries in the year 2000 was over 25 years (UNDP 2002, 152). In poor countries each year, half a million women die in childbirth, at rates 10 to 100 times those in industrial countries (UNDP 1997, 3). The Joint United Nations Programme on HIV/AIDS (UNAIDS) estimates that 40 million are now infected with HIV, including 2.5 million children.[1] Containing this epidemic—even providing basic health care—requires infrastructures that are far too often lacking in poor countries. It is clear that enormous disparities in health and health care still very much define our global order.

Such disparities have not gone unnoticed through time. A number of responses, from bilateral aid missions to multilateral World Bank efforts, have attempted to reduce global disparities in health with mixed results. But, some of the more successful ventures have come in the field of health. Albert Schweitzer and Tom Dooley elevated the status of the medical profession through their widely acclaimed work in Africa and South East Asia. Other committed individuals—William Larimer and Gwen Mellon, Bernard Kuschner, Jonathan Mann, and Paul Farmer—have continued that tradition. Health workers from CARE, the International Committee of the Red Cross, and the United Nations (UN) have worked in some of the world's worst humanitarian crises over the past 50 years. A group of French physicians, Medecins Sans Frontieres (MSF), changed the way we respond to disasters. A handful of physicians and scholars at Partners In Health changed the way the world treats tuberculosis. Teams of World Health Organization (WHO) public health officers conquered smallpox. Schweitzer, MSF, Amnesty International, and several specialized UN agencies have won the Nobel Peace Prize. "All of these people have placed a higher calling above personal comfort, professional advancement, or material acquisition. In so doing, they have tapped into the ethical, faith-based roots of our profession, where the art of medicine intersects with the highest aspirations of man."

Stories of people and organizations involved in this work have percolated down through the medical profession like surreal dreams. For most health providers, this realm has remained distant and seemingly inaccessible. "Mainstream" medicine has averted its gaze, concentrating on worthy but different priorities. Most individual health providers have followed suit, though not for a lack of interest. Many have expressed at least a modicum of interest in working internationally. Whether inspired by stories of Schweitzer, Farmer, or Dooley, or perhaps knowing someone who had served abroad, they have expressed to me a wish to reconnect with the ideals that first drew them to a career in health care, or to give something back in exchange for all they have derived from their work in the field.

Despite such interest, however, opportunities to serve abroad have long been hard to find, and relatively few providers have engaged. In one of the few surveys to date, Johns Hopkins' Dr Timothy Baker found that only 0.32% of physicians and 0.12% of nurses surveyed had been active in international health prior to the study's publication in *JAMA* in 1984 (Baker et al 1984, 502). While such dismal numbers have likely increased slightly over the past 20 years, it is time for a far wider swath of the medical profession to consider engaging where they are most needed, and for the ideal of international health service to move into the mainstream of the medical profession.

A logical first step is to make it easier for health providers to engage. That is the chief purpose of this book and its prequel *Awakening Hippocrates: A Primer on Health, Poverty, and Global Service*, both of which fill a void long known to those who have tried to do this work. For many people, the first step is to call the Peace Corps, then MSF or other well-known NGOs, where they frequently fail to find the opportunity they are looking for, and stop their search. Those who do serve abroad often do so with little advance preparation, with little research into the "critical reflections" that should inform this kind of work. Much of the literature surrounding this work describes charitable, short-term endeavors rather than justice-based work designed cooperatively with those in the host countries. The history of international health service is full of stories of people who went abroad with the best intentions but did little to help—or even harmed—those they sought to aid. This book will help you think about these issues and provide the practical information you need to get there.

Why This Book?

In 1987, I worked as a fourth-year medical student for one month in Makiungu Hospital in Tanzania. During that time, I saw for the first time the harsh realities of extreme poverty, and experienced what Dr Tom Dooley bluntly called, "the stink and misery in which idealism must rub its nose" (Fischer 1997, 171). Despite the harsh environment, I loved my time there and saw a beauty of a people trapped by poverty and circumstance. I learned valuable lessons about working with the poor, coming to see them as people first and not as objects of my own benevolence or charity. I began to see their problems as *our* problems. The experience transformed me and redirected my life path.

While in Tanzania, it became painfully clear to me that the rich world had insufficiently dealt with the problems of global poverty and inequality. During the next seven years of residency and school loan repayment, I frequently returned to the questions that had been raised in Tanzania. I planned a return to East Africa but found it difficult to find the right opportunity. A friend, oncologist Barbara Bjornson, directed me to Father Bill Fryda with whom I worked in Nairobi's Nazareth Hospital for three months in 1994. However, I saw that there was no single book that oriented health providers to service, covered the core topics that anyone serving the poor should consider, and listed the organizations that would send them. It struck me that such a book could significantly increase the ranks of those who regularly serve internationally. So, in 1994, I began to compile information on organizations that send health providers abroad to serve.

As several students, volunteers, and I gathered information on service opportunities, it became clear that much more information was needed. Thousands of health providers had served internationally, but it was not clear that all had served well. So the text on service opportunities evolved into something larger, explaining the sources of global inequality, and the stories of some who had modeled ethical service abroad. The data collection and background research work in the mid to late 1990s became the first "program" of an NGO called Omni Med.

I founded Omni Med (loosely translated from the Latin meaning *health care for all*) in 1998, and was soon joined by several committed physicians, all sharing a passion to make a difference through health volunteerism. Since that time, we have been sending health providers (over 100 trips as of late 2005) to developing countries to teach and serve, as well as developing innovative programs, always in cooperation with local providers and government officials. Underlying our work is a program philosophy that states that all people have a right to health and quality health care; and that all health professionals, by their very involvement in the profession, share an ethical imperative to make quality health care broadly accessible to all people, regardless of their nationality or income. Our work at Omni Med has provided me plenty of opportunities to understand what is important in international health work.

How This Book Is Designed and How to Use It

Since so few medical providers work internationally on a regular basis, I thought it would be important for those interested to first understand some larger concepts at play in our world. As such, I wrote a somewhat lengthy text that looked at health, poverty, and the larger role of the health profession through history. That was originally part one of this text, with part two, the text you now hold, being dedicated to the more pragmatic aspects of global health service.

Because of the length of the material, the editors at the American Medical Association wisely decided to cut the original text in half, with part one becoming the text, *Awakening Hippocrates: A Primer on Health, Poverty, and Global Service,* and part two becoming what you are now holding. I have long believed that health providers serving abroad need a basic understanding of the constraints under which the poor of our world live their lives, in part so that we do not blame them for their poverty, and in part so we can design programs that work with them to craft solutions. Far too many mistakes have been made through history because one or both points were ignored. Powerful though unseen forces course through the lives of the poor, consigning them at birth to poverty, disease, suffering, and, far too often, an early death. I outlined these "forces of disparity" in detail in *Awakening Hippocrates,* and strongly encourage all who venture to serve abroad to read it, though I will summarize some of its key points in the Introduction that follows.

Before volunteering, providers should also undertake a "critical reflection" on issues that will affect them and those they will serve. They must understand some basic but important points about culture, service, personal health, and physical dangers involved, and try to listen to the muted voices of the poor. In considering such work, many questions will arise, such as, What shots will I need? How safe is it to bring my family? How can I possibly get the time away from work to do this? Which organization will offer me the best opportunity? All these questions are addressed in the chapters that follow.

Our focus in *A Practical Guide to Global Health Service* is on direct action. The first two chapters outline how one safely and effectively engages in this realm. We review how to overcome such common obstacles as fear, time and money constraints, familial and work obligations, and inertia. Other pragmatic discussions follow on travel, booking cheap flights, securing passports, obtaining visas and health insurance, and reducing health risks while flying. We also review the importance of culture and how we can best prepare ourselves ahead of time to both gain and give the most during our service time, however long it lasts. We cover some more practical concerns, such as shipping or transporting drugs and medical supplies. This section also covers health and safety concerns, including road accidents, commonly acquired illnesses like traveler's diarrhea, more "tropical" illnesses like malaria, and other concerns known to dissuade some from engaging.

Chapter 4 represents the culmination of over 10 years of work by many people. The Omni Med Database of International Health Service Opportunities may well be the most comprehensive of its kind. Since 1994, over 20 students, volunteers, and I have compiled data on roughly 240 organizations that send health personnel abroad. We have checked Web sites, sent e-mails, called and visited many, and sent out well over 3000 questionnaires to compile the data. We outline some practical suggestions for researching organizations in the database, and explain how best to judge each one. Following the database, there is a cross-indexing section in Chapter 5 that should make the research far easier and less time-consuming. Through this database, you should be able to narrow and focus your search, then quickly find the right fit for you. Chapter 6 lists many other important organizations that work internationally. Some are civil society organizations, such as Jubilee 2000, Amnesty International, or Fifty Years is Enough, that try to influence the public and political leaders on issues of great importance to the global poor. Others perform specific functions like sending medical supplies abroad or responding to disasters. All, however, are of importance to our larger purpose of creating a more just world.

Those who read this book and then serve internationally will have fully taken advantage of what it offers. I welcome your comments on organizations (see www.omnimed.org); we will likely expand subsequent editions to include your feedback. There are hundreds of organizations interested in channeling your energies into life-saving actions abroad. This book's fundamental purpose is to make those initial steps easier and much better informed.

As was the case in *Awakening Hippocrates,* it is my sincere hope that you will use this text wisely, in a manner that will assist those who need you. We stand at the dawn of the new millennium, filled with possibility and hope. We in the health profession can be stewards of a new age of reasoned compassion. Ours is a unique position in the world and in the societies of man. I urge you to make full use of the information that follows, reflect on the critical questions, and finally, act. Whether through the political process, any of the civil service organizations involved in these struggles, or, best of all, directly through international service, there is no shortage of opportunities for you. You have only to choose.

Endnote

1. For more information see the UNAIDS Web site at www.unaids.org.

Introduction

Why Should We Do This Anyway?

Martin Luther King, Jr, once said, "The racial problem in America will be solved to the degree that every American considers himself personally confronted with it" (Cloud 1996). We can extend a similar analogy to the problem of global health inequality. This problem too will only be solved to the degree to which each of us feels personally confronted by it—particularly those of us in the health profession. That remains difficult if the overwhelming majority of health providers remain secluded away in the relative comfort of the industrialized world.

It is only through an active engagement with the poor that our perspectives can evolve. Gustavo Gutierrez, the father of liberation theology, once advised people to forget the "head trip" of studying the problems of the poor and take a "foot trip" to work among them (Brown 1990, 50). Only through such engagement, he argued, can we begin to work with them toward solutions. Poverty remains the most important killer in the world, and the best way to understand it is to work with those who live under its yoke.

While working abroad, we may also acquire the tools needed to affect political change here at home. The forces that serve to maintain current global disparities in health are both powerful and largely invisible. Many stem directly from decisions made by governments in the United States and other industrialized countries. Yet, doctors, administrators, nurses, and other workers in the profession remain widely respected. When they speak, the public usually listens. If more health providers would take a role in attacking the global inequalities in health, great change would result. Influencing the levers of power in the United States may more greatly affect change for the global poor than an army of doctors volunteering their services abroad.

In that process, we may also save the lives of some of our young soldiers. As this was being written in 2005, a steady drumbeat of killed or wounded young American soldiers returning home from Iraq echoed through the United States. It is fitting to ask whether there is anything that we, as individuals, can do to reduce such conflicts. A 1994 Central Intelligence Agency study found that "state failure"—defined as war, genocide, or disruptive regime changes—followed three common characteristics in a given country: lack of democracy, lack of "openness" of an economy, and a rising infant mortality rate (Sachs 2001a, 187). In other words, societies that fail to listen to their people, close themselves off from the world, and don't care for their most vulnerable, tend to fail, producing war or chaos. Failed states inevitably become "seedbeds of violence, terrorism, international criminality, mass migration and refugee movements, drug trafficking, and disease" (187). This same study, which tracked 113 cases of state failure between 1957 and 1994, also found that state failure preceded every instance of US military intervention abroad since 1960. While the perpetrators of the horrific attacks on September 11, 2001, may have been wealthy Saudis, their Al Qaida associates found sanctuary in the impoverished, failed state of Afghanistan. To prevent war, we might look more closely at means to bring health and stability to poor countries abroad. We might even revisit the concept of a US International Health Service Corps, albeit one primarily focused on training and education (Baker and Quinley 1987, 2622; US Congress 1987; Kindig et al 1984, 10).

We can best effect change by sharing our knowledge, our wealth, and our most valuable resource of all, our people. Perhaps nowhere is this as important as through those who care for the sick. In the Millennial Survey of 1999, people around the world rated "good health" as their number one concern, reflecting long held patterns.[1] From my research on the rise of health in the industrialized world, it is clear that the transfer of knowledge among nations has contributed more than any other factor to steady increases in life expectancies everywhere.

In the process of addressing such global inequalities, those who undertake this work will share some great experiences. During the last 17 years, I've traveled to Africa, Central and South America, and Asia. I've hitchhiked through East Africa, played in piano bars in Europe and Asia, and scaled Mayan ruins in the jungles of Central America. Along the way, I've met some remarkable people, seen some of the wonder of the world, and come to better understand myself and the nature of man. I have been able to look back on the culture of my birth and see it clearly for the first time. Living and working abroad has enriched my life and that of my family beyond anything else I can imagine. While I want my fellow providers to serve internationally because there is such dire need and because we are ethically compelled to do so, I also want more providers to share in a truly uplifting experience. Most who go wonder why it took them so long to get involved.

Some clinicians may ask: why should those of us who are comfortable, after years of hard work reaching a certain position in the health profession, bother with those who are suffering? We can find answers from a variety of sources. Christianity, Judaism, Islam, and almost every other faith share world views rooted in social justice. Each commands its adherents to care for the poor while creating a just world order. A branch of Christianity called Liberation Theology compels its adherents to follow the scriptures and *act* to free the poor from their oppression. Similarly, the expanding paradigm of human rights informs us that each person has a birthright to life, health, education, freedom, and the dignity that comes from membership in the human race.

Albert Schweitzer searched world theology and philosophy, ultimately arriving at the principle, "Reverence for Life," which compels each of us to care for all of the life around us, including people not within our traditional realm of concern. He added a message to the comfortable,

> Just as the wave cannot exist for itself, but is ever a part of the heaving surface of the ocean, so must I never live my life for life itself, but always in the experience which is going on around me. It is an uncomfortable doctrine which the true ethics [of Reverence for Life] whisper to my ear. You are happy, they say; therefore you are called upon to give much (Schweitzer 1949, 321).

From a practical perspective, the summons is equally strong. Acquired immunodeficiency syndrome (AIDS), multidrug resistant tuberculosis (MDR-TB), and many other infectious pathogens that arise from poverty ultimately threaten all of humanity. We ignore such lessons at our own peril. Paul Farmer has written extensively on the microbial links that still connect the poor with the affluent, "despite all the barriers our age has set up to separate them" (Kim et al 2000, xiv). Farmer also found the following passage, written almost a century ago by physician and writer William Budd, warning of the dangers of typhoid,

> This disease not seldom attacks the rich, but it thrives among the poor. But by reason of our common humanity we are all, whether rich or poor, more nearly related here than we are apt to think. The members of the great human family are, in fact, bound together by a thousand secret ties, of whose existence the world in general little dreams. And he that was never yet connected with his poorer neighbor, by deeds of charity or love, may one day find, when it is too late, that he is connected with him by a bond which may bring them both, at once, to a common grave (Budd 1931, 174).

When we consider that MDR-TB, human immunodeficiency virus (HIV), Ebola, and Lassa have all freely traversed international borders, we should reconsider just how "other" they are who are most commonly afflicted. The idea that one group of people can remain isolated from any other group should have long ago expired. Severe acute respiratory syndrome (SARS) should have destroyed any remaining illusions. The next plague, the one that will inevitably follow AIDS, is just one short airplane flight away. The sooner we embrace all of humanity, the better our prospects for long-term survival will be.

There is yet one more compelling reason for this undertaking: to dispel widely held beliefs about poor people that say, "People are poor because they are lazy, stupid, or immoral. They simply need to pull themselves up by their bootstraps and get a job." One does not have to look far to find those with such beliefs. However, the reality is far different from the mythology surrounding poverty. People are poor for reasons that are complex and largely invisible to those of us who live in relative comfort in the wealthier countries. Most people are not, in fact, poor chiefly due to their own faults. "Some are lazy, some hard working, some good and some bad, but the overwhelming majority of people are poor because the array of forces aligned against them is utterly insurmountable." For those of us venturing to work among them, it is important to try, at the outset, to understand the constraints under which they live their lives. It is far easier to find fault and abandon rather than to understand complex issues and engage, and the default mode for many through the years has been to blame the victims for the problems they face. As such, it is easier not to "waste" the money, or spend the time and energy required on those deemed somehow unworthy. People may find other reasons to avoid this work, but it should not be because those most in need don't warrant the effort.

Charity and Justice

Dr King once wrote, "The moral arc of the universe is long, but it bends toward justice." I picture this "moral arc" as a tangible reality, consisting of increasing degrees of righteousness, clarity of purpose, and importance to the poor as we move toward its end. Inherent within such an arc lie the ideals of both charity and justice. Charity is a core principle both in Judaism and Christianity, and is one of the five pillars of Islam. It conveys a love of man for fellow man, or benevolence, often manifested through acts of kindness to those in need. *Charity* is also the term that best describes much of the medical literature on international health service.

Most of the medical service work that we read about is worthwhile, though constrained by a lack of perspective. In the realm of "charity," those who give to the less fortunate are, by wide agreement, doing good work. Their motives and their methods, however, are rarely questioned. Author Christopher Hitchens wrote, "The rich world likes and wishes to believe that someone, somewhere, is doing something for the Third World. For this reason it does not inquire too closely into the motives or practices of anyone who fulfills, however vicariously, this mandate" (Hitchens 1997, 49). Because the givers are doing good works, their methods remain beyond reproach. The history of charitable endeavors abroad is littered with the harm that results from well intended, though poorly informed people who undertake such work. Even the large bi- and multilateral donors have made huge errors due to a lack of perspective. Program designs often accomplish far less than they could have had the founders only thought more broadly at their inception. Further, by following subconscious "charitable" notions, we may even become trapped by a blinding self-righteousness, unable to hear criticism from the oft-muted voices of those with the greatest stakes involved. We may fail to search out deeper root causes to the harsh realities we see; even exonerate ourselves after learning that we are very much complicit in maintaining orders of inequality.

Most of the focus of charitable work remains on the giver. A typical medical mission reported in the literature describes how a group of health providers provided care in a poor setting, left, and then expressed thanks for the opportunity to call a place like the United States "home." Those they cared for remain poor, unfortunate people, unable to help themselves. The "poor" thus remain mere passive recipients of the benevolent acts of the more fortunate.

While charity has its place, it is important to reflect on our motivations for undertaking such work. We must look behind the veil of humanitarianism to understand how our own motivations might clash with the needs and desires of those whom we hope to serve. How might we turn the noble impulse of "charity" into something more powerful?

Let's take a deeper look at the point in Dr King's "moral arc" where it bends "toward justice." Justice is a fundamental concept in our worldview, defined as "the use of power and authority to uphold what is right, just, or lawful" (Merriam-Webster 1991). Just such a process did occur during the framing of the Universal Declaration of Human Rights in the aftermath of World War II. Yet the concept of justice requires more work than that of a charitable act. Charity focuses our attention on the comfortable, familiar domain of the giver, while justice demands that we focus our attention on the unseemly and disturbing world of those on the receiving end. In charity, we can send some surplus supplies abroad, or we can give our time and skills to those in need. But, to arrive at justice, we are required to take a far more arduous journey. We need to understand the needs and desires of the poor as well as the forces that constrain their hopes or very existence. Such understanding does not come easily. "Many of the answers to the most pressing questions lie buried deep under common presuppositions that we rarely challenge. The very recordings of our society preclude an honest assessment for the majority of us."

The basic question, "Why are they poor?" answers the question, "Why are they sick?" and requires that we understand the complex worlds of trade relations, history, racism, sexism, foreign aid flows, development, governance and global financial flows, among others, all of which conspire to perpetuate poverty. Only through such work can we understand what is real in the world. At such a time, many of the arguments that historically blame the victims fall away. We can then target our efforts at the forces most responsible, crafting solutions while working directly with those in poor communities.

This is a tall order for the medical profession. We have long viewed the world through the comfortable position of providing life-enhancing care on a daily basis. Ours is truly a profession that allows us to do well while doing good work. That we care for the sick, and do so with such competence, provides us with sufficient moral cover. We can hear of others responding to the ills of the world and consider ourselves involved, if only through our daily work. Yet, there is far more required of us, both abroad in poor settings, and at home in the corridors of power.

On Transformation

"One of the more powerful products of working with the poor is the personal transformation that often results. Within the realm of international service work among the poor, such stories are legion." The sheer power of the experience is sufficient to change hearts and minds. We may more readily understand the concept of transformation by turning to some of our more celebrated political leaders. We know Franklin D. Roosevelt as the compassionate president who launched the New Deal, Social Security, and the Four Freedoms—the "touchstone" of the Universal Declaration of Human Rights (Glendon 2001, 176). When he contracted polio, according to biographer Doris Kearns Goodwin, he "came to empathize with the poor and the underprivileged, with people to whom fate had dealt a difficult hand" (Goodwin 1994, 16). Eleanor Roosevelt added, "Anyone who has gone through great suffering is bound to have a greater sympathy and understanding of the problems of mankind." Robert F. Kennedy underwent a similar transformation upon the assassination of his brother. Following the deep melancholy that engulfed him after the fall of "Camelot," the transformed Attorney General actively sought out the poor of America, touring shacks of the rural South, meeting with migrant workers and marginalized people of color, in the process attracting armies of the dispossessed until his untimely death at age 42 (Johnson 2005).

More pertinent to our task here, Dr Tom Dooley grew up a wealthy aristocrat in St Louis, aspiring to become a society obstetrician. However, seeing up close the misery of Vietnam's refugees tapped a faith-based wellspring within him, transforming his remaining life into a resolute struggle against poverty and illness in South East Asia. Paul Farmer, similarly, found the suffering and premature dying of the poor in rural Haiti more than he could bear. Such injustice has driven him to work for decades in poor communities around the world, always seeking a means to improve their health and quality of life. Poverty and the devastation wrought by AIDS have had a similar transformative effect on U2 frontman Bono, former US Secretary of State Colin Powell, economist Jeffrey Sachs, and others (Behrman 2004, 265). In each of these stories, the sheer power of harsh experience proved enough to transform the individual. There may be no more passionate or potent force than that unleashed by those who have been transformed.

Through the experience of service, I have no doubt that more Paul Farmers will emerge, and hundreds of people will rededicate a portion of their clinical lives. Health providers widely share the trait of compassion. It is impossible to do this work well without it. As such, health providers form the ideal cohort to reach out into the world to bring the experience of poverty home to a slumbering electorate. In the process, they can send out ripples of change that can reverberate powerfully throughout our country and our world.

World Orders Old and New

When we look at our world, we see only that which is shown to us. Americans live in the world's richest country and learn about the world primarily through a media heavily slanted toward coverage of American concerns, particularly those in the realm of popular culture. It is understandable why typical American perceptions of the world are quite distant from the reality. Travelers from the United States who first experience life in a poor country commonly hear perspectives on America that they find shocking. These views come from the other side of history, from those who for the most part remain powerless and voiceless. But to truly understand what life is like for the poor whom we hope to serve while abroad, we need to dig deep beneath our presuppositions. We need to enter their world with eyes and minds open.

Those who have already spent time abroad will have come to understand the reasons for such views already. For the uninitiated, such matters still seem distant, unconnected to the immediate task at hand. Yet the poor know all too well the importance of a host of forces, many invisible, that dominate their lives. International trade policy, foreign aid, globalization, World Bank and International Monetary Fund (IMF) policies, militarism, racism, sexism, and history itself comprise tangible realities that directly affect the quality and duration of life for so many of the world's poor. An in-depth discussion of each of these forces is beyond the reach of this book, but suffice it here to at least provide an overview of how these forces work and wreak their particular destruction on the lives of the poor.

Yesterday

To even the most casual observer of our world, there are clear dichotomies in wealth, literacy, life expectancy, and infant mortality, to name a few. Yet any analysis of the world order must start at the beginning, to where things began to diverge. History, more than any other factor, has shaped current world orders. Through its lingering effects, history is very much alive, though largely forgotten by and invisible to those in rich countries who benefit most from its alteration.

A first casualty to the mythology of history is that of the interconnected nature of things. There is no "American" history in isolation, just as there is no European, Asian, or African history in isolation. There is but one history—a tangled, interdependent, and ongoing world history in which the dominant powers of the day compete for raw materials and cheap labor. In the process, the dominant powers erase the histories of the conquered while enshrouding their own histories in mythology. When Europeans first arrived in the New World in the fifteenth century, they found a continent populated by countless tribes like Inca, Maya, Aztec, Sioux, and Apache, each with their own complex social orders and long histories; Europeans did not find the mostly empty continent so often depicted in history books. The Europeans called these diverse peoples "Indians," whose immediate fate included genocide, disease, and marginalization for the few who survived the initial onslaught. According to current best estimates, 95% of the New World population succumbed to the invading armies and microbes (Diamond 1999, 210). In addition to their advanced technologies, the invading Spaniards carried with them the microbes against which none of the indigenous peoples of the New World had immunity. Smallpox, measles, influenza, typhus, diphtheria, malaria, mumps, pertussis, plague, tuberculosis, and yellow fever claimed many more lives than genocide.

The legacy of this epic clash is readily apparent to those who travel anywhere in the Americas or the Caribbean. Those with the highest infant mortality rates, maternal mortality rates, and unemployment, and the lowest levels of literacy, per capita income, and life expectancy tend to be indigenous people, the direct descendents of those crushed by the invading Europeans. After indigenous people, the group with the next worst indices tends to be those of African origin, many the direct descendents of the 10–15 million slaves transported from Africa to the New World during the fifteenth through nineteenth centuries.

Slavery comprises another one of the major forces shaping human history and the current world order. In addition to accelerating the development of European powers and New World economies, slavery changed the population makeup of most of the Western Hemisphere (Farmer 1994, 62). It raised port cities from Liverpool to Lisbon and altered the dynamics of power in Africa, Europe, and the New World.

Ultimately, slavery was about the sacrifice of human lives in a relentless drive for wealth and power. It set in motion forces that have long since polarized societies everywhere, helped to fuel a civil war in the United States, and set back the continent of Africa for generations. Its reverberations still affect us all, and the racism that fueled it at its peak has declined but never abated.

From a health perspective, one of the more salient lessons from history is that, for most of human history, people didn't live as long as they do today. Advances in nutrition and public health, along with the steady improvements in standards of living through economic growth that followed the Industrial Revolution (1790–1850) allowed Europe and the United States to dramatically improve the quality and duration of life for their people. By the year 1900, life expectancy in the United States had reached age 47, which is slightly better than that of sub-Saharan Africa today (United Nations Development Program [UNDP] 2005, 253; Centers for Disease Control and Prevention [CDC] 2002; 1999). Today Americans live on average to age 77. Many of the technological breakthroughs of the rich world have diffused to the developing world, sparking dramatic improvements in the health and longevity of the global poor, narrowing but not closing the sizable gap in human development.

Two centuries ago, great disparities in wealth did not exist; everyone was poor. In 1820 the income gap between the world's richest country, the United Kingdom, and the poorest region, Africa, was four to one. Two centuries of highly uneven economic growth and technological development has produced our modern, unequal world. Today, the gap between the world's richest country, the United States, and the world's poorest region, Africa, has increased to twenty to one (Sachs 2005, 28).

Following the cataclysm of World War II, the rich countries began the process of "developing" the poor countries, pouring in roughly $1 trillion in "aid" over the next six decades ("How to Make Aid Work" 1999). The United States' involvement in development dates back to Harry Truman's inaugural address in 1949, in which he called for a "worldwide effort for the achievement of peace, plenty and freedom" (Hancock 1989, 69). Previously, few Americans had taken much notice at all of the enormous disparities that had come to characterize the world.

While the epic battles of World War II raged on, delegates from 44 allied countries, led by Franklin D. Roosevelt, began the process of constructing a new world order, characterized by peace and cooperation. The United Nations became the centerpiece of this new world order, as did three UN entities: the IMF, World Bank, and the General Agreement on Tariffs and Trade (GATT), the precursor to the World Trade Organization (WTO). Because the world monetary system had been widely cited as a principal cause in the economic collapse that led directly to World War II, delegates created the IMF to stabilize world currency and prop up unstable economies. The World Bank became the principal leader of "development," charged with helping poor countries rise up out of poverty. The GATT agreement was the third piece of the delegates' plan, and for nearly a half-century governed international trade until replaced by the WTO in 1995.

The reconstruction of Europe, largely accomplished by the United States' Marshall Plan, opened the era of foreign aid. Inspired by the Marshall Plan's success,

FDR's "four freedoms" and Allied war rhetoric that all men should be free, the rich nations embarked on a 60-year quest to "develop" the poorest countries. To date, the rich world has transferred $1 trillion to the poor countries, with surprisingly little to show for it. Because most foreign aid has served the political, strategic, and economic interests of the donors, it is not surprising that so many efforts abroad have failed, at times spectacularly. In lieu of becoming the helping hand to pull many developing countries out of deadly "poverty traps," aid has become for many yet another cross to bear.

A most noticeable failure of "development" occurred during the 1960s–1980s when many of the world's poorest countries sank deeply into debt through unrestrained rich country bank lending, led and sanctioned by the World Bank. This nearly caused the collapse of the global monetary system in the 1980s debt crisis. The poorest citizens within these countries have since paid back some of this debt through Bank- and IMF-sponsored structural adjustment programs (SAPs), in which poor country economies cut basic services like education and health, and realign their economies toward export-oriented growth. While economic growth is the most potent engine to lift developing nations out of poverty, the SAPs were too brutally implemented. Millions of poor people felt the loss of basic services and most health indices have worsened since. Many countries are still saddled with crushing debt burdens, and many still pay more to foreign creditors than on the health and education of their citizens.

Within the realm of global health service, however, some glimmering rays of light have emerged. The non-governmental organization (NGO) community has expanded and spread its influence all over the developing world. NGO funding nearly doubled in the past decade, from $6.4 billion in 1995 to an estimated $12.3 billion in 2002 (Organization for Economic Co-Operation and Development [OECD] 2004, 134). The end of the Cold War spurned ever increasing faith and funding in those NGOs that could effectively render aid abroad, even as internal conflicts and complex humanitarian emergencies increased throughout the developing world. As NGOs have expanded their roles, the rich world's governments have receded. It has been a mixed blessing at best.

Some of the more storied efforts from within the health community have long inspired those who venture to join their ranks. Albert Schweitzer was a gifted musician, theologian, and philosopher who gave up three prosperous careers along with his status as a rising star among Europe's intellegencia to become a doctor in West Africa, where he labored for the next five decades. Schweitzer's philosophy, "Reverence for Life," compels each of us to care for all of the life around us, including those not in our traditional realm of concern. President John F. Kennedy called him "the towering moral figure of the twentieth century," and Schweitzer's call for people to serve where most needed is one that we can and should still heed today. His lifetime of work was rewarded with a Nobel Peace Prize in 1952.

Similarly, Tom Dooley was a wealthy American born in St Louis in 1927, who aspired to become a "society obstetrician," catering to St Louis' finest—and wealthiest. However, Dooley's service in "Operation Passage to Freedom" in Vietnam in the late 1950s deeply moved him. He saw the "filth and wretchedness, and stink and misery," of the Vietnamese refugees under his care, but also "their fineness, their magnificence, and their valiant, valiant faith" (Mahon 1998, 19). Dooley was a man transformed, and he became an icon for Americans of the Eisenhower era. He became a celebrated author, regularly appearing on popular television shows of the day like Jack Paar's *Tonight Show*, and was voted one of the 10 "most admired" men in the world in the *Reader's Digest* annual 1959 ranking (Fischer 1997, 4). He gave the remaining years of his life to service, succumbing to malignant melanoma at age 34. Ironically, his wake was held just as his friend, John F. Kennedy was sworn in as President. Kennedy later cited Tom Dooley as the inspiration for the United States Peace Corps.

Today

Now, more than any other time in history, we understand the problems of the developing world. Through CNN, the Internet, enhanced telecommunications, and air travel, we also have more immediate access to the global poor. Those who once existed in our peripheral vision only are now immediately before us, all the time. Yet we see their poverty and sickness solely at our discretion. Far too often, we turn away. Yet our charge remains to understand them and what robs them of their voice, their agency, and their very lives.

The single most important factors in determining how long and how well one will live today are the country where one is born and the socioeconomic strata that one is born into. Poverty itself is not a force of nature; it is a construct of man. The larger world orders that state that one person will live in luxury until a ripe old age while another is born into harsh poverty and will die young is called structural violence. When we look at our modern world, we can readily discern the "forces of disparity" responsible for maintaining such orders of inequality.

These forces of disparity include some already elucidated above, including history and poverty. Yet there are other, more clandestine forces at work. Throughout history, the most discriminated against group has been women. The modern face of poverty is distinctly feminine, and those who suffer and die most often in our world are women and the children wholly dependent upon them. Ancient patriarchal society structures have continued in much of the modern world, in which women lack the right to hold land, work for a wage, hold elective office, or agitate for basic rights. The UN reported that 70% of the 1.3 billion living in extreme poverty in 1995 were women, as were two thirds of the world's 900 million illiterates and 60% of those without access to primary school (UNDP 1995, 4). Many never make it that far. Economist Amartya Sen has estimated that, due to sex-selective abortions and female infanticide, there are over 100 million fewer women worldwide than would be expected based on standard gender-specific birth ratios (UNDP 1995, 35; Sen 1993, 46).

Global trade may well be the most potent vehicle for ending extreme poverty. Certainly economic growth rates of 8–9% per year will continue to propel millions of Chinese and Indians out of poverty in the coming years. Yet for those who live in the less favored developing countries, like Haiti, Papua New Guinea, and most of sub-Saharan Africa, trade becomes yet another obstacle in their path.

In September 2003, a young South Korean farmer named Lee Kyoung Hae climbed a barricade during demonstrations at a WTO meeting in Cancun, Mexico, and held aloft a sign reading "WTO kills farmers" (Vidal 2003). He then plunged a dagger into his chest and died in the arms of his friends. While his death was dramatic, he became in reality just one more victim of global trade imbalances and rigged policies. While rich countries provide roughly $60–80 billion annually in aid to the poor countries, these same rich countries provide roughly $350 billion in annual subsidies to their farmers (UNDP 2005, 129). As a result, these farmers, many of whom work for large agro-businesses like Archer Daniels Midland, can drop their price of their goods on world markets and flood developing country markets with cheap imports. Poor farmers can't compete, and their families starve. Wealthy multinational companies prompt the rich countries to support such subsidies and impose tariffs, greatly aiding their business ventures. Because these rich countries call the shots at the WTO, such policies won't readily change. What options do poor farmers have?

When poor countries export to rich countries, they face tariff barriers of $100 billion, almost twice as much annually as foreign aid expenditures in recent years (Oxfam 2002, 5). The *New York Times* noted the irony of the situation in a September 2003 article on the WTO talks in Cancun, "Africans find this double attack of subsidies and tariffs especially maddening since they have been told they should trade their way out of poverty, not look for foreign aid" (Becker 2003). One agricultural expert from Sierra Leone said, "For Africa, it's a major problem. . . . People can't better themselves if they can't feed themselves, and farmers are being driven off their land" (Becker 2003). The irony is not lost on the poor, who have vocally denounced the trade policies of rich nations for decades.

Other forces acting on the current world stage include rising militarism and ineffective governance in the least developed countries. Far too many poor governments spend more on their militaries than on the health and education of their people. Further, ineffective government initiatives in trade, banking, infrastructure development, health, and education act as a brake on economic growth and provide little incentive for foreign direct investments, which can radically effect change, as shown by both China and India. Inequality itself is a pathological force acting in the world, with the richest nations using power and money to increase their political and strategic influence around the world. The wealthiest countries dictate the terms of aid, trade, debt repayment schemes, and economic restructuring for the poor countries. In global forums, power increasingly shifts from the "one country, one vote" system at the UN to the "one dollar, one vote" system of the World Bank and the IMF (Sachs 2005, 286).

A clear concern for those in developing countries is the strong preference of rich countries, particularly the United States, to spend far greater sums on their militaries than on development. The Bush administration's fiscal year 2005 military budget called for $430 billion in expenditures, not including the costs of the ongoing conflicts in Iraq and Afghanistan (Corbin and Pemberton 2004). This amount also does not include the amount of the federal debt incurred through military spending, which would add at least another $100 billion, nor does it include military retirement pay, veterans' benefits, foreign military aid, the space program, peacekeeping, and other expenditures (Center for Defense Information [CDI] 2002, 34). These additional costs brought the 2005 fiscal year defense and defense-related budget to more than $600 billion, with additional funds required for Iraq and Afghanistan. In 2004 the United States spent 30 times more on the military ($450 billion) than on foreign aid ($15 billion) (Sachs 2005, 329). In his book, *The Sorrows of Empire*, author Chalmers Johnson wrote, "We now station innumerably more uniformed military officers than civilian diplomats, aid workers, or environmental specialists in foreign countries—a point not lost on the lands to which they are assigned (2004, 4). Although the Bush administration rightly elevated development to the third pillar of national security, along with defense and diplomacy, it seems that development remains a weak and poorly funded pillar (USAID 2002, iv).

Infectious disease comprises yet another entity that affects those in poor countries far more than those in rich countries. While the rich world has nearly eradicated deaths from infectious illnesses such as malaria and tuberculosis, and dramatically reduced childhood deaths from commonly acquired infectious agents that cause diarrhea and pneumonia, the same is not true in developing nations. Malaria causes roughly 1 million deaths annually, nearly 250 times as many deaths in the world's poorest countries as in the richest countries (WHO 1999, 51). Roughly 2 million die each year of tuberculosis, of whom 98% live in developing countries (WHO 2004). As anthropologist and physician Paul Farmer wrote, "Tuberculosis is thus two things at once; a completely curable disease and the leading cause of young adult deaths in much of the world" (Farmer 1999, 185). While rich countries have had cures to such diseases for over 50 years, most of the poor remain without access to treatment.

The HIV/AIDS epidemic comprises a pathogenic force in and of itself. Every day, AIDS claims 8000 lives, with over 28 million deaths thus far, a number that exceeds the total of combatant deaths in the entire twentieth century (Behrman 2004, xi). Some estimates place the number of those afflicted by AIDS at 250 million by the year 2025, with a projected death toll that will likely exceed the total number of people who have died in all of history's wars (149 million) since the first century. In the worst hit countries, with HIV prevalence at 20% of the population, annual economic growth (gross domestic products [GDP]) has slowed by 2.6 points, a drag that even rich industrialized countries could not long tolerate ("The Cost of AIDS" 2004). Perhaps no other infectious entity has so dramatized the dichotomies in our modern world than HIV. Those with the ability to pay for anti-retrovirals survive while those lacking the means perish, often leaving young children behind. By the end of this decade, there will likely be 25 million AIDS orphans (Behrman 2004). Only recently have rich countries begun to engage the epidemic seriously.

A host of health providers are at work in our world seeking to reduce such glaring disparities in longevity and health. Paul Farmer is a physician and anthropologist who turned a small clinic in the Central Highlands of Haiti into a model hospital.

Borrowing from liberation theology, Farmer designed systems in which poor people became empowered to improve their own health. The NGO Farmer founded, Partners In Health, has become a model for how to provide competent treatment for MDR-TB and HIV/AIDS in resource-poor settings. Paul has also made significant contributions to the fields of medicine and anthropology by analyzing the underlying structures that propagate poverty, and thus foster poor health. While the field of anthropology had chosen to focus its attention on the "culture" of those in poor places, Paul Farmer called attention to the impact of unjust trade practices, untreated infectious diseases, politically motivated embargos, and the pathogenic forces of inequality itself. He has received virtually every humanitarian award available, including a MacArthur "Genius" grant and a Heinz award. President Clinton recently suggested that he be nominated for the Nobel Peace Prize.

Jim Yong Kim was Paul Farmer's partner in the founding of Partners In Health, and helped to grow the organization into a multi-million dollar NGO with considerable global impact. Partners In Health espouses a philosophy of creating a "preferential option to the poor," working in Haiti, Peru, and many other locales. Jim challenged WHO policy for treatment of MDR-TB and, together with Farmer, helped to change the way the world treats multi-drug resistant tuberculosis. Jim briefly left Partners In Health to direct the WHO's "3 by 5" campaign, which sought, albeit unsuccessfully, to bring anti-retroviral therapy to 3 million people by the end of 2005. Jim also received a MacArthur award, among other honors.

Other modern day health providers give us further incentive to serve. Father Bill Fryda designed Nairobi's St Mary's Hospital along with its Kenyan staff and has turned this hospital into a model for the developing world. Situated at the edge of Kibera Slum, which is home to roughly 800,000 people, St Mary's offers competent affordable health care to those who previously had none. Dr Tom Durant spent a lifetime working in refugee camps in the aftermath of the world's worst complex humanitarian disasters, seeing the "power of the human spirit" in the most desolate of places. Similarly, Dr Peter Allen, a dentist in Belize, has spent most of his professional life seeking to improve life for those in his adopted country. People such as these inspire those who have been more reluctant to engage the problems directly.

Tomorrow

For the first time in history, we have the knowledge and resources to truly heal the world. In just one generation, we could end extreme poverty and dramatically improve the health of the poor—but only if we summon the will to do so. Following 60 years of often-ineffectual development aid to the poor nations, we now hold a blueprint for change. Leaders from 189 countries gathered at the UN headquarters in New York in September 2000, and agreed on a series of eight specific millennium development goals (MDGs), all of which impact health and target their results for the year 2015. The MDGs may represent the best vehicle yet for the rich world to correct the ills of those in poor countries by taking aim at the root causes of illness through carefully constructed, clear, and achievable targets.

Despite a sluggish response from the world's wealthiest countries to the MDGs thus far, there is still reason for optimism. In recent years, there have been a number of positive signs that the discourse on global poverty is changing, particularly in the United States. Conservative senator Jesse Helms, who for years had reduced single-handedly US foreign aid budgets, apologized for not doing more to help those with HIV/AIDS for so long (Eaton and Etue 2002, 60). US foreign aid budgets have increased more under President George W. Bush than any US president since Kennedy, and foreign aid is now seen as the "third pillar" of US national security (USAID 2002, iv). The most recent addition to US foreign aid, the Millennial Challenge Account (MCA), offers a new and interesting paradigm for giving foreign aid. Only those countries that demonstrate the capacity to use aid dollars effectively will receive aid dollars in the future. The MCA will add a full $5 billion to annual US aid tallies starting in 2006 if fully funded, though full funding now seems unlikely given the large US budget deficits ("Between Hope and Hope" 2005). Such a process, however, combined with the strict eligibility requirements for inclusion, suggests that the business of aid may well be changing—and considerably for the better.

Other large-scale, recent initiatives like the Global Alliance for Vaccines and Immunization (GAVI), represent interesting means of addressing global health disparities. Led by the Gates Foundation, GAVI's genius may be in stitching together industry, foundation, academic, and government bodies to produce a whole larger than the sum of its parts. Another group effort, the Global Fund, specifically targets three infectious disease entities: HIV, TB, and malaria. It has received widespread praise thus far and comprises humanity's best chance to halt the AIDS epidemic. The UN Commission that created the Global Fund estimated that increasing rich country health donations by $22 billion per year by 2007 could save 8 million lives per year (Sachs 2001a, 16). In the end it comes down to money; it always has.

In his 2003 State of the Union address, President Bush announced a five-year $15 billion program for global AIDS relief, called the President's Emergency Plan for AIDS Relief (PEPFAR). Despite considerable shortcomings, including large allocations to a few countries, restrictions on condom distribution, requirements that recipients purchase expensive US-made anti-retroviral medications, and an overly strong emphasis on abstinence, the program signals a positive development for the world's richest country. American leadership on global health is critical; without US leadership, little will happen. That is all the more reason to feel optimistic about the recent changes in Washington, particularly while conservative Republicans, a group traditionally hostile to foreign aid, control both ends of Pennsylvania Avenue.

In addition to the leadership in Washington, an eclectic group of people has begun to lead the global charge to end extreme poverty. Jeffrey Sachs is widely viewed as one of the world's most respected and influential economists. For years, he has been a passionate and vocal advocate for ending extreme poverty, largely by scaling up rich world "aid" to the poorest countries. Sachs chaired the UN Commission on Macroeconomics and Health, which created the Global Fund, and has argued in *The Economist, New York Times*, and everywhere else that rich governments simply must give more. Allied with Kofi Annan, Sachs has significantly changed the terms of the debate on global AIDS, foreign aid, and debt relief. No longer content asking the world community for incremental increases in funding, Sachs has been out front, demanding billions. During a conference at the American Academy of Arts and Sciences on May 2, 2002, he said, "We have faked it for a generation. Rich people do everything to say, 'It's not about money.' But the whole international debate is about money. It's *all* about money" (Sachs 2002). Sachs has been joined by U2's front man Bono, who was nominated for the 2005 Nobel Peace Prize for his tireless work on AIDS, foreign aid to Africa, and debt relief. Others that have engaged in the larger political fight include the late Pope John Paul II, Kofi Annan, former Presidents Clinton and Carter, former US Secretary of State Colin Powell, and Senate Majority Leader Bill Frist.

In a July 2005 meeting in Gleneagles, Scotland, the world's richest countries (the G-8) agreed to an outright cancellation of the debts of the poorest 18 countries, totaling $40 billion, in the Heavily Indebted Poor Countries (HIPC) initiative. During the Gleneagles Summit, UK Prime Minister Tony Blair persuaded the world's most powerful leaders to double aid to Africa by 2010. While many pledges were mere reiterations of past, broken promises, the increased attention and large-scale debt relief were nonetheless welcome. Such complete debt forgiveness was unprecedented, and bodes well for future movements to relieve unsustainable debt burdens in the world's poorest countries. Of even greater importance, world leaders have taken positive, though decidedly tentative steps toward changing the fundamental nature of foreign aid, from strategic and self-serving to humanitarian and transformational. Of note, the One Campaign in the United States and the One World Campaign in the United Kingdom spurred worldwide attention, and more people than ever before are now focused on these issues.

For health providers, these issues should now command our attention as never before. We now have more opportunities to engage in these struggles and directly serve through hundreds of committed NGOs or lobby the political powers through other civil society organizations. NGOs like Fifty Years is Enough, the Jubilee 2000 Campaign, Physicians for Human Rights, among others, have worked with activists and scholars such as Jeff Sachs to change the tone of the debate and steer the rich countries toward dealing with these problems directly. NGOs, like Health Volunteers Overseas (HVO), Partners In Health, Operation Smile, Project Hope, Catholic Relief Services (CRS), CARE, and hundreds of others, work directly in developing countries to provide care and or training for local health providers. Literally hundreds of NGOs have opportunities for health providers who would like to directly engage in this struggle by serving overseas.

Informal estimates of medical students indicate that serving internationally is one of the most popular pursuits in medical schools across the country today. It will only increase in the future, and more leaders in international health will emerge. Tomorrow's health providers may well see international health move into the mainstream of the US medical profession, and become a staple in the education of our medical students. The Peace Corps has been sending recent college graduates to developing countries for over 40 years. Its 2004 budget totaled $323 million (Congressional Research

Service [CRS] 2004, 23). Couldn't doctors also be of use? (Baker and Quinley 1987, 2622; US Congress 1987; Kindig and Lythcott 1984, 10) Prior governmental efforts to integrate US physicians into international health have failed, but changing times and a markedly increased demand should prompt a renewed effort.

In the end, the poor simply can't wait for a few inspirational leaders to emerge. It will take a greater effort by a much larger percentage of the medical profession to effect change. The smaller individual efforts by thousands more health providers may prove collectively more effective in the long run than the heroic efforts of just a few. There are certainly plenty of good models out there through which health providers can engage, both in direct service and training. History teaches us that no group of physicians—no matter how wise and dedicated—could ever replace the basic engines of better health, namely, better nutrition, effective public health measures (clean water, basic sanitation, basic education, and universal vaccinations), and the rising prosperity afforded by economic growth. However, many programs, including ours at Omni Med, have proven the efficacy of sending health providers abroad to teach. Even those with no prior international experience have made a considerable impact.

The struggle to lift the world's poor out of their "poverty traps" and improve their basic health is an old one. In the end, it will not come down to a mere understanding of the problems at hand, even as they become increasingly soluble with each passing year. Despite the emerging technologies that ever more enhance our ability to see clearly into the darkest corners of our modern world, the most compelling answers will still come from the oldest of sources. Religion provides a clear moral direction for many of the world's people, and is the backbone of human rights. Ultimately, the ills of the world stem less from preconceived orders of nature than the willful intentions of man. Only through ethics, rooted in religion, can we hope to amend unjust world orders that date back centuries.

The Universal Declaration of Human Rights (UDHR) stands as a pinnacle of human aspirations, deriving its core principles from the world's most influential religions. Comprised of the fundamental strivings of humanity and conceived in the aftermath of humanity's darkest hour—World War II—the document rings with an eloquence that radiates truth. Our essential longings are truly universal. Our love for our children, desire for peace, health, security, a decent job, and happy family life are similar across lines of race, faith, gender, and time. Only through a gradual acceptance of the universality of our quest will we one day be able to address these concerns for all people. Within just two pages of its preamble and 30 articles, the declaration concisely expressed centuries of human aspirations. In its opening strains, the declaration states:

> Recognition of the inherent dignity and of the equal and inalienable rights of all members of the human family is the foundation of freedom, justice and peace in the world. . . . All human beings are born free and equal in dignity and rights.

The UDHR has become a road map for many who work in the realm of international health. Increasingly, NGOs frame their work and mission statements borrowing language and ideas from international human rights law. Jonathan Mann used the UDHR to lobby the UN and rich governments to take on AIDS, a practice that many will emulate in other realms.

Perhaps our best times are still ahead of us. For so many of the world's people, life is short, dominated by poverty, sickness, and insecurity. But we in the health profession can become important catalysts of change. Ultimately, motivations to work to improve the life of the poor come from a far deeper place, when each of us contemplates what is most important to us in life. Those questions are never easily answered, but few who become fully engaged in this work come to regret it. Quite to the contrary, work of this nature is often cited as the most valuable of life experiences. And that should come as no surprise. This work resonates with the core teachings of the three monotheistic religions, as well as virtually all others. The concerns of the least of those among us should truly be our own. By insisting that all people attain the fundamental human rights that are both their birthright and a demand of virtually all of the major world religions, we can improve health for the world's people. By taking action ourselves, we can directly effect change. We can at least take the critical first steps required to engage the problem, to find a reason to care.

In what follows here, you will find the means to engage in this realm. It is my sincere hope that a significant number of health providers will choose to bring their skills and talents to where they are most needed. Ultimately our aversion to tackle directly the root causes of global extreme poverty poses the gravest of threats to humanity. We are a strange people, abounding in the wealth and technologies and skills to solve all of these problems, yet we engage them with only a fraction of our potential. Ultimately, we reap what we sow, and if current dichotomies of wealth and health continue, ours will indeed be a bitter harvest. We are all connected far more than we are inclined to think, and our efforts to save our foreign brethren may one day save us as well.

Endnote

1. For more information see the Gallup-International Web site at www.gallup-international.com.

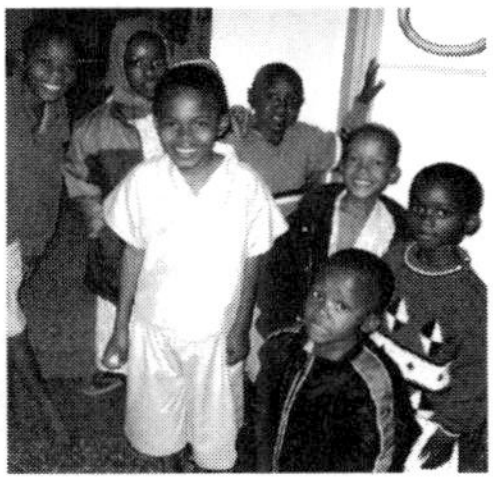

Chapter 1

Overcoming Obstacles: Cultural and Practical Guidelines

True generosity consists precisely in fighting to destroy the causes which nourish false charity. False charity constrains the fearful and subdued, the "rejects of life," to extend their trembling hands. True generosity lies in striving so that these hands—whether of individuals or entire peoples—need be extended less and less in supplication, so that more and more they become human hands which work and, working, transform the world.

—Paulo Freire

There are two overwhelming barriers in this country [the United States]: People think there are no solutions other than what we are doing, and that we are doing enough.

—Jeffrey Sachs

There's a natural mystic blowing through the air;
If you listen carefully now you will hear.
This could be the first trumpet, might as well be the last:
Many more will have to suffer,
Many more will have to die—don't ask me why.

—Bob Marley

There are a host of obstacles that keep people from serving internationally. This book should eliminate one of them—the lack of information. However, a number of obstacles become insurmountable for many, causing them to miss out on what is often a life-changing experience. Among the most important obstacles are planning, fear, time, money, inertia, and familial obligations. We explore each of these issues in this chapter, emphasizing aspects of travel to the developing world that many people overlook. Culture poses the greatest, if most invisible of challenges to those who venture abroad. We review important aspects in preparation for culture and the inevitable culture shock that affects so many. We also review the stories of those who have served well, and discuss some simple behaviors that can turn a routine health mission into something far more important both to the volunteer and to those served. Finally, we review some of the practical considerations, like the value of short-term versus long-term volunteers; the particulars of passport, visa, and health insurance; a few points about packing; and donating or transporting medical supplies (something people should consider well ahead of time). Taken together, the material in this chapter should help any health volunteer prepare properly. In the next chapter, we will cover matters of travel, health, and safety.

People traveling to poor countries need some basic information to ensure a safe stay. I will cover all of those basic points here, as well as many additional points to ensure a more cost-effective and productive stay. For those interested in reading further in the realm of "third world" travel, one book covers the essentials of this so-called independent travel better than any other, *The Practical Nomad: How to Travel Around the World*, by Edward Hasbrouck (2000). This book is not just for those planning around-the-world trips, it is for anyone traveling to the developing world. I have never met Mr Hasbrouck and have no incentive for recommending his book. However, he writes beautifully and covers most of the practical and logistical matters that routinely confront the international health service traveler: booking airfares; securing visas, passports, and insurance; packing soundly; overcoming cultural barriers; among others. The 80-page resource section at the back of the book alone is worth the cover price. Some of the suggestions that follow here come directly from his book. In addition to Hasbrouck's book, I recommend you find the relevant *Lonely Planet* or *Rough Guide* books for the given destination. There are other series available, but none match these two for scope and detail. We have used the *Rough Guide* series in our Belize program for years with good results.

Disclaimer

It is important for me to state at the outset here that this entire section is designed to augment your other pre-travel preparations. In no way should it replace your planned visits with a travel clinic beforehand and afterward, or your own reading. Nor should it dissuade you from conducting your own research—some of it through sources that I will cite as we move through this chapter. What follows is culled from my own experience, from feedback from those who have gone through Omni Med programs, from a review of medical literature, and from an invaluable course I attended called "Intensive Update in Clinical Tropical Medicine and Traveler's Health," by the American Society of Tropical Medicine and Hygiene (ASTMH). I encourage all who have a real interest in this realm to consider such a course for themselves or the longer, degree-oriented programs sponsored by ASTMH. Please be advised that I am neither an expert in travel medicine nor an anthropologist. I offer the following only in the spirit of helping those destined for parts unknown to have a safer and healthier stay. So, read broadly, make clear plans with the nongovernmental organization (NGO) or group that will sponsor you, and get to a traveler's clinic at least four to six weeks before you go.

Also note that the following is not intended to frighten the potential volunteer into staying comfortably at home. The risks involved in traveling to poor settings are, in my opinion, offset by the rewards incurred through service and travel, and by the overriding moral imperative that motivates us from the beginning. Every day we do far more risky things than travel abroad. There are over 40,000 road fatalities in the United States every year, though few of us avoid driving (Kristoff 2004). As in driving, there are a number of things one can do to markedly decrease the likelihood that something bad will happen. Such is the case here as well.

Planning

This is where most people make their first mistake. It takes time to plan experiences of this sort. In addition to extensive reading, be sure to leave yourself plenty of time to find an organizational match, and then properly cover the logistics of your trip. Most people should allow at least six months to prepare for their trip, one year for longer sojourns. When I planned my three-month stay in East Africa in 1994, it took nearly four months just to find the right opportunity. Factor in that it can take weeks to months for mail to reach remote mission sites, if it gets there at all. While the Internet has reduced communication time dramatically, many poorer locales have sporadic Internet access or none at all. The resource section in Part 2 of this text should markedly reduce your search time, but there is still a lot to do.

In addition to the time required to actually find the right organizational fit and location, you will need time to book a flight, visit a travel clinic, secure the correct travel documents, and properly prepare yourself mentally for life in a strange culture. The more in advance you book your flight, the cheaper it will be. Travel agents like Edward Hasbrouck recommend booking flights three to six months in advance, and longer in advance for travel during December or other peak seasons (Hasbrouck 2000, 247). Most authorities advise visiting a travel clinic at least four to six weeks before you plan on leaving, earlier if you are going long term. Some vaccines, such as hepatitis A and B, rabies, and Japanese B encephalitis, require a full month of immunizations. The full immunization course for hepatitis B is six months, so the non-immune might well plan this first.

Overcoming Obstacles

Fear

For many considering overseas service, fear remains the most daunting obstacle. Stories of humanitarian workers targeted, of volunteers killed by land mines or road accidents, of others returning with malaria or other dreaded tropical illnesses cause many to postpone or even cancel their sojourns. There is certainly an element of truth giving rise to such fears. However, the overwhelming majority of people who have traveled to and served in poor communities abroad do so with either no illness at all or merely that of the nuisance variety, such as traveler's diarrhea. Further, many of them return again, overwhelmed by the power of the experience.

Some simple measures, like those we will cover here, can markedly increase the safety for everyone who travels abroad. Yet fear is an irrational animal, and one that thrives on misunderstanding and ignorance. The US media doesn't help, attracting viewers by playing on their fears. It is little wonder that so much of the developing world seems such a frightening place to those who have never traveled there. Most poor countries receive attention only when overcome by war, terrorism, or natural disasters.

As Edward Hasbrouck has noted, most of travelers' fears are unfounded, and many of the travelers he has served as a travel consultant focus their questions on air safety, terrorism, and exotic disease. He writes,

> Statistically speaking, however, these questions say more about travelers' fears than about the actual dangers of travel. Travel by land or water is far more dangerous than travel by air; serious injury—most often from road accidents—is much more likely than serious illness; most violent crime is economic, with no obvious political content and no relation to terrorism; hygiene and behavior have more effect on travel health than do inoculations; and government advisories are a poorer indication of violence than daily newspapers (2000, 373).

US media outlets succeed in frightening us about all things foreign while covering in depth every airline crash anywhere in the world. No wonder so many people fear flying. Similarly, every terrorist attack receives broad coverage leaving many people convinced that terrorists lurk around every corner of the developing world. While terrorist attacks have increased in recent years, achieving an ignoble pinnacle on September 11, 2001, the risk of dying at the hands of a terrorist remain just a tiny percentage of those of dying while driving your car. There are many "tropical" illnesses for which one must take precautions, but the likelihood of acquiring any of them while abroad remains small.

Fortunately, there is a sizable literature that covers the risks of those who travel to developing countries. The most valuable information comes from studies of Peace Corps volunteers (PCVs) because these people travel to remote rural areas and live under conditions most similar to those that health volunteers may well find in hospitals or clinics in the developing world. By 2002, over 170,000 PCVs had served in 136 countries over 42 years. In its 2002 Annual Safety Report, over 99% of the PCVs felt safe where they worked and 97% where they lived (US Peace Corps

2002). In 1985, the Peace Corps developed an epidemiological surveillance system to monitor its 5500 volunteers in 62 countries around the world (Bernard et al 1989, 220). They found that the most common problems encountered were diarrheal illnesses, injuries, bacterial skin infections, and dental problems. By contrast, malaria, schistosomiasis, and hepatitis were uncommon. The Peace Corps prepares its recruits well, and they have stayed healthy as a result. Anyone planning on traveling to the developing world should learn this lesson from the Peace Corps. You can be safe while traveling and working abroad—but you have to prepare.

While data such as this may reassure some, others will no doubt remain convinced that international health work is simply too dangerous. I still recall vividly the concerns I had when first traveling to East Africa—the fear that flowed ever so freely from the great unknown. The first step is to inoculate our fears with knowledge, which these two chapters should do. Then, you should talk with those who have gone before you. Find the organization in Chapter 3 that most appeals to you and ask to speak with some people who have already served. People who do this work usually like to talk about their experiences and will no doubt provide some reassurance.

Time

More than people in any other society, we Americans seemingly abhor being away from our jobs. Unlike the Europeans who regard time off as a right, Americans still view theirs as a privilege. In fact, there is no legal obligation for US employers to provide vacation time ("A Great Time" 1999). The typical US worker takes just two weeks off each year while those in Italy, France, Sweden, Denmark, and Germany take four to five weeks off (Verespej 1999). According to the International Labor Organization, Americans work an average of nine more weeks per year than their European counterparts, when average hours per workweek are factored in (Sanders 2003). Australians commonly take 6 to 12 months to pursue other interests. When I traveled across the United States for two months in 1982, I met as many Australians in the youth hostels as Americans. Step one for many Americans is to overcome strongly ingrained cultural recordings that lead us to believe that we should not go away. For many doctors and other highly motivated people in health care, that may take some doing. It's OK—it's all right to go.

Many health providers, however, understandably find it difficult to get away from the obligations of clinical practice. With the knowledge that a number of their patients feel comfortable with them only, many providers feel that they are violating sacred covenants by going away, particularly for long periods of time. There is certainly merit in such concerns, and only the individual provider can weigh the pros and cons involved. However, when factoring in our larger global responsibilities, one can certainly find sufficient moral justification to serve outside one's traditional practice realm. I believe that we have an ethical obligation to do so.

Through the years, I have sought interesting and creative ways through which individual providers, practice groups, or hospitals have integrated an international component into their practices. Most of the approaches stemmed from the efforts of just a few interested people. While such practices remain novel, they are well within reach of those willing to put in the time and effort, as the following examples demonstrate. If there are no programs similar to those that follow where you work, consider starting one. Most of the individuals cited in the pages that follow have provided contact information (available in the endnotes) and agreed to offer advice if contacted.

Many providers have first tried their hand in international medicine through short-term service missions. For most, it is the best way to try out such an experience and there are a host of organizations in Part 2 of this text that offer such opportunities. See Chapter 5 for programs with short-term opportunities; we will discuss the pros and cons of short-term service shortly. Keep in mind that many of those who have gone on to long-term service started through a short-term foray.

Omni Med For eight years now, I have run an NGO, Omni Med, that sends health providers to several developing countries on short-term educational missions. Given our educational focus, we have been able to provide a unique opportunity for short-term service to those with no prior international health experience, while simultaneously offering ongoing educational programs that help local health providers update and improve their clinical skills. Of the 100-plus trips that we have sponsored thus far, I have yet to hear of anyone that regretted going abroad. In fact, most people rave about their experiences, and we now have detailed questionnaires dating back to 1999 that prove the efficacy of this approach. Colleague and Omni Med member Dr John O'Brien offered this commentary about his work in Belize. "Every day in Belize," he says, "is the equivalent of a month at home in terms of learning and life experiences. You are just bombarded with new and different insights into how medicine is practiced elsewhere, and have a unique opportunity to look back at health care in the United States—both the good and the bad. The experience also provides insights into American foreign policy, global trade, foreign aid, culture, poverty, and life in a developing country. Your senses are overwhelmed by new and fascinating things, while you are making a difference in the world. From both a professional and personal standpoint, it is an extraordinarily rich experience."

Another colleague, Dr Ed Wyman, was a veteran of Hospital Albert Schweitzer in Haiti and a host of other international locales during his long career in orthopedics. During a visit with me to Nairobi's St Mary's Hospital in 2001 he said, "I can never understand why people *don't* do this. They just have no idea of what they are missing." Several of the physicians who served through our programs have gone on to found new programs, all of which afford them the opportunity to return to the same place once or twice annually while maintaining busy clinical schedules.

Some physicians find that they can most effectively serve by regularly returning to the same site for brief periods. Dr Tom Antkowiak is another orthopedic surgeon who has worked in a number of hospitals abroad. Following an initial visit to St Mary's Hospital in Kenya in 2002, Dr Antkowiak has made a number of return trips and has become the de facto orthopedic surgeon for the hospital. During his regular visits, he operates on any outstanding orthopedic cases and teaches local surgeons in the process.

Dr Joseph Bowlds Dr Joseph Bowlds is an ophthalmologist and administrator from the Lahey Clinic who has traveled annually to the same area in El Salvador for 15 years through an NGO called the Salvadoran Rural Health Association, also known as ASAPROSAR.[1] Given the confines of a busy schedule, Dr Bowlds spends just 10 days in El Salvador each year. However, unlike most short-term volunteers, he and the others at ASAPROSAR have been able to learn of specific needs and help locals meet them, slowly but progressively, year after year. In the beginning, a former Peace Corps volunteer, Eloise Clawson, RN, and a neuropsychologist, Dr Alan Gruber, began a relationship with Dr Vicki Guzman, an impressive Salvadoran physician. Together they were able to develop a health initiative for the poor in the region of Santa Ana. Through word of mouth, more health providers became involved, including Dr Bowlds. When he first traveled to El Salvador in 1989, Dr Bowlds and six other volunteers performed eye exams and distributed eyeglasses and medications.

Over time, a number of groups came together to help Dr Guzman develop her vision for a community health center, which now includes ambulatory surgery. One group in particular, the United Church of Christ in Norwell, has contributed substantial funds for 20 years. Dr Bowlds helped procure medical equipment, office furniture, and supplies from the Lahey Clinic, Symms Hospital, and elsewhere, ultimately helping to build and then outfit Dr Guzman's clinic in 1999, which now serves 30,000 people.[2] In addition to distributing eyeglasses, Dr Bowlds now brings surgical teams, operating on over 100 patients annually over the past few years. Through modest charges for eye exams, ASAPROSAR now employs a well-trained Salvadoran ophthalmologist, who works part-time throughout the year.

By committing time, skill, and resources, in addition to collaborating with several other groups, this committed network of goodwill has helped an extraordinary Salvadoran physician create a comprehensive health center in El Salvador. In the process, Dr Bowlds has introduced many of his colleagues to this work, many of whom have returned and/or helped to fund the construction of the clinic. Those who feel they don't have time for this work should heed Dr Bowlds' example. He has combined a full-time clinical-administrative position with substantive international work for 15 years. By developing collaborative relationships and understanding local needs, Dr Bowlds greatly enhanced his impact. He terms this work "immensely rewarding" and garners a special pleasure in sharing his enthusiasm with colleagues, well over 100 of whom have accompanied him to El Salvador through the years.

Hospital Albert Schweitzer Hospital Albert Schweitzer (HAS), the creation of Dr Larimer and Gwen Mellon in Haiti, has become a periodic home for many health providers.[3] Although I have never been there, I know several who have and I understand it is quite an impressive place. Rhena Schweitzer Miller (Albert Schweitzer's daughter) who spent many years working internationally with her physician husband called this hospital the best she'd seen in the developing world; it has short-term opportunities (one-month minimum) for many types of clinicians. Many providers have returned following their initial visit. The Peach Tree Orthopedic Group in Atlanta has sent orthopedic surgeons there three to four times yearly since the hospital opened in 1956. One HAS repeat volunteer and alumni director, Dr Robert Moses, cited the value of the many short-term volunteers who have worked there through the years. Those with a specialty skill teach while there, and many have either returned for additional service, donated money, or recruited other donors. Plus, he adds, "The short-termers re-energize the place." HAS has a strong long-term staff of 17–20 physicians who can accommodate short-term help. In addition, their orientation program allows it to use the short-term volunteers effectively.

Shortly after the Mellons opened HAS, they realized that they needed help in pediatrics. Dr and Mrs Mellon met with Drs Bob McGovern and Florence (Skeets) Marshall, who had just completed their pediatric residencies at Cornell. "They agreed to set up a pediatric practice in New York and another one for Dr Mellon in Haiti," said partner Dr Duane Dowell.[4] "Then they went home to look on the map to see where Haiti was." Their plan was one of the most viable and interesting models I have yet seen, in which "Practice A" in New York helped to fund "Practice B" in Haiti. Drs McGovern and Marshall at first rotated between the two practices every other year until Dr Phillip Eskes joined, replaced by Dr Dowell in 1968. The model worked continuously from 1957 until 1980, with one of three physicians spending one full year in Haiti each year. They changed on September 1 to coincide with the children's school year, and all physicians convened in New York every August to review their overall plans. According to Dr Dowell, medical director of HAS from 1999–2004, the model worked well. The practices in both New York and Haiti were "fun" and rewarding, while their families all gained from the experience. All three of Dr Dowell's children recall the experiences "fondly" and have worked internationally—two are in medicine.

The only downfall to the practice was that they as a practice group were, according to Dr Dowell, "overly altruistic." They were one of the few practices on Long Island that accepted Medicaid at the time and often undercharged. Dr Dowell feels that they could have continued far longer had they only had a more sound business model. How many physicians now in more lucrative practices could adopt such a model, or even send one member abroad for just a few months per year?

Dr Edmund Browne In yet another innovative approach to working abroad, Dr Edmund Browne began a long-term relationship with the Mopan Clinic in the town of Benque Viejo in Western Belize in 1986. He had visited Belize in October of 1984 and found a "crying need for help," so he approached the Minister of Health. Having been burned many times before by those pledging aid from the United States, the Ministry at first turned him down. Undaunted, Dr Browne rented a house, bought a pick-up truck, hired a housekeeper, and then recruited physician volunteers to staff the clinic, ultimately gaining the full trust and support from the Ministry. In time the clinic grew to become one of the best equipped in Belize. Typically, there were two physicians on staff at all times, one long-term (one year) and one short-term (one to three months). In time, they incorporated two medical students per month, all living together, staffing the clinic and visiting the surrounding villages year-round. Long-term volunteers received $200/month, while short-term volunteers paid their own way in full. Students paid $125/month to defer expenses. Dr Browne visited the clinic five to six times yearly, met with the appropriate officials in Belize, and regularly sent medical supplies. While he was able to raise $7,000 to $10,000 per year, he paid most of the annual $50,000 cost out of personal funds. From the first year of operations, he was deluged with requests and never had openings unfilled over the eight years in which he ran the clinic, up until his retirement from medicine.

I heard of Dr Browne's work through my visits to Belize and spoke with him on the phone several times. Even through the imperfect medium of the telephone, it was easy to hear his sincerity, his passion, and his fond recollections of this work. Those who knew him in Belize recalled him fondly—several used the word "saint." He became the godfather to a child of Dr Ramone Figueroa, a Belizean physician and a high-ranking minister. Dr Browne recalls with pride the satisfaction he felt upon seeing a medical student volunteer later return to the Mopan Clinic as a physician volunteer. The volunteers all loved their time and, according to Dr Browne, "99% of them were good people." Similar to the experiences of those in other programs, Dr Browne recalls that most volunteers felt they had received far more than they had given. Like other similar programs, the Mopan Clinic relied on collaboration between several groups. St John's College in Belize City, the Jesuit International Volunteer Program, the Ministry of Health in Belize, even the bi-annual volunteer service opportunity publication in *JAMA* all played important roles.

Ultimately, however, like so many programs, it was one person who dedicated his time and funds to develop something that made a difference. I visited the Mopan Clinic during a Belize trip in 2002, and found a shell of what had once been. There was no commemorative plaque, and none of the people who had worked with Dr Browne's group in the 1980s and 1990s remained. However, ask any older person in Benke Viejo about Dr Browne and they will invariably smile and tell a story or two. His legacy lives on through those who received the gift of better health through his and his many volunteers' efforts. For those feeling time pressures, Dr Browne's model represents another opportunity to serve well. He was able to fully staff a clinic with physicians and students for eight years while maintaining a busy surgical practice in the United States. Again, it just takes time, money, and passion, with the latter paving the way for the former.

Additional Options Many hospital or provider networks have service options available for their employees—here are a few examples:

- The Southern California Permanente Medical Group (a member of Kaiser-Permanente) has an "extended medical service leave" program through which physicians can take up to three months off every five years with half-pay.[5] The original design, still in existence, allows physicians to take leaves to serve abroad so they gain "the opportunity to broaden their experience and see other parts of the world by working in under-served areas."
- Since 1993, the Lahey Clinic in Burlington, Massachusetts, has run a program called "Global Outreach" through which employees receive full airfare

coverage for short-term medical missions abroad. Run by an enterprising woman named Patricia Newton, the program raised several hundred thousand dollars through golf tournaments, road races, local business support, and sales of a Global Outreach Cookbook, which includes donated recipes from well-known local restaurants.[6] Two hundred people, some recurrently, have gone on 85 missions over 12 years, as of November 2005.

- The Caritas health system, in which I work, has a sabbatical program in which employees can take off unpaid leaves of absence for any number of reasons, including international health service. Many academic centers also offer sabbaticals and other forms of assistance for those interested in service.

Whatever program you choose, you should not let time become the chief obstacle. There are enough different program models out there that you can try this work during normally allotted vacation time. For those with families, consider meeting up at the end of the working portion of your trip, as occasionally happens in our Belize program. Some programs will accommodate families as well, though rarely for short-term work. A local orthopedic surgeon-internist couple, Glen and Susan Crawford, have taken their children to several countries on short-term missions, including Tanzania, India, and Bhutan (Greene 2003). There are ways to do this; you just have to find the best way for you.

Money

For many who would like to get involved, money remains another daunting obstacle. Money carries the additional burden of being among the most sensitive of subjects. Americans will talk about sexual indiscretions and family secrets on national television—just don't ask us what we earn. Such tendencies make it difficult for many to hold honest discussions about one of the chief obstacles in the path of service. However, there is simply no way around it. Work of this nature is far from a lucrative endeavor—we simply need to be a little creative to get there.

Whether people feel the weight of a mortgage, student loans, education costs for children, medical bills, or a plethora of other expenses, we must recognize the weight of real financial obligations. Few international service programs will cover costs for those who serve short-term, and most longer service programs will cover only a comparable wage for the host country, which is small by American or European standards. Even salaried clinical positions abroad typically require an element of sacrifice, but work of this nature usually does. Having run an NGO for eight years, I am well acquainted with just how difficult it is to keep such programs alive. In the United States, it remains extremely difficult for small NGOs with programs overseas to secure funding. Because most programs run on limited budgets and operate in countries with miniscule expenditures in the health sector, those who get involved should recognize up front that they will rightly be asked to give something back. But US health providers are comparatively well paid—in my opinion, we should offer our services.

In discussing such matters, I fully recognize that the financial positions of various members of the health profession are not equal. Physicians and those in top positions of health administration have far greater financial leeway to volunteer their services abroad than do paramedics, technicians, or many nurses. However, in my experiences, the amount of money earned—or lack thereof—does not pose the chief obstacle to serving abroad or domestically. In the immediate aftermath of the fall of the World Trade Center Towers in New York during that horrible time of September 2001, steel workers, firefighters, and health personnel of all kinds volunteered their services for long periods of time. Few of these people were wealthy. Similar patterns hold true internationally. I have long suspected that rising incomes may even inversely correlate with tendencies to serve. Those who keep finances in perspective may indeed have more opportunity than those who earn more money but feel obligated to spend it all. The late Dr Tom Durant, who spent a lifetime working in refugee camps throughout the world, once told me that the reason so many of his physician colleagues could never accompany him on his international travels was that they had become slaves to their lifestyles. They didn't believe that they could afford the missed income and additional expenditures that international service work demands. When large homes, expensive cars, private schools, summer homes, and fine clothes become essential, then perhaps they are right. Ultimately, however, it comes down to perspective.

Some of the most impressive work I have seen internationally has come from lay people following their passion. A small group of Rotarians in Orange Walk, Belize, and Hingham, Massachusetts, figured out how to transport valuable medical equipment from the United States to Belize. Subsequently, the Hingham Rotary group, under the leadership of Richard Bridges, became the most important element in transporting millions of dollars of relief supplies to Honduras, ravaged by Hurricane Mitch in October of 1999. The individuals involved were simply working men and women who had the passion to make a difference—and did so magnificently.

The first step in deciding if you can afford to take the time off to serve is to figure out your priorities. How important is this to you? More specifically, what things would you rather put your time and money toward? We can take that question one important step further by asking, "If you had one year left to live, how would you spend your time and money?" Would you change any of your priorities, or would you keep things just as they are now? The question will be different for students and those still in training than for those many years out of training or retired. But they are questions we all need to answer eventually.

These are difficult question for everyone, and quite often pushed aside by the rush of every day. Periodically, books come along that move such questions to the forefront and get many people to change their priorities, even their lives. Let me suggest four such books. The first, *Your Money or Your Life: Transforming Your Relationship with Money and Achieving Financial Independence* by Joe Dominguez and Vicki Robin (Viking 1992) was a national bestseller in the early 1990s and has maintained its relevance ever since.[7] The authors make the simple claim that "money is something that we choose to trade our life energy for" (Dominguez and Robin 1992, 54). As such, we need to view all of our expenses in terms of the hours of work required for purchase. For example, a dedicated clothes shopper may well become less so when forced to face the hours of work each new item requires. The authors challenge the readers with the following, "Was this expenditure of life energy in alignment with my values and my life purpose?" (184) For a number of people who followed this book's recommendations, many "things" lose their value when compared to the hours, even years spent to acquire them. Realigned priorities, often in the form of service, offer so much more value than many of the things we are convinced we "need." The authors present a road map for financial independence and allow the reader to pursue that which he or she really wants to do.

In *First Things First: To Live, to Love, to Learn, to Leave a Legacy* (Simon & Schuster 1994), Steven Covey similarly asked readers to prioritize things in their lives, to be sure their life orientations were aligned with their most strongly held convictions, those, as he says, that are facing "true north." Covey noted that far too often, "we've painstakingly climbed the 'ladder of success' rung by rung—only to discover as we reached the top rung that the ladder is leaning against the wrong wall" (Covey et al 1994, 20). Covey offers a simple process through which people can prioritize things in their lives in accordance to their deepest held convictions. While this may seem at first blush distant from financial concerns, consider that many never find international health service because they have not taken the time to figure out their values. Those in the medical profession will often find a connection with the ideals that first interested them in the profession. How valuable is that?

Another useful book in this genre is Viktor Frankl's *Man's Search for Meaning* (Simon & Schuster 1959). Frankl spent three years in Auschwitz, Dachau, and other concentration camps during World War II and witnessed unconscionable cruelty of man to man. He also viewed how some seemed to rise above the deplorable conditions by maintaining their basic humanity. Simple acts of kindness like caring for another gave meaning to the lives of those often destined to die. Frankl's "logotherapy" became widely applied and remains useful for us today. Are we truly pursuing a life filled with meaning and purpose? Many health providers would answer a resounding "yes" to that question, though in the era of managed care, 15-minute patient visits, and productivity-oriented repayment schemes, many have questioned whether they still have control over their professional lives. Could there be something more out there?

The Millionaire Next Door: The Surprising Secrets of America's Wealthy by Thomas J. Stanley and William D. Danko (Longstreet Press 1996) is another useful book. These two authors surveyed a number of US millionaires and found some common qualities about saving money, and saving money will give more people an opportunity to serve. Many will simply not do so unless they can afford to. More accurately, they will not until they *feel* that they can afford to. Because so much of our financial status is based on perceptions of what is and is not needed in life, books of this genre are invaluable tools to find the release to pursue activities that one values, like service. Pursuing such work may force some to reconsider their priorities in life. Do you really need some of the material acquisitions that you have sought? Would you not feel a greater sense of fulfillment if you could replace certain baubles with relationships to those in other lands, and the enriching experiences that can create a whole new meaning in life for you?

My family and I have adopted a number of the above ideas into our lifestyle. I last worked full time in 1992—in the years since I have worked more hours at Omni Med gratis than I have as an ER physician for a salary. Yet I would not trade the richness this other life has brought to my family and me. We simply never bought into the ideology that states that one requires a lot of material things to be happy. By saving and living frugally, my wife and I look forward to an early transition to working internationally and providing a unique educational experience to our children.

Medical students and residents will want to look for travel assistance through a number of programs out there, often at the school or residency program. The American Medical Student Association (AMSA) and the Global Health Education Consortium (GHEC) have developed a resource guide for medical students and residents, available on the AMSA Web site (www.amsa.org/resource/amsarc/creative/creative.cfm). AMSA estimates that the typical six-week elective costs $2500, which most students fund themselves (American Medical Student Association 2004). When I traveled to Tanzania as a fourth-year medical student in 1987, I simply borrowed it all. I had huge loans from George Washington University School of Medicine at the time already, and my experience in Tanzania added just a small amount to my total debt. More importantly, I had suspected that this would be an experience worth the extra costs—and it was.

On a more pragmatic basis, we can look at the comparative costs and the potential savings involved. For those who worry whether they have sufficient funds to go, consider that short vacations are far more expensive than longer ones, an analogy with relevance for short-term and long-term service trips. The average six-month overseas trip budget for someone constantly traveling is only three times that of the average two-week trip budget, far less than the time differential would suggest (Hasbrouck 2000, 13). This makes sense as airfares and hotel stays comprise the largest expenses, and those traveling longer tend to stay in less expensive accommodations. Most people working in clinical settings abroad will spend little or nothing for room and board during their stay, and the cost of living in most developing countries is very low. In fact, it is difficult to spend a lot of money in many poor countries. During my three trips to East Africa, I paid only for airfare and some nominal travel expenses afterward, but almost nothing for daily living expenses. Be sure to subtract the differential between what you would have spent at home and what little you will spend abroad when calculating the cost of overseas work—it adds up. Further, there are tax breaks available for those who work abroad, such as converting individual retirement accounts (IRAs) into Roth IRAs during a year in which salary is less, amounting to considerable tax savings later on (510).

While none of these considerations may outweigh the "opportunity costs" of the lost income you would have otherwise generated, I can only ask that you weigh all factors into your final decision. First, recall the "ethical imperative" that we all share, and try to remember just where your considerable good fortune came from. Second, consider how life-changing an experience this work can be and try to put a dollar value on it. Why else would so many people who first try this work return repeatedly and what would such an experience actually be worth? Third, put finances into perspective. While there are certain things that we can only acquire through money, use some of the above resources to help you align your own expenses with your values. You may see opportunities that now elude you. Finally, factor in that most trips abroad cost less than an average vacation to a resort in someplace warm. They are far more enriching and educational, and may even become a regular part of your life. Experiences like those offered in Part 2 of this text are well within reach for a majority of health providers in the United States and Europe. While some may have truly pressing financial obligations that constrain them, most people can find the means to do this if they really try.

Inertia

Many people have not yet planned an international health experience primarily because it has been too difficult to do so. Inertia is a trait common to us all, and there is no shortage of reasons why one simply can't get around to planning such an excursion. However, this book should eliminate one of the more daunting obstacles for many people. Most of what you need to plan an international health experience will be found within these pages. If not, there are sufficient references where you can find answers to remaining questions or concerns. If you still find it difficult to motivate or find the right incentive, I suggest that you leaf through the organizations in Chapter 3 that most appeal to you. Call them up and ask to speak with people who have gone through them previously. Because the overwhelming majority of those who have gone on both short-term and long-term service missions will highly recommend it to others, you just may find the final push you need. As previously stated, planning will take time, so you should begin your inquiries well in advance. However, vacations also take time to plan, and an experience through one of the organizations listed in Chapter 3 of this text could well become one of your most valued life experiences. Make the time and plan—it's worth it.

Family Matters

Many health workers don't embark on such trips because of concerns about family. Given the dangers of treacherous roads, illness, or political unrest, many forego what could be a life-changing experience for the entire family. At each locale in which I have worked, I have encountered those who brought their entire families with them. In 1987, I met a carpenter from Ireland who brought his wife and five children to rural Tanzania for a year. The youngest was still in diapers and the mother taught all the kids through home schooling. They were a joyous and quite well adjusted bunch. That description fits most of the families I have encountered during my work experiences abroad. The risks of illness are real, but for the most part can be avoided.

Many people worry about children missing school during travel excursions, particularly for long periods abroad. However, there is no better education for young and eager minds than that available from living in another culture, particularly in a developing country. There is also no better way to learn another language than immersion, and children learn language most easily. Because the world is increasingly interconnected, what better education to offer a young person than to show him or her the world as it really is? Those who have lived abroad as children or young adults often recall the experience as the best times of their lives, despite the frequent hardships that such experiences entail.

Dr James Meyer Dr James Meyer was an intern in the transitional program at St Elizabeth's Medical Center in Boston where I met him during his ER block in the early summer of 2002. As of this writing, he is a radiologist in training at Baystate Medical Center in Springfield, Massachusetts. James' father was an internist who moved the family from their comfortable environs in Massachusetts to Dominica for James' fifth and sixth grade years. While in Dominica, James hunted with friends in the jungle, went spear fishing, had his own farm animals, and lived a life so radically different from his prior one that the experience, as he says, "changed me." The experience pulled his family together and showed him a side of life that he has never forgotten. His father was the sole physician for one half of the island, and he worked hard to care for patients and build up the hospital. His mother started a library, and was "very involved" in community development.

Because his family was so oriented toward a service ethic, he says, "I just assumed that everyone thought similarly, that it was a common fabric of our society. The idea that people should all pull themselves up by their bootstraps was completely foreign to me. I thought everyone cared for the poor." The experience of living abroad shaped him and his siblings, making them, in his words, "philosophical and altruistic." It also attracted him to medicine.

Like that of many others, the experiences of James and his family were not all positive. Given his clinical and other administrative responsibilities, James' father "worked to the bone," which took its toll on the family. Subsequent long-term work experiences in India and Nepal caused James to feel "rootless," envying those with family and friends rooted in one place. Keep in mind that James and his family lived in a number of different places, more so than those who do this work for a year or two, or regularly return to the same place. Still, James reflects on his experiences as "definitely a net positive," and like so many others, would not trade them. Author Robert Kohls reviewed a number of studies of "third-culture kids," those who grow up overseas as children of military personnel, missionaries, or diplomats (Kohls 1996, 112). In short, they become more independent, mature faster, are more sophisticated and cosmopolitan, and are far more knowledgeable about the world. Despite the psychological challenges of the common perceptions of "rootlessness," Kohls writes, "virtually all of them, once they are grown, say they would not trade their international growing-up experience for anything else" (112).

There is a certain value in seeing the world as it is—particularly when young and impressionable. So many Americans turn away from the problems of the world. In some ways, it is easier to not know, to simply avoid looking at the poorest countries and the people who inhabit them. However, such is a dangerous tendency that is inconsistent with reality, and the lessons available to a child who sees the world for what it is are invaluable and permanent. They are impossible to replicate in the classroom.

The Merry Seven Dr Steve and Kayleen Merry have led extraordinary lives by any standard, with work excursions in Côte d'Ivoire (1990–1991), Uganda (1995–1998), and Togo (2002–2003) thus far. French commandos evacuated their family of seven out of Côte d'Ivoire on September 29, 2002, just 10 days after civil war broke out. Fortunately, none of their family was harmed. They had just arrived one month earlier with plans to start a Family Practice Residency at Hôpital Baptiste, with plans to stay for 10 years. They spent the next year working at a mission hospital just two countries over in Togo. Steve is a gifted family practitioner whom I worked with in 1992–1993. Kayleen is a teacher, writer, and mother of five, who grew up in Côte d'Ivoire, the daughter of medical missionaries. Her father was a general surgeon, and her mother a nurse who raised four of Kayleen's six siblings there until evacuated by United Nations (UN) troops following an outbreak of violence in 1961. Rebels held Kayleen's father and uncle (an obstetrician) under house arrest for days while detaining her mother, pregnant with Kayleen, and other siblings at the border. Many of the other missionaries were killed during the uprising. The family subsequently moved to Côte d'Ivoire, where Kayleen's parents continued to work until their retirement in 1992. Despite such traumatic beginnings, all six siblings have worked in Africa—five have made it their primary home.

Kayleen was born in Côte d'Ivoire, and considers it her true home. She finds it more difficult to leave Africa than the United States, where her parents now reside. For her, growing up in Africa meant sacrifice, but also a rich life without all the "distractions" of television, sports, and club activities that dominate US culture. Like the rest of her family, she "fell in love with" the people of Côte d'Ivoire, and loved the pace of life there. Echoing the comments of most who have lived in Africa, she recalls how people there are much better at living in the moment, enjoying the little they have, and leading a relationship-based existence that adds a richness she finds lacking in the United States. In Africa, people make the best out of their circumstances. Instead of sitting in front of a TV, they talk to each other. The cultural differences from the United States are stark, and they permeate every aspect of life, from the way you raise your children to a heightened awareness one has of the presence of God. For her, the social justice perspective is invaluable, and one that permeates every aspect of life. "[Life in Africa] offers an entirely different perspective," she says. "Once you have lived in the Third World, you are never the same."

Life in West Africa is not without its share of risks. The Merry's have lost several friends in road accidents, while others have died at the hands of insurgents. Yet Kayleen puts it all in perspective—none of the risks have proved enough to dissuade them from returning. It becomes just another part of the terrain. One learns to minimize risks, she says, "avoid driving at night, and avoid taking public transportation when possible." However, she adds, "there are risks wherever you live." Snakes comprise her one great fear, following a bite at age six. She now checks "fanatically" under beds and makes sure the kids always wear shoes and use flashlights when outside walking at night.

Dr Steve Merry feels that the choice to bring a family abroad is a highly individual thing, though he "absolutely" feels it is a net positive experience. He recommends waiting until after the first year, because so many vaccinations are completed by then, though he and Kayleen left for Côte d'Ivoire when their youngest was only four months old. Steve echoes most language development experts who advise language training as early as possible. His own children learned some of the Ewe tribal dialect of Togo, which he expects will help them to learn other languages later on. Their two oldest children became fluent in French at age eight during a language immersion program in Quebec, Canada. When the Merrys arrived in Quebec in September 2001, Steve and Kayleen made the difficult decision to place the twins in French public school. As Steve says, both failed miserably at first because they understood no French. But by year's end, they had adapted well and had gained an immeasurable amount of confidence. At the end of their year, daughter Marielle received the highest score in her third grade class while brother Matthew placed second in a class entirely taught in French.

Echoing others I have spoken to, Dr Merry feels that the experiences abroad have been largely mixed, though net strongly positive. The time away certainly "helped to really pull the family together." He also feels that it instilled a "quiet confidence" in their children. As he says, "They have been through some difficult times abroad, they've weathered some storms. So when confronted with obstacles at home, they deal with them." While his kids may feel somewhat "out of it," not knowing popular styles and cultural icons, they have done something that most kids find "cool," which more than makes up for their losses. Steve does note that each transition has required that the kids "grieve" the loss of certain friends, places, and possessions, including the family dog. But, by keeping lines of communication open and being supportive of their children, they have done well. Both missionaries, Steve and Kayleen hope that the experiences abroad will instill a broader Christian social justice perspective that will guide their children through life.

Many parents ask when the best time is to bring their children abroad. The answer depends mostly on the parents themselves. One physician serving in Western Belize felt that the ideal time was roughly from ages 5 to 10. In his opinion, older kids want to be with their friends and younger kids may miss out on much of the value of the experience. Some, like the Merrys, feel that earlier is better. Whatever age one goes, however, it is important for all family members to be well aware of the adjustments each member must go through. Everyone will experience some degree of culture shock, and the stresses are real. As such, families contemplating serving abroad should pay particular heed to the many cultural considerations involved. Nowhere else in this work is the landscape so treacherous and so misleading.

A few additional points about families warrant mention. It is important that both the clinician and spouse find fulfilling activities while abroad. If one spouse works long clinical hours and the other sits alone at home, there will be problems. Kids can study, via home schooling if necessary, but will need more time of each parent. Be sure to include time for regular family discussions when planning such a venture. Women should also be aware that many societies in our world are patriarchal.

For an independent, career-oriented American woman, there may be some real adjustments involved.

Be aware that shorter-term stays abroad may be difficult for families, though some families, like the Crawfords mentioned earlier, do fine. Kayleen Merry recommends that families spend at least a full year to fully benefit from the experience. She recalled one family that came to Togo for two months and had a disastrous experience; the father, a physician, worked all the time, and the wife and children never fully adjusted. It takes time for most people to adapt to the vast cultural differences, which supports the idea of longer sojourns. Also, it is more disruptive for children to leave from the middle of a school year than to spend one full school year abroad. Once children have lived abroad, the acclimation time is less and the adjustment less difficult.

Most of the families I have interviewed for this book or encountered abroad have found international experiences a net positive. Those who have lost a loved one, or those who have found themselves under attack or in extreme danger may well feel otherwise. However, it is important to place the relative risks in perspective. Most people do this work safely and gain experiences that remain among their most cherished.

Cultural Considerations

Many who travel abroad overlook the importance of adjusting to a new and strange culture, yet such considerations are paramount. Most who remain in a foreign culture for longer than a few weeks will experience some degree of culture shock, and all who stay longer will experience it. Some people adapt better than others, but everyone can benefit from preparation beforehand. Over the past seven years, every physician traveling through one of our programs for the first time has received a copy of Robert Kohls' *Survival Kit for Overseas Living* (Intercultural Press 1996). This 132-page book covers all the essentials of culture and may be the most important book you read before going—it is short enough to read on the plane en route if necessary. Some of what follows comes directly from it. I highly recommend it to everyone traveling and working abroad, where the most difficult challenges encountered remain largely invisible, encoded in culture.

Culture is in us and all around us, embedded in our mannerisms, language, beliefs, actions, rules of law, governance, patterns of socializing, and any number of subconscious ways in which we go through our daily lives. Kohls writes that culture is "an integrated system of learned behavior patterns that are characteristic of the members of any given society. Culture refers to the total way of life of particular groups of people. It includes everything that a group of people thinks, says, does, and makes—its systems of attitudes and feelings" (Kohls 1996, 23). We don't see American culture because we live in it every day. However, those who come to the United States recognize its distinct characteristics immediately, as the French nobleman Alexis de Tocqueville did in the eighteenth century.[8] Nearly 200 years later, much that de Tocqueville observed in American culture remains: our hurried pace, informality, loudness, respect for the law, strong work ethic, frugality, aggressiveness, tendency to criticize our government, and lack of clear class boundaries. To this list

Robert Kohls adds: boastful, disrespectful of authority, ignorant of other countries, materialistic, superficial, friendly, punctual, and confident we have all the answers (Kohls 1996, 9). When we go abroad, we immediately see differences from our own culture, and, often for the first time, may recognize both good and bad aspects of our own culture.

In my experience, the most valuable traits one can carry to another country are *flexibility, adaptability, a sense of humor*, and a willingness to *lower expectations.* I ask each physician who comes through our programs to decide ahead of time if he or she can handle the myriad problems that inevitably arise: missed connections, rides on the public bus, no electricity, no running water, lack of dependable communication, and having everything run late. If they think they would find these things overly troublesome, then I advise them to strongly consider doing something else. Kohls adds the *ability to fail* as another valuable trait. In short, do not expect things to go as they do at home. Lower your expectations, roll with the challenges that inevitably come your way, and learn to laugh both at yourself and the situations that frustrate you. Those who are naturally curious, inquisitive, outgoing, friendly, and open tend to adapt more readily to new and strange cultures, while those who are more rigid, and expect much from themselves and those around them, become more readily frustrated.

One of the chief pitfalls integrated within every culture is a set of "recordings" of which most of us remain blissfully unaware. By recordings, I mean the set of images, Hollywood stereotypes, media portrayals, and water cooler gossip about certain ethnic or national groups, including our own, that inform our opinions of them and of us—often subconsciously. In a trait common to many cultures through history, people within a given society have considered themselves somehow superior, and foreigners of all types inferior. This is called ethnocentrism, and it remains alive and well within US culture today. These strong cultural recordings reinforce our own superior images and remain key obstacles to functioning well in other societies, particularly those that are predominantly poor. Racial recordings compound problems for many unaware they harbor such ideas.

Such ethnocentric ideas are enshrined in the very terms of development. In earlier times, Europeans considered Native Americans, as indigenous inhabitants elsewhere, "savages" and "primitive," annihilating them by the tens of thousands. Through time we have collectively made significant advances in understanding different cultures. Anthropologists have found complexities in all cultures, even those that on the surface seem "primitive." We have finally come to understand that those cultures that differ from our own are not necessarily inferior, they are simply "other." The terms have evolved to reflect such understanding. In lieu of primitive, poor countries became "underdeveloped," or "developing." While such terms were an improvement over earlier descriptions, they remain inherently judgmental, implying that these countries were becoming "just like us" in the industrialized world. There is really no ideal term to describe poor countries, and I use "developing" and "poor" interchangeably throughout this text. Whatever term one chooses, the point is to remain aware that we all carry subconscious "recordings" about the people in these countries that can prove destructive. We each need to raise our own awareness of the problem. For Americans, that means to try to see ourselves as others see us.

We should always remember: that which we value, others may not. For example, while Americans value frugality, another culture may value keeping one's word. Americans commonly make promises like "I'll send you pictures," or "Come up and visit us any time." Many foreigners have expressed surprise at how few Americans actually keep such "promises." While most Americans believe in hard work, others value the advantages of an unhurried pace, leisure time, and time with family.

"Culture shock" is a widely used term that describes the psychological discomfort that inevitably follows the transition to living in a culture markedly different from one's own. Two aspects warrant mention (Kohls 1996, 89). First, culture shock stems from the experience of regularly facing a belief system that threatens your "unconscious" belief that your values, assumptions, and behaviors are right. Second, culture shock does not hold the immediacy the term implies. Rather, it evolves slowly from many cumulative events that are difficult to pinpoint. What at first delights in its difference may later become annoying and frustrating. In time, the cumulative differences become disorienting and cause stress or "shock."

For some this comes out in the form of increased irritability, or anger toward host nationals. Others become depressed, withdrawn, or dependent on alcohol or other substances. Some become the dreaded, complaining ex-pat that seeks out newcomers to share in his disdain for all things local, while others simply abandon their stay, overwhelmed by vague incompatibilities in a hundred different realms, each impossible to identify. So, it is well worth taking some proactive steps ahead of time.

One of the best cures for the initial culture shock is to learn as much as possible about the host country. We have been sending health volunteers to eight program sites throughout Belize since January 1999, and have developed quite an effective orientation program. In addition to Kohls' book, we provide all of our Belize program volunteers with copies of the *Rough Guide to Belize* (Rough Guides 2004), with recommended readings on history, arts, and politics. We also provide a nice cultural summary written by a former Peace Corps volunteer, and our program director in Belize, Mrs Loretta Garcia Palacio, hosts all new volunteers for an orientation dinner. By having a basic understanding of the host country, a visitor's questions are better informed, and locals are invariably pleased that one has made an effort to learn about their country.

Because so much of a culture is encoded in its language, one should make every effort to learn at least some of the local language, particularly for longer visits. You can also learn a lot by simply talking with people. During my travels, I query cab drivers, shopkeepers, security guards, and anyone else who can give me insight into the country. There is no one who can't teach you something about the politics, history, popular culture, music, and heroes and heroines of a country. The more you know beforehand, the more you will derive from the experience and the easier you will find the transition.

It helps considerably to befriend those who have gone before you. Most NGOs have entire communities of ex-pats who will be more than willing to help you adjust. However, beware that each individual handles such transitions differently, and not all handle it well. Be particularly leery of those who focus on the deficiencies of the host country. Such individuals have not made the transition well themselves and are a poison in the well that one should avoid.

When culture shock does set in, it is important to deal with it directly and not put it off until later when you "have the time." Talk with trusted ex-pats, and try to pinpoint some of the various components to your frustration. Bring along a book such as Kohls' and follow the steps outlined within. Plan time for a getaway to the places of beauty that so many poor countries have in abundance. Most importantly, give yourself plenty of leeway. Americans are known for setting unattainable goals and often feel frustrated working in environments where things don't work as they do at home. I counter such feelings by constantly reminding myself that my own frustrations are small compared to those who spend their entire lives working against the difficulties imposed by poor infrastructure, lack of technology, lack of social and/or political freedoms, and disease burdens unknown to me at home. My own frustrations quickly diminish.

One final word about culture shock: it occurs all over again when you return home. I recall returning home from a life-changing experience in Tanzania only to find that I could not talk about it with most people. The only person who really understood was then my brother-in-law, Tom Hanson. He had served a tour of duty in Vietnam and had seen similar levels of poverty and even worse suffering. No one else seemed to understand. Our conversations made my re-entry far easier. Similarly, upon returning from Kenya in 1994, I recall just how much advertising there was in the United States, and just how busy everyone seemed. Fortunately, my wife joined me at the end, so she understood. Because my terms abroad had been just 6 weeks and 14 weeks, respectively, my re-entries had been relatively easy. However, those who spend longer time away will have more difficult re-entries. Much of what works for entering a foreign land also works for the return home again. It may help for those returning home to talk with others who have been to the same country, gone through the same program, or plan on doing so. You may find solace in the conversation and give those at home an infusion of infectious enthusiasm. I have found through the years that people returning home can't wait to talk about their experiences with someone who understands what they just experienced. They always inspire me and remind me just how important the work is.

On Serving Well

Dr Chris Hudson was a fourth-year medical student at the Mayo Clinic when he decided to spend one month working with Rev Dr Bill Fryda at Nazareth Hospital in Kenya.[9] Although I never met him, I understand that Chris is a gregarious person, at once engaging, funny, and passionate—he certainly comes across that way on the phone. While at Nazareth, he learned the name of everyone on the hospital grounds while asking each to teach him some Swahili, which most did gladly. He became enormously popular while there, prompting a large send-off party when his month ended. He then decided to delay his residency and returned to Nazareth for one year, during which time he became one of the most beloved figures to ever visit. I began my three-month stay there in 1994 just one year after he left and was amazed by the number of people who still asked about him. I was from the United States, so did I know him? I half expected to walk out to the main gate one morning and find a statue erected in his memory, such was the impact he had.

As I asked more questions, I learned that Chris had been one of those outgoing people that everyone naturally likes. However, the impression he left seemed far greater than mere popularity alone; this was something deeper. What he had brought to Nazareth had seemed to resonate with something deeply held, maybe even a need on the part of the people who worked there. This is all conjecture on my part, but I think that people held him in such high esteem because he learned their names and asked them for their help. Learning names is such a simple thing. Yet how many of us know the names of everyone in the workplace? A person's name is their embodiment of self in an often-faceless world. Even more so for the poor, so often beaten down by their encounters with the world. Far too many of those encounters produce feelings of worthlessness, particularly those that involve foreigners. Paulo Freire argues that much of the "horizontal violence" we see in poor countries, such as "necklacing"—setting tires around victims necks afire in Africa, is a result of individuals lashing out at each other because they cannot lash out at those who oppress them (Freire 1970, 44). When someone of a visiting doctor's status takes the time to learn one's name, it carries a special significance.

Dr Hudson visited patients in their homes and asked them to teach him all about their lives. He engaged people on their own terms and then took the near unprecedented step of asking for their help. In so doing, he reversed traditional roles. Most health providers come to poor countries to administer aid or help the needy. What is far too often overlooked in the process is the inherent dignity shared by all people, even those who must beg for their very existence. Some have dignity and perhaps nothing more. When they are respected, when they are sought after for their counsel, their knowledge, some of that dignity is restored. They again become human, and gain an added sense of purpose. While Dr Hudson was expert in providing medical care, those he queried were expert in local culture and language, sought after by the doctor, valuable in that which only they could provide. Most visiting physicians said hello and went about their business. This doctor went well beyond that, engaging them on their own terms and learning much in the process.

During a visit to Guatemala in 1997, I learned of another visiting physician who had gone out into the cornfields to see where local villagers worked, asking them to teach him how they plant their fields, and later visiting their homes. He had brought along his harmonica and introduced an entire village to American blues. By engaging people as equals, by expressing interest in how they lived and asking them to teach him how to cultivate crops, he, similarly, had restored their sense of dignity. Again, the local people had been asked their opinions and had been valued as teachers. *They* had something to teach, something valued by an outsider. And that mattered.

Perhaps the most powerful application of this ideology, if we can call it that, comes from Partners In Health (PIH), the NGO founded by Paul Farmer and Jim Kim. Farmer recognized early on that the poor people in Haiti's Central Plateau wanted to help themselves and were fully capable of doing so. Following principles from liberation theology, Farmer, Kim, and others began to train local people to become community health workers, giving out medications, performing basic health checks, and collecting data. By involving local, uneducated peasants (uneducated due to their poverty; and peasants is the name they call themselves), the PIH group empowered local communities to lead their own struggles against tuberculosis and AIDS. The results of those endeavors have been widely reported in the medical literature, as by author Tracy Kidder (2002). Such themes caught the attention of the centers of power in the World Health Organization (WHO), and elsewhere in the UN. PIH took their model to Peru, Mexico, and elsewhere, and the WHO is currently working to export this model to additional sites. Simply by empowering poor people, Farmer and others turned those that others look down on into soldiers of health, valuable co-workers in the ongoing battle against disease in "resource poor" settings. Theirs is a lesson we can all learn from.

I belabor the above mainly because one of the chief historical flaws of "development" work has been the tendency of "experts" from rich countries to bring solutions with them, while ignoring and marginalizing the poor they allegedly serve. There is an extensive literature addressing such concerns, and history is replete with examples of failed "development" in the hands of the large bi- and multilateral donors. Those who have succeeded in developing countries, including Albert Schweitzer, Tom Dooley, Paul Farmer, Father Bill Fryda, and others, have done so because they learned to work with locals to craft solutions to problems often deemed intractable. Dooley and his corpsmen integrated themselves into the local communities, attended the weddings and funerals, and used the housing built for them as a hospital while living in huts as the local villagers did. Father Fryda has developed a Kenyan staff and Partners In Health a Haitian one. More importantly, all of these programs sought active input from locals in assessing needs, creating means to affect change, and delivering care. Such actions ensure long-term efficacy and survival. While such principles seem common sense, many programs have made this most fundamental of mistakes.

Observations of Paulo Freire For those interested in serving in poor communities, the Brazilian educator Paulo Freire holds some important lessons for us to consider. First off is the universal importance of self-worth. Freire once wrote about the poor, "So often do they hear they are good for nothing, know nothing and are utterly incapable of learning anything—that they are sick, lazy and unproductive—that in the end they become convinced of their own unfitness. Almost never do they realize that they, too, 'know things' they have learned in their relations with the world and with other women and men" (Freire 1970, 45). As such, the previous examples illustrate our potential to restore a sense of dignity to those whom we will serve. We can broaden such concerns to educational encounters as well. For years, I have been advising volunteers in our programs that part of our mission is to bolster the confidence of local providers, who far too often see themselves as inferior clinicians. It is worth remembering that many of the people you will encounter abroad have deeply instilled notions of inferiority reinforced through countless encounters with visiting foreigners. It never hurts to give some positive reinforcement. However, most visitors—including ours—to poor countries are amazed at just how much local providers are able to do with so little (Gawande 2003, 2383). Many visiting clinicians find themselves learning much from their hosts. Indeed, few US or European clinicians have seen many of the tropical illnesses that local providers recognize so readily. Even the best-trained Western physicians initially flounder.

Second, as I stressed in the introduction, people are poor due to forces beyond their control. It is critical that we realize this when we engage them. As Freire writes,

> If what characterizes the oppressed [the poor] is their subordination to the consciousness of the master, as Hegel affirms, true solidarity with the oppressed means fighting at their side to transform the objective reality which has made them these 'beings for another.' The oppressor [us] is solidary with the oppressed only when he stops regarding the oppressed as an abstract category and sees them as persons who have been unjustly dealt with, deprived of their voice, cheated in the sale of their labor—when he stops making pious, sentimental, and individualistic gestures and risks an act of love. True solidarity is found only in the plentitude of this act of love, in its existentiality, in its praxis. To affirm that men and women are persons and as persons should be free, and yet to do nothing tangible to make this affirmation a reality, is a farce (1970, 31).

Third, Freire correctly cautions us to beware of our own impulses and hidden motivations. Those of us from wealthy countries carry with us the subconscious beliefs and ideals that inform who we are, and who the oppressed classes are. As such, we may truly want to help the poor, but may be hamstrung by subconscious beliefs that do not allow us to fully trust them. As Freire writes, "A real humanist can be identified more by his trust in the people, which engages him in their struggle, than by a thousand actions in their favor without that trust" (Friere 1993, 42). As such, we must constantly re-examine ourselves. Are we fully aware of our own biases and prejudices? Are we able to fully engage people in the struggle for their betterment on their own terms, and in a full partnership with them?

Far too many interactions through history have stressed the ideas of the donors and ignored the recipients, as discussed above. Freire terms this "cultural invasion," and cautions against the tremendous harm this can cause. Referring to so many well-intentioned people from afar, Freire writes:

> They see themselves as 'promoters' of the people. Their programs of action (which might have been prescribed by any good theorist of progressive action) include their own objectives, their own convictions, and their own preoccupation. They do not listen to the people, but instead plan to teach them how to 'cast off the laziness which creates underdevelopment.' To these professionals, it seems absurd to consider the necessity of respecting the 'view of the world' held by the people. The professionals are the ones with a 'world view.' They regard as equally absurd the affirmation that one must necessarily consult the people when organizing the program content of educational action. They feel the ignorance of the people is so complete that they are unfit for anything except to receive the teachings of the professionals (1993, 136).

Contrary to popular myth, most people do not want to depend on the largess or expertise of others; they prefer to help themselves. When Mother Theresa's Missionaries of Charity proposed setting up operations in Anacostia, a dense urban ghetto in Washington, DC, the local residents resented that anyone would consider them "helpless and abject Third Worlders." Just before Mother Theresa was to hold a press conference, a group of black men invaded her office. According to assistant Rathy Sreedhar, "They were very upset. . . . They told Mother that Anacostia needed decent jobs, housing and services—not charity. Mother didn't argue with them, she just listened" (Hitchens 1997, 10). These men said what most people feel, including those in developing countries. Rather than charity, people want inclusion in decisions that affect them, and prefer to work *with* those who are there to help, rather than *for* them.

When I first traveled to Belize in 1997, I had a clear idea of what I thought would be an ideal program. However, after touring the country and talking with doctors, nurses, and administrators, it soon became clear that they wanted something far different. Ultimately, our program design came largely from Belizean health providers, as have virtually all of the modifications since inception. It is run by Loretta Garcia Palacio, a Belizean national, and coordinated by locals at each of eight sites. Whatever modicum of success we have had over the years no doubt stems from local input and control. Our programs in Guyana and Thailand also follow cooperative designs that have ensured their success. Similar sentiments run through a number of successful organizations, including Partners In Health and St Mary's Hospital in Kenya.

In closing this section, I want to share an e-mail sent by one of my colleagues from the Kellogg Fellowship. Several people in my fellowship group read Freire's *A Pedagogy of the Oppressed* (1970) at the same time, generating an impassioned discussion group. One of them was a community activist from Vermont named Ellen Kahler, whose own perspective warrants repeating,

> It is the intentions and belief systems behind our actions that need to be constantly examined. Many well-intentioned people try to help people for the wrong reason and/or do so in a patronizing, paternalistic or condescending way. The effect is that the very people we are trying to help are actually being hurt (oppressed) more by our actions . . . because the unspoken message is that they are not capable of doing it themselves, are not intelligent, or worse, not as human. If we are going to put ourselves in situations where we are 'helping' people, we need to have in our hearts—and display in our actions and with our words—that we do so in such a way that . . . helps to empower that person to recognize for themselves that they have innate worth and that their experiences are valuable and should be acknowledged as such.

Ultimately, it is not just the service we render, but the manner in which we relate to all those around us. Anyone who has spent time abroad can tell you at least one story of a volunteer whose time in a foreign country seemed painfully long to everyone involved. Mr Austin Flores worked as a high school principle in Southern Belize and recalls a volunteer teacher who came from England to spend a year teaching at the school. Upon arrival, he found that the water, electricity, and phone in his home were not working. He demanded immediate action and stormed off to school. Upon arriving home, he became irate that nothing had been done. Mr Flores reminded him, "This is Belize. We said we would get to it, we just didn't say when." After three days of constant complaining about the missing services, Mr Flores finally had to tell him. "You sir, are really missing just one thing . . . England. Why don't you go home."

It is worth repeating that international volunteers must be *flexible*, *adaptable*, maintain a sense of *humor*, *lower expectations*, and show an *ability to fail*—at least for a while. This ensures the right preparation for the inevitable lapses that occur in virtually all international programs. You simply cannot expect things to work as they do at home in the United States or Europe. Ultimately, by reflecting on culture, and adapting yourself to the inevitable change, you will grow and will make your own transitions less of a burden to those with whom you will work while abroad.

Practical Considerations

Short-term vs Long-term Volunteers

There has been a long-running debate on the relative value of short-term vs long-term volunteers among those who do work of this nature. While those with specific skills like ophthalmologists, dentists, or maxillo-facial surgeons can easily find short-term programs that will put their surgical skills to good use, most other specialists and generalists alike contribute most through short-term visits by teaching. Those who go on short-term trips to provide clinical care may become more of a resource drain. Consider the drain on your workplace if you had a series of high-maintenance (let's be honest) physicians, each with his or her own set of adjustment issues, each unfamiliar with the local illnesses, medications, hospital patterns, local culture, and language. It takes most people several weeks to adjust, some far longer. Some programs, such as Haiti's Hospital Albert Schweitzer, have been able to develop orientation and supervisory programs to maximize short-term volunteers in clinical work. For many others, however, the short-term volunteers take more than they give, which is why many programs require three- to six-month minimum stays.

Because many people first enter this work through short-term programs, consider looking through the various programs with short-term openings in Chapter 3 of this text. Then, query those who have gone before you. Ask if you will you be able to contribute something of value in your proposed time period. If not, find another program. There are good program models out there, like HAS, Health Volunteers Overseas, and ours at Omni Med. The "acid test" of this work is whether one leaves behind as much as one gains from the experience.

Passports

One of your first steps in planning to go abroad is to secure your passport, an essential travel document that a full 85% of Americans lack (Hasbrouck 2000, 13). If you are one of them, you have work to do, starting at least four to six months before you plan to leave. It can take up to two months to complete a passport application process by mail, and several more weeks to secure a visa, for which a passport is a prerequisite. The Passports page on the US Department of State Web site (http://travel.state.gov/passport/passport_1738.html) has all of the information you will need to apply. You can also apply in person at any post office or in any Department of State Passport Agency office. Please note that many countries will not allow you in unless your passport is valid for a full six months after your planned date of *departure* from that country. The best advice is to look at your passport right now while you are thinking about it and check the expiration date. If you have no passport or need to renew, do it now. When you travel abroad, make a note of the nearest US embassy or consulate and keep either an expired passport or a photocopy of your current passport packed separately so you can quickly renew it if the need should arise.

Visas

A visa is an authorization given by a country to allow you in. It usually comes in the form of a stamp or piece of paper inserted into your passport specifying dates the host government is allowing you to stay. Obtaining a visa is a time-consuming, overly bureaucratic process, though a necessary one. Remember that there are no laws requiring countries to allow you in. The decision is an arbitrary one and is completely up to the authorities of each country. Even a legitimate visa does not guarantee that you can enter a given country. They can honor it or not as they see fit. Further, many countries will require that you have proof of sufficient funds while there, a return airline ticket, proper immunizations such as for yellow fever, and no entries in your passport from countries they consider hostile to theirs.

To apply for a visa, you will need a valid passport, two to three photos, a processing fee often paid through cashier's checks or certified money orders, and time. Most visas require three weeks to process and should be done through Federal Express with an enclosed, pre-paid FedEx return envelope—you will, after all, be sending your passport. Apply in person if possible, but, because most consulate offices are in Washington, DC, most people apply by mail. You should send it overnight and call the next day to check its status. For those who find such processes overly cumbersome, there are visa services that will make things far easier. I have found their charges worth the savings in time and aggravation. Express Visa Service Inc (www.expressvisa.com) has an excellent Web site with all forms and entry requirements spelled out clearly. Cost for visa processing ranges from $75 to $125. Travel the World Visas offer comparable services and rates (www.world-visa.com). Both of these companies can also help you secure or renew a passport. There are many companies that offer similar services available through the Internet or travel agents.

Before moving on to health insurance, it is worth adding in some perspective on dealing with "foreign" authorities in both the United States and in other countries. Edward Hasbrouck points out that, for many privileged North Americans, the experience of submitting to a governmental authority is a difficult one. Our fierce independence and rejection of authority comprise key parts of our cultural makeup and may prove particularly troublesome while abroad. The first step is to recognize that you are not in control, and that any attempts to exercise authority or prove your self-perceived worth will fail miserably. Attempts to take control of a situation at a border or an airport may remind those in charge, particularly those in former colonies, of the imperialist impulses that proved so destructive in the past. In short, such confrontations "push all the wrong buttons of the postcolonial psyche" (Hasbrouck 2000, 371).

Many Americans carry with them a subconscious attitude of world dominance for which our country is known and disliked. While not stated, many Americans traveling abroad project this attitude through a thousand subconscious actions. While we may think we are keeping our thoughts to ourselves, those who staff the customs offices, border crossing stations, and security checkpoints abroad have seen this all before and will read us clearly, as if we were shouting our frustrations aloud. As such, it is best to adjust your attitude ahead of time. Better to continually remind yourself that you are not in charge, your entry comes solely at the discretion of those with whom you are currently dealing, and that you really are happy to be there, even at customs.

One might even view such experiences as the learning opportunities that they are. On a regular basis, most of the world's people have to accept far worse than those of us in Europe and the United States ever experience. To quote Hasbrouck again, "Situations of dependence, inferior status, and lack of privilege may be, for Northerners, among the most important learning experiences of world travel" (Hasbrouck 2000, 371). Instead of locking horns in a futile effort to demonstrate your status, adopt as much a posture of supplication as you can muster. By showing genuine respect and deference, you will be far more likely to pass through unscathed.

When a soldier casually pointed his rifle at me during routine questioning in Tanzania in 1987, I initially felt a mixture of fear and indignation. Yet protest and escalation never help in such situations; I remained calm and respectful, just as anyone should in similar situations. Our efforts should be to change the underlying forces that cause soldiers to point rifles in the first place, not challenge the individual soldiers and border personnel who are merely doing their jobs.

Insurance

The final practical matter at hand is insurance. For international travel, there are three types of insurance one should consider: health, medical evacuation, and trip cancellation. Many will find themselves lulled into a false sense of security thinking that their US health insurance will cover them internationally. For some, that will prove a costly mistake. You should first check with your insurance plan to see if you are covered abroad, and if so, for how long. Health insurance policies change frequently, with tendencies toward less coverage, not more. Once you find where the holes in your coverage are, you might then consider supplemental travel health insurance for the duration of your time abroad.

Medical evacuation insurance is not covered by most US health insurance plans. To charter an air ambulance after an accident or catastrophic medical illness develops while abroad can run upwards of $20,000. While many conditions will respond to local treatment or can await transport via a commercial airliner, some people do become critically ill while abroad. Most people should have this coverage, particularly those considering more dangerous activities while abroad, working in higher risk settings, or with pre-existing serious medical conditions.

The final insurance, that of trip cancellation, may be the most useful and least acquired. Only 3% of Americans traveling abroad purchase any, according to one insurance executive (Cohen 2000). The most common form this insurance takes is that of trip cancellation or interruption. The cost is typically 4%–6% of the cost of the airline tickets (Daniel 2002). Those with elderly parents or relatives with medical problems should strongly consider such policies. Because most trips are booked months in advance, it is not uncommon for a sudden illness or death of a relative to force a cancellation or delay in travel plans. Such insurance is cheaper when purchased directly through the company rather than through a travel agent, and can influence decisions to return home in the event of a crisis, at least by removing concerns over lost finances. Many companies offer "comprehensive" plans that include components of all three insurance types. Some companies include Global Care in Massachusetts, Travelex of Omaha, Nebraska, The Travelers of Hartford, CSA Travel Protection in San Diego, and Travel Guard International in Wisconsin (Cohen 2000). I have found Wallach & Company (www.wallach.com; 800-237-6615) reliable.

A Word About Packing

Most of us give little thought to what we bring with us. For a number of years, I followed a similar, painful ritual of throwing all that I thought I might need into a bag at the last possible minute, and then rushing off to the airport. Longer overseas stays would push me to pack earlier, though with precious little more thought. Yet there is much to gain from planning what you will bring with you, and to following the axiom "when in doubt, leave it out." Pat Mattheisen annually teaches a course on "traveling lightly" at Boston's Center for Adult Education (Daniel 2002). Pat startles her class by hoisting two soft-sided carry-on bags for her and her husband's annual three-week trip to Europe. While a trip to Europe will markedly differ from a longer trip to a poor country, her basic points are worth repeating.

First, make a checklist of all that you will need ahead of time. Many NGOs will make recommendations for you, but the goal remains to keep it light. Wear wrinkle-free clothing, which wears better, and plan to wash clothes frequently. While Ms Mattheisen advises travelers to include some black clothing, which hides stains better, keep in mind that light clothing absorbs less heat and will be more comfortable. Remember that you can often pick up items you need in host countries, though you should inquire ahead of time if going to a rural or extremely poor region. In addition to the usual items, I add the following to my list: a Swiss army knife, suntan lotion, plenty of plastic bags in various sizes, a small flashlight, nail clippers, photocopies of essential documents packed separately, "flight socks" and a neck pillow for long flights, sunglasses, DEET-containing repellent, and a small water purifier for more rural trips.

Finally, a word about the packer. Few give much thought to their physical conditioning prior to traveling abroad. However, from a number of years spent treating minor musculoskeletal injuries in the emergency department, I can tell you that those most frequently affected by annoying muscle strains are those who do not regularly exercise. Because most people will be unable to pack lightly, they will have to carry heavy luggage in awkward positions, at times for long periods of time. Many will transport bulky medical supplies as well, adding to the load. Even moderate exercise and light weight-lifting routines can prevent some injuries by enhancing muscle tone and flexibility. It's a good idea for general cardiovascular health anyway (Carnethon et al 2003, 3092), so consider adopting an exercise routine in advance of any significant international travel. Spare yourself the annoying injuries that may color your first few weeks abroad.

Donating or Transporting Medical Supplies

Most people who venture overseas for medical work will bring medical supplies, drugs, or medical books with them. Others will ship some such supplies overseas. Because the history of medical supply donations is riddled with good intentions gone awry, it is well worth consideration ahead of time. Every new natural disaster brings with it stories of inappropriate or unusable donations from afar, many conferring considerable tax write-offs for the donors. And any official or health worker in a developing country who has worked with foreigners will be able to tell at least one story of useless donations that required time and effort to sort through and dispose of. We have seen similar problems in our work in Belize.

The former medical director of the Karl Heusner Memorial Hospital in Belize City, Dr Frances Smith, once went on Belize national television to denounce a large shipment of donations publicized as worth over $300,000 that had arrived amid much media fanfare. After sorting through the donations, Dr Smith pronounced most of the supplies "useless." The drugs had expired, the medical equipment was beyond repair, and the time and salary expense required to sort and repair the materials involved soon exceeded the value of the entire shipment. Dr Smith rightly told the media that such donations create problems because the general public erroneously expects such donations to improve their health care. When it does not, they blame the doctors and other medical staff at the hospitals. Dr Smith told of other donations that often were worthless: old ambulances, outdated equipment beyond the local capacity to repair, drugs far beyond their expiration dates, and dialysis equipment for a country lacking the infrastructure required to use it. In the end, the real benefactors are the donors, who receive generous tax write-offs for donations whose real value is often artificially inflated.

Part of the problem stems from the tax deductions that many governments grant to those who make "charitable" donations abroad. It is often cheaper to ship outdated equipment abroad than pay someone to remove it and properly dispose of it. I once received a call from a dentist who wanted to donate his outdated dental operatory (light, chair, and drilling equipment). He did not want to pay the high costs for removal and disposal, so he asked if I could come and "just take it away," which would also provide him with a substantial tax deduction. Keep in mind that there are laws that dictate just how such equipment must be removed and disposed of, which accounts in part for the high cost of its removal. Because it is very expensive to ship overseas ($7,000–$8,000 per container from the United States to East Africa for example), one can quickly see why some choose to simply donate their equipment and leave details to others. Unfortunately for many abroad, some donate mainly for the tax deductions, and less for the good their donations may render abroad. Anyone planning to ship materials abroad should be sure the shipment complies with locally stated requests, is serviceable in country, and works properly.

Those who aspire to coordinate larger shipments undertake a huge task, often with little understanding at the outset. Following the devastation of Hurricane Mitch in 1999, local groups all over the Boston area collected donations of all sorts, though few had any idea how to actually transport the items from Boston to Central America. It was a local Rotarian named Richard Bridges who, with help from the members of the Hingham Rotary Club, ultimately arranged for transportation to Honduras aboard C-130 military transport planes, secured with the help of Massachusetts Senators Kerry and Kennedy. Mr Bridges had worked in shipping to Central and South America for years so was one of the few who actually knew all that was involved. In the end, they managed to ship millions of dollars worth of supplies. Anyone considering putting together a large shipment should first do some research. For the past five years, we have worked with a very efficient company, MedShare International (www.medshare.org; 770-323-5858) based in Lithonia, Georgia, to get supplies to Kenya. Another NGO named Missionary Expediters has a useful publication titled: "How to Plan your Shipment."[10] This short monograph answers all relevant questions about packing, documentation, inventory, trucking, departure port, international carriage, arrival port, customs clearance, and onward carriage. From my experiences in transporting drugs and supplies, I strongly suggest that people follow through on these various sources. This is a complex and demanding business with many pitfalls—do not take it lightly.

Drug donations have a long history of misadventures as well. Following the 1988 earthquake in Armenia, less than half the donated drugs were relevant to the emergency situation, while 5000 tons of donated drugs took 50 people a full six months to sort (Hogerzeil et al 1997, 737). During Eritrea's war for independence in 1989, many inappropriate donations delayed proper assistance: seven truckloads of expired aspirin tablets took six months to burn while 30,000 half-liter bottles of an expired amino acid infusion could not be disposed of locally due to its acrid smell (WHO 1999, 1). A Harvard study found that between 10% and 42% of donated drugs were not high-priority items listed either by the recipient country or the WHO (Abelson 1999). Many such drugs then require scarce personnel and funding resources for proper disposal.

Due to many such stories, the WHO, in cooperation with a number of NGOs, developed guidelines for drug donations in 1996, updated in 1999 (WHO 1999, 1), which anyone transporting or shipping drugs abroad should review. The report outlines some commonsense approaches to drug donation that stress four "core principles:"

- **Maximum benefit to the recipient.** All donations should be based on expressed need and unsolicited donations discouraged.
- **Respect for wishes and authority of the recipient.** In other words, be aware that it is the local authorities and personnel who will become the ultimate arbiters of any donations, so one should follow established guidelines that make their work easier and conform to local standards.
- **No double standards in quality.** In short, why should the poor not receive the same quality of medications that those in the industrialized world receive? Drugs should arrive at the destination with more than one year before expiration (some say six months), unless clearly agreed to by the recipient. No free samples, no vague labels, and language congruency when possible. According to the WHO guidelines, "if the quality of an item is unacceptable in the donor country, it is also unacceptable as a donation."
- **Effective communication between donor and recipient.** Those in developing countries best know their needs, what works and what doesn't. It rarely if ever makes sense to bring drugs or supplies just because you have them. It always makes sense to ask ahead of time what is most needed and useful.

On each of my visits to East Africa, I have carried medications and supplies with me, as do many who travel abroad for clinical work. It is often cheaper for a visitor to transport such supplies than to pay a courier or freight-forwarding company to ship them—even when additional costs of the excess baggage are factored in. Passengers departing from the United States may check two pieces of luggage through. Size and weight limits vary between airlines, though they are usually between 60 and 70 lbs (27 and 32 kg) (Hasbrouck 2000, 399). International standards are less, with 44 lbs (20 kg) per person customary. It is best to clarify the weight or baggage limit ahead of time with the airline, as well as to transport those items most needed by the host site.

Beware of the inspectors at the destination site. In Kenya, security officers often require bribes to allow donated medical items through. While I can't advise visiting health professionals to stuff dollar bills into envelopes as I did, I can share one other anecdote. One enterprising woman from Kenya packs all of her donated medical supplies in the bottom of a green duffel bag, then places bras, panties, women's toiletries, and other such items at the top. When the security officers start pulling out these items, she feigns profound embarrassment, which usually prompts them to move on to the next passenger.

A word of caution is in order. Be very clear with the NGO you will be working with about exactly what you are transporting into the country and what the customs are. You could find your items confiscated, a hefty penalty assessed, or you could be detained. Even though you may feel indignant that you are there to help and these supplies should not be subject to bribes, remember that you are still a guest in this country and must follow their laws, just as immigrants to the United States or European countries must follow the laws there.

In this chapter, we have reviewed some means to overcome the chief obstacles of serving overseas. The reader should now have a sense of how to proceed at the outset, how to serve effectively, and how to negotiate the treacherous landscape of culture. Although we have broached the subject of fear in the preceding, we have not addressed the best way to keep fear at bay. In the next chapter, we will review clear steps to reduce risks and stay healthy through every part of your experience, no matter of what duration.

Endnotes

1. For more information see the ASAPROSAR Web site at www.thegreenresource.com/asaprosar.
2. Dr Joseph Bowlds is now retired from active clinical work, though continues to travel to El Salvador each year. He can be reached at Joseph H. Bowlds, MD, 6 Wildwood Drive, Peabody, MA 01960-7914, and through e-mail at jhbowlds@massmed.org.
3. For those interested in a position at HAS, see the Hospital Albert Schweitzer Haiti Web site at www.hashaiti.org. The mailing address (as of March 2004) is: Medical Director, Hôpital Albert Schweitzer, c/o Lynx Air, P.O. Box 407139, Fort Lauderdale, FL 33340. See also Chapter 3 of this text for more details.
4. Contact Dr Dowell through the HAS Web site (www.hashaiti.org) or through Hertha Isaac in the Sarasota office at the Grant Foundation, 1360 Whitfield Ave, Sarasota, FL 34243, phone: 941-752-1525, e-mail: herthaisaac@hashaiti.org.
5. For more information see the Southern California Permanente Medical Group Rules and Regulations, Section 6, pgs 8–9. Also see *Historical Review of the Southern California Permanente Medical Group* (pgs 59–60) by Raymond M Kay, MD. Those interested should contact Dr William Cory at william.c.cory@kp.org.
6. Contact Patricia Newton at the following address: Assistant Director of Philanthropy, The Lahey Clinic, Burlington, MA 01805, phone: 978-744-3928, e-mail: patricia.a.newton@lahey.org.
7. For more information about their programs, see the New Road Map Foundation Web site at www.newroadmap.org/default.asp.
8. Information from *Democracy in America* by Alexis de Tocqueville, published by Penguin Books in1956, written in 1835–1840.
9. Contact Dr Chris Hudson at the following address: 705 East Oak Street, Fremont, MI 49412.
10. For more information see www.solvenet.com or call 800-299-6363.

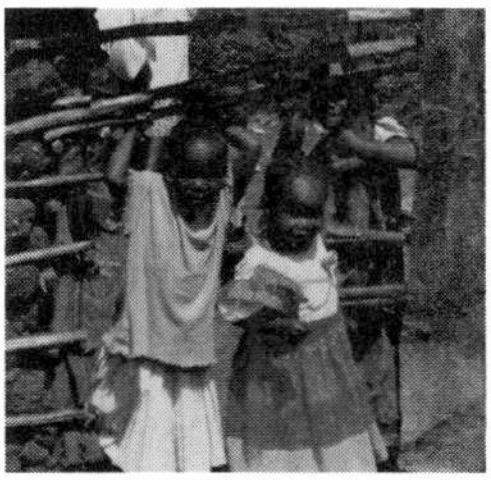

Chapter 2

Travel, Health, and Safety Guidelines

Chance favors the prepared mind.

—Louis Pasteur

The cool, cool river sweeps the wild, white ocean
The rage of love turns inward to prayers of devotion
And these prayers are the constant road across the wilderness
These prayers are the memory of god, the memory of god
And I believe in the future we shall suffer no more
Maybe not in my lifetime but in yours I feel sure
Song dogs barking at the break of dawn
Lightning pushes the edges of a thunderstorm
And these streets, quiet as a sleeping army
Send their battered dreams to heaven, to heaven
For the mother's restless son
Who is a witness to, who is a warrior
Who denies his urge to break and run

—Paul Simon

We can best care for others by first caring for ourselves—particularly our health. That is best achieved by proper preparation. There are a number of vaccinations and pre-travel preparations that can make a difference; we will review them here. In addition, because most people will get to their destination by flying, we will review some common practical and health matters related to flying, such as finding the best fares and avoiding barotraumas, infections, blood clots, and jet lag. Because so many people avoid work of this sort because of fear, we review how one best avoids the main dangers: violence, crime, and the biggest danger of all—road travel. We then cover the most common health problems involved: from the common traveler's diarrhea, to the more exotic ailments such as schistosomiasis. We cover at length just how one avoids getting malaria and other mosquito-borne illnesses, and spend some time on the environmental pitfalls that commonly afflict travelers such as mountain sickness and water-related health problems. Because HIV is so common in much of the developing world, we review commonsense prevention strategies, as well as the prophylactic regimens that every health provider should take along with them. We end with a potpourri of other travel recommendations and summarize the chapter with a list that any traveler could personalize. In short, there is no reason why you can't travel to a developing country, render effective service, and return home safely, albeit changed by the experience.

Some General Health Considerations

There are significant health risks in poor countries. These stem chiefly from poverty and all it engenders: poor water supplies, poor or absent sanitation, contaminated food sources, dangerous roads, and a lack of health infrastructure. While those most affected are the abundant poor who call such places home, there is plenty of risk to go around, some of which is inevitably shared by those who visit and work in such environs. Some of the health risks stem from the fact that many of the world's poor countries lie in tropical or sub-tropical zones, where insect and microbial life thrives. It is an unusual experience for North Americans or Europeans to find worms in their stools or migrating along under their skin or conjunctiva, or to see a fly maggot emerging from a hole in their skin. Yet these are common experiences for those who live in such zones. Just two different types of worms, roundworms (*Ascaris lumbricoides*) and hookworms (*Ancyclostoma duodenale* and *Necator amereicanus*), infect 1.3 and 1 billion people worldwide, respectively, with enormous morbidity, particularly for children.

Although injuries and deaths from road accidents pose the greatest risk to anyone who works in a developing country, the overwhelming majority of people who travel and work abroad do so safely. The risk posed by terrorism, crime, land mines, and violence depends on the situation, but remains small overall. The same is true for infectious health problems. A Swiss group reviewed the monthly incidence of health problems per 100,000 travelers to tropical regions and found that four infectious diseases stood out. Over the course of an average month, the average traveler acquired the following diseases: traveler's diarrhea (TD) (30%), malaria (3%), hepatitis A (0.3%), and typhoid fever (0.03%) (Behrens et al 1994). All of these are largely preventable if one follows current recommendations. The concerned should take comfort in the fact that over two thirds of those surveyed acquired no illness at all during a full month in the tropics. Your risk can be still lower if you merely follow some simple guidelines.

Pre-Travel Planning/Vaccines

There is one source that I highly recommend to anyone traveling to the developing world. "The Traveler's Pocket Medical Guide and International Certificate of

Vaccination" (www.travelclinic.com.au/order-form.htm) is a compact, passport-sized pocket medical guide that reviews most of the common travel-related illnesses (Leggat 2001). It can fit comfortably in your neck pouch or wherever you keep your passport. It is 48 pages and weighs just 1.3 ounces, with a durable plastic cover that will withstand sweat or rain, and should last years. It also contains the yellow fever form with a listing for all of your vaccinations. It covers everything from traveler's diarrhea to malaria to altitude sickness and swimming hazards, with commonsense treatments for common illnesses. I advise people to order one well in advance and pick up some of the recommended medications before departure. Most of the recommendations are similar to what I advise here, though some medications differ due to its Australian source.[1] Per unit cost is $7.43 plus shipping.

Try to get to a travel clinic at least four to six weeks before departure, eight weeks for longer trips. The immunizations you will need depend on a host of factors, including where you are going and for how long, the season, and the type of travel and work (ie, more secure, urban work or more risky work in the bush). Studies have shown that most unvaccinated travelers return home safely, acquiring none of the illnesses against which we routinely immunize. Those unvaccinated for hepatitis A are just 0.3%–0.6% likely to contract it per month, while 0.08%–0.24% contract hepatitis B and just 0.03% contract typhoid.[2] Given potential side effects to all vaccines, it is up to you to decide which ones you should receive. However, most vaccines are safe and effective, and the diseases they protect us against are often deadly or debilitating. It is best to review each one with a travel medicine expert, and I encourage people to receive all of the recommended vaccinations.

Standard vaccinations include tetanus-diptheria toxoid, measles, polio (for endemic areas), pneumococcal, and influenza. Influenza is very common in travelers, and respiratory illnesses are among the most commonly acquired illness of any kind during travel. Flu vaccines are widely available, and new intranasal preparations are available for 5- to 50-year-olds. Several other immunizations are standard depending on destinations. Everyone should receive both the hepatitis A and hepatitis B vaccines. They are safe and highly effective. Health care workers should all have hepatitis B vaccination already. Hepatitis A is the least serious of the viral hepatitis strains, yet can occasionally cause fulminant illness requiring liver transplantation. There is no reason to assume such risk given such a safe and near universally effective vaccine. Its efficacy has largely replaced immune globulin, the prior standard for prevention of hepatitis A.

The need for several other vaccinations depends upon the destination. Yellow fever vaccination is required for entry into certain countries, though is live and therefore comprises a risk to the elderly or immunocompromised. You should obtain the appropriate forms at the time of vaccination, and show them upon arrival. Typhoid vaccination is roughly 70% effective and wise to receive. Typhoid fever, caused by *Salmonella typhi,* can cause debilitating illness, including intestinal perforations that cause bowel adhesions and later, obstruction. Travelers to Asia should avoid the Japanese encephalitis vaccine unless very high risk; disease incidence in travelers is low and vaccine-related morbidity is high. One should also consider vaccinations against Meningococcus (meningitis) and Varicella ("chicken pox," far more serious in adults). While most people won't need rabies vaccine before leaving, they should have a low threshold to receive it after any potential exposure; rabies is near universally fatal once symptomatic and extremely difficult to diagnose. Exposure to infected animals, particularly bats, and certain animal bites warrant postexposure treatment. Because the rabies virus infects the central nervous system, the closer the bite is to the spinal chord (ie, face, trunk), the less time one has to receive immunization following a bite; review this with your doctor before leaving. I would advise health providers, particularly doctors, to follow the advice of those in traveler's clinics on all these matters. Don't do this yourself. This is a constantly evolving area that warrants consultation with an expert.

Getting There Safely

Speaking of Flying

The next step of your travel preparation involves purchasing your ticket and taking your flight. There are ways to acquire cheaper tickets, and there are health dangers inherent in air travel, though not always well publicized. Because most people will travel to their service destination through the air, it is well worth reviewing this portion of your trip in some detail.

Booking Flights

The airline industry follows a complex set of rules and procedures designed to get you to your destination while simultaneously helping you part with the largest possible amount of money. They are very good at both aspects. Since my first trip to Tanzania in 1987, I have made over 20 subsequent trips to developing countries. While that qualifies me as a novice in some circles, it has given me an appreciation for the complexity of the airline industry. I have booked flights after exhaustive searches on-line, used travel agents, and contacted airlines directly. We have even worked out arrangements with American Airlines in Belize and North American Airlines in Guyana, through which our volunteers receive discounted airfares, gifts for which I am ever grateful. Yet, in my experience, there is simply no substitute for a knowledgeable travel agent who works with consolidator fares.

Contrary to popular mythology, you can't beat the travel agent's fares—a travel agent, that is, who specializes in international "independent" travel through consolidators. While most travel agents specialize in cruises, all-inclusive stays, or more common deluxe forms of travel, travel agents who know developing world destinations are more rare and invaluable. Specifically ask for a "discounter" agent (Hasbrouck 2000, 233). In addition to being able to offer perspectives from those who have recently traveled to a given country, they can get you fares cheaper than anything you can find on your own, including those available on-line. They do this through "consolidator" fares, in which the agent reimburses you a percentage of the discount they receive off the face value of the ticket. For most international travelers, this option represents the most flexible and cheapest means for travel, second only to using frequent flier miles. For those who are students or faculty, booking student fares is another means of inexpensive flights, though more restrictive and occasionally more expensive than consolidator tickets.

Health Considerations During Your Flight

The airline industry transports roughly 2 billion people per year (Gendreau and DeJohn 2002, 1067). As such, there is a lot of accumulated experience in airline travel and we can now cite a growing literature to review common problems associated with flying—in particular with long flights. There are five particular health issues worth reviewing: flight anxiety, cabin pressure and humidity, risk of blood clots, risk of infection, and jet lag.

Fear of Flying

The most important step in taking a long distance flight is getting on the plane. Yet for many people, this is a daunting task. Because an airline crash anywhere in the world immediately becomes front-page news, it is not surprising that some people are paralyzed by a fear of flying. The reality, however, is that airplanes are the safest form of travel. Massachusetts Institute of Technology's Dr Arnold Bennett calculated that between 1975 and 1994, each time someone boarded a commercial airliner, the risk of dying was 1 in 7 million.[3] By contrast, the risk of dying each time someone got in their car was 1 in 368,000, roughly 19 times higher. Despite the horror of September 11, 2001, commercial airliners remain the safest of all travel options. That should provide reassurance to the worried. However, many fears calm with time, conversation, or short-acting benzodiazepines like Ativan or Xanax.

Cabin Pressure, Oxygen, and Humidity

Most commercial airliners travel at cruising altitudes of 35,000 to 43,000 feet, where atmospheric pressure, oxygen, and relative humidity are considerably lower than at sea level (Johnston 2001, 385). To compensate, airlines pressurize cabins, though only to an average equivalent of an elevation of 5000 to 8000 feet (Gendreau and DeJohn 2002, 1067). For passengers, this relative "high altitude" forces an inevitable encounter with Boyle's law, which informs us that as atmospheric pressures fall (with rising altitude), gases expand. Problems develop mainly from gases trapped in fixed spaces like sinuses, middle ears, teeth, and the abdominal cavity. For most healthy people, minor abdominal or ear discomfort is common during takeoff and landing. Yet for those with colds and blocked eustachian tubes, the pain from gases expanding in an inner ear (aerotitis media) or in a sinus (barosinusitis) can make the flight seem interminable. Yawning, sneezing, or swallowing can help, as can chewing gum. Infants can gain relief by sucking on pacifiers or nursing. Gentle Valsalva maneuvers such as closing the nose with thumb and finger and exhaling gently with the mouth closed may also help. For those with prior difficult experiences or colds, Afrin nasal drops or spray in both nostrils one-half hour before takeoff works best, though oral decongestants such as long-acting Sudafed may suffice in minor cases. Those with high blood pressure or allergies should first consult their physicians. Patients with casts placed within 48 hours should have them bivalved (cut on one side to allow for tissue expansion) and those with recent surgical procedures should consult their surgeon but often wait up to two weeks before flying after general procedures and two days following laparoscopic surgeries (Johnston 2001, 385).

Low levels of oxygen and low humidity comprise two other components of the cabin that may produce discomfort. Although oxygen reductions in flight are minimal, they may be significant for those who require higher ambient oxygen pressures, such as those with heart or lung disease. Because of high regulatory standards, most airlines provide oxygen and will not allow patients to bring their own supply. The cabin's humidity is also significantly lower than that found at sea level, causing eye or mucosal irritation for many. Plan on drinking water during the flight, avoid wearing contact lenses, and consider nasal saline spray and/or Natural tears for long flights. Because eye blinking stimulates meibomian gland secretions, which in turn moisten the eyes, more frequent blinking should help.

Alcohol is best avoided during flights for a number of reasons. Alcohol is a diuretic (causes fluid loss through urination), so it worsens the already dry conditions. Alcohol has also been shown to be a contributing cause to at least a fourth of the increasingly common episodes of in-flight air rage (Gendreau and DeJohn 2002, 1067). My wife is a former FBI agent who once arrested a man at Boston's Logan Airport. His unruly behavior had caused the Paris to Miami flight to divert and land prematurely, an increasingly common occurrence. Naturally, alcohol was a key factor. As we review shortly, alcohol also contributes to formation of clotting during long flights, by "thickening" the blood through diuresis, as well as causing us to shift our bodies less frequently than we ordinarily would.

Risk of Infections Aboard Aircraft

Cases of transmission of multidrug-resistant tuberculosis (MDR-TB) among airline passengers in the early 1990s received wide media attention, prompting wider concerns about the risk of acquiring infections while flying (Kenyon et al 1996, 933). The most notable case involved a 32-year-old Korean woman who infected up to 15 other passengers on flights while she was symptomatic with cavitary tuberculosis, an illness that killed her just 13 days after her last flight. Most of those exposed sat within two rows of her during a long flight, and no one outside her section of the aircraft was infected, proving the relative safety of recirculated cabin air (933). Another case documented a flight attendant with pulmonary tuberculosis that likely infected several coworkers and passengers during a contagious phase of tuberculosis lasting six months (Driver et al 1994, 1031). Other infectious pathogens shared during air travel include Meningococcal meningitis (Centers for Disease Control and Prevention [CDC] 2001a, 485), severe acute respiratory syndrome (SARS) (Olsen et al 2003, 2416), influenza, measles, and the common cold (Driver et al 1994, 1031). As such, an anxious public, particularly worried about press reports of "Ebola with wings," a common moniker for MDR-TB, prompted researchers to study the risk of getting sick while flying and to study whether the "circulating air" aboard planes was a concern.

The subsequent studies have produced mostly good news. While there is always a risk of acquiring an infection during a flight, it is remarkably low (Wenzel 1996, 981; Zitter et al 2002, 483). In fact, according to Dr Richard Wenzel, modern cabin air is "remarkably clean" (1996, 981). Most modern aircraft circulate 50% of the cabin air through the jet engines (482°F [250°C]), and then through particulate matter filters, which remove most pathogens. The combination of downward air circulation and frequent air exchanges in cabins (every 3 to 4 minutes vs every 5 to 12 minutes in offices and homes) renders airline cabin air significantly less bacteria laden than comparable air in city buses, shopping malls, or airline terminals (Driver et al 1994, 1031). While transmission of infectious pathogens does occur in flight, it is far less common than we would anticipate, given the large number of people traveling by air. Sitting in a college classroom poses greater risk.

Many deadly infections have quietly passed through terminals and aircraft unshared. An influenza outbreak affecting 59% of the passengers did occur aboard an airplane in 1979 (Driver et al 1994, 1031). However, this occurred during a three-hour delay for takeoff during which the ventilation system was off. It is likely that the attack rate would have been lower with less waiting time and an operating ventilation system. Passengers have boarded international flights carrying the deadliest of viruses, including two with Lassa, though neither infected any of the 280 combined fellow passengers (Wenzel 1996, 981).

Given the rise of MDR-TB worldwide, and the difficulty treating it, we should stay vigilant for those highly infectious. "Because TB is largely a disease of poverty, however, we are far more likely to encounter cases of active TB among the patients we serve than on the planes that bring us to them." To his credit, one editorialist from the *New England Journal of Medicine* did state, "investing in the control of infection in other countries could lead to great dividends at home," a perspective depressingly absent from far too many mainstream journal articles (Wenzel 1996, 981; Farmer 2001, 208). Ultimately, the risk of infection aboard aircraft is no larger than that of any confined space over time. It is not the cabin air that should concern us; rather, it is the health of our immediate neighbors, and there is usually little we can do about that. However, standard measures of hand washing and avoiding touching the eyes, nose, or mouth should help decrease the likelihood of acquiring certain viruses. The risk of infectious pathogens such as TB may depend more on our response to the spread of this infection everywhere. Without adequate attention, acquisition on planes may become the least of our worries.

Blood Clots and Air Travel

Over the long, anxious hours of the London Blitz of 1940, terrified Londoners huddled together in the cramped spaces of bomb shelters beneath the city streets, often immobile for hours on end. An astute British surgeon named Keith Stinson noted a six-fold increase in fatal pulmonary embolisms (PE) during September and

October 1940 compared to the same two-month period in the previous year. He rightly concluded that the cramped quarters had predisposed people to clot formation (Stinson 1940, 744). His 1940 *Lancet* article echoed Dr Virchow's earlier elucidation of the cause of blood clots, the classic triad of venous stasis (blood not moving through veins), hypercoagulability (increased clotting in blood), and endothelial injury (an injury to the inside lining of blood vessels that triggers clotting). When these three components come together, blood clots occasionally form, most commonly in the veins of the legs, either superficial or deep. Because the deep veins of the legs most commonly produce severe local problems or emboli, they are the most feared. Such a clot is called a deep venous thrombosis (DVT). A small percent of these clots can then break off and travel to the lungs causing PEs, which block blood flow to some areas of the lungs and can prove fatal. A more recent war, this time in Iraq, again brought the dangers of Virchow's triad to prominence when NBC reporter David Bloom died suddenly of a pulmonary embolism after sitting for days in the narrow confines of a tank advancing on Baghdad.[4] Desert conditions causing dehydration and long periods of sitting with legs folded under him likely combined to cause a fatal clot in this otherwise healthy 39-year-old man.

For years, studies in the medical literature have shown that the prolonged immobility of lengthy flights causes clot formation, giving rise to the term "economy class syndrome" (Symington and Stack 1977, 138). Lest those in business and first class relax, however, more clots occur in economy class mainly because more people sit there (Dalen 2003, 22674). Over the last three decades of the twentieth century, there were over 100 case reports of flight-induced PE in the medical literature (Perry 2000). One 28-year-old "bride-to-be" died suddenly of a PE soon after disembarking a 12-hour Sydney to London flight in 2000, in a case that garnered worldwide attention. This and other episodes of flight-induced clots have produced a rash of lawsuits against several major airlines (Wong 2003). Judging by the medical literature, the airlines have much to worry about.

A study published in *Chest* in 1999 first proved a conclusive link between travel and clot formation (Ferrari et al 1999, 440). A group that had recently traveled more than four hours was more than four times more likely to have a clot than a group with no travel history. Another study found that over a three-year period PE was the second most common cause of death in the long distance traveler (Isayev et al 2002, 960). A well-designed trial from France found that those who traveled over 6200 miles by air had three times more PEs than those who flew 3100 miles (Lapostolle et al 2001, 779). Another trial in Spain later confirmed that the risk of PE markedly increased as the flight time lengthened (Perez-Rodriguez et al 2003, 2766). One trial found deep venous clot formation in 10% of passengers on flights averaging 24 hours (Scurr et al 2001, 1485), while nurses at one hospital near Heathrow Airport report seeing one flight-related DVT per week ("News Feature" 2001, 116).

Given the pathophysiology involved, it follows that flying is the most dangerous form of travel, as the literature suggests. Prolonged immobilization is a given, and compression of popliteal veins against the edges of seats may produce endothelial injury. Further, the relatively low humidity of the cabins produces dehydration, producing a concentration of blood. Decreased oxygen tension and ambient cabin pressure impair the body's ability to lyse clots and may even induce clotting (Ansell 2001, 828). Accumulation of fluid in the legs (called edema) compresses veins, which may further produce clotting. The resultant clot in the legs usually causes local problems for the legs, with occasional PE, or even more rarely, stroke in those with congenital holes in their hearts, a phenomenon known as Patent Foramen Ovale (PFO) (Isayev et al 2002, 960).

Before anyone becomes overly concerned, however, we should note that the overall incidence of serious flight-induced clots is extremely low. Over a seven-year period in one of the world's busiest airports, investigators found only 56 cases of "severe" PE out of 135 million passengers (Lapostolle et al 2001, 779). Certainly some cases were missed, but even doubling the number would still produce a very low overall incidence. Another study in Madrid found just 16 PEs in 41 million people over six years (Perez-Rodriguez et al 2003, 2766). Other studies have found that we form clots all the time, but very few of these prove to be of any significance. Sitting in front of a computer screen for hours on end may also cause clot formation in those with risk factors.

So, if flying can trigger potentially fatal, though rare, complications from clotting, just how risky is it? A series of five studies (and counting) under the heading LONFLIT has compiled the best evidence to date, allowing us to answer the question. Appropriately, all of these trials first separated subjects into those at high risk and low risk for clotting. The authors defined "high-risk" patients as those having a prior history of DVT, a clotting disorder, cancer within the prior two years, limitation of mobility due to bone or joint problems, recent surgery, obesity, or large varicose veins. While oral contraceptive use was not included as high-risk, it should have been; these agents are known, along with pregnancy, to increase the risk of clot formation (Belcaro et al 2002, 635). One trial found that oral contraceptives combined with air travel increased the risk of clotting by a factor of 14 (Martinelli et al 2003, 2771).

In the first LONFLIT trial, the authors found no clots in low-risk subjects while 2.8% of "high-risk" subjects developed DVTs during long flights averaging 12.4 hours (Belcaro et al 2001, 369). While a higher percentage (4.8%) of high-risk subjects developed either superficial or deep clots, we focus on the deep clots only because these carry the real risk. Superficial clots rarely lead to real problems and are readily treated with aspirin and warm compresses. In a pattern reproduced in all subsequent studies, almost all clots (94.7%) formed in passengers sitting in non-aisle seats. This makes sense because aisle passengers have less "restricted motion" than their non-aisle counterparts. They also have to get up every time anyone in their row has to get up, providing less continuous time for clot formation. LONFLIT1 proved that there was a significant risk of clot formation in high-risk passengers during long (10–15 hour) flights, particularly for those not in aisle seats.

LONFLIT2 randomized 833 high-risk subjects into a control group and a group that wore elastic compression stockings (Below-knee, Scholl, Flight Socks, with maximum compression of 25 mm Hg of pressure at the ankle) during long (10–15 hour) flights (Belcaro et al 2001, 369). While 19 subjects (4.5%) in the control group developed DVTs, only one (0.24%) did in the group that wore the compression stockings. The authors concluded that by simply wearing elastic stockings on long flights, high-risk subjects could reduce their risk of DVT by a factor of 18.5. In this second study, 76% of DVTs formed in subjects in non-aisle seats. Instructions given to both groups included the following: move often (three minutes every hour); drink water (at least one glass every two hours); stretch the limbs every hour for two minutes; do not keep baggage under the space under the seat; avoid salty snacks; and wear comfortable clothes.

LONFLIT3 took the prophylaxis question one important step further (Cesarone et al 2002, 1). This study compared two treatment options for the high-risk subjects, aspirin and low-molecular-weight heparin (LMWH) (enoxaprine). A third group receiving no treatment formed the control group. Roughly 100 subjects comprised each group, and no one wore elastic stockings. In the control group, four subjects (4.82%) developed DVT, while in the aspirin group, three (3.6%) subjects developed DVT. In the LMWH group, no one (0.00%) developed DVT. No side effects developed in subjects taking one dose of enoxaprine (1000 IU per 10 kg body weight) prior to the flight. The authors concluded that one dose of enoxaprine is an effective prophylactic against clot formation for high-risk patients taking long flights. However, the authors felt that the evidence may well be lacking to recommend this to all high-risk passengers without contraindications, though this may well change with time. Individuals should consult their primary care or travel clinic physician for individual recommendations.

LONFLIT4 found that flight stockings prevented edema and clot formation in low-medium risk subjects (Belcaro et al 2002, 635). The "medium risk" subjects included the above-mentioned three women taking oral contraceptive agents, who comprised all but one of the four DVTs found in the study. This study also proved that flight socks markedly decrease edema formation, a complication that can cause significant discomfort, usually in flights five hours or longer. LONFLIT5 confirmed that flight socks prevent clot formation in high-risk subjects and are well tolerated (Belcaro 2003, 197).

Given the above, we could summarize the current state of our knowledge as follows. The overall risk of clot formation for most people is low, though occasional news stories of fatal PEs will continue to send shock waves through the traveling public. Those in the "low-risk" group, comprised of all those lacking "high-risk" traits, should feel reassured that their risk of developing a clot while flying remains very low. However, because low-risk subjects do occasionally develop serious clots, it is worth following some simple measures: stay well hydrated, avoid alcohol and salty snacks, periodically move about the cabin, stretch or exercise the lower legs in the seat, wear loose-fitting clothing, and avoid crossing the legs. Choosing an aisle seat will also help. Flight Socks are inexpensive, well tolerated, and proven to decrease both edema and clot formation, so even low-risk subjects should consider them on longer flights. Some low-risk people, such as athletes with bruised or torn muscles predisposed to clotting, should consider flight socks (Wong 2003). Remember also that longer flights mean higher risk, a fact that low-risk people should consider. I fall in this category and find the socks comfortable, sparing me the occasional edema, which is not.

For those in the "high-risk" group, some form of clot prophylaxis is warranted. All of the above measures apply, and this group should consider purchasing and wearing Scholl's Class I Flight Socks, or the United States' equivalent "Travel Compression Socks," available at www.easygoing.com/travelsox.html (800-675-5500) and from the United Kingdom at www.aviation-health.org/shop/catalog.asp?Cat=2#AP15. Medical supply stores in the United States and many airport shops also stock them. The decision to take enoxaprine is an individual one and should be made in consultation with the primary care or travel clinic physician. People with bleeding disorders should likely avoid such therapy and one should factor in the considerable risk of road accidents at the destination site. Enoxaprine is short-lived (12–24 hours depending on dosing), so one could simply delay any potentially dangerous travel or other activities upon arrival by 12–24 hours.

This is an area that receives considerable attention given the general population's proclivity for long distance travel. The largest ongoing research effort is the World Health Organization's (WHO) Research Into Global Hazards of Travel (WRIGHT) Program, a four-year investigation started in June 2001, which should be published in early 2006.[5] Until this and other research clarifies remaining questions, it remains best to follow the simple measures outlined above and ask the right questions at the travel clinic before you board a plane.

Jet Lag

Those who cross multiple time zones soon find themselves in a place familiar to those of us who routinely do shift work, as I have done for the past 13 years in the emergency department. Following the readjustment of our body clocks, it is not uncommon to feel nausea, fatigue, irritability, headache, and just plain lousy, all while being unable to sleep at night. The root of this misery lies in the pineal gland, and its chief inducer of sleep, melatonin. When we stay up all night or travel through several times zones we disrupt our usual circadian rhythms, which are based on exposure to daylight. For the traveler, symptoms are more severe when traveling east, and with more time zones crossed. Typically, it takes one full day to adapt for each time zone crossed.

Given the extent of modern travel, as well as the large numbers of people who do shift work, there are a host of antidotes to this common affliction. I have always found that exercise helps adjusting sleep-wake cycles, something widely recommended (Kozarsky 1998, 305). Running a few miles following either a night shift (after sleeping through the next afternoon) or a time zone change always helps both my general feeling and my ability to adapt. Napping also helps. Trying to get to bed closer to what will be the usual time at the destination during the days to weeks beforehand can also help considerably, as does readjusting meal times according to anticipated schedules.

Many seasoned travelers use short-acting benzodiazepines like Ambien or Sonata to sleep on the plane en route. I have also tried these measures and found them helpful. Benadryl in small doses such as 25 to 50 mg will induce short periods of sleep for many. Melatonin has grown in popularity due to its short duration and efficacy. Given its central role in inducing sleep, it has been shown to restore normal sleep patterns to the blind, who are commonly afflicted with insomnia (Arendt 2000, 1114). Doses of 3–5 mg taken at 6–7 p.m. in the days before traveling eastward, followed by bedtime dosing for about four days after arrival can help considerably (Kozarsky 1998). For westward travel, just take it at bedtime for four days after arrival. Because melatonin is not approved by the Food and Drug Administration in the United States, it should be used with caution, if at all. Melatonin is currently marketed as a dietary supplement, allowing the manufacturers to get by with considerably less scrutiny than that given most US pharmaceuticals. As such, the active ingredient will be inconsistent from one bottle to the next. That manufacturers have also made some unsubstantiated claims of melatonin's "miraculous potential" also warrants concern (Arendt 2000, 1114). Many impurities have been found in the product and there certainly is a precedent for over-the-counter medications causing harm. Keep in mind that melatonin does have a hangover effect, as do many other sleep agents. Best to try out any agent well before a trip to learn the potential side effects and see if it works for you.

One final word on sleep-inducing agents during flights warrants mention. Any medication that induces sleep will also reduce overall movement, and may therefore increase the risk of clotting. Those in high-risk groups for clot formation should review this with their physician. The added risk may well outweigh the benefits of additional sleep.

Dangers: Road Travel, Conflicts, and Crime

Road travel, conflict, land mines, and crime comprise some of the risks of traveling and working in the developing world. We start by looking at general mortality causes for all those who travel. Over 30 million Americans travel abroad each year, mostly to Europe and popular destinations in the Caribbean and Mexico (Hargarten and Baker 1991, 622). Roughly 1200 Americans die overseas each year while traveling for any purpose.[6] Not unexpectedly, most US deaths abroad occur in older travelers, with cardiovascular diseases the most common cause, roughly half. Because most US travelers visit Mexico, and Europe, that is where most of the deaths occur. The risk of death rises with travel to less developed countries (622). None of this is surprising.

What is most striking about studies on travel-related fatalities is the high incidence of traumatic causes. In the above study, "unintentional injury" accounted for a full 22% of deaths, typical of the US tourist population. Of these, motor vehicle accidents accounted for the highest percentage. Drownings was next, followed by homicides and suicides. By contrast, infectious disease caused just 1% of all deaths, though many such deaths might well be delayed until return and would have been missed.

With these figures as background, we can now look at more relevant data, courtesy of the US Peace Corps. In perhaps the most important study for anyone considering international health work, Hargarten and Baker studied fatalities in US Peace Corps workers from 1962 through 1983 (Hargarten and Baker 1985, 1326). This study represents a more accurate assessment of risk for the traveler to the developing world, because most Peace Corps volunteers (PCVs) are young and not expected to import fatal illness with them. Their deaths reflect the true risks posed by life in poor regions.

When Hargarten and Baker reviewed the 185 deaths over this 21-year period, they found that 70% were caused by "unintentional injury." Motor vehicle crashes (MVCs) caused more than one-third of overall deaths and over half of the unintentional deaths. One-third of these MVC deaths were due to motorcycle crashes. Most of the motor vehicle crashes occurred at night, and three deaths that occurred in trucks resulted from the PCV riding in the back, either through ejection or crush injuries sustained in a rollover. Most deaths occurred when the PCV was using private means of transportation. Deaths due to drowning, suicide, and homicide may well reflect a young, active population often isolated in rural settings for two years at a time.

It should be little surprise that road travel constitutes the greatest risk to those who travel in developing countries. By its very nature, road travel can be dangerous. Highway crashes in the United States claim over 40,000 lives and cause 3.5 million injuries each year (National Transportation Safety Board [NTSB] 1998). Every day, road accidents claim 1000 lives around the world (Hasbrouck 2000, 380). In developing countries, travel is considerably more dangerous. Most developing countries lack the uniform safety standards that we in the industrialized world take for granted. Largely unnoticed but effective means of improving US roadway safety include: drunk-driving laws, legitimate driver's licenses, guard rails, energy-absorbing barriers, seatbelt laws, airbags, child safety seats, commercial driver's licenses that bar untrained drivers, heavy truck brakes, highway bridge maintenance, road maintenance, car inspections,, and many more. These all have come about because of the NTSB in the United States and equivalent agencies in other rich countries. Many or all of these unseen protections are lacking in poor countries, where driving is often a terrifying experience. Animals and slow-moving vehicles like tractors share the roads with cars, making driving more dangerous. When unskilled and impatient drivers pull around slower moving vehicles or livestock, tragedy occasionally follows. Everyone I know who has spent time in the developing world has at least one story about travel. I too have had a few close calls at high speed. So take heed. The greatest health risk abroad comes from getting into a car or, still worse, getting on a motorcycle.

In my experience, people in many poor countries drive overly fast with a recklessness that would give even a Boston driver pause. For example, many of the public bus and *matatu* drivers in greater Nairobi are young, fearless, testosterone-fueled males that typify drivers in a number of countries. It was not uncommon for these men to take incredible chances to pass slower-moving trucks on divided two-lane roads. Every ride was an experience, and we saw a number of victims of road crashes in Nazareth Hospital. In fact, victims of road crashes, many critically injured, are common visitors to emergency departments and clinics in all developing countries. I had a recent experience driving along the Western Highway in Belize where two cars were passing each other simultaneously from the opposite direction in my lane in the rain. I narrowly missed a crash only by slowing down quickly and getting far off the road's shoulder. One of the government drivers for our Belize program crashed in 2003 head long into a truck while passing a slower-moving car. In this horrific accident, his Cuban physician passenger was killed instantly and he was hospitalized for several weeks with multiple fractures to the legs, pelvis, and arms. Two years earlier, I had asked him to slow down while he drove our group along the Northern Highway from Orange Walk to Belize City. I think he had been insulted by my request, but he slowed down and we arrived safely.

The point of all of this is not to frighten you out of traveling anywhere, but rather to make you aware of the biggest risk of international travel—driving, particularly in poor countries with lax safety standards and many bad drivers. Yet there are ways to minimize your risks. First of all, make arrangements with the nongovernmental organization (NGO) or sponsoring group to assure safe travel once you arrive. Specifically ask which roads are most dangerous and when—the locals always know. Drive with those who you know or those who come recommended to you whenever possible. If someone is driving recklessly, forget about cultural sensitivities. Speak up and save your life first; worry about offending people second. Always avoid traveling at night, particularly weekend nights when alcohol flows freely. As much as possible, avoid traveling when it rains. Rain combines with oil to form a slick that causes many accidents, particularly early on after the rain starts. Because many vehicles in developing countries are older and poorly repaired, they leak more oil. Combine this with dust that settles in on highways in rural areas and you have a recipe for a crash. In addition, many poor countries have single-lane, divided highways that markedly increase risk.

Naturally, there are other forms of transportation available while traveling abroad. When choosing public transportation, find out all you can about reputations, accident history, overloading, and other factors beforehand. Public transportation in some countries is extremely dangerous and should be avoided. In others, travel on buses may prove safer as collisions between buses and cars favor the former. Many trains and ferries have provided service for years, though most suffer from overloading. In general, flying is safest, trains are next safe, and public road transport such as buses or smaller vans are least safe. Daily newspaper stories tell of ferries capsizing, buses crashing, or trains derailing, often killing scores of people in a single horrific accident. Because boats, trains, and buses are generally old, poorly maintained, and hopelessly overcrowded, it is no surprise that these occur with such regularity. It is yet one more cost of being poor. It is best to inquire from your hosts as to the safest forms of transportation in a specific region. Better yet, inquire before you leave and arrange for someone to pick you up at the airport. In my experience, the safest transport abroad comes through friends and colleagues.

Humanitarian and Civilian Targets

Naturally, the risk of any international medical work depends mostly on the type of travel and the nature of the work involved. For those signing up with Medecins Sans Frontieres (MSF), the Red Cross, Care, or other relief organizations to work in complex humanitarian emergencies, which include conflict, refugee movements, and natural disasters, the overall risk is higher. Similarly, working in a region with high concentrations of land mines like Cambodia, Angola, Sudan, or Afghanistan, or in countries with political instability adds in a whole other layer of risk.

For those traveling to zones of conflict, keep in mind that the rules of the game have changed considerably in recent years. The nature of conflict has changed, with civilians increasingly targeted and humanitarian workers increasingly employed by governments in lieu of their own soldiers. Images of US soldiers dragged through the streets of Mogadishu did not support the concept of the US military as peace broker. Increasingly, governments have shuttled that role to NGOs. The results are predictable, with over 380 humanitarian workers killed in zones of conflict between 1985 and 1998 alone (World Health Organization [WHO] 2002, 218). As Oxfam president Raymond C. Offenheiser said, "Governments are backing away from their responsibilities, and leaving aid agencies to fill the void. No government wants to see its soldiers die on CNN. But when an aid worker gets killed, there's no political heat. It is just another tough luck story in some unhappy place" (Nickerson 1997).

In recent years, those "unhappy" places are legion, as are the tragic stories that inevitably spring from them. While there are no official tallies, most NGOs find that the numbers of aid workers kidnapped, raped, or killed have "soared." CARE lost 44 humanitarian workers in Somalia alone while UN agencies such as UNICEF has seen its death rates increase from one per month a decade ago to one per week more recently (Nickerson 1997). The United States, United Nations, and European Union have mostly stood idly by when there have been internal conflicts or genocides. As Offenheiser said, "Their policy, if you want to call it that, has been to look away from the worst horrors—the slaughters in Rwanda or Bosnia—then look to the NGOs to clean up" (Nickerson 1997).

As the events of September 11, 2001, and attacks in Kenya, Bali, Russia, Great Britain, Spain, and Turkey have made perfectly clear, some will make political points by claiming innocent lives. Terrorist acts, however, occurred long before al Quaida burst onto the international scene. Rebels from Peru's Shining Path guerrilla movement killed seven people in Lima, Peru, in 1986 (McNeil 1999). Islamic militants killed 71 people, including 60 tourists, in the "Valley of the Kings" in Luxor, Egypt, in 1997, another in a long series of attacks dating back to the early 1990s (Sennott 1997). Militants have long sought to replace Hosni Mubarak's secular rule in Egypt with an Islamic state, often resorting to terror as a means to make statements (Jehil 1997). Ugandan rebels killed eight tourists in 1999 while bandits robbed and raped students and teachers along a notorious stretch of highway in Guatemala in 1998 (McNeil 1999). While it is clear that there are considerable risks traveling and working abroad, some perspective is required. First, those who choose to work in complex humanitarian emergencies must recognize the risks involved. While many consider the adrenaline rush and the immediacy of the work rewarding, one should factor in the opinions of those who have sustained significant injuries from land mines, gunshots, or other forms of violence. This type of work certainly fits some hardy soles out there and, like most others, I have great respect for all of them. But please make a clear calculation of risk and benefit ahead of time. If this is what you really want to do, then take the appropriate precautions, talk with a number of people who have gone before you, and be clear you understand how best to remain safe while performing your job. Many people may want to try their hand in a program that offers teaching or direct clinical care before jumping into more risky work, and most programs that put clinicians in harm's way prefer those with prior international experience.

As for the risk of a terrorist attack on those who are traveling in developing countries, keep in mind that, apart from Iraq, the number of events such as the above is vanishingly small, particularly when compared to the number of those who travel to all parts of the world each year. Horrible things do happen without warning, like the September 11 tragedies. However, many events occur in areas known to be high risk, often with State Department warnings posted ahead of time. A long series of attacks on both local Egyptians and tourists had predated the killings at Luxor. The Shining Path had long been active in Peru before the attacks and the stretch of highway in Eastern Guatemala was known to be dangerous long before the teachers and students made their plans.

While there are real dangers out there, keep in mind that perceptions often trump reality, particularly in US culture in which mass media plays upon our fears to sell its sponsors' wares. In 1991, I traveled to Dublin, Ireland, for a six-week visiting clerkship at St Vincent's Hospital. While preparing for my trip, I was struck by the number of people who cautioned how dangerous it was in Ireland, given the well-known strife between IRA and Protestant factions. I was leaving the "safe" environs of Boston, and residency at Boston City Hospital to go to a country "at war" according to many. However, a cursory review of available mortality data shows that in 1992, just 89 people died in the whole of Ireland as a result of the conflict (Sutton 1994). By contrast, there were 152 homicides in Boston alone around the same time.[7] There were nearly 24,000 homicides in the United States during the same year.[8] Because the US population in 1992 was 73 times larger than that of Ireland, we would expect 329 killings if Ireland were equally dangerous. Obviously, it was not. Again, some perspective is in order. Those Americans inclined to attribute all violence to problems overseas should recall that we live in one of the world's most violent countries, something not lost on foreigners coming here. Of note, in 1993, nine foreign tourists were killed in South Florida, many through carjackings at or near the airports. For a brief but significant period of time thereafter, Germany put Florida on its "don't go" list (McNeil 1999).

Land mines remain another very real concern for those planning to work in certain countries. According to the NGO Landmine Action, there are over 85 countries with active mines, with the worst affected including Afghanistan, Angola, Bosnia,

Cambodia, Iraq, Laos, Mozambique, Somalia, Sri Lanka, and Sudan.[9] Many NGOs, including the 1997 Nobel Peace Prize co-recipient International Campaign to Ban Landmines, can provide information on risks of mines in service destinations.[10] It is well worth checking the potential for land mines in any country you plan to visit, given the enormous risks they pose.

Crime remains a another formidable foe to those planning to serve abroad. Carjackings have become increasingly common in Nairobi, though far from the commonplace occurrence they are in such locales as South Africa. Arms tend to follow drug traffic, leading to more dangerous locales throughout the Caribbean, South and Central America, and Asia. In Belize, the national jail in Hattieville is increasingly filled with young toughs deported from the United States for gang-related activities. Unfortunately, they carry their knowledge of gang tactics back home and criminal activities soon escalate in both frequency and violence. As US culture spreads through the world via movies and television shows, other countries become more dangerous places. As such, it is best to always be prepared, and always remain fully aware of your surroundings. Ask locals about areas to avoid, when it is safe to travel to certain areas, and how reliable the local police are. Because my father was a policeman, it took me a while to get used to the idea that in Kenya the police can't be trusted. That is true in a number of poor countries. The same is often true of soldiers, even more so.

While one can do little more than avoid major violence whenever possible, one can take a more active role in avoiding petty theft. While many travelers wear waste belts holding passports, money, and other valuables, I have always seen those as advertisements to thieves. Waist belts or neck pouches that one wears under the clothes are far safer and considerably less inviting. I always carry two wallets as well. One carries my cash, license, credit card, and health insurance card. The second is my "decoy" wallet, containing some cash, and old library, insurance, and other cards. If robbed, this is the one I'll hand over. As long as it holds sufficient cash, it should do. I keep my real wallet thin and tucked into a front pocket where it is hard to see and harder to remove. Others have recommended sewing Velcro over pockets to prevent theft. The loud ripping sound associated with Velcro serves notice of an intruder.

Because wallets, passports, and other valuables are frequently lost or stolen, it is wise to photocopy everything in your wallet or pouch before departure, and leave a copy with someone you can contact in an emergency. Carry only essentials with you; leave the nonessentials at home. And don't bring jewelry or expensive watches—leave it all home.

Specific Health Concerns

Traveler's Diarrhea

Traveler's diarrhea (TD) comprises the most common of travelers' illnesses, accounting for 64% of all illnesses affecting tourists (Virk 2001, 831). Various studies have reported that from 30% to 60% of travelers to developing countries will become sick from TD (De Bruyn et al 2002), accounting for over 7 million cases per year (Adachi et al 2000, 1079). The largest study to date screened 30,369 people vacationing in Jamaica and found an attack rate of 23.6% (Steffen et al 1999, 811). Naturally, those going to less developed areas than the all-inclusive tourist resorts of that study have higher attack rates. The Peace Corps found that over 95% of their volunteers developed diarrheal disease annually, although they live and work "in a style comparable to their host-country coworkers" that no doubt increases their risk (Bernard et al 1989, 1079). The most important risk factors for developing TD are the destination, time of year, type of travel, and the age and eating habits of the traveler (Ramzan 2001, 665).

Most who read this have previously become acquainted with the clinical symptoms. By definition, TD involves the passage of at least three unformed stools in a 24-hour period. Most infected undergo a self-limited course that resolves within three to four days, while 10% of cases last longer than seven days.[11] TD usually comes on abruptly, and is occasionally associated with vomiting (in 15%), abdominal cramping, or low-grade fever (De Bruyn et al 2002). More severe cases involve bloody diarrhea (dysentery), high fevers, abdominal pains, or a prolonged course. Bacteria cause most episodes of TD, with enterotoxigenic *E. coli* (ETEC) the organism most often responsible. Other frequent causative organisms include *Campylobacter, Salmonella,* and *Shigella. Vibrio parahemolyticus* is a frequent cause from seafood in Asia. Viruses cause few cases while parasitic causes such as *Entamoeba, Giardia, Cryptosporidium, Cyclospora,* and intestinal helminthes (worms) become more important the longer one stays in poor, endemic areas.[11]

Prevention For years travelers to developing countries have heard the following axiom: "boil, bottle, or peel." Because most TD comes from bacteria transmitted by the fecal-oral route, it is best prevented through careful screening of food and water and good hygiene. First, avoid drinking water that is not in a sealed bottle or purified by boiling, filtration, or iodine. Be careful of vendors selling unpurified tap water in capped, though unsealed, bottles, a scam I once watched unfold in Nairobi. Always look for a seal, though carbonated beverages, beer, and wine are usually safe. Bottled water is available in many developing countries, but travel to rural or impoverished settings may require a filter or iodine. I have carried a PUR water filter during travel to Africa and more remote settings. They are available through a number of on-line sites and camping stores, lightweight and inexpensive, roughly $100 for the Scout or other similar model. Another alternative is to boil water for at least 10 minutes or add drops of iodine and let stand for 10 to 20 minutes (Cohen 2000, 5). Those with a history of thyroid disease should avoid the latter. I prefer the filter mainly because the iodine adds a terrible aftertaste. Be careful to avoid brushing your teeth with contaminated water. I usually place a towel over the sink as a reminder to use bottled water for teeth brushing, even in many cities abroad. Ice cubes, salads, and peeled fruit are common sources of contamination. Be sure to ask hosts about food and water sources, peel fruit yourself, and be sure milk products are pasteurized. Wash your hands with soap and water before each meal. Also be sure meat is fully cooked; and avoid raw seafood, despite its allure. Despite the attraction of many enticing aromas, it is wise to avoid street vendors. Private homes, restaurants and vendors offer increasingly risky meals in that order.[11]

Most people will not require ongoing prophylaxis with antibiotics. Simply following the commonsense measures outlined above will markedly decrease the likelihood of getting sick. Further, antibiotics have potential side effects and propagate antibiotic resistance. However, for some, prophylaxis with antibiotics may well make sense. For those with immunosuppression such as transplant recipients, those taking corticosteroid medications like prednisone, or chronic medical conditions such as inflammatory bowel disease, as well as those who are on shorter, time-sensitive trips, prophylactic regimens of a flouroquinolone antibiotic (Cipro 500 mg once daily, Norflox 400 mg once daily, or Ofloxacin 300 mg once daily) have been shown to be the most effective (Ramzan 2001, 665; Virk 2001, 831). Other regimens, including doxycycline 100 mg once daily (beware photosensitivity reactions) and bismuth salicylate (Pepto Bismol) (beware those with aspirin allergies and bleeding tendencies) taken four times daily, have proven effective. Bactrim is best for children who should not take either doxycycline or the flouroquinolones. Again, these agents should rarely be taken prophylactically.

Treatment Because at least half of those who travel to developing countries will develop TD at some point, the first rule is to be prepared. I first encountered TD in 1987 while hitchhiking to Makiungu Hospital through rural Tanzania, hardly the best place for it to strike. Fortunately, I had packed a roll of toilet paper in a plastic bag, which kept it dry in the torrential rains that ever so greatly enhanced the experience. I recommend that anyone with rural travel plans keep a small roll in a plastic bag as well; such is a fixture in my day-pack while abroad.

When TD does strike, the first consideration should be rehydration, particularly because so many developing countries lie in tropical or sub-tropical zones. A good rule of thumb is to try to match stool output with fluid intake. A mild case may warrant little to moderate rehydration with any type of liquid while a severe case warrants aggressive rehydration with appropriate solutions. The WHO has devised oral rehydration solution (ORS) packets with the correct balance of electrolytes that are widely available in many developing countries. Pedialyte is also widely available. You can make a safe and effective ORS by mixing 8 teaspoons of sugar (a handful) with 1 teaspoon of salt (a pinch) into 1 liter of *clean* water (Werner and Sanders 1997, 42). Be particularly careful to properly rehydrate infants and children, who are far more susceptible to "dehydration" from diarrheal illness. Again, use either prepackaged solutions or clean water with ORS packages or homemade remedies. Breast-feed infants if possible. Those traveling with young children will want to review treatment options with their health providers well before their departure.

Many people carry anti-motility agents such as loperamide (Imodium) with them. This has been shown to be safe and effective for mild to moderate cases. The standard dose is 4 mg after the first loose stool, then 2 mg after each loose stool to a total of 16 mg per day. However, avoid these agents if diarrhea is associated with bloody stools or fever.

A large number of studies have demonstrated the efficacy of antibiotics in TD (De Bruyn et al 2002). Prompt treatment with either a floroquinolone in adults or trimethoprim-sulfamethoxazole (Bactrim) in children can reduce the illness duration from three to five days to less than one to two days (Guerrant et al 2001, 331). One study found that a single dose of Ciprofloxacin reduced symptoms of mild TD by roughly one day over a group that took placebo (50.4 hours to 20.9 hours) (American College of Physicians 1995, 43). The study authors included only mild cases, excluding patients with bloody stools, fever, or severe diarrhea. Although azithromycin, doxycycline, aztreonam, and Bactrim have all been effective, the flouroquinolones (like Cipro) remain the drugs of choice, despite increasing resistance worldwide (Virk 2001, 831). Those with more severe illness will require longer, three- to five-day treatment regimens. People should seek medical help if symptoms fail to resolve after a few days of treatment with antibiotics (Adachi et al 2000, 1079).

In sum, it remains best to avoid becoming ill by following the preventive measures outlined above. Carry toilet paper in your pack when traveling rurally. When ill, use appropriate rehydration, anti-motility agents, and antibiotics in relation to the degree of illness, as per the following summary (Adachi et al 2000, 1079). For mild cases, defined as one to two stools/24 hours, use no therapy or use loperamide or bismuth preparations alone. For mild to moderate cases, defined as more than two stools/24 hours with or without "distressing" symptoms, use appropriate rehydration, loperamide, or bismuth preparations, and a single dose of a flouroquinolone (Cipro 500-750 mg once orally; or Norfloxacin 800 mg once orally; or Levofloxacin 500 mg once orally). Because this class of antibiotics should not be used in pregnancy or children, consider either TMP-SMZ (Bactrim 2 double-strength tablets once, TMP 5 mg/kg once) for children or Azithromycin (1000 mg once) for adults unable to take flouroquinolones. If symptoms persist after 24 hours, continue antibiotics for three days, with Cipro 500 mg twice daily, or Norfloxacin 400 mg twice daily, or Levofloxacin 500 mg once daily. For severe cases, which include more than six stools/24 hours, fever or bloody stools, avoid usage of anti-motility agents, and use the above flouroquinolone regimen for three to five days. Some resistant cases of *Campylobacter* may respond to Azithromycin (Guerrant et al 2001, 331). Because bismuth preparations bind any of the flouroquinolones, avoid mixing these drugs.

Respiratory Ailments

After TD, respiratory ailments comprise the most commonly acquired illnesses among travelers. The elderly or those with underlying respiratory ailments should consider the pneumovax vaccine. Everyone should consider influenza vaccine prior to travel, because long travel exposes individuals to those infected with influenza, particularly in the close confines of airport waiting areas or planes. Despite widespread practices to the contrary, antibiotics offer no benefit for acute bronchitis in younger people with no underlying lung disease or other serious illnesses (Gonzales and Sande 2000, 981; Bent et al 1999, 62; Fahey et al 1998, 906). Be sure to first distinguish bronchitis from the more serious bacterial pneumonia (Metlay et al 1997,

1440). It is rare for those with pneumonia to have normal vital signs and a clear lung exam (Gonzales and Sande 2000, 981). Inhalers improve symptoms for many people afflicted with the post-infectious inflammatory changes in their airways. Those with a tendency to wheeze following upper respiratory infections should bring an inhaler and Spacer with them.

Malaria

Malaria is the world's most important parasitic disease, causing 300-500 million infections and over 1million deaths annually (Kain and Keystone 1998, 267). Complications from malaria kill a child every 30 seconds (Fradin and Day 2002, 13). Only HIV and TB cause more infectious deaths annually. It remains endemic throughout most of Africa, Asia, the Middle East, Hispaniola (Haiti and the Dominican Republic), Central and South America, and Oceania. Malaria used to infect North Americans from Montreal to Miami—at least 1 million soldiers suffered from malaria during the US Civil War (Garrett 1994, 48). It was not until the 1950s that the United States achieved full eradication, though there have been sporadic outbreaks since, including one in Palm Beach, Florida, in 2003 (2003, 2931). A WHO-led campaign for global eradication of malaria from 1955 to 1976 failed miserably, and malaria continues to exact an enormous toll annually, chiefly among the poor (Epstein 1999, 2).

Roughly 30,000 travelers from industrialized countries contract malaria each year (Virk 2001, 831). Malaria is by far the most common cause of fever in the returning traveler (Magill 1998, 445). It is also the infectious entity most likely to kill the traveler to endemic regions. Malaria is more lethal in US travelers due to their non-immune status, with near 100% febrile illness produced. Case fatality rates are high when infected travelers return home due to missed diagnosis, unreliable diagnostic testing, and a general lack of familiarity among US health providers (King 2002, 1256). Malaria is a miserable and often lethal illness, though an entirely preventable one. There is simply no excuse for a health provider going to a malarious region unprepared.

From 1985 to 2001, the CDC received reports of 10,100 cases of malaria among US civilians. More recent reports estimate 1200–1500 cases per year (Newman et al 1999, 15), though even these are likely gross underestimates (Kain and Keystone 1998, 267). Of these, 58% came from Africa; 18% from Asia; 16% from the Caribbean, Central, or South America; and 7% from other parts of the world.[12] This included 70 fatalities, almost all due to *P. falciparum* (94%), mostly from sub-Saharan Africa (74%). In 2000, only 483,000 US residents traveled to sub-Saharan Africa while 27 million traveled to other countries where malaria is endemic. So, even though 56 times more people traveled to other world regions, a full 71% of the fatalities came from sub-Saharan Africa. This illustrates one of the most important points about malaria. While there are four subtypes that cause malaria, by far the most dangerous is *P. falciparum.* Travelers are far more likely to acquire it in sub-Saharan Africa due to the fact that it is higher there, and transmitted in both rural and urban areas.

Malaria is caused by one of four species of the intraerythrocytic protozoa *Plasmodium*: *P. falciparum, P. vivax, P. ovale,* and *P. malariae* (Strickland 2000a, 614). The female *Anopheles* mosquito spreads malaria by transmitting the protozoa through her salivary glands during a bite. Once inside the human host, the protozoa replicate, infecting red blood cells. When the young protozoa mature, they cause the red blood cells to rupture, causing fever, anemia, low oxygen levels, and, in severe infections, death. When the *Anopheles* mosquito bites an infected person, the micro protozoa enter the mosquito and the process repeats. In both *P. vivax* and *P. ovale,* the protozoa may become dormant in the liver, where they survive long-term and cause relapsing infections. These forms require a two-week course of Primaquine for eradication.

Clinical Clinical manifestations of malaria depend on the strain, with *falciparum* by far the worst (Strickland 2000a, 614). Because the other three strains are rarely fatal, we will consider *falciparum* here. The incubation period is 10–14 days, sometimes longer. Many patients have prodromal symptoms such as malaise, myalgia, headache, anorexia, and fever for a few days before the acute attack begins. Then patients have classic rigors with chattering teeth, followed 30–60 minutes later by fever, often 104–106°F, profuse sweating, headache, myalgias, malaise, nausea, vomiting, or cough. This "hot" stage lasts two to six hours, then the cooling down stage lasts two to three hours. The term *tertian malaria* refers to the life cycle of *falciparum* and *vivax* malaria in which the schizonts rupture every 48 hours. The patient may look well in between fevers. For the first several days, however, fevers occur daily. Gastrointestinal symptoms including diarrhea, nausea, vomiting, and abdominal pain are not uncommon. Serious clinical sequellae of malaria include: cerebral malaria (altered mental status), acute renal failure (Blackwater fever), pulmonary edema (high respiratory rate, and chest X-ray findings), severe anemia, and stillbirth.

Laboratory diagnosis is the key. A thick smear will show the parasite clearly in most cases of *P. falciparum.* The relative parasitemia will determine the ease of detection. A 5% parasitemia is high, meaning that 5% of all red blood cells are infected. Thin smears allow identification of species. Most patients with *falciparum* malaria will be positive on the first smear. Serology is available though rarely needed.

Risk of Acquiring Malaria A number of factors determine how likely it is that one will contract malaria while abroad. Certainly, the destination is important. Seven areas account for two-thirds of reported malaria cases worldwide: Africa, India, Brazil, Sri Lanka, Vietnam, the Solomon Islands, and Columbia (Kain and Keystone 1998, 267). Travelers to West Africa are 240 times more likely to acquire malaria than those who go to Central America, while only 1 in 12,254 travelers to Thailand will acquire malaria. Remember, however, that malaria prevalence fluctuates with weather patterns, mass migrations, wars, natural disasters, and economic downturns. Resistance to various treatment regimens also changes frequently, such that it is important to have updated information when deciding on appropriate prophylaxis. The CDC (www.cdc.gov) and WHO (www.who.int) update travel recommendations frequently, and travel clinics also monitor disease patterns, adjusting treatment accordingly.

Other factors that directly affect the risk for acquiring malaria include the type and duration of travel/work, whether one will spend time in urban or rural areas, and the season of travel. Naturally, those who work in rural areas with more exposure to bites during rainy seasons are at higher risk. The MSF worker out in the field is far more likely to contract malaria than is a businessman on a short trip to Nairobi. Those who are out during peak biting times, dusk to dawn, also incur higher risks. Those visiting areas following natural disasters that involve flooding (more breeding sites and higher mosquito populations) or disruption of anti-malarial measures such as spraying incur higher risk as do those who work with refugees or in war zones. Host immune response also factors in, with those who have never been previously exposed at highest risk.

Malaria Prevention There are many commonsense measures that can markedly decrease the risk of acquiring malaria. Keep in mind that these apply to other mosquito-borne diseases as well, including yellow fever, Japanese encephalitis, dengue fever (transmitted by a day-time biting mosquito), and West Nile fever. While people have acquired malaria through blood transfusions (Mungai et al 2001, 1973), shared needles, and visits to international airports, most people still get it through the evening and night bites of the female *Anopheles* mosquito. Therefore, the best way to cut your risk is to limit the mosquitoes' opportunities to bite you. Start by curtailing activities that bring you outside in the evenings or at night, if possible. Wear long pants and long-sleeved shirts during evening and night hours. Many places in tropical and subtropical locales cool down sufficiently in the evening to make such clothing comfortable. You should also spray clothing with permethrin, a mosquito retardant that is available in most camping stores or online. Once sprayed on fabrics, it will remain effective for at least two weeks (Fradin 1998, 931). Lightweight travel tents are available through campmore.com or Long Road Travel. I set up my tent (3 lbs) everywhere in East Africa during my second sojourn there in 1994. Consider spraying the room with insecticide before retiring and looking for mosquitoes about the room before bed.

Many available products will repel mosquitoes. One study compared DEET, Citronella, soybean oil, and others (Fradin and Day 2002, 13). Subjects applied the various products to an arm, inserted it into a mosquito-filled cage, and then counted the minutes until the first bite. Contrary to popular mythology, "Skin So Soft" proved useless, protecting subjects' arms for a mere 9.6 minutes. By contrast, preparations that contain DEET lasted for hours, prompting the authors to call it "the gold standard." The higher the DEET concentration, the longer the protection, as follows: 4.75% DEET—1½ hours of protection; 6.65% DEET—2 hours; 20% DEET—4 hours; 23.8% DEET—5 hours. The protective effect plateaus at concentrations of 50%. The 3M Corporation developed a slow-release, polymer-based 35% DEET preparation called HourGuard that is now standard issue for all US military personnel. This is available from Amway Corporation in New York (800-544-7167) (Fradin 1998, 931). Neither garlic, vitamin B6, nor repellant-laden wristbands provided any protection.

Many worry about potential toxicity of DEET-containing preparations, but the overall risks are small. Despite estimates of over 8 billion applications globally, including use by 38% of the US population, there have been fewer than 50 case reports of adverse effects since 1960, and most of these were due to incorrect application (Fradin and Day 2002, 13). Of note, however, most of those adverse effects have occurred in children, with encephalopathy in 14, three of whom died. Here again, most involved incorrect applications. The American Academy of Pediatrics currently recommends that children receive no more than 10% DEET-containing preparations to ensure safety (Fradin 1998, 931). Despite such caveats, however, DEET is a remarkably safe product when used correctly. The Environmental Protection Agency concluded, "normal use of DEET does not present a health concern to the general US population." Apply to exposed skin only, not to hands, and use concentrations of 35% or less. Some kids may need patch testing first, to assure no adverse reactions. Pregnant women should see a travel specialist prior to departure, but can safely use DEET following specific guidelines. It will irritate the eyes, so avoid contact. Because DEET damages plastics, one should exercise care when applying near eyeglasses, watches, or synthetic fibers.

The final barrier to malaria prevention remains the most daunting to travelers. Chemoprophylaxis against malaria constantly evolves as new medications appear and old ones become less effective through emerging resistance. By the time you read this, some recommendations may well change, so consult the CDC or WHO Web sites or visit a travel clinic for current recommendations. Many people have questioned the need for prophylaxis at all, while media reports have heightened concerns of prophylaxis with one particular drug, mefloquine. While visitors on brief trips to urban areas in malarious zones may well be fine without prophylaxis, most people require it. In fact, it may prove life saving. According to the CDC, none of the 21 people who died from malaria in the United States and Canada in 2000 had taken prophylactic treatment against malaria (CDC 2001b, 597). Just as important as taking prophylaxis is taking the correct prophylaxis. *P. falciparum* resistance to chloroquine treatment has spread widely in recent years. Yet some people still take chloroquine as prophylaxis in resistance zones. In 2001, the CDC reported that seven people had died since 1992 after taking chloroquine for travel to sub-Saharan Africa, a peak zone of chloroquine-resistant *P. falciparum* (597). Alarmingly, of 4685 malaria cases among returning US travelers reported to the CDC in 1992–2001, 19% took inappropriate prophylaxis while 56% took none at all (597).

There has been sufficient experience to date to confidently say that taking an effective anti-malarial prophylactic works and works extremely well.[13] For those traveling to areas with chloroquine-sensitive strains of malaria of any species, chloroquine remains the drug of choice. Take it once weekly, starting one week before leaving, during the stay, and for four weeks upon return. It is quite bitter tasting, and will induce vomiting, as I learned, if taken on an empty stomach. Chloroquine is safe for kids but is highly toxic if overdosed. As little as 500 mg can kill a one-year-old, so be sure to keep it out of reach of children. For areas of chloroquine resistance, there are essentially three choices, mefloquine (Larium), atovaquone-proguanil (Malarone), and doxycycline. Primaquine can also be used but is less effective.

Mefloquine is the mainstay of prophylaxis in chloroquine-resistant areas due to its efficacy (90–100%) and weekly dosing schedule. It has been saddled with bad press and is quite a difficult drug for some to take. I was one of the few who had to stop when last in Kenya due to disruptive nightmares. Following reports of homicides among returning US soldiers and other neuro-psychological problems, mefloquine now carries contraindications against prescribing to those with a history of depression, anxiety, psychosis, or major psychiatric disorders; also against those with a history of seizures. Despite this, however, studies have found mefloquine reasonably well tolerated. In one series, only 5% of 483 patients had to discontinue it, mostly due to neuropsychiatric problems, though nearly one third reported adverse effects (Overbosch et al 2001, 1015). Given the usual difficulties of culture shock, homesickness, and the other stresses of transitions involved in serving in poor communities, one should be aware of the potential problems related to this drug. Colleague Dr/Rev Bill Fryda, who has spent over 20 years in East Africa, states that neither he nor many other long-term ex-pats in East Africa recommend it. Those on shorter visits might well consider using another agent like atovaquone/proguanil (Malarone) and those on longer trips should have a back-up plan in place. Of note, there are now chloroquine- and mefloquine-resistant areas, along the borders of Thailand, Cambodia, and Myanmar (Burma) (Virk 2001, 831). For travel to these areas, doxycycline or atovaquone/proguanil remain the standard of care. Doxycycline is effective and cheap but requires daily dosing and causes photosensitivity reactions. It can also cause an erosive esophagitis if a pill gets stuck there; so drink lots of fluids after taking pills. Atovaquone/proguanil is very well tolerated but expensive and requires daily dosing. In the same study mentioned above with mefloquine, only 1.2% of patients had to discontinue this drug for any reason, and just 14% reported any side effects. It is ideal for shorter trips to chloroquine-resistant areas.

Some people have self-medicated at the onset of fever, or relied on personnel at host sites in developing countries for treatment. Those who self treat may do so inappropriately, taking potentially toxic medications unnecessarily, or not taking appropriate medication soon enough when they do have malaria. If people do decide on this course, recognize that this is a temporizing measure only, and they should quickly seek medical help as soon as possible (Kain and Keystone 1998, 267). While there are certainly a host of knowledgeable health personnel all over the world, neither the diagnosis nor treatment of malaria is assured anywhere. Studies have shown laboratory diagnosis of malaria in developing countries is often lacking, with false positives up to 75% and false negatives up to 20%, leading to inappropriate or no treatment (Keystone 2003). As such, it may be wise to continue on treatment even if the malarial smears are "negative," depending on how confident you are about the skill of the laboratory personnel. I worked with outstanding technicians during my stays in Africa, and trusted them fully—they taught me a lot. Yet there is a broad range of variability in labs everywhere. Just factor this into your decision on how to proceed.

There have also been reports of fake or counterfeit drugs in developing countries, leading to treatment failures. So, it is most often worth the additional expense to purchase the full course of medications for malaria treatment prior to departure. For those who return home ill with malaria, there is no guarantee of effective treatment awaiting them. Due in part to the unfamiliarity most US clinicians have with malaria, it is often missed, or treatment is delayed, occasionally with fatal consequences (CDC 2001b, 597). Similarly, limited blood-smear testing in US labs limits the ability to diagnose it properly (King 2002, 1256). Due to decreasing use of IV quinidine in cardiac dysrrhythmia management, this most valuable drug for treating severe malaria may be difficult to find in a timely fashion. IV quinine, the standard in most of the developing world, remains unavailable in the United States.

Treatment *P. falciparum* malaria is a medical emergency. It rapidly infects red blood cells, lyses them, causes capillary leaking, and ultimately end organ failure from a lack of oxygen. Bad outcomes occur because the patient delays seeking treatment, the diagnosis is missed, or the treatment chosen is incorrect. Prompt diagnosis often allows oral therapy and produces a good outcome. Delayed diagnosis often leads to intravenous treatment and produces a bad outcome. For those who develop a febrile illness while abroad, seek medical care as soon as possible. If care is not immediately available, consider the following regimens for treatment of *P. falciparum.*[14] In chloroquine-sensitive areas, use chloroquine (Aralen) 1 gm orally, then 500 mg orally 6 hours later, then 500 mg orally at 24 and 48 hours. Be absolutely certain there are no resistant strains before following this regimen. In chloroquine-resistant areas, use atovaquone/proguanil (Malarone), two adult tablets two times daily for three days. Those with kidney disease or those taking Malarone as prophylaxis already should avoid this regimen (King 2002, 1256). Alternatives include quinine sulfate 650 mg every eight hours for three days plus doxycycline 100 mg twice daily for seven days. Fansidar is another alternative though used far less frequently.

P. falciparum can rapidly escalate into a fatal illness. I once had three cases on the ward in Kenya die within hours of admission, all from *P. falciparum* cerebral malaria. The CDC recommends against self-treatment for good reason. Seek medical help as soon as you become ill with a febrile illness, particularly if working in sub-Saharan Africa. For those who show signs of end organ damage such as altered mental status, rapid respiratory rate, or dark urine, begin intravenous quinine (quinidine gluconate if in the United States) as soon as possible.

The bottom line is, exercise appropriate behaviors, such as limiting exposure by wearing long-sleeved shirts and long pants; spraying clothing, bed nets, and exposed skin areas with repellants; and taking area-specific malarial prophylaxis. With appropriate precautions, few serving in endemic areas should contract it. This is one illness that, with proper preparation, can almost always be avoided.

Sexually Transmitted Diseases

It may seem pure common sense to advise travelers to refrain from unprotected intercourse, particularly during travel to poor countries that tend to have high endemic rates of HIV and hepatitis B. However, travelers often have a sense of anonymity that may lead to more promiscuous behaviors (Ryan and Kain 2000, 1716). Some studies have shown that 25%–50% of travelers engage in sexual activities with locals, other tourists, or commercial sex workers, though these studies primarily reflect sexual activities in young backpackers (Virk 2001, 831). Concerns of HIV infection seem surprisingly lacking. Long-term European workers in developing countries have HIV prevalence rates 100 to 500 times higher than similar populations in Europe, and up to half of European workers living in sub-Saharan Africa have reported casual sexual encounters with African partners (Ryan and Kain 2000, 1716). One study of Peace Corps volunteers found that less than one-third used condoms regularly, even though many served in areas with high HIV seroprevalence (Moore et al 1995, 795). Other larger trials have shown similarly dangerous patterns among international travelers. While men traveling abroad have shown patterns of condom usage similar to that practiced at home, women tend to adopt the practices of their partners, often increasing the risk of infection (Bloor et al 1998, 1664). All health providers should have hepatitis B vaccination and those so inclined should use condoms in every sexual encounter. Condoms purchased in developing countries are often unreliable, so bring a supply with you as needed (Virk 2001, 831). Because both HIV and hepatitis are both readily transmitted through tattooing and body piercing, one should avoid both of these activities while abroad. Finally, women traveling alone should beware of the very real risk of rape. A colleague is treating a woman who acquired HIV in East Africa after a game park guide raped her. Be careful and travel with others when possible.

Environmental Concerns

Because many who visit developing countries take advantage of the natural wonders that so many locales offer, it is important to consider briefly some of the ailments common to such environments. Most people will encounter extremes of heat beyond what they are used to at home, so remember to drink plenty of fluids. It can take several days to truly acclimate to hotter environments, so curtail heavy physical activities if possible just after arrival. Use sunscreen with 15 SPF or higher and wear light-colored clothing, a hat, and sunglasses. Keep in mind that many medications, including some over-the-counter ones, can block sweating or produce hyperthermia in other ways. Be careful with allergy medications, sleep aids that contain Benadryl, and antidepressants. Be sure to read the precautions on the labels of any medications you take with you.

A lot of people who travel to developing countries hike or trek, as I did up Mount Kilimanjaro in Tanzania in 1987. Just like me then, many are wholly unprepared for the potential dangers of altitude. Acute mountain sickness (AMS) is a common though unpredictable disorder afflicting those who ascend too rapidly or too high. Counterintuitively, people over 50 are less susceptible than those younger, and physical fitness is not protective (Hackett and Roach 2001, 107). One study noted a 22% incidence of AMS at 7000–9000 feet and 42% over 10,000 feet (107). Most people with AMS experience nausea, headache, dizziness, and fatigue. When people push through these symptoms, they are at risk for the more serious altitude syndromes of high-altitude pulmonary edema (HAPE) or high-altitude cerebral edema (HACE), both of which can prove fatal within hours. Both are caused by hypoxia (low oxygen)-induced capillary leakage and subsequent edema (swelling) in the lung or brain, respectively. The best way to prevent any form of altitude sickness is gradual ascent, though acetazolamide (Diamox at 125 mg twice daily starting three days prior to hitting the target altitude) has proven helpful, and is more effective than steroids like dexamethasone. Treatment depends on severity of symptoms, though rapid descent is common to all syndromes. Supplemental oxygen and positive-pressure (Gammow) bags may prove lifesaving.

Many tropical locations in the Caribbean, Africa, Oceania, and Asia offer the possibility of diving or swimming, which includes a host of pleasures and accompanying dangers. Drowning still represents one of the most common causes of fatality in travelers. In the Peace Corps, there were 26 deaths due to drowning in 21 years; drowning comprised nearly one in five deaths and was the second leading cause of death after motor vehicle and motorcycle accidents (Hargarten and Baker 1985, 1326). Those who swim in unfamiliar environments may be unaware of prevailing currents, rip tides, and other dangers. Some drowning deaths involve alcohol, never a great idea around water. Other deaths come through boating accidents. In a US Park Service study of 48 water-related deaths in 1989, the single factor common to all was the failure to wear a lifejacket (Hargarten 1991).

Divers have their own set of risks and it seems obvious that one's first experience with diving should not come in a country that lacks proper dive instruction and supervision. Given time constraints, some people go immediately from a dive to a flight. Yet, one should follow established tables for flying after diving, which advise waiting 24 hours after multiple dives or any dive requiring decompression. Because mefloquine has become standard malarial prophylaxis in chloroquine-resistant areas, concerns have surfaced about its potential impact on those who dive. Monitor any neuro-psychiatric symptoms closely and consider timing dives away from weekly dosing of mefloquine, when drug concentrations are at their peak. The Divers Alert Network, or DAN, offers valuable advice, maintaining a 24-hour emergency advice line at 916-684-8111. Non-emergency advice is available at 916-684-2948.

There are some sea creatures that all swimmers should pay attention to (Kozarsky 1998, 305). Sea urchins are small, round, spiny creatures that deposit their painful spines in your unsuspecting foot. Consider wearing protective rubber shoes (most sporting goods stores carry them) designed for use in water. But if you do step on one of these creatures, immerse the foot in hot water and carefully try to remove the spines. I recently gave a third-year medical student the opportunity to remove a large number of these spines from the foot of a returned traveler; it took well over an hour to get many, though not all, of them out. Keep in mind that what looks like a spine may actually be dye only and most of these will work their way out on their own. Consider an X-ray if there is a possibility that a spine has entered a joint, which may warrant surgical removal. Some coelenterates (jellyfish) can inflict painful stings when swimmers inadvertently contact their tentacles. Their larvae can get under bathing suits and cause an itchy rash. These are best rinsed with seawater or vinegar. Because the nematocysts remain in the bathing suit, throw it away. Many beaches in the United States with such infestations have jugs of vinegar available, though such may not be the case in developing countries. Any wound that occurs in the water may become infected with gram-negative rods of *Vibrio* species. Therefore, antibiotic coverage should be broader spectrum, like a quinolone such as Cipro.

Schistosomiasis

Schistosomiasis ("snail fever" or "bilharzias") is a common parasitic infection caused by trematodes (a worm) endemic in Africa, Asia, the Caribbean, and South America. Over 200 million people worldwide are infected (Kozarsky 1998, 305). It is transmitted by a swimming cercaria (larval form) that travels from the snail host to those wading or swimming in freshwater, penetrating their intact skin to cause a variety of syndromes. "Swimmer's itch" is the most common ailment, an intense itch caused two to six days after the cercaria penetrate the skin. From there, the maturing worms may penetrate intestine, bladder, or lungs to cause acute and chronic illness, including portal hypertension, central nervous system lesions, intestinal scarring, and both bladder and colon cancer, though many people remain asymptomatic for long periods. I cared for several people with complications from schistosomiasis in Kenya in 1994. The CDC reported two cases in unsuspecting Peace Corps workers who contracted the disease while swimming in Lake Malawi (CDC 1993, 565). One developed visual loss and seizures from central lesions and the other incontinence and leg weakness from T11 lesions. The first fully improved while the second retained some gait weakness and required periodic self-catherization, at age 26. Subsequent testing of expatriates around Lake Malawi found a full 33% positive for schistosomal antibody. The point of all of this is not, "don't go to Africa." Rather, avoid freshwater swimming or wading while you're there, particularly in slow-moving or stagnant pools of water. Immediately toweling off or applying isopropyl alcohol after freshwater contact in endemic areas may also be protective. Returning travelers from endemic areas should also consider follow-up schistosomal antibody testing in travelers' clinics. This illness is treated easily enough with praziquantel, but is easily missed, with potentially devastating consequences.

Risk of HIV and Hepatitis B and C in Endemic Settings, Needle-stick Injuries

In impoverished settings internationally, the one risk that targets health workers specifically is infection with blood-borne pathogens from the workplace. Needle-stick injuries, splashes to mucosal surfaces, exposure to blood during deliveries and surgeries all increase the risk of HIV, hepatitis B and C, Lassa, Ebola, and other hemorrhagic fever viruses endemic to some tropical regions (Sagoe-Moses et al 2001, 538). Currently there is little effective treatment for hepatitis C and only supportive treatment for Lassa, Ebola, and others. However, there is an effective vaccination for hepatitis B (which all health providers should now have) and effective treatment for occupational exposure to HIV. It is well worth considering such risks ahead of time and preparing for a potential exposure.

Common sense dictates that the risk of acquiring any of these blood-borne pathogens rises along with the endemic rate of infection in the local population. In sub-Saharan Africa, HIV and hepatitis B and C are all endemic, with high prevalence rates in many poor settings around the world (Sagoe-Moses et al 2001, 538). Some regions of sub-Saharan Africa have HIV prevalence rates in adults up to 40%.[15]

Although HIV prevalence in many poor countries is high, the occupational risk of health providers acquiring HIV in these countries remains largely unknown. Ninety percent of the *documented* HIV infections stemming from occupational exposures come from the developed world, despite producing only 4% of the global HIV burden (Sagoe-Moses et al 2001, 538). By contrast, while over 70% of the cases of HIV in 2000 were in sub-Saharan Africa, only 4% of the occupational HIV infections come from the same region. This paradox stems from the little surveillance available in poor countries. Many don't report infections because there is no testing or treatment available.

As in occupational settings at home in the United States or Europe, the most effective prophylaxis comes through maintaining universal precautions, including the following: maintaining extreme diligence in handling needles and other sharp instruments, never recapping needles, always wearing gloves around blood and other body fluids, wearing a gown and mask with a face shield during procedures, and exercising strict hand-washing immediately following any exposure. Because there is a safe and effective vaccine against the potentially lethal hepatitis B, there is no reason to travel to an endemic area unvaccinated. In one study, 61.2% of schoolchildren in Ghana carried markers of hepatitis B infection (Martinson et al 1996, 278). Similarly, one should receive a tetanus booster prior to departure if the last booster was more than 10 years earlier.

Of concern to anyone working in poor areas with high prevalence rates of HIV and hepatitis B and C is that many of the safety practices common to industrialized countries are lacking. Due to limited health budgets, many health facilities reuse syringes, requiring further handling. Given the common cultural belief that only injections can cure, many unnecessary injections increase the occupational exposure for health workers in such settings. There is rarely the means for proper disposal of hazardous waste, and protective items such as gowns, gloves, facemask, and shields are only sporadically available and frequently recycled. I recall being covered in blood during a delivery in Tanzania as a medical student in 1987; there were no gowns available.

For health workers, the risk of acquiring HIV or hepatitis in poor locales is probably much higher than in most comparable settings in the developed world. As such, it makes sense to be prepared. Health providers should update their vaccinations against hepatitis B and tetanus prior to departure. For HIV, it makes sense to inquire about available HIV prophylaxis at the hospital or clinic you will visit or consider bringing a prophylactic "needle-stick" regimen with you. The good news is that the overall risk of acquiring HIV through a needle stick appears to be small. As of December 2001, the CDC had reported only 57 documented cases of HIV transmitted by occupational exposure in the United States, with another 138 "possible" exposures, despite over 380,000 needle-stick injuries in US hospitals every year (Gerberding 2003, 826). Overall risk of HIV conversion from a needle-stick injury (percutaneous exposure) is just 0.3%, while that of HIV conversion following a mucous-membrane exposure is just 0.09%. The risk of conversion from exposure to non-intact skin is too low to be assessed. Because saliva contains low levels of HIV, the risk from bites or spit is low unless contaminated with blood. The risk of sero-conversion rises with hollow-bore needle injuries, when the device causing injury was clearly contaminated with blood, when the device had been used to puncture a vein or artery, when the device inflicts a deep injury, or when the source patient dies within two months after exposure (Cardo et al 1997, 1485).

Following an exposure, treatment should follow two parallel tracks. First, if the source patient is HIV-positive or likely so, begin a course of empiric treatment for HIV with at least two antiretroviral medications, possibly three if severe exposure or known resistance patterns to certain medications exist locally. Naturally, prophylactic regimens should avoid medications with known local resistance. Prophylaxis should start as soon as possible after exposure. Such treatments are highly effective. The CDC found an 81% reduction in HIV conversion through post-exposure treatment with zidovudine (Busch et al 1995, 91). Factors that influence the rates of transmission following post-exposure treatment include: the amount of viral inoculum, the interval between the exposure and onset of treatment, the duration of treatment, and the drugs used (Gerberding 2003, 826).

Second, find out all that is available about the source patient. In some settings it may well be impossible to perform HIV testing. If the source HIV status is unknown, one should follow established guidelines based on the type of exposure, the likelihood of HIV positivity in the source, and the HIV resistance patterns of the immediate region, if known. A history and physical examination may well show the likely presence of HIV: weight loss, fevers, malaise, persistent diarrhea, or other opportunistic infections, generalized lymphadenopathy (lymph nodes), rash, wasting, thrush (whitish growth in the mouth), hairy leukoplakia (a corrugated, whitish appearance to the lateral aspects of the tongue), among other findings. If the patient is known to be HIV-positive, one should find out if there is a known viral titer, and if the patient is receiving medications. Because local treatment patterns at your potential service site are known already, you should consult an infectious disease or travel medicine expert beforehand and devise the most logical prophylaxis regimen before departure.

There are many prophylactic treatment regimens available, and one should tailor the regimen to local resistance patterns that typically result from the available local antiretrovirals. The most commonly used regimen employs zidovudine (Retrovir) plus lamivudine (Epivir) in a combination tablet called Combivir taken twice daily for four weeks, but other regimens may better fit different regions (Gerberding 2003, 826). Stop only if the source patient tests negative. Current recommendations are to start the regimen as soon as possible following the exposure. In deeper inoculums or higher-risk settings, one may well consider adding a third drug, most commonly Indinavir or Nelfinavir. One should follow standard blood-borne pathogen precautions while working abroad and be prepared for the unexpected. Prophylactic regimens should be clarified beforehand, not in the panicked aftermath of a serious exposure. The CDC updates current recommendations at www.cdc.gov/travel/travel.html, while University of California at San Francisco maintains a hotline phone number that can field questions at 888-448-4911. Similarly, University of California at Los Angeles maintains a Web site at www.needlestick.mednet.ucla.edu. The CDC's Dr Julie Louise Gerberding wrote a nice summary in the *New England Journal of Medicine* in February 2003, available at *NEJM* 2003; 348:826-833.

Other Considerations

For those with medical problems, it is wise to fully prepare before departure. For those who require routine medications or injectables like insulin, a physician's letter may help assuage quizzical customs agents (Virk 2001, 831). Given the difficulty of finding reliable medications in some developing countries, it is also wise to bring a full supply of required medications with you. The same holds true for contact lens wearers, who may find it difficult to find correct cleaning and storing solutions. Given the dry, dusty conditions found in many locations, as well as the difficulty of treatment in the event of an eye emergency, contacts are often best left at home. Those who do bring them should also consider bringing along a prescription for a topical antibiotic such as Ocuflox or Tobrex ophthalmic ointments in case of an eye infection. A small pocket mirror can also come in very handy.

Potpourri

Over many years of traveling abroad, I have compiled a list of suggestions that may well help those new to the area. Everyone with any significant travel experience has his or her own favorites. These come in no particular order and may or may not help given the relative travel experience of the reader. But here they are anyway: Everyone traveling to a developing country should consider investing in a backpack, preferably one with a detachable daypack. (Never leave the daypack attached when out of your sight—it will be stolen.) I have used the same Jansport World Traveler for over a decade. In your pack, you should consider carrying a Swiss army knife (though not in your carry-on), which comes in handy in a number of situations, from opening bottles or cans to spreading peanut butter on the road. I am a staunch believer in plastic bags. I usually keep several folded up in the bottom of my pack and place any fluids, such as suntan lotion, in plastic bags in preparation for the inevitable leak. Muddy shoes, damp clothes, and other liquids all remain separate from my dry clothes given a ready supply of plastic bags. My watch has a built-in alarm clock and timer, to get me up on time and track my approximate running distances. I bring powdered laundry detergent with me, and wash clothes as I go, which serves to lighten the load. A retractable clothes line often comes in handy. Finally, I never go anywhere without a small flashlight (with spare batteries), which seems to come in handy at least once each trip. Because I read every night in bed, I often bring a small reading light with me.

As befits a section titled "potpourri," one should be careful not to leave clothes drying outside in areas endemic with the bot fly—found mainly in Africa and South and Central America. These flies lay eggs in clothing, after which the larvae migrate through intact skin to grow, producing a syndrome called myiasis. These later comprise the "something is moving under my skin" that terrifies so many travelers. You can prevent infection by ironing clothes, a common practice in many locales. Once infected, treatment is by suffocating the larvae by applying Vaseline to the opening in the skin.

Resources for Travelers

Years ago, I received an audio training tape from a group called G.W. Associates. The $10 tape, called *Living Media,* gave clear, step-by-step instructions to those returning from international experiences on how to contact the local media and raise awareness of international issues. I view such work as critical and encourage everyone traveling abroad to use this great resource: G.W. Associates/Director Peter Wirth: 315-476-3396; 702 S. Beech Street, Syracuse, NY 13210; www.accucom.net/pwirth/.

The American Society of Tropical Medicine and Traveler's Health has compiled a *Clinical Consultants Directory* that lists physicians with expertise in tropical medicine and traveler's health. The directory is available on-line at www.astmh.org. It makes sense for anyone traveling to a developing country to at least write down a few names and numbers for emergencies. Many NGOs have a wealth of expertise and local connections for emergencies. However, arrival at the destination often does not place you immediately into the welcome embrace of your hosts. When I traveled to Tanzania as a medical student in 1987, it took 10 full days of public transportation and hitchhiking before I finally arrived at Makiungu Hospital in Singida, in the middle of the country.

Medical Kit

All travelers to developing countries should bring a medical kit with them. This can prove even more valuable to the trained health professional in rural settings. There are many standard recommendations for what to include in the kit, but individuals should adapt the kit to the circumstances of the trip. Someone going to a city would have markedly different needs than someone going to a refugee camp or rural outpost. A basic kit contains Tylenol, aspirin, ibuprofen, an antibiotic for diarrhea, anti-diarrheals such as loperamide, an antihistamine, antimalarials, medication for sleep if needed, insect repellent, a water purifier or iodine tablets, cold-sinus medication, sunscreen, antiseptics, gauze, soap towelettes, and topical antibiotic such as Bacitracin (Kozarsky 1998, 305). Also carry personal medications with you. Many drug stores carry pre-made kits that work fine.

Summary of Travel, Health, Cultural, and Safety Recommendations

We have covered a lot of ground in the past two chapters, and I hope you are now clearer about how to prepare for life in a developing country. The risks are certainly real, but can be reduced significantly by following simple guidelines. Let me offer here a summary of the more salient points:

- Order *The Traveler's Pocket Medical Guide and International Certificate of Vaccination* from The Travel Clinic in Australia and document all vaccinations in the back (www.travelclinic.com.au).
- Book flights well in advance through a consolidator.
- Plan your in-flight experience well, with bottled water and clot prophylaxis as indicated.
- Obtain current passport, visa, and all necessary travel documents well in advance.
- Pick up Edward Hasbrouck's *The Travel Nomad* well in advance, available at www.practicalnomad.com or in bookstores.
- Pick up Robert Kohls' *A Survival Kit for Overseas Living* and reflect on the importance of cultural preparations ahead of time.
- Get to a travel clinic two months prior to departure, earlier if a longer trip, and get proper immunizations. Follow up there after your trip, if sufficiently "remote."
- Properly plan your in-country travel. Remember, road trauma is the greatest risk of all for international travel.
- Bring medications for traveler's diarrhea, including loperamide and a course of a flouroquinolone antibiotic (like Cipro) or Bactrim for kids; avoid raw or uncooked foods, be sure any dairy products have been pasteurized, and bring a water filter or iodine tablets to purify all water if remote or rural travel is planned. Avoid salads, fruits that you don't peel yourself, and bottled water lacking an intact seal.
- Plan your malarial prophylaxis, including DEET, permethrin (for clothes and bedding), a lightweight tent for more rural travel, prophylactic medications, and emergency treatment options.
- Assemble a travel medical kit.
- Make photocopies of your passport, visa, and health insurance information. Leave one set of copies at home with someone you can contact in an emergency and pack another separately from your actual documents.
- Prepare a medical regimen for needle-stick or other occupational exposure to HIV-contaminated blood, and bring the correct medications with you if not available locally.
- Be careful in the tropical or subtropical sun; use sunscreen, a hat, and sunglasses and drink plenty of fluids.
- Prepare for any other travel, swimming, diving, trekking, or mountain climbing.

Endnotes

1. For more information see the Travel Clinic Web site at www.travelclinic.com.au, or write to the Travel Clinic at 263 Glen Eira Road, North Caulfield, Melbourne, 3161/ Victoria, Australia. Phone: (61 3) 9528 1222. E-mail: travel@travelclinic.com.au
2. Information from "Immunizations for Travel," an American Society of Tropical Medicine and Traveler's Health (ASTMH) course by Dr David Freedman, San Diego, October 2003.

3. For more information see the Anxieties.com Web site at www.anxieties.com/7Fear_of_flying_safety.htm.
4. For more information see the MSNBC Web site at http://msnbc.msn.com/id/3079105.
5. For more information see the World Health Organization's WRIGHT Project Web site at www.who.int/cardiovascular_diseases/wright_project/en/.
6. Information from "Epidemiology of Travel-Related Deaths" by Stephen W. Hargarten, available on the Travel Medicine Advisor Web site. See www.travelmedicineadvisor.com for subscription availability.
7. Information from "Police-Probation Teams Address Juvenile Violence in Boston Through Operation Night Light," an article summarizing a forum held on March 1, 2002, downloaded from the Web site www.ojp.usdoj.gov/eows/forumcj3.htm.
8. I couldn't find an exact tally, so I multiplied the 1992 US population of 255,029,699 (US census data) by the annual homicide rate from 1974–1992 of 9.3 killings per 100,000 people to arrive at the estimate of 23,718. The latter figure of 9.3/100,000 comes from a homicide study published in an MIT journal in 1994, available on the MIT Web site at http://web.mit.edu/newsoffice/tt/1994/aug17/37717.html.
9. Information from the Landmine Action Web site at www.landmineaction.org.
10. For more information see the International Campaign to Ban Landmines Web site at www.icbl.org.
11. For more information about traveler's diarrhea, see the Centers for Disease Control and Prevention Web site at www2.ncid.cdc.gov/travel/yb/utils/ybGet.asp?section=dis&obj=travelers_diarrhea.htm&cssNav=browseoyb.
12. For more information about malaria, see the Centers for Disease Control and Prevention Web site at www2.ncid.cdc.gov/travel/yb/utils/ybGet.asp?section=dis&obj=index.htm&cssNav=browseoyb.
13. For appropriate dosing schedules, see the Medical Letter Web site at www.medletter.com.
14. Information from "Drugs for Parasitic Infections" on the Medical Letter Web site www.medletter.com.
15. For more information see the UNAIDS Web site at www.unaids.org/EN/Resources/Epidemiology/EPI_Search.asp.

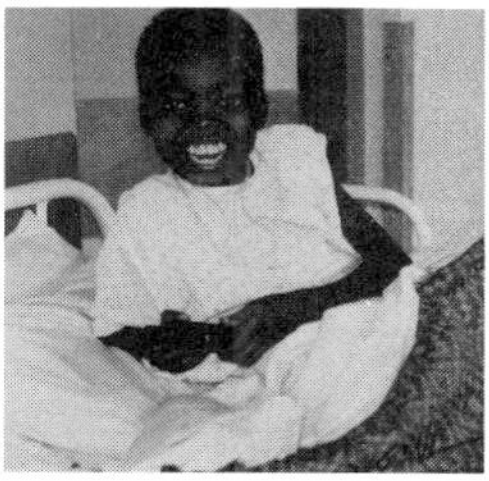

Chapter 3

The Omni Med Database of International Health Service Opportunities

It struck me as inconceivable that I should be allowed to lead such a happy life while I saw so many people around me struggling with sorrow and suffering. . . . The thought came to me that I must not accept this good fortune as a matter of course, but must give something in return.

—Albert Schweitzer

And when the broken hearted people, living in the world agree

There will be an answer, let it be

For though they may be parted, there is still a chance that they will see

There will be an answer, let it be

—John Lennon and Paul McCartney

Let no one be discouraged by the belief there is nothing one man or one woman can do against the enormous array of the world's ills—against misery and ignorance, injustice and violence. . . . Few will have the greatness to bend history itself; but each of us can work to change a small portion of events, and in the total of all those acts will be written the history of this generation. . . . It is from the numberless diverse acts of courage and belief that human history is shaped. Each time a man stands up for an ideal, or acts to improve the lot of others, or strikes out against injustice, he sends a tiny ripple of hope, and crossing each other from a million different centers of energy and daring, those ripples build a current which can sweep down the mightiest walls of oppression and resistance.

—Robert F. Kennedy

The following database is the culmination of over 10 years of work by a number of people, including staff, students, volunteers, and me at Omni Med. We sent out several thousand detailed questionnaires to nongovernmental organizations (NGOs) that send health volunteers both domestically and abroad. We then poured over Web sites and made hundreds of telephone calls to check the data. Patricia Newton and her staff in the philanthropy office at the Lahey Clinic graciously helped to coordinate our efforts before Omni Med existed. Since Omni Med's founding in 1998, a series of incredible people have updated our information and expanded the database. Three worked at Omni Med before going to medical school; two are there now; two are in computer sciences and another in public health. I would be quite remiss not to offer my profuse thanks here to each of them, in order of when they worked with us, starting in 1996: Ted Kordis, Dr Jamie McCabe, Maggie Zraly, Dr Doreen Ho, Dr Ian McClure, Fran Wang, Phillip Choi, and Yioula Sigounas. Ted Kordis designed the initial database in 1996, and Fran Wang further expanded it to its present, user-friendly form. Peter Cuomo is an attorney who worked with us during the winter and spring of 2005, carefully updating and expanding all of the information that follows; we were fortunate to have him. While I have read over each organization and edited all that follows, the database would not exist were it not for the dedicated people who nurtured it along all of these years. Any errors are my responsibility alone. This may well be the most comprehensive and detailed listing of international health service opportunities anywhere; it certainly took long enough to put it together.

Let me first share some impressions gleaned over 10 years of reading through brochures, Web sites, and questionnaire responses. First, the most striking feature of the NGOs depicted in that text is the humanity that shines through their mission statements. There are a lot of good people trying to do good work, in many cases at great personal expense. Judging by their program depictions, most are succeeding. That a world of poor people should forge connections with the world's most talented and privileged health care providers seems a predetermined fait accompli. Nearly one third of the organizations in our database have religious underpinnings; most welcome practitioners of any faith. The NGO I run is secular, as are most involved in this work. Yet most organizations follow an ethical premise that clearly resonates with faith-based values, even when not overtly stated.

Second, the breadth of the NGOs in operation is striking. Some send surgical teams to repair cleft palates or excise cataracts. Others offer dental care. Still others send medical supplies. Some focus all of their efforts on training, others entirely on direct service. Many combine health service work with environmental, agricultural, or economic activities. Several see health work as part of their ministerial outreach, and others perform clinical services while operating chiefly in the policy or human rights realm. Anyone interested in international health service can now easily find an opportunity.

Finally, it is easy to admire the heroic efforts I read about in the organizational literature we have compiled through the years. Few in the NGO community earn high wages for doing this work. Many people volunteer their time and, despite the usual pressures from jobs, tuitions, mortgages, and family obligations, still make this happen. Through the years, I have talked with many such people and derive great pride through the affiliations. They are the beating heart of the medical profession and offer the truest moral direction for our future. A conversation with any of them should inspire those who hesitate for any reason.

How to Use This Database

First, flip through some of the organizations in the following pages and get an idea of what's here. Read the mission statements and see what information they have supplied to us. See if any jump out at you. Next, turn to Chapter 4 and find the answers to the questions that are important to you. We asked organizations for a lot of information and much of that is reproduced here. Then follow these simple steps:

1. Find the list of the organizations that are looking for those from your specialty area (see page 304). We surveyed opportunities for virtually all physician specialty areas, as well as for dentists, hospital administrators, nurse practitioners, nurses, nurse mid-wives, optometrists, pharmacists, technicians, social workers, and many more. In total, we sought opportunities for 28 physician specialty areas and 22 non-physician, allied health areas. Most of the medical profession is represented here, so you should be able to find several organizations that are seeking your services.
2. Find the list of organizations that work in the world region (see page 348) in which you are most interested in working, if you have one. By cross matching the first two lists, you will quickly reduce your search to the organizations that may well prove the best match for you.
3. Turn to the "Minimum Time Available" section (see page 301) and find all of the organizations that accept people for the time period you seek. If you have limited time, find the list of organizations that send health providers for less than two weeks.
4. Look through Chapter 4 at the list of the questions we asked of all these organizations. The lists include organization responses on whether they accept the following: couples in which one or both spouses are health providers; families with children; pre-medical and college students; medical students; other health professional students; doctors in training; health care personnel who are and are not US citizens; and health personnel with no prior experience in developing countries.

Once you have narrowed your search down to a few organizations, then read the mission statements and search their Web sites. Write to them and ask them to send you their literature if they have any. Search on-line to learn whatever you can about them. Then contact them directly. Talk to representatives at each NGO and ask to talk with at least three volunteers who have gone through their programs. At Omni Med, we ask all of our volunteers to respond to queries from perspective volunteers. No one has ever refused and most enjoy the opportunity to share their experiences. I recognize that I am biased in favor of our program designs, though I do try to give both the good and bad of what I understand to be our volunteers' experiences. However, there is no substitute for talking to those who can give you an unbiased opinion of what working for an NGO in a certain region is like.

Because people have radically different experiences based on the season, political climate, personnel present at the time, and a host of other variables, it is always wise to talk with more than one. The longer your planned work experience and the more rural or difficult it may be, the more extensive your research should be ahead of time.

Because there are many different program models out there, there is no simple set of questions that will cover all that you will need to know. The questions we asked each of the NGOs in this chapter is a good place to start, but there is more you should seek. For the past seven years, we have asked our Omni Med volunteers to fill out detailed questionnaires on virtually all aspects of their service experiences abroad. Because our programs focus on education and training, we ask each volunteer to answer several questions about the efficacy of the teaching at the end of their experience. We also question the health providers in Belize and Guyana (eg, the "learners" in our programs) about how much they are getting out of it, so we can make changes where needed. I have modified some of these questions here; they may or may not be relevant to you, but they should give you some ideas of what might be important to ask ahead of time:

- Upon their departure, do volunteers in your program typically feel that they made a significant contribution?
- Do they recommend your program to others?
- What do your volunteers say they gain from the experience of working with you?
- What do local health providers and other local people say are their most pressing needs generally and their most pressing health needs?
- What is the safety record? Any problems to date? Are there problems with crime?
- How does one get to the program or hospital? Is there transportation provided and how safe is the travel in that region?
- Do people have opportunities to interact with locals outside of the immediate hospital or clinic? Do they develop an understanding about the host culture during their stay and how it differs from home?
- Why do people want to go? What are their motivations? What do they typically hope to accomplish during their stay?

The database contains NGOs of almost every kind. Some are partly clinical and partly evangelical; some have health as a small part of their overall function while some work exclusively in the field of health. I have no doubt that the vast majority of organizations that follow here are good. However, I cannot vouch for them all. To do so would be presumptuous on my part and a bit dangerous. I have worked internationally long enough to know that, alongside NGOs like Partners In Health and Health Volunteers Overseas, there are NGOs with ulterior motives and less than exemplary practices. A few organizations shouldn't be doing this work at all. By asking a lot of questions and talking to those who have gone through the NGO before you, you should be able to eliminate the few NGOs that are questionable.

We have complete data for over 280 organizations, though this is quite a dynamic sector. NGOs come and go, change names, locations, programs, and even their basic missions. Despite updating the information frequently, there will no doubt be some dated information in what follows here. Partly, that is due to the realities of publishing. We last updated the database information in the spring and summer of 2005, so some of the information has no doubt changed. Further, we solicited information on a wide range of questions, though we could not include all of the responses here. Specifically, questions on language and religion requirements and specific region and country destinations had to be omitted due to space considerations. (You will notice that there are Notes within most organizational descriptions. Simply track the respective number to the corresponding number under the Notes heading.) In time, we will develop a Web-based searchable database and may include CD-ROMs in future versions of this text. In the meantime, those requiring further information can check on the status of the database at www.omnimed.org.

Ultimately, you will choose a program based on what is most important to you. The overwhelming majority of organizations that follow do good work and will provide you with an effective opportunity to serve. The good news is that there are many options available and finding the right organization or locale is easier than it ever has been before. The opportunity to make a real difference in the world lies before you. Let us start here.

ACCESS

Continents Served
Africa ☐ Asia ☑ Europe ☐ The Americas ☐

Countries Served
India

Address: **'Chandana Nilaya',169 Ramdev Gardens, K.K. Halli, St. Thomas Town P.O. Box 4223, Bangalore 560084 India**

Phone: **918025431610** FAX:

E-Mail: **thomasswaroop@yahoo.co.in** Web:

Mission: church-based organization

Placement opportunities for . . .

People of only certain faiths? *1*	Yes
Couples: both are health providers?	Yes
Couples: only one is a health provider?	No
Families with children?	No
Medical students?	Yes
Pre-medical or college students?	Yes
Other health professional students?	Yes
Doctors in training?	Yes
Health personnel who are US citizens?	Yes
Health personnel who are non-US citizens?	Yes
Health personnel with no prior experience in developing countries?	Yes
Health personnel who are not current members of your organization?	Yes

Organization/Service Specifics:

Size of the Organization's Staff:	11-20
Number of providers sent or received/year:	1-2
Minimum term of assignment: *3*	4 weeks
Maximum term of assignment:	1 year
Is funding available for travel?	No
Are room and board provided? *2*	No
Is any other funding available?	No
Is training provided or available?	Yes
Is a language other than English required?	No

Health Professionals Placed:

Physicians:

Internal Medicine GPS & PCP; Pediatricians

Allied Health Professionals:

Nutritionists & Dieticians; Public Health Specialists, Epidemiologists and Health Educators; Social Workers

Notes

1. Protestant; *2.* But arrange at visitors cost; *3.* 4-12 weeks.

Action Against Hunger

Continents Served
Africa ☑ Asia ☑ Europe ☑ The Americas ☑

Countries Served

Afghanistan	Angola	Argentina
Armenia	Azerbaijan	Bolivia
Burundi	Cambodia	Chad
Colombia	Congo	East Timor
Ethiopia	Georgia	Guatemala
Guinea	Haiti	Honduras
Indonesia	Ivory Coast	Kenya
Laos	Liberia	Malawi
Mali	Myanmar (Burma)	Nicaragua
Niger	Pakistan	Palestine
Philippines	Sierra Leone	Somalia
Sri Lanka	Sudan	Tajikistan
Uganda	Zambia	Zimbabwe

Address: **247 W. 37th Street, Suite #1201, New York, NY 10018 U.S.A.**

Phone: **(212) 967-7800** FAX: **(212) 967-5480**

E-Mail: **info@aah-usa.org** Web: **www.aah-usa.org**

Mission: Action Against Hunger directly delivers emergency aid and longer-term assistance to people suffering from the dire consequences of natural disaster or man-made crisis. Our mission is to save lives by combating hunger, disease, and the crises threatening the lives of helpless men, women, and children. There is a minimum one year commitment, while there is no maximum. Funding is provided and French or Spanish may be required depending on the place of service.

Placement opportunities for . . .

People of only certain faiths?	No
Couples: both are health providers?	Yes
Couples: only one is a health provider?	Yes
Families with children?	No
Medical students?	No
Pre-medical or college students?	No
Other health professional students?	Yes
Doctors in training?	No
Health personnel who are US citizens?	Yes
Health personnel who are non-US citizens?	Yes
Health personnel with no prior experience in developing countries?	Yes
Health personnel who are not current members of your organization?	Yes

Organization/Service Specifics:

Size of the Organization's Staff:	21-50
Number of providers sent or received/year:	21-50
Minimum term of assignment:	1 year
Maximum term of assignment:	
Is funding available for travel?	Yes
Are room and board provided?	Yes
Is any other funding available? *1*	Yes
Is training provided or available?	Yes
Is a language other than English required? *2*	Yes

(continued)

Health Professionals Placed:

Physicians:

Physicians; Internal Medicine GPS & PCP; Pediatricians

Allied Health Professionals:

Nurse Practitioners; Nurses; Nutritionists & Dieticians; Public Health Specialists, Epidemiologists and Health Educators; Water/Sanitation Specialists

Notes

1. Monthly stipend ranging from $800-$1400; *2.* French or Spanish may be required depending on the country of service.

Adventist Development and Relief Agency International

Continents Served

Africa ☑ Asia ☑ Europe ☑ The Americas ☑

Countries Served

Address: **12501 Old Columbia Pike, Silver Spring, MD 20904-6600 U.S.A.**

Phone: **(301) 680-6380** FAX: **(301) 680-6370**

E-Mail: **Ron.Mataya@adra.org** Web: **www.adra.org**

Mission: Adventist Development and Relief Agency (ADRA) supports communities in need through a portfolio of cooperative activities, providing assistance in acute or chronic distress situations to achieve long-term developmental solutions. Enhancing indigenous capacities to sustain the environment, child health, and the equitable treatment of women reflects the humanitarian character of God. The length of stay and type of health care provider needed varies from trip to trip.

Placement opportunities for . . .	
People of only certain faiths? *1*	No
Couples: both are health providers?	Yes
Couples: only one is a health provider?	Yes
Families with children?	Yes
Medical students?	Yes
Pre-medical or college students?	Yes
Other health professional students?	Yes
Doctors in training?	Yes
Health personnel who are US citizens?	Yes
Health personnel who are non-US citizens?	Yes
Health personnel with no prior experience in developing countries?	Yes
Health personnel who are not current members of your organization?	Yes

Organization/Service Specifics:	
Size of the Organization's Staff:	51-100
Number of providers sent or received/year:	11-20
Minimum term of assignment:	varies
Maximum term of assignment:	varies
Is funding available for travel?	No
Are room and board provided?	Yes
Is any other funding available? *2*	Yes
Is training provided or available?	
Is a language other than English required?	No

Health Professionals Placed:

Physicians:

Allied Health Professionals:

Notes

1. Seventh-Day Adventists are preferred; *2.* Depends according to funding of project.

Africa Inland Mission, International

Continents Served

Africa ☑ Asia ☐ Europe ☐ The Americas ☐

Countries Served

Central African Rep. Chad Kenya Mozambique Uganda

Address: **P.O. Box 178, Pearl River, NY 10965-0178 U.S.A.**

Phone: **(845) 735-4014** FAX: **(845) 735-1814**

E-Mail: **go@aimint.org** Web: **www.aim-us.org**

Mission: Africa Inland Mission is an evangelical, non-denominational mission agency, working in partnership with the church to place individuals of the Protestant faith in short- and long-term appointments. It focuses on countries in Africa, the islands of the Indian Ocean, as well as the United States. Language requirements are specific to each country. Volunteers are required to make a two-month commitment and raise their own financial support.

(continued)

Placement opportunities for . . .		Organization/Service Specifics:	
People of only certain faiths? *1*	Yes	Size of the Organization's Staff:	>200
Couples: both are health providers?	Yes	Number of providers sent or received/year:	21-50
Couples: only one is a health provider?	Yes	Minimum term of assignment:	8 Weeks
Families with children?	Yes	Maximum term of assignment:	
Medical students?	Yes	Is funding available for travel?	No
Pre-medical or college students?	Yes	Are room and board provided?	Yes
Other health professional students?	Yes	Is any other funding available?	No
Doctors in training?	Yes	Is training provided or available?	Yes
Health personnel who are US citizens?	Yes	Is a language other than English required? *2*	Yes
Health personnel who are non-US citizens?	Yes		
Health personnel with no prior experience in developing countries?	Yes		
Health personnel who are not current members of your organization?	Yes		

Health Professionals Placed:

Physicians:

Anesthesiologists; Family Practitioners; General Surgeons; Internal Medicine GPS & PCP; OB/GYN; Orthopedic Surgeons; Pediatricians; Psychiatrists

Allied Health Professionals:

Dentists; Medical Technicians (lab, X-ray, etc); Nurse Midwives; Nurses; Physical & Occupational Therapists; Psychologists

Notes

1. Volunteers must be Protestant; *2.* Language requirements are dependent on the country of service.

African Inter-Mennonite Mission

Address: **1013 Division Street, PO Box 744 Goshen, IN 46527-0744 U.S.A.**

Phone: **(574) 535-0077** FAX: **(574) 533-5275**

E-Mail: **aimm@aimmintl.org** Web: **www.aimmintl.org/home.htm**

Continents Served

Africa ☑ Asia ☐ Europe ☐ The Americas ☐

Countries Served

Botswana; Burkina Faso; Egypt; Kenya; Lesotho; Rwanda; Senegal; South Africa; Zaire (DemRepCongo)

Mission: AIMM sends committed Christians to live, learn, and serve among the peoples of Africa. We seek to have a servant's heart while recognizing our responsibilities to be stewards of the Gospel. Medical personnel are requested to work in rural hospitals, encourage a Public Health Care program and train practical nurses. A certificate in Tropical Medicine is required.

Placement opportunities for . . .		Organization/Service Specifics:	
People of only certain faiths? *1*	Yes	Size of the Organization's Staff:	0-5
Couples: both are health providers?	Yes	Number of providers sent or received/year:	1-5
Couples: only one is a health provider?		Minimum term of assignment:	0
Families with children?	Yes	Maximum term of assignment:	3 years
Medical students?	No	Is funding available for travel?	No
Pre-medical or college students?	No	Are room and board provided? *2*	varies
Other health professional students?	No	Is any other funding available?	No
Doctors in training?	No	Is training provided or available?	No
Health personnel who are US citizens?	Yes	Is a language other than English required? *3*	Yes
Health personnel who are non-US citizens?	Yes		
Health personnel with no prior experience in developing countries?	No		
Health personnel who are not current members of your organization?	No		

Health Professionals Placed:

Physicians:

Physicians

Allied Health Professionals:

Nurses

Notes

1. We are a Mennonite organization; *2.* Would need to negotiate room and board; *3.* French.

Africare

Continents Served	
Africa ✔ Asia ☐ Europe ☐ The Americas ☐	

Countries Served

Angola	Benin	Central African Rep.
Chad	Egypt	Ethiopia
Ghana	Guinea	Guinea-Bissau
Kenya	Liberia	Malawi
Mali	Mozambique	Niger
Senegal	Sierra Leone	South Africa
Tanzania	Uganda	Zambia
Zimbabwe		

Address: **Africare House, 440 R Street, NW, Washington, DC 20001-1935 U.S.A.**

Phone: **(202) 462-3614** FAX: **(202) 387-1034**

E-Mail: **africare@africare.org** Web: **www.africare.org**

Mission: Quite simply, Africare helps Africa. Over the course of its 30 years in existence, Africare has become a leader among private, charitable US organizations assisting Africa. Africare's self-help programs assist Africans in broad areas including food, water, the environment, health, private-sector development, governance and emergency humanitarian aid, with a special focus on the growing African AIDS crisis. Volunteers can serve for 2-3 year terms. French or Portuguese may be required depending on the place of service.

Placement opportunities for . . .		Organization/Service Specifics:	
People of only certain faiths?	No	Size of the Organization's Staff:	51-100
Couples: both are health providers?	Yes	Number of providers sent or received/year:	6-10
Couples: only one is a health provider?	Yes	Minimum term of assignment:	2 years
Families with children?	Yes	Maximum term of assignment:	3 years
Medical students?	Yes	Is funding available for travel?	Yes
Pre-medical or college students?	No	Are room and board provided?	Yes
Other health professional students?	Yes	Is any other funding available?	Yes
Doctors in training?	No	Is training provided or available?	No
Health personnel who are US citizens?	Yes	Is a language other than English required? *1*	Yes
Health personnel who are non-US citizens?	Yes		
Health personnel with no prior experience in developing countries?	No		
Health personnel who are not current members of your organization?	No		

Health Professionals Placed:

Physicians:

Allied Health Professionals:

Administrative Health Positions; Nutritionists & Dieticians; Paramedics; Public Health Specialists, Epidemiologists and Health Educators; Social Workers; Water/Sanitation Specialists

Notes

1. French or Portuguese may be required depending on the place of service.

Aid for International Medicine

Continents Served	
Africa ✔ Asia ✔ Europe ✔ The Americas ✔	

Countries Served

Afghanistan	Bhutan	China
Ethiopia	Nepal	South Africa
St. Lucia	Thailand	Vietnam

Address: **PO Box 119, Rockland, DE 19732 U.S.A.**

Phone: **(302) 655-8290** FAX: **(302) 655-0487**

E-Mail: Web:

Mission: Aid for International Medicine (AIM) is an independent, non-profit, privately funded philanthropic organization that was founded in 1965 for the purpose of advancing medical aid and medical education throughout the world where members of the board have personally served and documented the need. Volunteers must fund themselves for a minimum of 1 week service trips, although often longer. Through the years, AIM has developed training programs, provided direct clinical care, shipped over $8 million in medical supplies, and served as a liaison between local health providers and US funders. Founder and president Dr John Levinson has over 40 years of experience and AIM still provides services worldwide.

(continued)

Placement opportunities for . . .		Organization/Service Specifics:		
People of only certain faiths?	No	Size of the Organization's Staff:		0-5
Couples: both are health providers?	Yes	Number of providers sent or received/year:	*2*	1-5
Couples: only one is a health provider?	Yes	Minimum term of assignment:		1 week
Families with children?	No	Maximum term of assignment:		none
Medical students?	No	Is funding available for travel?		No
Pre-medical or college students?	No	Are room and board provided?		No
Other health professional students?	Yes	Is any other funding available?	*1*	No
Doctors in training?	No	Is training provided or available?		No
Health personnel who are US citizens?	Yes	Is a language other than English required?		No
Health personnel who are non-US citizens?		Yes		
Health personnel with no prior experience in developing countries?		Yes		
Health personnel who are not current members of your organization?		Yes		

Health Professionals Placed:

Physicians:

Physicians; Anesthesiologists; Cardiologists; Emergency Medicine Physicians; Family Practitioners; General Surgeons; Infectious Disease Spec.; Internal Medicine GPS & PCP; OB/GYN; Orthopedic Surgeons; Plastic/Hand/Reconstructive Surgeons

Allied Health Professionals:

Nurse Practitioners; Nurses; Physician Assistants

Notes

1. All volunteers must provide their own funding. *2.* Health professionals needed not completed by NGO, best estimates provided.

Ak' Tenamit

Continents Served

Africa ☐ Asia ☐ Europe ☐ The Americas ☑

Countries Served

Guatemala

Address: **Apartado postal # 2675. Zona 1 Ciudad de Guatemala, Guatemala, C.A.**

Phone: **(502) 254-1560** FAX: **(502) 254-3346**

E-Mail: **info@aktenamit.org** Web: **http://aktenamit.org/main.htm**

Mission: While respecting Mayan culture and tradition, international volunteers and Kek'chi/Guatemalan staff of the Guatemalan Tomorrow Fund work together to develop and implement grass-roots programs in health, education, and income-generation in over 40 isolated villages. Programs include a 24-hour clinic, vaccination campaigns, women's health programs, and preventative health education, among others. There are no religious requirements. While Spanish is not required for volunteers, it is helpful.

Placement opportunities for . . .		Organization/Service Specifics:		
People of only certain faiths?	No	Size of the Organization's Staff:		21-50
Couples: both are health providers?	Yes	Number of providers sent or received/year:		21-50
Couples: only one is a health provider?	Yes	Minimum term of assignment:		4 weeks
Families with children?	No	Maximum term of assignment:		
Medical students? *1*	Yes	Is funding available for travel?		No
Pre-medical or college students?	No	Are room and board provided?		Yes
Other health professional students?	Yes	Is any other funding available?		No
Doctors in training?	Yes	Is training provided or available?		No
Health personnel who are US citizens?	Yes	Is a language other than English required?	*2*	No
Health personnel who are non-US citizens?		Yes		
Health personnel with no prior experience in developing countries?		Yes		
Health personnel who are not current members of your organization?		Yes		

Health Professionals Placed:

Physicians:

Physicians; Emergency Medicine Physicians; Family Practitioners; Gastroenterologists; Infectious Disease Spec.; Internal Medicine GPS & PCP; OB/GYN; Oral Surgeons; Pediatricians

Allied Health Professionals:

Dental Hygienists; Dentists; Nurse Midwives; Nurse Practitioners; Nurses; Paramedics

Notes

1. 3rd and 4th year medical students only; *2.* Spanish is helpful.

Albert Schweitzer Fellowship

Continents Served
Africa ☑ Asia ☐ Europe ☐ The Americas ☐

Countries Served
Gabon

Address: **330 Brookline Avenue, Boston, MA 02215 U.S.A.**
Phone: **(617) 667-5111** FAX: **(617) 667-7989**
E-Mail: **info@schweitzerfellowship.org** Web: **www.schweitzerfellowship.org/**

Mission: Each year since 1978, the Albert Schweitzer Fellowship has selected over 90 US medical students to spend three months working as Fellows at the Albert Schweitzer Hospital in Lambarene, Gabon. The mission of the Albert Schweitzer Fellowship is to develop Leaders in Service: individuals who are dedicated and skilled in addressing the health needs of underserved communities, and whose example influences and inspires others. We achieve this through an interdisciplinary, service-learning model for fostering moral and professional development. This model combines mentored, entrepreneurial, community-based service projects; a curriculum that emphasizes values and leadership; structured opportunities for individual and group reflection; lifelong fellowship with service-oriented colleagues

Placement opportunities for . . .		Organization/Service Specifics:	
People of only certain faiths?	No	Size of the Organization's Staff:	0-5
Couples: both are health providers?	No	Number of providers sent or received/year:	1-5
Couples: only one is a health provider?	No	Minimum term of assignment:	3 months
Families with children?	No	Maximum term of assignment:	3 months
Medical students?	Yes	Is funding available for travel?	Yes
Pre-medical or college students?	No	Are room and board provided?	Yes
Other health professional students?	No	Is any other funding available?	Yes
Doctors in training?	No	Is training provided or available?	Yes
Health personnel who are US citizens?	Yes	Is a language other than English required? *1*	Yes

Health personnel who are non-US citizens?	Yes
Health personnel with no prior experience in developing countries?	Yes
Health personnel who are not current members of your organization?	Yes

Health Professionals Placed:

Physicians:

Allied Health Professionals:

Notes

1. French.

Aloha Medical Missions (AMM)

Continents Served
Africa ☐ Asia ☑ Europe ☐ The Americas ☑

Countries Served

Bangladesh	Cambodia	China
Laos	Nepal	Philippines
United States	Vanuatu	Vietnam

Address: **1314 South King St., Suite 503, Honolulu, HI 96814 U.S.A.**
Phone: **(808) 593-9696** FAX: **(808) 591-1266**
E-Mail: **info@alohamm.org; alohamm@lava.net** Web: **www.alohamm.org**

Mission: Aloha Medical Mission provides medical care to the poor in Asia. All specialties are welcome, although there is a particular need for ophthalmologists, plastic surgeons, and anesthesiologists. A large number of the physicians who volunteer with AMM are either Filipino-American or residents of Hawaii. Two week trips must be funded by the volunteer. There are no language or religious requirements.

Placement opportunities for . . .		Organization/Service Specifics:	
People of only certain faiths?	No	Size of the Organization's Staff:	0-5
Couples: both are health providers?	Yes	Number of providers sent or received/year:	101-150
Couples: only one is a health provider?	Yes	Minimum term of assignment:	2 weeks
Families with children?	No	Maximum term of assignment:	2 weeks
Medical students?	Yes	Is funding available for travel?	No
Pre-medical or college students?	Yes	Are room and board provided?	No
Other health professional students?	Yes	Is any other funding available?	No
Doctors in training?	Yes	Is training provided or available?	No
Health personnel who are US citizens?	Yes	Is a language other than English required?	No

Health personnel who are non-US citizens?	Yes
Health personnel with no prior experience in developing countries?	Yes
Health personnel who are not current members of your organization?	Yes

(continued)

Health Professionals Placed:

Physicians:

Physicians; Anesthesiologists; Cardiologists; Dermatologists; Emergency Medicine Physicians; Endocrinologists; Family Practitioners; Gastroenterologists; General Surgeons; Hematologists; Oncologists; Infectious Disease Spec.; Internal Medicine GPS & PCP; Nephrologists; OB/GYN; Ophthalmologists; Oral Surgeons; Orthopedic Surgeons; Otolaryngologists; Pathologists; Pediatricians; Plastic/Hand/Reconstructive Surgeons; Psychiatrists; Pulmonary Specialists; Urologists

Allied Health Professionals:

Administrative Health Positions; Dentists; Nurse Practitioners; Nurses; Nutritionists & Dieticians; Paramedics; Pharmacists; Physical & Occupational Therapists; Physician Assistants; Podiatrists; Respiratory Therapists

Notes

Amazon-Africa Aid and Fundacao Esperanca

Address: **PO Box 7776, Ann Arbor, MI 48103 U.S.A.**

Phone: **(734) 769-5778** FAX: **(734) 769-5779**

E-Mail: **info@amazonafrica.org** Web: **www.amazonafrica.org/volunteer.html**

Continents Served

Africa ☐ Asia ☐ Europe ☐ The Americas ☑

Countries Served

Brazil

Mission: Amazon-Africa Aid supports the Fundação Esperança, a Brazilian nonprofit organization that has been providing health and education to the inhabitants of the Amazon for over 30 years. Every year, volunteer physicians and dentists from around the world join with local doctors and dentists to provide quality care to the needy in the region. We rely heavily on volunteer and donor support.

Placement opportunities for . . .	
People of only certain faiths?	No
Couples: both are health providers?	Yes
Couples: only one is a health provider?	Yes
Families with children?	No
Medical students?	No
Pre-medical or college students?	No
Other health professional students?	No
Doctors in training?	No
Health personnel who are US citizens?	Yes
Health personnel who are non-US citizens?	Yes
Health personnel with no prior experience in developing countries?	Yes
Health personnel who are not current members of your organization?	Yes

Organization/Service Specifics:		
Size of the Organization's Staff:		6-10
Number of providers sent or received/year:		21-50
Minimum term of assignment:		3 weeks
Maximum term of assignment:		2 months
Is funding available for travel?		No
Are room and board provided?		Yes
Is any other funding available?		No
Is training provided or available?		Yes
Is a language other than English required?	*1*	No

Health Professionals Placed:

Physicians:

Physicians; Dermatologists; Family Practitioners; General Surgeons; Internal Medicine GPS & PCP; OB/GYN; Ophthalmologists; Pediatricians

Allied Health Professionals:

Dentists

Notes

1. Spanish or Portuguese helpful for Brazil program.

Amazon-Africa Aid Organization (3AO)

Address: **PO Box 7776, Ann Arbor, MI 48103 U.S.A.**

Phone: **(734) 769-5778** FAX: **(734) 769-5779**

E-Mail: **info@amazonafrica.org** Web: **www.amazonafrica.org**

Continents Served

Africa ☐ Asia ☑ Europe ☐ The Americas ☑

Countries Served

Brazil

Mission: The Amazon-Africa Aid Organization (3AO) is dedicated to improving the human condition by providing technical and financial aid to impoverished regions around the world. The Amazon African Aid Organization supports a health clinic run by the Funadação Esperança. The health clinic depends on volunteer dentists and physicians to provide care for the needy people of the Amazon. Volunteers can serve for 3-week to 3-month assignments. Room and board is provided. The programs in Africa are currently being re-examined.

(continued)

Placement opportunities for . . .		**Organization/Service Specifics:**	
People of only certain faiths?	No	Size of the Organization's Staff:	0-5
Couples: both are health providers?	Yes	Number of providers sent or received/year:	21-50
Couples: only one is a health provider?	Yes	Minimum term of assignment:	3 weeks
Families with children?	No	Maximum term of assignment:	3 months
Medical students?	No	Is funding available for travel?	No
Pre-medical or college students?	No	Are room and board provided?	Yes
Other health professional students?	Yes	Is any other funding available?	No
Doctors in training?	Yes	Is training provided or available?	No
Health personnel who are US citizens?	Yes	Is a language other than English required?	No
Health personnel who are non-US citizens?	Yes		
Health personnel with no prior experience in developing countries?	Yes		
Health personnel who are not current members of your organization?	Yes		

Health Professionals Placed:

Notes

Physicians:

Physicians; Anesthesiologists; Cardiologists; Dermatologists; Family Practitioners; Gastroenterologists; General Surgeons; Hematologists; Oncologists; Infectious Disease Spec.; Internal Medicine GPS & PCP; OB/GYN; Ophthalmologists; Oral Surgeons; Orthopedic Surgeons; Pediatricians; Plastic/Hand/Reconstructive Surgeons; Urologists

Allied Health Professionals:

Dentists; Physical & Occupational Therapists

American Baptist Board of International Ministries

Address: **P.O. Box 851, Valley Forge, PA 19482 U.S.A.**

Phone: **(610) 768-2164**
(800) 222-3872

FAX: **(610) 768-2088**
(610) 768-2115

E-Mail: **bimvolunteers@abc-usa.org**

Web: **www.internationalministries.org/**

Continents Served

Africa ✔ Asia ✔ Europe ✔ The Americas ✔

Countries Served

Dominican Republic, Haiti, India, Nepal, Nicaragua, Rwanda, Thailand, United States

Mission: The mission of International Ministries is to glorify God in all the earth by crossing cultural boundaries to make disciples of Jesus Christ. We need people called upon to spread the word of Christ around the world. We have volunteer opportunities in missions for both teams and individuals available through International Ministries. We receive requests from our partners and missionaries throughout the world for volunteers to assist in their ministry and have numerous health care possibilities, specifically in Africa, Asia, Europe, and Latin America.

Placement opportunities for . . .		**Organization/Service Specifics:**	
People of only certain faiths? *1*	Yes	Size of the Organization's Staff:	>200
Couples: both are health providers? *2*	No	Number of providers sent or received/year:	51-100
Couples: only one is a health provider? *2*	No	Minimum term of assignment:	2 weeks
Families with children? *2*	No	Maximum term of assignment: *5*	none
Medical students?	No	Is funding available for travel? *3*	varies
Pre-medical or college students?	No	Are room and board provided? *3*	varies
Other health professional students?	Yes	Is any other funding available?	No
Doctors in training?	No	Is training provided or available?	No
Health personnel who are US citizens?	Yes	Is a language other than English required? *4*	No
Health personnel who are non-US citizens?	No		
Health personnel with no prior experience in developing countries?	Yes		
Health personnel who are not current members of your organization?	Yes		

Health Professionals Placed: *6*

Physicians:

Physicians; Anesthesiologists; Cardiologists; Emergency Medicine Physicians; Pediatricians; Radiologists

Allied Health Professionals:

Nurses; Physician Assistants

Notes

1. Baptist; *2.* Possibly. Some positions in conjunction with other orgs; *3.* Varies depending on position; *4.* Sometimes; *5.* Usually 3 months; *6.* Many other specialties depending on needs.

American College of Nurse-Midwives

Address: **8403 Colesville Rd, #1550, Silver Spring, MD 20910 U.S.A.**

Phone: **(240) 485-1830** FAX: **(240) 485-1818**

E-Mail: **info@acnm.org** Web: **www.midwife.org**

Mission: The mission of the American College of Nurse-Midwives Department of Global Outreach is to improve the lives of women and their families by expanding the ability of health care providers to offer effective, appropriate care through policy development, institutional strengthening, services education, and research. Paid consultants can serve from 2 weeks to three years. Opportunities to volunteer are available with preference given to nurse-midwives. French or Spanish is required for volunteers serving in some countries.

Continents Served

Africa ✔ Asia ✔ Europe ✔ The Americas ✔

Countries Served

Belize	Benin	Bolivia
Botswana	Burkina Faso	Burundi
Cambodia	Cape Verde	
Central African Rep.		El Salvador
Ethiopia	Gabon	Gambia
Ghana	Guatemala	Guinea
Haiti	Honduras	India
Indonesia	Ivory Coast	Kenya
Lesotho	Liberia	Malawi
Malaysia	Mali	Mauritania
Mexico	Morocco	
Mozambique	Nepal	Nicaragua
Nigeria	Peru	Philippines
Romania	Rwanda	Sierra Leone
Somalia	South Africa	Swaziland
Switzerland	Tanzania	Uganda
Vietnam	Zaire (DemRepCongo)	
Zambia	Zimbabwe	

Placement opportunities for . . .

People of only certain faiths?	No
Couples: both are health providers?	No
Couples: only one is a health provider?	No
Families with children?	No
Medical students?	No
Pre-medical or college students?	No
Other health professional students?	Yes
Doctors in training?	No
Health personnel who are US citizens?	Yes
Health personnel who are non-US citizens?	Yes
Health personnel with no prior experience in developing countries?	No
Health personnel who are not current members of your organization?	Yes

Organization/Service Specifics:

Size of the Organization's Staff:	6-10
Number of providers sent or received/year:	6-10
Minimum term of assignment:	2 weeks
Maximum term of assignment:	3 years
Is funding available for travel?	Yes
Are room and board provided?	Yes
Is any other funding available? *1*	Yes
Is training provided or available?	No
Is a language other than English required? *2*	Yes

Health Professionals Placed:

Physicians:

OB/GYN

Allied Health Professionals:

Nurse-Midwives; Nurse Practitioners; Nurses; Public Health Specialists, Epidemiologists and Health Educators

Notes

1. Projects are mostly funded by USAID, WHO, UNICEF, The World Bank, and other donor agencies; *2.* French or Spanish may be required for some assignments.

American Jewish World Service

Address: **45 West 36th St., 10th Floor, New York, NY 10018-7904 U.S.A.**

Phone: **(800) 889-7146** FAX: **(212) 736-3463**

E-Mail: **ajws@ajws.org** Web: **www.ajws.org**

Mission: AJWS is an independent non-profit organization founded in 1985 to alleviate poverty, hunger, and disease among the people of the world. AJWS provides humanitarian aid, technical support, emergency relief, and skilled volunteers to grassroots project partners. While AJWS does provide direct health services, they generally emphasize training local health workers and professionals and working on public health projects. AJWS has a summer volunteer program called the International Jewish College Corps. They encourage people in and just out of college to apply to this program.

Continents Served

Africa ✔ Asia ✔ Europe ✔ The Americas ✔

Countries Served

Afghanistan	Argentina	Belize
Benin	Brazil	Cambodia
Chile	Dominican Republic	
Ecuador	El Salvador	Ethiopia
Gambia	Ghana	Guatemala
Haiti	Honduras	India
Israel	Kenya	Malawi
Mali	Mexico	Namibia
Nepal	Nicaragua	Nigeria
Peru	Philippines	Senegal
South Africa	Thailand	Togo
Uganda	USSR, former	Venezuela
Vietnam	Yugoslavia, former	
Zambia	Zimbabwe	

(continued)

Placement opportunities for . . .		**Organization/Service Specifics:**	
People of only certain faiths? *1*	Yes	Size of the Organization's Staff:	6-10
Couples: both are health providers?	Yes	Number of providers sent or received/year:	6-10
Couples: only one is a health provider?	Yes	Minimum term of assignment:	1 month
Families with children?	No	Maximum term of assignment:	1 year
Medical students?	Yes	Is funding available for travel?	Yes
Pre-medical or college students?	No	Are room and board provided?	No
Other health professional students?	Yes	Is any other funding available?	Yes
Doctors in training?	Yes	Is training provided or available?	No
Health personnel who are US citizens?	Yes	Is a language other than English required? *2*	No
Health personnel who are non-US citizens?	Yes		
Health personnel with no prior experience in developing countries?	Yes		
Health personnel who are not current members of your organization?	Yes		

Health Professionals Placed:

Physicians:

Physicians; Cardiologists; Emergency Medicine Physicians; Family Practitioners; Infectious Disease Spec.; Internal Medicine GPS & PCP; OB/GYN; Ophthalmologists; Pediatricians; Psychiatrists

Allied Health Professionals:

Administrative Health Positions; Nurse Midwives; Nurse Practitioners; Nurses; Nutritionists & Dieticians; Physician Assistants; Public Health Specialists, Epidemiologists and Health Educators; Water/Sanitation Specialists

Notes

1. Volunteers must be Jewish;
2. Language requirements may depend on the assignment.

American Leprosy Missions Inc.

Address: **1 ALM Way, Greenville, SC 29601 U.S.A.**
Phone: **(800) 543-3135** FAX: **(864) 271-7062**
E-Mail: **amlep@leprosy.org** Web: **www.leprosy.org**

Mission: Working with its sister organization, Leprosy Mission International, American Leprosy Missions is a non-denominational Christian ministry providing care to people in 20 countries in Africa and Asia with leprosy and related disabilities. Case-finding, diagnosis, community development, and physical and vocational rehabilitation are among the chief goals of the organization's outreach projects. Leprosy Mission International and American Leprosy Missions seek Christian nurses, physicians, public health/development workers, physiotherapists, occupational therapists, and podiatrists for short to long term (3 months to lifetime) stays, providing training and transportation for participants.

Continents Served

Africa ☑ Asia ☑ Europe ☐ The Americas ☐

Countries Served

Bangladesh	Bhutan	Chad
Congo	Ethiopia	Guinea
India	Indonesia	Laos
Mozambique	Nepal	Niger
Nigeria	Papua-New Guinea	Sudan
Thailand	Uganda	

Placement opportunities for . . .		**Organization/Service Specifics:**	
People of only certain faiths? *1*	Yes	Size of the Organization's Staff:	>200
Couples: both are health providers?	Yes	Number of providers sent or received/year:	>200
Couples: only one is a health provider?	Yes	Minimum term of assignment:	3 Months
Families with children?	Yes	Maximum term of assignment:	life
Medical students?	Yes	Is funding available for travel?	Yes
Pre-medical or college students?	Yes	Are room and board provided?	Yes
Other health professional students?	No	Is any other funding available? *2*	Yes
Doctors in training?	No	Is training provided or available?	Yes
Health personnel who are US citizens?	Yes	Is a language other than English required? *3*	Yes
Health personnel who are non-US citizens?	Yes		
Health personnel with no prior experience in developing countries?	Yes		
Health personnel who are not current members of your organization?	Yes		

Health Professionals Placed:

Physicians:

Physicians; Dermatologists; General Surgeons; Ophthalmologists

Allied Health Professionals:

Nurses; Physical & Occupational Therapists; Podiatrists; Public Health Specialists; Epidemiologists and Health Educators

Notes

1. Volunteers must be Christian;
2. Funding is sometimes available;
3. Language requirements depend on the project.

American Physicians Fellowship for Medicine in Israel

Continents Served

Africa ☐ Asia ☑ Europe ☐ The Americas ☐

Countries Served

Israel

Address: **2001 Beacon Street, Suite 210, Boston, MA 02135 U.S.A.**

Phone: **(617) 232-5382** FAX: **(617) 739-2616**

E-Mail: **apl@apfmed.org** Web: **www.apfmed.org**

Mission: The key purpose of Medical Volunteers On-Call for Israel (an American Physicians Fellowship [APF] program) is to provide medical assistance to Israelis during crises as well as during peacetime. APF was organized to staff Israeli hospitals with American physicians when their Israeli counterparts performed required military duty. APF remains the only organization designated by the State of Israel to maintain such a volunteer registry. MVI provides on-call training with four courses offered each year in Israel. The courses are offered in association with the Ministry of Health and Israeli Defense Forces Medical Branch and volunteers may attend meetings with senior officials from those agencies. After training the participants become eligible to serve in Israeli hospitals. Participants will also meet with fellow doctors at the hospitals and receive briefings on psychological preparedness and receive protocols on providing treatment while dealing with stress/terror.

Placement opportunities for . . .	
People of only certain faiths?	No
Couples: both are health providers?	Yes
Couples: only one is a health provider?	No
Families with children?	No
Medical students? *2*	Yes
Pre-medical or college students?	No
Other health professional students?	No
Doctors in training?	Yes
Health personnel who are US citizens?	Yes
Health personnel who are non-US citizens?	Yes
Health personnel with no prior experience in developing countries?	Yes
Health personnel who are not current members of your organization?	Yes

Organization/Service Specifics:	
Size of the Organization's Staff:	0-5
Number of providers sent or received/year: *1*	
Minimum term of assignment: *3*	
Maximum term of assignment: *3*	
Is funding available for travel?	Yes
Are room and board provided?	Yes
Is any other funding available?	
Is training provided or available?	Yes
Is a language other than English required?	No

Health Professionals Placed: *3*

Physicians:

Allied Health Professionals:

Notes

1. Medical personnel listed in the APF database will be contacted to respond to medical emergencies after a request by the Israeli Ministry of Health; *2.* 3rd or 4th years depending on need; *3.* Depends on need, please contact APF for more info.

American Refugee Committee

Continents Served

Africa ☑ Asia ☑ Europe ☑ The Americas ☐

Countries Served

Bosnia and Herzegovina, Guinea, Kosovo, Liberia, Macedonia, Pakistan, Rwanda, Serbia and Montenegro, Sierra Leone, Sudan, Thailand, Uganda, Yugoslavia, former

Address: **430 Oak Grove Street, Suite 204, Minneapolis, MN 55403 U.S.A.**

Phone: **(612) 872-7060** FAX: **(612) 607-6499**

E-Mail: **archq@archq.org** Web: **www.archq.org**

Mission: The American Refugee Committee (ARC) provides multisectoral assistance to hundreds of thousands of uprooted people in Africa, Asia and Europe with programs providing assistance in primary health care delivery (including reproductive health services), improved water and sanitation, shelter reconstruction, micro-credit schemes, environmental rehabilitation and psychosocial services. ARC works with local communities and their leaders to build their capacity to care for themselves.

(continued)

Placement opportunities for . . .		Organization/Service Specifics:	
People of only certain faiths?	No	Size of the Organization's Staff:	>200
Couples: both are health providers?	Yes	Number of providers sent or received/year:	21-50
Couples: only one is a health provider? *1*	Yes	Minimum term of assignment:	1 year
Families with children?	No	Maximum term of assignment: *5*	
Medical students?	No	Is funding available for travel?	Yes
Pre-medical or college students?	No	Are room and board provided? *2*	Yes
Other health professional students?	Yes	Is any other funding available? *3*	Yes
Doctors in training?	No	Is training provided or available?	Yes
Health personnel who are US citizens?	Yes	Is a language other than English required? *4*	Yes
Health personnel who are non-US citizens?	Yes		
Health personnel with no prior experience in developing countries?	No		
Health personnel who are not current members of your organization?	Yes		

Health Professionals Placed:

Physicians:

Physicians; Emergency Medicine Physicians; Family Practitioners; Infectious Disease Spec.; Internal Medicine GPS & PCP; OB/GYN; Pediatricians; Psychiatrists

Allied Health Professionals:

Administrative Health Positions; Medical Technicians (lab, X-ray, etc); Nurse Midwives; Nurse Practitioners; Nurses; Physician Assistants; Public Health Specialists, Epidemiologists and Health Educators; Water/Sanitation Specialists

Notes

1. Sometimes available; *2.* Room only; *3.* Medical insurance and monthly stipend; *4.* French may be required for some, but not all, assignments; *5.* Usually 1 year assignments with renewable contracts.

Amigos de las Americas

Address: **5618 Star Lane, Houston, TX 77057 U.S.A.**

Phone: **(800) 231-7796** FAX: **(713) 782-9267**

E-Mail: **info@amigoslink.org** Web: **www.amigoslink.org/**

Continents Served

Africa ☐ Asia ☐ Europe ☐ The Americas ☑

Countries Served

Costa Rica, Dominican Republic, Honduras, Mexico, Nicaragua, Panama, Paraguay

Mission: Amigos de las Américas (AMIGOS) creates opportunities for young people to excel in leadership roles promoting public health, education and community development. Founded in 1965, AMIGOS is a non-profit organization that provides exceptional leadership training and volunteer service opportunities in the United States and Latin America. AMIGOS' youth-led programs and strong partnerships with international development, non-profit, and government agencies distinguishes it from other international experiences.

Placement opportunities for . . .		Organization/Service Specifics:	
People of only certain faiths?	No	Size of the Organization's Staff:	11-20
Couples: both are health providers?	No	Number of providers sent or received/year:	>200
Couples: only one is a health provider?	No	Minimum term of assignment:	4 weeks
Families with children?	No	Maximum term of assignment:	8 weeks
Medical students?	No	Is funding available for travel? *1*	Yes
Pre-medical or college students?	Yes	Are room and board provided?	Yes
Other health professional students?	Yes	Is any other funding available?	No
Doctors in training?	No	Is training provided or available?	Yes
Health personnel who are US citizens?	No	Is a language other than English required? *2*	Yes
Health personnel who are non-US citizens?	No		
Health personnel with no prior experience in developing countries?	No		
Health personnel who are not current members of your organization?	No		

Health Professionals Placed:

Physicians:

Allied Health Professionals:

Notes

1. All expenses except for domestic transportation are included in the program fee; *2.* Some Spanish.

Anderson University School of Nursing

Address: **1100 E. 5th Street, Anderson, IN 46012 U.S.A.**

Phone: **(765) 641-4390** FAX: **(765) 641-3095**

E-Mail: **akoepke@anderson.edu** Web: **www.anderson.edu**

Continents Served

Africa ☐ Asia ☑ Europe ☐ The Americas ☑

Countries Served

Belize, Honduras, India, Korea, South, United States, USSR, former

Mission: Anderson University is a Christian program committed to providing a variety of clinical experiences in varied settings including churches. The emphasis is on inter-cultural nursing care, including a three week senior experience in another culture. Funding and training is provided. There are no language restrictions.

Placement opportunities for . . .		Organization/Service Specifics:	
People of only certain faiths?	No	Size of the Organization's Staff:	11-20
Couples: both are health providers?	No	Number of providers sent or received/year:	21-50
Couples: only one is a health provider?	No	Minimum term of assignment:	
Families with children?	No	Maximum term of assignment:	
Medical students?	No	Is funding available for travel?	Yes
Pre-medical or college students?	No	Are room and board provided?	No
Other health professional students?	Yes	Is any other funding available?	No
Doctors in training?	No	Is training provided or available?	Yes
Health personnel who are US citizens?	Yes	Is a language other than English required?	No
Health personnel who are non-US citizens?	Yes		
Health personnel with no prior experience in developing countries?	Yes		
Health personnel who are not current members of your organization?	No		

Health Professionals Placed:

Physicians:

Allied Health Professionals:

Nurse Practitioners; Nurses

Notes

Ann Foundation Inc

Address: **20 Old Shelter Rock Road, Roslyn, NY 11576 U.S.A.**

Phone: **(516) 570-0088** FAX: **(516) 570-0088**

E-Mail: **ann@annfoundation.org** Web: **www.annfoundation.org**

Continents Served

Africa ☑ Asia ☑ Europe ☐ The Americas ☑

Countries Served

Haiti, India, Uganda

Mission: The Ann Foundation is a nonprofit nonsectarian organization dedicated to providing healthcare, educational, and other humanitarian aid to children in need worldwide. It is concerned with the welfare of children who suffer from a range of physical and other disabilities with a focus on less developed countries. Volunteer medical care providers are needed to share their skills and knowledge.

Placement opportunities for . . .		Organization/Service Specifics:	
People of only certain faiths?	No	Size of the Organization's Staff:	0-5
Couples: both are health providers? *1*	Yes	Number of providers sent or received/year:	11-20
Couples: only one is a health provider? *1*	Yes	Minimum term of assignment:	8 days
Families with children?	No	Maximum term of assignment: *1*	variable
Medical students?	Yes	Is funding available for travel?	No
Pre-medical or college students?	Yes	Are room and board provided?	No
Other health professional students?	Yes	Is any other funding available?	No
Doctors in training?	No	Is training provided or available?	Yes
Health personnel who are US citizens?	Yes	Is a language other than English required?	No
Health personnel who are non-US citizens?	Yes		
Health personnel with no prior experience in developing countries?	Yes		
Health personnel who are not current members of your organization?	Yes		

(continued)

Health Professionals Placed: *1*

Physicians:

Allied Health Professionals:

Notes

1. Contact Ann Moideen for details on how you might be able to contribute to current and upcoming missions.

APUSAN-USA

Continents Served

Africa ☐ Asia ☐ Europe ☐ The Americas ☑

Countries Served

Nicaragua

Address: **International Studies & Programs, University of Nebraska Medical Center, Omaha, NE 68198-5735 U.S.A.**

Phone: **(402) 559-2924** FAX: **(402) 559-2923**

E-Mail: **sepirtle@unmc.edu** Web: **www.unmc.edu/isp**

Mission: In September 1994, a new medical clinic opened its doors in a poverty ridden neighborhood in Managua, Nicaragua. Aptly named "Los Chavalitos" ("street kids"), the clinic's focus is on pediatric, family panning and pre-natal care. Students in the health professions are invited to participate in an international health elective with Los Chavalitos clinic. Due to the public health emphasis on the clinic, non-clinical, as well as clinical electives are available. A minimum stay of four weeks is recommended.

Placement opportunities for . . .

People of only certain faiths?	No
Couples: both are health providers?	Yes
Couples: only one is a health provider?	Yes
Families with children?	No
Medical students?	Yes
Pre-medical or college students?	Yes
Other health professional students?	Yes
Doctors in training?	Yes
Health personnel who are US citizens?	Yes
Health personnel who are non-US citizens?	Yes
Health personnel with no prior experience in developing countries?	Yes
Health personnel who are not current members of your organization?	Yes

Organization/Service Specifics:

Size of the Organization's Staff:	6-10
Number of providers sent or received/year:	1-5
Minimum term of assignment:	4 weeks
Maximum term of assignment:	6 month
Is funding available for travel?	No
Are room and board provided?	No
Is any other funding available?	No
Is training provided or available?	Yes
Is a language other than English required? *1*	Yes

Health Professionals Placed:

Physicians:

Physicians; Internal Medicine GPS & PCP; OB/GYN; Orthopedic Surgeons; Pediatricians

Allied Health Professionals:

Nurses; Social Workers

Notes

1. Spanish.

Archdiocesan Health Care Network for Catholic Charities

Continents Served

Africa ☐ Asia ☐ Europe ☐ The Americas ☑

Countries Served

United States

Address: **924 G St., NW, Washington, DC 20001 U.S.A.**

Phone: **(202) 772-4364**
(202) 772-4300 FAX: **(202) 772-4408**

E-Mail: **luxiong@catholic charitiesdc.org** Web: **www.catholic charitiesdc.org**

Mission: Every year in Washington, DC, and surrounding Maryland counties Catholic Charities of the Archdiocese of Washington serves 80,000 men, women, and children through 50 social service programs at 26 community sites. Our programs assist all needy members of our community, regardless of race, religion, or national origin. We have a network of specialty health care providers and always need physicians, nurses, dentists, and other heath care personnel to donate their valuable time to homeless and uninsured patients. *(continued)*

Placement opportunities for . . .

People of only certain faiths?	No
Couples: both are health providers?	Yes
Couples: only one is a health provider?	
Families with children?	
Medical students?	
Pre-medical or college students?	
Other health professional students?	
Doctors in training?	
Health personnel who are US citizens?	
Health personnel who are non-US citizens?	
Health personnel with no prior experience in developing countries?	
Health personnel who are not current members of your organization?	

Organization/Service Specifics:

Size of the Organization's Staff:	>200
Number of providers sent or received/year:	151-200
Minimum term of assignment:	
Maximum term of assignment:	
Is funding available for travel?	
Are room and board provided?	
Is any other funding available?	
Is training provided or available?	No
Is a language other than English required?	No

Health Professionals Placed: *1*

Physicians:

Physicians; Anesthesiologists; Cardiologists; Dermatologists; Emergency Medicine Physicians; Endocrinologists; Family Practitioners; Gastroenterologists; General Surgeons; Hematologists; Oncologists; Infectious Disease Spec.; Internal Medicine GPS & PCP; Nephrologists; Neurologists; Neurosurgeons; OB/GYN; Ophthalmologists; Oral Surgeons; Optometrists; Orthopedic Surgeons; Otolaryngologists; Pathologists; Pediatricians; Plastic/Hand/Reconstructive Surgeons; Psychiatrists; Pulmonary Specialists; Radiologists; Urologists

Allied Health Professionals:

Administrative Health Positions; Dental Hygienists; Dentists; Nurses; Nutritionists & Dieticians; Physical & Occupational Therapists; Podiatrists; Prosthetists; Psychologists

Notes

1. Our health care needs are met by referrals to our volunteer network and encompass all areas.

Armenian EyeCare Project

Continents Served

Africa ☐ Asia ☑ Europe ☐ The Americas ☐

Countries Served

Armenia

Address: **337 East Bayfront Road, Newport Beach, CA 92662 U.S.A.**
or PO Box 4275, Laguna Beach CA 92652

Phone: **(949) 675-5767** FAX: **(949) 673-2356**

E-Mail: **aecpt@eyecareproject.com** Web:

Mission: To make 21st century eye care available and affordable to every Armenian. Volunteers can serve between 10 days and 1 month. Armenian or Russian would be helpful, but neither is required.

Placement opportunities for . . .

People of only certain faiths?	No
Couples: both are health providers?	Yes
Couples: only one is a health provider?	
Families with children?	No
Medical students?	Yes
Pre-medical or college students?	Yes
Other health professional students?	No
Doctors in training?	No
Health personnel who are US citizens?	Yes
Health personnel who are non-US citizens?	Yes
Health personnel with no prior experience in developing countries?	Yes
Health personnel who are not current members of your organization?	Yes

Organization/Service Specifics:

Size of the Organization's Staff:	0-5
Number of providers sent or received/year:	51-100
Minimum term of assignment:	10 Days
Maximum term of assignment:	1 Month
Is funding available for travel?	No
Are room and board provided?	Yes
Is any other funding available?	No
Is training provided or available?	No
Is a language other than English required? *1*	No

Health Professionals Placed:

Physicians:

Ophthalmologists

Allied Health Professionals:

Notes

1. Armenian or Russian would be helpful.

Armenian Social Transition Program

Continents Served			
Africa ☐	Asia ☑	Europe ☐	The Americas ☐

Countries Served
Armenia

Address: **3750 14 Sundukyan Yerevan, Armenia**

Phone: **(374) 127-2785**
(374) 127-3176 FAX: **(374) 127-2743**

E-Mail: **eabrahamyan@padco.am** Web: **www.padco.am**

Mission: The Armenia Social Transition Program (ASTP) is supporting the Government of the Republic of Armenia (GOA) in its efforts to introduce primary health care reforms. Primary health care reforms are a key component of the government plan to reform and improve the health sector. ASTP is sponsored in part by USAID and seeks experienced primary care physicians to train and precept Armenian physicians.

Placement opportunities for . . .		Organization/Service Specifics:	
People of only certain faiths?	No	Size of the Organization's Staff:	51-100
Couples: both are health providers?	No	Number of providers sent or received/year:	11-20
Couples: only one is a health provider?	No	Minimum term of assignment:	1 month
Families with children?	No	Maximum term of assignment:	18 months
Medical students?	No	Is funding available for travel?	Yes
Pre-medical or college students?	No	Are room and board provided?	Yes
Other health professional students?	No	Is any other funding available? *1*	Yes
Doctors in training?	No	Is training provided or available?	No
Health personnel who are US citizens?	Yes	Is a language other than English required? *2*	No
Health personnel who are non-US citizens?	Yes		
Health personnel with no prior experience in developing countries?			
Health personnel who are not current members of your organization?	Yes		

Health Professionals Placed:

Physicians:

Physicians; Emergency Medicine Physicians; Family Practitioners; Infectious Disease Spec.; Internal Medicine GPS & PCP; OB/GYN; Pediatricians

Allied Health Professionals:

Notes

1. $1000/month stipend;
2. Russian or Armenian helpful.

ASAPROSAR: The Salvadoran Association for Rural Health

Continents Served			
Africa ☐	Asia ☐	Europe ☐	The Americas ☑

Countries Served
El Salvador

Address: **210 Whiting Street, Suite 6, Hingham, MA 02043-3729 U.S.A.**

Phone: **(781) 740-1855** FAX: **(781) 383-8117**

E-Mail: **alangruber@aol.com** Web: **www.FriendsOfASAPROSAR.org**

Mission: Provision of eye health services to poor rural inhabitants of El Salvador, in conjunction with Salvadorian Association for Rural Health. Service trips are 2 weeks long. There are no language or religious requirements.

Placement opportunities for . . .		Organization/Service Specifics:	
People of only certain faiths?	No	Size of the Organization's Staff:	0-5
Couples: both are health providers?	Yes	Number of providers sent or received/year:	21-50
Couples: only one is a health provider?	Yes	Minimum term of assignment:	2 weeks
Families with children?	No	Maximum term of assignment:	2 weeks
Medical students?	No	Is funding available for travel?	No
Pre-medical or college students?	No	Are room and board provided?	No
Other health professional students?	No	Is any other funding available?	No
Doctors in training?	No	Is training provided or available?	Yes
Health personnel who are US citizens?	Yes	Is a language other than English required?	No
Health personnel who are non-US citizens?	Yes		
Health personnel with no prior experience in developing countries?	Yes		
Health personnel who are not current members of your organization?	Yes		

(continued)

Health Professionals Placed:

Physicians:

Anesthesiologists; Ophthalmologists; Optometrists

Allied Health Professionals:

Nurses

Notes

Associate Reformed Presbyterian Church, World Witness

Continents Served

Africa ☐ Asia ☑ Europe ☐ The Americas ☐

Countries Served

Pakistan

Address: **1 Cleveland St., Suite 220, Greenville, SC 29601-3696 U.S.A.**

Phone: **(864) 233-5226** FAX: **(864) 233-5326**

E-Mail: **johnH@worldwitness.org** Web: **www.worldwitness.org**

Mission: Christian Hospital, through the support and organization of World Witness, has served the bustling city of Sahiwal, Pakistan, and its surrounding areas for the past 82 years. Each day, through the doors of this medical haven come the blind, sick, and lame, seeking healing in a land where only the most wealthy receive quality health care. Other hospitals exist in the area, but Christian Hospital is the only one where the poor can receive quality, compassionate care. The open admission policy means no one is turned away for the inability to pay. Lengths of service vary from 2 weeks to life. Health care providers must be Christian in order to serve through World Witness.

Placement opportunities for . . .	
People of only certain faiths? *1*	Yes
Couples: both are health providers?	Yes
Couples: only one is a health provider?	Yes
Families with children?	Yes
Medical students?	Yes
Pre-medical or college students?	No
Other health professional students?	Yes
Doctors in training?	Yes
Health personnel who are US citizens?	Yes
Health personnel who are non-US citizens?	Yes
Health personnel with no prior experience in developing countries?	Yes
Health personnel who are not current members of your organization?	Yes

Organization/Service Specifics:	
Size of the Organization's Staff:	0-5
Number of providers sent or received/year:	1-5
Minimum term of assignment:	2 weeks
Maximum term of assignment:	unlimited
Is funding available for travel?	No
Are room and board provided?	No
Is any other funding available?	No
Is training provided or available?	
Is a language other than English required?	No

Health Professionals Placed:

Physicians:

Physicians; Anesthesiologists; General Surgeons; Neurosurgeons; Orthopedic Surgeons; Plastic/Hand/Reconstructive Surgeons; Urologists

Allied Health Professionals:

Notes

1. Providers must be of the Christian faith.

Associazione Italiana 'Amici Raoul Follereau'

Address: **Via Borselli 4-6 Bologna, 40135 Italy**

Phone: **39051433402** FAX: **39051434046**

E-Mail: **info@aifo.it** Web: **www.aifo.it**

Mission: AIFO is an Italian Non-Governmental Development Organisation (NGDO) based in Italy and with the head office in Bologna. AIFO provides support to projects in developing countries, without any discrimination on the basis of color, race, religion, gender, etc. AIFO has no political or religious aims of any kind. The majority of projects supported by AIFO deal with leprosy control at national levels or integrated in to primary and community health care settings. AIFO also provides emergency relief in areas where they are already working with local partners. Volunteers can serve between 3 weeks and 1 year. Portuguese or French may be required for certain countries.

Continents Served

Africa ☑ Asia ☑ Europe ☐ The Americas ☑

Countries Served

Angola	Bangladesh	Brazil
Cape Verde	China	Comoros
Congo	Egypt	Eritrea
Ethiopia	Ghana	Guinea
Guinea-Bissau	Guyana	India
Indonesia	Kenya	Liberia
Mongolia	Mozambique	
Myanmar (Burma)		Nepal
Pakistan	Papua-New Guinea	
Somalia	Sudan	Vietnam
Zaire (DemRepCongo)		Zambia
Zimbabwe		

Placement opportunities for . . .

People of only certain faiths?	No
Couples: both are health providers?	Yes
Couples: only one is a health provider?	Yes
Families with children?	Yes
Medical students?	No
Pre-medical or college students?	No
Other health professional students?	No
Doctors in training?	No
Health personnel who are US citizens?	Yes
Health personnel who are non-US citizens?	Yes
Health personnel with no prior experience in developing countries?	Yes
Health personnel who are not current members of your organization?	Yes

Organization/Service Specifics:

Size of the Organization's Staff:		21-50
Number of providers sent or received/year:		11-20
Minimum term of assignment:		3 weeks
Maximum term of assignment:		1 year
Is funding available for travel?		Yes
Are room and board provided?		Yes
Is any other funding available?	*1*	Yes
Is training provided or available?		Yes
Is a language other than English required?	*2*	Yes

Health Professionals Placed:

Physicians:

Physicians; Dermatologists; Infectious Disease Spec.

Allied Health Professionals:

Physical & Occupational Therapists; Prosthetists

Notes

1. A salary and housing are provided; *2.* Portuguese or French may be required for certain countries.

Bairo Pite Clinic

Address: **P.O. Box 259, Dili, East Timor**

Phone: **(670) 723-4873** FAX:

E-Mail: **volunteer@bairopiteclinic.org.tp** Web: **http://bairopiteclinic.tripod.com/**

Continents Served

Africa ☐ Asia ☑ Europe ☐ The Americas ☐

Countries Served

East Timor

Mission: Primary health care is a top priority for the Bairo Pite Clinic; upwards of 600 patients are seen each day. The clinic also makes mobile visits to the remote and often-neglected mountainous areas, and receives patients from all over the country. Volunteers are needed for all aspects of health care and to possibly help train Timorese medical students.

(continued)

Placement opportunities for . . .	
People of only certain faiths?	No
Couples: both are health providers?	Yes
Couples: only one is a health provider?	No
Families with children?	No
Medical students?	Yes
Pre-medical or college students?	Yes
Other health professional students?	Yes
Doctors in training?	Yes
Health personnel who are US citizens?	Yes
Health personnel who are non-US citizens?	Yes
Health personnel with no prior experience in developing countries?	Yes
Health personnel who are not current members of your organization?	Yes

Organization/Service Specifics:	
Size of the Organization's Staff:	11-20
Number of providers sent or received/year:	6-10
Minimum term of assignment:	4 weeks
Maximum term of assignment:	1 year
Is funding available for travel?	No
Are room and board provided?	No
Is any other funding available?	No
Is training provided or available?	No
Is a language other than English required? *1*	No

Health Professionals Placed:

Physicians:

All physician specialties

Allied Health Professionals:

All allied health professionals

Notes

1. Portuguese or Indonesian desirable.

Baptist General Conference

Address: **202 S. Arlington Heights Rd., Arlington Heights, IL 60005 U.S.A.**

Phone: **(800) 323-4215** FAX: **(847) 228-5376**

E-Mail: **chansen@baptistgeneral.org** Web: **www.bgcworld.org/index.html**

Continents Served

Africa ☑ Asia ☐ Europe ☐ The Americas ☐

Countries Served

Cameroon Ethiopia Ivory Coast

Mission: The Baptist General Conference is a group of churches (currently about 875 of them) that cooperate to help people in the U.S. and other countries hear and understand the good news of Jesus Christ as it is explained in the Bible. The Baptist General Conference needs both short- and long-term workers. Health care workers needed for international missions primarily in the African continent.

Placement opportunities for . . .	
People of only certain faiths? *1*	Yes
Couples: both are health providers?	Yes
Couples: only one is a health provider?	Yes
Families with children?	Yes
Medical students?	Yes
Pre-medical or college students?	Yes
Other health professional students?	Yes
Doctors in training?	Yes
Health personnel who are US citizens?	Yes
Health personnel who are non-US citizens?	Yes
Health personnel with no prior experience in developing countries?	Yes
Health personnel who are not current members of your organization?	Yes

Organization/Service Specifics:	
Size of the Organization's Staff:	>200
Number of providers sent or received/year:	11-20
Minimum term of assignment: *2*	6 months
Maximum term of assignment:	career
Is funding available for travel? *3*	
Are room and board provided? *3*	No
Is any other funding available? *3*	No
Is training provided or available?	Yes
Is a language other than English required? *4*	No

Health Professionals Placed:

Physicians:

Physicians

Allied Health Professionals:

Nurses; Pharmacists

Notes

1. Baptist; *2.* 2-3 months in Cameroon; *3.* Funding often available for long-term volunteers; *4.* Sometimes a foreign language is needed depending on assignment.

Baptist Medical and Dental Mission International

Continents Served			
Africa ☐	Asia ☐	Europe ☐	The Americas ☑

Countries Served

Honduras; Nicaragua

Address: **11 Plaza Drive, Hattiesburg, MS 39402 U.S.A.**

Phone: **(601) 544-3586** FAX: **(601) 544-6508**

E-Mail: **katrina@bmdmi.org** Web: **www.bmdmi.org/**

Mission: Baptist Medical and Dental Mission International is a non-profit Christian organization that exists to spread the message of salvation through the free grace of Jesus Christ, as well as to meet the needs of impoverished people on the foreign field through medical-dental volunteer mission teams, children's homes, Christian schools, and benevolence programs.

Placement opportunities for . . .

People of only certain faiths? *1*	Yes
Couples: both are health providers?	Yes
Couples: only one is a health provider?	Yes
Families with children?	Yes
Medical students?	Yes
Pre-medical or college students?	Yes
Other health professional students?	Yes
Doctors in training?	Yes
Health personnel who are US citizens?	Yes
Health personnel who are non-US citizens?	Yes
Health personnel with no prior experience in developing countries?	Yes
Health personnel who are not current members of your organization?	Yes

Organization/Service Specifics:

Size of the Organization's Staff:	21-50
Number of providers sent or received/year:	>200
Minimum term of assignment:	1 Week
Maximum term of assignment:	life
Is funding available for travel?	No
Are room and board provided?	No
Is any other funding available? *2*	No
Is training provided or available?	Yes
Is a language other than English required?	No

Health Professionals Placed:

Physicians:

Physicians

Allied Health Professionals:

Dentists; Nutritionists & Dieticians; Physical & Occupational Therapists

Notes

1. Must profess Christ as personal savior; *2.* Each volunteer is responsible for their own costs.

Baptist Medical Missions International

Continents Served			
Africa ☑	Asia ☑	Europe ☑	The Americas ☑

Countries Served

Bolivia	Brazil	Burkina Faso
Cape Verde	Dominican Republic	
El Salvador	Ghana	Guatemala
Haiti	Honduras	Jordan
Mexico	Nicaragua	Philippines
Russia	Togo	Ukraine

Address: **PO Box 30910, Little Rock, AR 72260 U.S.A.**

Phone: **(501) 455-4977** FAX: **(501) 455-3636**

E-Mail: **bmaam@bmaam.com** Web: **www.bmaam.com**

Mission: Baptist Medical Missions International (BMMI) provides competent medical, dental, and other health care in underserved areas of the world with the hope of sharing the Gospel and establishing new churches. BMMI seeks evangelical Christians for relatively short-term (1-6 week) stays in countries around the world. There are no language restrictions, although Spanish and French are desirable for some assignments. Funding is unavailable with the exception of limited funds for room/board.

Placement opportunities for . . .

People of only certain faiths? *1*	No
Couples: both are health providers?	Yes
Couples: only one is a health provider?	Yes
Families with children?	No
Medical students? *2*	No
Pre-medical or college students?	No
Other health professional students?	No
Doctors in training?	Yes
Health personnel who are US citizens?	Yes
Health personnel who are non-US citizens?	Yes
Health personnel with no prior experience in developing countries?	Yes
Health personnel who are not current members of your organization?	Yes

Organization/Service Specifics:

Size of the Organization's Staff:	0-5
Number of providers sent or received/year:	151-200
Minimum term of assignment:	1 weeks
Maximum term of assignment:	6 weeks
Is funding available for travel?	No
Are room and board provided? *3*	Yes
Is any other funding available?	No
Is training provided or available?	No
Is a language other than English required? *4*	Yes

(continued)

Health Professionals Placed:

Physicians:

Physicians; Anesthesiologists; Cardiologists; Dermatologists; Emergency Medicine Physicians; Endocrinologists; Family Practitioners; Gastroenterologists; General Surgeons; Hematologists; Oncologists; Infectious Disease Spec.; Internal Medicine GPS & PCP; OB/GYN; Ophthalmologists; Oral Surgeons; Optometrists; Orthopedic Surgeons; Otolaryngologists; Pediatricians; Plastic/Hand/Reconstructive Surgeons; Psychiatrists; Urologists

Allied Health Professionals:

Administrative Health Positions; Dental Hygienists; Dentists; Medical Technicians (lab, X-ray, etc); Nurse Midwives; Nurse Practitioners; Nurses; Nutritionists & Dieticians; Paramedics; Pharmacists; Physical & Occupational Therapists; Physician Assistants; Podiatrists; Prosthetists; Public Health Specialists, Epidemiologists and Health Educators; Respiratory Therapists; Social Workers; Water/Sanitation Specialists

Notes

1. Volunteers are predominantly Evangelical Christians; *2.* Medical students may occasionally go on short-term trips; *3.* Room and board are provided on a limited basis; *4.* Spanish and French are desirable for certain assignments.

Baptist Mid Missions

Address: **7749 Webster Road, P.O. Box 308011, Cleveland, OH 44130-8011 U.S.A.**

Phone: **(440) 826-3930** FAX: **(440) 826-4457**

E-Mail: **info@bmm.org** Web: **www.bmm.org/**

Mission: Baptist Mid Missions is an independent Baptist fundamental faith mission agency with around 1000 career missionaries in over 50 nations, with a variety of ministries including medical clinics and hospitals in areas underserved by government and commercial hospitals. Hospitals are in Haiti, CAR, Chad, Bangladesh, plus clinics in Ghana, Liberia, and Chad. All personnel are sent out by independent Baptist churches, including career workers and volunteers for 2 weeks to 2 years.

Continents Served

Africa ☑ Asia ☑ Europe ☑ The Americas ☑

Countries Served

Australia	Austria	Bangladesh
Botswana	Brazil	Cambodia
Central African Rep.		Chad
Chile	Dominican Republic	
Ecuador	Ethiopia	Finland
France	Germany	Ghana
Guam	Guyana	Haiti
Honduras	Hong Kong	India
Ireland	Italy	Ivory Coast
Jamaica	Japan	Liberia
Mexico	Netherlands	New Zealand
Peru	Puerto Rico	Romania
Russia	Slovakia	Spain
St. Lucia	St. Vincent	Taiwan
Thailand	United Kingdom	
United States	Venezuela	Zambia

Placement opportunities for . . .

People of only certain faiths? *1*	Yes
Couples: both are health providers?	Yes
Couples: only one is a health provider?	Yes
Families with children?	Yes
Medical students?	Yes
Pre-medical or college students?	
Other health professional students?	Yes
Doctors in training?	Yes
Health personnel who are US citizens?	Yes
Health personnel who are non-US citizens?	Yes
Health personnel with no prior experience in developing countries?	Yes
Health personnel who are not current members of your organization?	Yes

Organization/Service Specifics:

Size of the Organization's Staff:	>200
Number of providers sent or received/year:	6-10
Minimum term of assignment:	2 weeks
Maximum term of assignment:	2 years
Is funding available for travel?	No
Are room and board provided?	Yes
Is any other funding available?	No
Is training provided or available?	No
Is a language other than English required?	No

Health Professionals Placed:

Physicians:

Physicians; Family Practitioners; General Surgeons; OB/GYN; Ophthalmologists; Otolaryngologists

Allied Health Professionals:

Dentists; Medical Technicians (lab, X-ray, etc); Nurse Midwives; Nurses

Notes

1. Protestant/Independent Baptist.

Beeve Foundation for World Eye and Health, The

Continents Served
Africa ☐ Asia ☑ Europe ☐ The Americas ☐

Countries Served
Fiji

Address: **PO Box 823, Verdugo City, CA 91046 U.S.A.**

Phone: **(818) 790-1005** FAX: **(818) 952-6445**

E-Mail: **beevefoundation@earthlink.net** Web:

Mission: The Beeve Foundation for World Eye and Health is a non-profit corporation dedicated to providing basic eye and health care to the remote island populations of Fiji and neighboring Pacific Island groups. The Foundation is committed to expanding the education of native medical practitioners through information exchange and experiential training. The principle upon which the Foundation is established is to provide physical, mental, and emotional health to those who otherwise have no access to modern medicine. Volunteers can serve for 1-3 weeks. The Beeve Foundation provides most funding for interested personnel. There are no religious or language requirements.

Placement opportunities for . . .		Organization/Service Specifics:	
People of only certain faiths?	No	Size of the Organization's Staff:	21-50
Couples: both are health providers?	Yes	Number of providers sent or received/year:	21-50
Couples: only one is a health provider?	Yes	Minimum term of assignment:	1 week
Families with children?	No	Maximum term of assignment:	3 weeks
Medical students? *1*	Yes	Is funding available for travel?	Yes
Pre-medical or college students?	No	Are room and board provided?	Yes
Other health professional students?	No	Is any other funding available? *3*	Yes
Doctors in training? *2*	Yes	Is training provided or available?	Yes
Health personnel who are US citizens?	Yes	Is a language other than English required?	No
Health personnel who are non-US citizens?	Yes		
Health personnel with no prior experience in developing countries?	Yes		
Health personnel who are not current members of your organization?	Yes		

Health Professionals Placed:

Physicians:

Physicians; Anesthesiologists; Dermatologists; Emergency Medicine Physicians; Endocrinologists; Family Practitioners; Infectious Disease Spec.; Internal Medicine GPS & PCP; OB/GYN; Ophthalmologists; Oral Surgeons; Optometrists; Pediatricians; Plastic/Hand/Reconstructive Surgeons

Allied Health Professionals:

Administrative Health Positions; Dental Hygienists; Dentists; Medical Technicians (lab, X-ray, etc); Nurse Midwives; Nurse Practitioners; Nurses; Nutritionists & Dieticians; Paramedics; Pharmacists; Physician Assistants; Podiatrists; Prosthetists; Public Health Specialists, Epidemiologists and Health Educators; Social Workers; Water/Sanitation Specialists

Notes

1. There may be some placements for medical students; *2.* There may be placements for doctors in training; *3.* There is some other funding available.

Ben-Gurion University of the Negev

Continents Served
Africa ☑ Asia ☑ Europe ☑ The Americas ☑

Countries Served

Belgium	Brazil	Canada
Ecuador	El Salvador	Ethiopia
France	Germany	India
Israel	Japan	Kenya
Mexico	Netherlands	Panama
Peru	Rwanda	South Africa
South Africa	Switzerland	Thailand
United Kingdom		United States

Address: **P.O. Box 653, Beer Sheva, 84105 Israel**

Phone: **972 864 00914** FAX: **972 762 60445**

E-Mail: **malkan@mail.bgu.ac.il or malkan@bgumail.bgu.ac.il** Web: **www.bgu.ac.il/**

Mission: Ben-Gurion University of the Negev was founded by the government of Israel of 1969. Its purpose: to act as a driving force in the development of Negev, a desert area comprising more than 60 percent of the country. The University was inspired by the vision of Israel's first prime minister, David Ben-Gurion, who believed that the country's future lay in the region.

(continued)

Placement opportunities for . . .		**Organization/Service Specifics:**	
People of only certain faiths?	No	Size of the Organization's Staff:	>200
Couples: both are health providers?	Yes	Number of providers sent or received/year:	1-5
Couples: only one is a health provider?	No	Minimum term of assignment:	0
Families with children?	No	Maximum term of assignment:	0
Medical students?	Yes	Is funding available for travel?	No
Pre-medical or college students?	Yes	Are room and board provided?	No
Other health professional students?	Yes	Is any other funding available?	No
Doctors in training?	Yes	Is training provided or available?	
Health personnel who are US citizens?	No	Is a language other than English required?	Yes
Health personnel who are non-US citizens?	Yes		
Health personnel with no prior experience in developing countries?			
Health personnel who are not current members of your organization?	Yes		

Health Professionals Placed:

Notes

Physicians:

Physicians; Anesthesiologists; Cardiologists; Dermatologists; Emergency Medicine Physicians; Endocrinologists; Family Practitioners; Gastroenterologists; General Surgeons; Hematologists; Oncologists; Infectious Disease Spec.; Internal Medicine GPS & PCP; Nephrologists; Neurologists; Neurosurgeons; OB/GYN; Ophthalmologists; Oral Surgeons; Orthopedic Surgeons; Otolaryngologists; Pathologists; Pediatricians; Plastic/Hand/Reconstructive Surgeons; Psychiatrists; Pulmonary Specialists; Radiologists; Urologists

Allied Health Professionals:

Administrative Health Positions; Medical Technicians (lab, X-ray, etc); Nurse Midwives; Nurse Practitioners; Nurses; Paramedics; Pharmacists; Physician Assistants; Prosthetists; Psychologists; Public Health Specialists, Epidemiologists and Health Educators; Respiratory Therapists; Social Workers

---

Board of World Mission of the Moravian Church

Address: **P.O. Box 1245, Bethlehem, PA 18016-1245 U.S.A.**

Phone: **(610) 868-1732** FAX: **(610) 866-9223**

E-Mail: **bwm@mcsp.org** Web: **www.moravianmission.org/**

Continents Served

Africa ☐ Asia ☐ Europe ☐ The Americas ☑

Countries Served

Honduras Nicaragua

Mission: The Board of World Mission is the overseas mission and support agency of the Moravian Church in America. It continues the work begun in 1745 by the Society for Propagating the Gospel, North America's oldest Protestant mission society. Active medical clinics are run in Honduras and Nicaragua.

Placement opportunities for . . .		**Organization/Service Specifics:**	
People of only certain faiths? *1*	Yes	Size of the Organization's Staff:	21-50
Couples: both are health providers?	Yes	Number of providers sent or received/year:	11-20
Couples: only one is a health provider?	Yes	Minimum term of assignment:	1 month
Families with children?	No	Maximum term of assignment:	6 months
Medical students?	Yes	Is funding available for travel?	No
Pre-medical or college students?	Yes	Are room and board provided?	Yes
Other health professional students?	Yes	Is any other funding available?	No
Doctors in training?	Yes	Is training provided or available?	Yes
Health personnel who are US citizens?	Yes	Is a language other than English required? *2*	Yes
Health personnel who are non-US citizens?	Yes		
Health personnel with no prior experience in developing countries?	Yes		
Health personnel who are not current members of your organization?	Yes		

Health Professionals Placed:

Notes

1. Protestant; *2.* Spanish.

Physicians:

Physicians; Dermatologists; Emergency Medicine Physicians; Family Practitioners; Infectious Disease Spec.; Internal Medicine GPS & PCP; Pediatricians

Allied Health Professionals:

Dentists; Medical Technicians (lab, X-ray, etc); Nurse Practitioners; Nurses; Pharmacists; Physician Assistants; Social Workers

Boston International Foundation for Medical Education

Continents Served			
Africa ✔	Asia ✔	Europe ✔	The Americas ✔

Countries Served

Address: **160 Heritage Lane, Weymouth, MA 02189-1061 U.S.A.**

Phone: **(781) 337-3933** FAX: **(617) 414-5315**
(781) 331-7926

E-Mail: **jjvitale@bu.edu** Web: **www.bifme.org/**

Mission: This foundation was established in January, 1996, by former and/or present faculty members at one of the three Boston based medical schools. Its purpose is to support senior medical students, medical and surgical residents and junior faculty from these schools, Harvard, Tufts and Boston University, who successfully complete a minimum two to six month elective at a foreign medical center acceptable to the foundation and the respective medical school administration. The financial support is intended to defray travel and living expenses. The Foundation believes that these individuals, early in their training and prior to becoming practicing physicians, who are willing to work along side and learn from their peers in providing health care to the less fortunate in less developed areas of the world, will make a significant contribution toward any initiative in achieving world peace. The experience provides useful and practical insight into the cultural, moral, and ethnic perceptions of health care of our multi-ethnic and multi-cultural society.

Placement opportunities for . . .

People of only certain faiths?	No
Couples: both are health providers?	Yes
Couples: only one is a health provider?	Yes
Families with children?	No
Medical students?	Yes
Pre-medical or college students?	No
Other health professional students?	No
Doctors in training?	Yes
Health personnel who are US citizens?	Yes
Health personnel who are non-US citizens?	No
Health personnel with no prior experience in developing countries?	Yes
Health personnel who are not current members of your organization?	No

Organization/Service Specifics:

Size of the Organization's Staff:	0-5
Number of providers sent or received/year:	1-5
Minimum term of assignment:	2 month
Maximum term of assignment:	indef
Is funding available for travel? *1*	Yes
Are room and board provided? *1*	Yes
Is any other funding available? *1*	Yes
Is training provided or available?	Yes
Is a language other than English required? *2*	Yes

Health Professionals Placed:

Physicians:

Physicians

Allied Health Professionals:

Notes

1. Fellowships, scholarships;
2. Depends on the country.

Boston University School of Medicine, Section of Preventive Medicine and Epidemiology

Continents Served			
Africa ✔	Asia ☐	Europe ☐	The Americas ☐

Countries Served
Cameroon

Address: **BU Medical Center, B-612, 715 Albany Street, Boston, MA 02118 U.S.A.**

Phone: **(617) 638-8074** FAX: **(617) 637-8076**

E-Mail: **munroproc@cs.com** Web:

Mission: Only open to students of BU School of Medicine. Dr Proctor is involved in a mission hospital in Cameroon, West Africa. Physician stays are relatively short term (1 month–1 year). No longer arranging overseas electives for medical students and/or hospital residents.

(continued)

Placement opportunities for . . .

People of only certain faiths?	No
Couples: both are health providers?	Yes
Couples: only one is a health provider?	Yes
Families with children?	Yes
Medical students?	Yes
Pre-medical or college students?	No
Other health professional students?	Yes
Doctors in training?	Yes
Health personnel who are US citizens?	Yes
Health personnel who are non-US citizens?	No
Health personnel with no prior experience in developing countries?	Yes
Health personnel who are not current members of your organization?	No

Organization/Service Specifics:

Size of the Organization's Staff:	11-20
Number of providers sent or received/year:	6-10
Minimum term of assignment:	1 Month
Maximum term of assignment:	1 Year
Is funding available for travel?	No
Are room and board provided?	Yes
Is any other funding available?	No
Is training provided or available?	No
Is a language other than English required?	No

Health Professionals Placed:

Physicians:

Physicians

Allied Health Professionals:

Notes

Bread for the World (Brot fur die Welt)

Address: **P.O. Box 10 11 42 70010 Stuttgart, Germany**

Phone: **(497) 112-1590** FAX: **0497112159288**

E-Mail: Web:

Continents Served

Africa ✔ Asia ✔ Europe ✔ The Americas ✔

Countries Served

Bosnia and Herzegovina, Liberia, Sudan, Yugoslavia, former

Mission: Bread for the World funds programs and projects of partner organizations in Africa, Asia and Latin America, on its mission to alleviate hunger and poverty. The overseas partners of Bread for the World primarily consist of churches and church-related groups, but also include cooperative societies and self-help groups which are engaged in projects that work towards justice for the poor.

Placement opportunities for . . .

People of only certain faiths?	No
Couples: both are health providers?	Yes
Couples: only one is a health provider?	Yes
Families with children?	Yes
Medical students?	No
Pre-medical or college students?	No
Other health professional students?	No
Doctors in training?	No
Health personnel who are US citizens?	No
Health personnel who are non-US citizens?	Yes
Health personnel with no prior experience in developing countries?	No
Health personnel who are not current members of your organization?	Yes

Organization/Service Specifics:

Size of the Organization's Staff:	101-150
Number of providers sent or received/year:	151-200
Minimum term of assignment:	depends
Maximum term of assignment:	depends
Is funding available for travel?	Yes
Are room and board provided?	Yes
Is any other funding available?	No
Is training provided or available?	No
Is a language other than English required? *1*	Yes

Health Professionals Placed:

Physicians:

Physicians

Allied Health Professionals:

Social Workers

Notes

1. French, etc.

Bridges to Community, Inc.

Address: **95 Croton Ave., Ossining, NY 10562 U.S.A.**

Phone: **(914) 923-2200** FAX: **(914) 923-8396**

E-Mail: **brdgs2comm@aol.com, or info@bridgestocommunity.org** Web: **www.bridgestocommunity.org**

Continents Served

Africa ☑ Asia ☑ Europe ☐ The Americas ☑

Countries Served

Kenya Nepal Nicaragua

Mission: Bridges to Community, established in 1992, operates from the conviction that we can renew and deepen our sense of responsibility for all of life, and thus become better informed and more proactive in our efforts to build a world that takes seriously the rights and needs of everyone while protecting our natural resources. Bridges to Community offers educational, service-oriented travel opportunities to Nicaragua. Bridges identifies and supports community-initiated projects that are aimed at empowering the local community to build a more promising future. Volunteer trips last for 10 days. There are no language or religious requirements, although some knowledge of Spanish is helpful.

Placement opportunities for . . .		Organization/Service Specifics:	
People of only certain faiths?	No	Size of the Organization's Staff:	11-20
Couples: both are health providers?	Yes	Number of providers sent or received/year:	21-50
Couples: only one is a health provider?	Yes	Minimum term of assignment:	10 days
Families with children?	No	Maximum term of assignment:	10 days
Medical students?	Yes	Is funding available for travel?	No
Pre-medical or college students?	Yes	Are room and board provided?	Yes
Other health professional students?	Yes	Is any other funding available? *1*	Yes
Doctors in training?	Yes	Is training provided or available?	
Health personnel who are US citizens?	Yes	Is a language other than English required? *2*	No
Health personnel who are non-US citizens?	Yes		
Health personnel with no prior experience in developing countries?	Yes		
Health personnel who are not current members of your organization?	Yes		

Health Professionals Placed: *3*

Physicians:

Allied Health Professionals:

Notes

1. There are limited scholarships available; *2.* Spanish is helpful for assignments in Nicaragua; *3.* No specific health professionals sought.

CAM International

Address: **8625 La Prada Dr., Dallas, TX 75228 U.S.A.**

Phone: **(800) 366-2264**
(214) 327-8206 FAX: **(214) 327-8201**

E-Mail: **info@caminternational.org** Web: **www.caminternational.org**

Continents Served

Africa ☐ Asia ☐ Europe ☑ The Americas ☑

Countries Served

Belize Costa Rica El Salvador
Guatemala Honduras Mexico
Panama Spain

Mission: CAM International establishes biblically based, culturally relevant, reproducing churches and equips leaders for future ministry work. CAM extends the Gospel to the whole world by engaging national churches for missions. CAM sends impact teams to provide needed services while continuing CAM's missionary work. Opportunites exist for medical personnel depending on impact team or specialized service needs.

Placement opportunities for . . .		Organization/Service Specifics:	
People of only certain faiths? *1*	Yes	Size of the Organization's Staff:	>200
Couples: both are health providers? *2*	No	Number of providers sent or received/year:	11-20
Couples: only one is a health provider? *2*	No	Minimum term of assignment:	1 week
Families with children? *2*	No	Maximum term of assignment:	career
Medical students?	Yes	Is funding available for travel?	No
Pre-medical or college students?	Yes	Are room and board provided?	No
Other health professional students?	Yes	Is any other funding available?	No
Doctors in training?	Yes	Is training provided or available?	No
Health personnel who are US citizens?	Yes	Is a language other than English required? *3*	Yes
Health personnel who are non-US citizens?	Yes		
Health personnel with no prior experience in developing countries?	Yes		
Health personnel who are not current members of your organization?	Yes		

(continued)

Health Professionals Placed:

Physicians:

Physicians

Allied Health Professionals:

Dentists; Nurse Practitioners; Nurses; Paramedics; Physician Assistants

Notes

1. Christian evangelical; *2.* Possibly depending on assignment; *3.* Spanish very helpful and is sometimes necessary.

Cameroon Baptist Convention Health Board

Address: **P.O. Box 1, Bamenda North West Province, Republic of Cameroon**

Phone: **(237) 348-1490** **(237) 776-4781** FAX: **(237) 348-1161**

E-Mail: **BBHCameroon@aol.com** Web:

Continents Served

Africa ☑ Asia ☐ Europe ☐ The Americas ☐

Countries Served

Mission: The Cameroon Baptist Convention Health Board seeks to assist in the provision of health care to all of those in need. We do so with an expression of Christian love and as a means of witness, in order that they might be brought to God through Christ. CBC runs 2 hospitals and 15 health centers and has openings for volunteer health care workers and programs for students. Some leadership positions have a religious requirement.

Placement opportunities for . . .	
People of only certain faiths? *1*	No
Couples: both are health providers?	Yes
Couples: only one is a health provider?	Yes
Families with children?	Yes
Medical students?	Yes
Pre-medical or college students?	No
Other health professional students?	Yes
Doctors in training?	Yes
Health personnel who are US citizens?	Yes
Health personnel who are non-US citizens?	Yes
Health personnel with no prior experience in developing countries?	Yes
Health personnel who are not current members of your organization?	Yes

Organization/Service Specifics:	
Size of the Organization's Staff:	>200
Number of providers sent or received/year:	21-50
Minimum term of assignment:	1 month
Maximum term of assignment:	2 years
Is funding available for travel?	No
Are room and board provided?	Yes
Is any other funding available? *2*	Yes
Is training provided or available?	Yes
Is a language other than English required?	No

Health Professionals Placed:

Physicians:

All physician specialties

Allied Health Professionals:

All allied health professionals

Notes

1. Must not be anti-Christian; *2.* Sometimes much needed volunteers get a stipend.

Campus Crusade for Christ International

Address: **100 Lake Hart Drive, Suite 1200, Orlando, FL 32832 U.S.A.**

Phone: **(407) 826-2864** **(407) 826-2000** FAX: **(407) 826-2851**

E-Mail: **Bill.Thomas@ccci.org** Web: **www.ccci.org**

Continents Served

Africa ☑ Asia ☑ Europe ☑ The Americas ☑

Countries Served

China	Hong Kong	Japan
Korea, North	Korea, South	Mongolia
Nigeria	Taiwan	Uganda
USSR, former		

Mission: Our Objectives are:
(1) to help expose every person in the world to the gospel; (2) to help win people to faith in Jesus Christ; (3) to help build them in their faith; (4) to help train them for ministry; (5) to help send them to win and disciple others. Volunteers can serve for short-term (2 week) assisgnments or longer term (3 years) assignments. There are no language requirements, but volunteers must be committed Evangelical Christians.

(continued)

Placement opportunities for . . .

People of only certain faiths? *1*	Yes
Couples: both are health providers?	Yes
Couples: only one is a health provider?	Yes
Families with children?	No
Medical students? *2*	No
Pre-medical or college students?	No
Other health professional students?	No
Doctors in training?	No
Health personnel who are US citizens?	Yes
Health personnel who are non-US citizens?	Yes
Health personnel with no prior experience in developing countries?	Yes
Health personnel who are not current members of your organization?	Yes

Organization/Service Specifics:

Size of the Organization's Staff:	>200
Number of providers sent or received/year:	1-5
Minimum term of assignment:	2 weeks
Maximum term of assignment:	3 years
Is funding available for travel?	No
Are room and board provided?	No
Is any other funding available? *3*	No
Is training provided or available?	Yes
Is a language other than English required?	No

Health Professionals Placed:

Physicians:

Physicians; Family Practitioners; Internal Medicine GPS & PCP; Radiologists

Allied Health Professionals:

Dentists; Public Health Specialists, Epidemiologists and Health Educators

Notes

1. Volunteers must be Evangelical Christians; *2.* There may be more future opportunities for medical and/or dental students; *3.* Everyone is responsible for their own funding. Training is provided to help with fundraising.

Canadian Society for International Health

Address: **1 Nicholas St, Suite 1105, Ottawa, Ontario, Canada K1N 7B7**

Phone: **(613) 241-5785** FAX: **(613) 241-3845**

E-Mail: **csih@csih.org** Web: **www.csih.org**

Continents Served

Africa ☑ Asia ☑ Europe ☑ The Americas ☑

Countries Served

Armenia	Azerbaijan	Bolivia
Croatia	Georgia	Guyana
Philippines	Russia	Ukraine

Mission: The Canadian Society for International Health, a national voluntary organization, facilitates and supports health and development activities around the world through the mobilization of Canadian and other resources. CSIH advocates for health policy and programming which contributes to global objectives of health for all, equity, and social justice through building partnerships with Canadian and other institutions and organizations. Volunteers can serve for 6-9 month terms. Internships are available for people under 30.

Placement opportunities for . . .

People of only certain faiths?	No
Couples: both are health providers?	No
Couples: only one is a health provider?	No
Families with children?	No
Medical students?	Yes
Pre-medical or college students?	Yes
Other health professional students?	Yes
Doctors in training?	No
Health personnel who are US citizens?	No
Health personnel who are non-US citizens? *1*	Yes
Health personnel with no prior experience in developing countries?	Yes
Health personnel who are not current members of your organization?	Yes

Organization/Service Specifics:

Size of the Organization's Staff:	11-20
Number of providers sent or received/year:	
Minimum term of assignment:	6 months
Maximum term of assignment:	9 months
Is funding available for travel?	Yes
Are room and board provided?	Yes
Is any other funding available? *2*	Yes
Is training provided or available?	Yes
Is a language other than English required? *3*	Yes

Health Professionals Placed:

Physicians:

None

Allied Health Professionals:

None

Notes

1. Canadian citizens or landed immigrants; *2.* There is an internship program for people under 30; *3.* Spanish may be required for some placements.

Canvasback Missions, Inc.

Continents Served			
Africa ☐	Asia ☑	Europe ☐	The Americas ☐

Countries Served
Caroline Islands; Marshall Islands

Address: **940 Adams St., Suite R, Benicia, CA 94510 U.S.A.**

Phone: **(800) 793-7215**
(707) 746-7828 FAX:

E-Mail: **mail@canvasback.org** Web: **www.canvasback.org**

Mission: Canvasbacks is a group of nondenomenational Christians that serves the tropical north Pacific. Doctors and dentists often serve in hospitals in Micronesia and the Marshall Islands, and most missions last two weeks. Clinics are conducted Monday through Friday while weekends are reserved for spiritual and recreational activities with the island people. Volunteers must be in good physical condition and will need to provide their own air transportation. In addition to general practictioners and dentists, physicians specializing in ophthalmology, orthopedic surgery, ENT, OB-GYN, and urology are always needed.

Placement opportunities for . . .	
People of only certain faiths? *1*	Yes
Couples: both are health providers?	Yes
Couples: only one is a health provider?	Yes
Families with children?	No
Medical students?	No
Pre-medical or college students?	No
Other health professional students?	Yes
Doctors in training?	No
Health personnel who are US citizens?	Yes
Health personnel who are non-US citizens?	Yes
Health personnel with no prior experience in developing countries?	Yes
Health personnel who are not current members of your organization?	Yes

Organization/Service Specifics:	
Size of the Organization's Staff:	11-20
Number of providers sent or received/year:	21-50
Minimum term of assignment:	2 weeks
Maximum term of assignment:	6 weeks
Is funding available for travel?	No
Are room and board provided?	Yes
Is any other funding available? *2*	Yes
Is training provided or available?	
Is a language other than English required?	No

Health Professionals Placed:

Physicians:

Physicians; Anesthesiologists; Dermatologists; Emergency Medicine Physicians; Family Practitioners; General Surgeons; Infectious Disease Spec.; Internal Medicine GPS & PCP; OB/GYN; Ophthalmologists; Orthopedic Surgeons; Pediatricians; Urologists

Allied Health Professionals:

Dental Hygienists; Dentists; Medical Technicians (lab, X-ray, etc); Nurse Midwives; Nurse Practitioners; Nurses; Physical & Occupational Therapists; Physician Assistants; Podiatrists; Social Workers; Water/Sanitation Specialists

Notes

1. Christian; *2.* Stipend provided in some cases.

Cape Cares

Continents Served			
Africa ☐	Asia ☐	Europe ☐	The Americas ☑

Countries Served
Honduras

Address: **1 River St., South Yarmouth, MA 02664 U.S.A.**

Phone: **(508) 394-2419** FAX:

E-Mail: **mldsy@juno.com** Web: **www.capecares.com**

Mission: Cape Cares is a group of caring volunteers who have donated their time and resources for the past 12 years to help elevate the lives of the poor and needy of Central America, specifically Honduras. We are internists, specialists, dentists, optometrists, chiropractors, nurse practitioners, nurse midwives, nurses, pharmacists, and lay people who all have devoted our time and energy on more than one occasion to these efforts. Volunteers can go on 1 week trips. Spanish is helpful, but not required.

Placement opportunities for . . .	
People of only certain faiths?	No
Couples: both are health providers?	Yes
Couples: only one is a health provider?	Yes
Families with children?	No
Medical students?	Yes
Pre-medical or college students?	Yes
Other health professional students?	Yes
Doctors in training?	Yes
Health personnel who are US citizens?	Yes
Health personnel who are non-US citizens?	Yes
Health personnel with no prior experience in developing countries?	Yes
Health personnel who are not current members of your organization?	Yes

Organization/Service Specifics:	
Size of the Organization's Staff:	0-5
Number of providers sent or received/year:	51-100
Minimum term of assignment:	1 week
Maximum term of assignment:	1 week
Is funding available for travel?	No
Are room and board provided?	Yes
Is any other funding available? *1*	Yes
Is training provided or available?	No
Is a language other than English required? *2*	No

(continued)

Health Professionals Placed:

Physicians:

Physicians; Emergency Medicine Physicians; Infectious Disease Spec.; Internal Medicine GPS & PCP; Ophthalmologists; Oral Surgeons; Pediatricians

Allied Health Professionals:

Dental Hygienists; Dentists; Nurse Practitioners; Nurses; Pharmacists; Physician Assistants

Notes

1. Volunteers pay a fee of $950. We try to raise the balance estimated at $400-$500 per volunteer expense; *2.* Spanish is not required, but it is helpful.

Cape Verde Care Agency, Inc.

Address: **120 Homestead St., Boston, MA 02321 U.S.A.**

Phone: **(617) 549-0360** FAX:

E-Mail: **ISilva1143@aol.com** Web: **www.capeverdecare.org**

Continents Served

Africa ☑ Asia ☐ Europe ☐ The Americas ☐

Countries Served

Cape Verde

Mission: CVC Agency Inc. aims to supply a broad range of medical, educational, and humanitarian services specifically to citizens of the west coast of Africa within the Archipelago of the Cape Verde Islands. It accomodates short term (1-2 weeks) stays for health care professionals but not students. There are no religious restrictions or language requirements.

Placement opportunities for . . .

People of only certain faiths?	No
Couples: both are health providers?	Yes
Couples: only one is a health provider?	Yes
Families with children?	No
Medical students?	Yes
Pre-medical or college students?	No
Other health professional students?	Yes
Doctors in training?	No
Health personnel who are US citizens?	Yes
Health personnel who are non-US citizens?	Yes
Health personnel with no prior experience in developing countries?	No
Health personnel who are not current members of your organization?	Yes

Organization/Service Specifics:

Size of the Organization's Staff:	6-10
Number of providers sent or received/year:	21-50
Minimum term of assignment:	1 Week
Maximum term of assignment:	2 Weeks
Is funding available for travel?	No
Are room and board provided?	Yes
Is any other funding available?	No
Is training provided or available?	No
Is a language other than English required?	No

Health Professionals Placed:

Physicians:

Not specified

Allied Health Professionals:

Not specified

Notes

Capiz Emmanuel Hospital

Address: **Roxas Ave., Roxas City, Capiz, 03600 Philippines, 5800**

Phone: **(036) 621-5608** FAX: **(036) 621-4761**

E-Mail: **emmanuel@captainweb.us** Web: **none**

Continents Served

Africa ☐ Asia ☑ Europe ☐ The Americas ☐

Countries Served

Canada, Kuwait, Saudi Arabia, Singapore, United Arab Emirates, United States

Mission: The Capiz Emmanuel Hospital is a non-stock, non-profit, private tertiary hospital, maintained by members of the Corporation through its governing body, the Board of Trustees. The hospital has a 100 bed capacity and is licensed by the Department of Health and Accredited by the Philippine Health Insurance Corporation. The hospital is situated in the City of Roxas, Profince of Capiz with 16 municipalities and 46 barangays, some of which are inaccessible to transportation facilities. It receives referrals from rural health units and other existing district and medicare hospitals in some municipalities.

(continued)

Placement opportunities for . . .

People of only certain faiths? *2*	No
Couples: both are health providers?	No
Couples: only one is a health provider?	No
Families with children?	No
Medical students?	Yes
Pre-medical or college students?	
Other health professional students?	No
Doctors in training?	No
Health personnel who are US citizens?	No
Health personnel who are non-US citizens?	No
Health personnel with no prior experience in developing countries?	No
Health personnel who are not current members of your organization?	No

Organization/Service Specifics:

Size of the Organization's Staff: *1*	101-150
Number of providers sent or received/year:	
Minimum term of assignment:	6 month
Maximum term of assignment:	1 year
Is funding available for travel?	No
Are room and board provided? *3*	Yes
Is any other funding available?	No
Is training provided or available?	Yes
Is a language other than English required?	No

Health Professionals Placed:

Physicians:

Physicians; Anesthesiologists; Cardiologists; Dermatologists; Endocrinologists; Gastroenterologists; General Surgeons; Hematologists; Oncologists; Infectious Disease Spec.; Internal Medicine GPS & PCP; Nephrologists; Neurologists; OB/GYN; Ophthalmologists; Orthopedic Surgeons; Pathologists; Pediatricians; Pulmonary Specialists; Radiologists; Urologists

Allied Health Professionals:

Administrative Health Positions; Dentists; Medical Technicians (lab, X-ray, etc); Nutritionists & Dieticians; Pharmacists; Physical & Occupational Therapists; Respiratory Therapists

Notes

1. Last information obtained on 11/02. No response to inquiries in 3/04 and 2/05; *2.* On equal footing, preference is given to Protestant applicants; *3.* There is a minimum charge for the room and board provided.

CardioStart International, Inc.

Address: **6110 Hartford St, Tampa, FL 33619 U.S.A.**

Phone: **(813) 689-3289** FAX: **(813) 685-9400**

E-Mail: **info@cardiostart.com** Web: **www.cardiostart.com/**

Continents Served

Africa ☐ Asia ☑ Europe ☑ The Americas ☑

Countries Served

Dominican Republic, El Salvador, Honduras, Iran, Nicaragua, Palestine, Peru, Philippines, Ukraine

Mission: CardioStart International provides heart surgery at no cost to people in need worldwide. The organization's volunteer teams perform complex heart operations and help provide instruction and education to assist the development of foreign doctors proficiency with heart and lung surgery and other related specialties. We also work to establish cardiac centers in areas with inadequate facilities including the Caribbean, eastern Europe, the Middle East, and Central America. The organization depends on volunteer medical staff and is in particular need of cardiologists, cardiac surgeons, and anesthesiologists. Missions typically last two weeks.

Placement opportunities for . . .

People of only certain faiths?	No
Couples: both are health providers?	Yes
Couples: only one is a health provider?	Yes
Families with children?	Yes
Medical students?	Yes
Pre-medical or college students?	Yes
Other health professional students?	No
Doctors in training?	Yes
Health personnel who are US citizens?	Yes
Health personnel who are non-US citizens?	Yes
Health personnel with no prior experience in developing countries?	Yes
Health personnel who are not current members of your organization?	Yes

Organization/Service Specifics:

Size of the Organization's Staff:	6-10
Number of providers sent or received/year:	51-100
Minimum term of assignment:	1 weeks
Maximum term of assignment:	3 weeks
Is funding available for travel?	No
Are room and board provided?	Yes
Is any other funding available?	No
Is training provided or available?	No
Is a language other than English required? *1*	No

Health Professionals Placed:

Physicians:

Anesthesiologists; Cardiologists; General Surgeons; OB/GYN

Allied Health Professionals:

Nurse Practitioners; Nurses; Physician Assistants

Notes

1. Bilingual health care providers are helpful.

Casa Clinica de la Mujer

Continents Served			
Africa ☐	Asia ☐	Europe ☐	The Americas ☑

Countries Served

Mexico

Address: **Campesina A.P. 81, Las Varas, Nayarit, 63715 Mexico**

Phone: **(523) 272-0184** FAX: **(523) 272-0184**

E-Mail: **info@mardejade.com** Web: **www.mardejade.com/index.php**

Mission: Mar de Jade is a vacation-retreat in Chacala, Mexico, and an hour north of Puerto Vallarta. Guests who choose to volunteer in the clinic program should come prepared to see how medicine is practiced in a very rewarding yet very different way from what they might be used to in their own country. We welcome students, and professionals from the varied fields of healthcare who are seeking to learn or share primary care diagnostic experience. This includes students or licensed allopathic practitioners as well as homeopaths, osteopaths, chiropractors, acupuncturists, rehab therapists and others. Clinic volunteers can expect to spend at least 16 hours a week with patient care, including two days at the clinic site plus attending patients from Chacala at Mar de Jade. In addition there are three hours of medical Spanish that include learning vocabulary, practicing interviewing the chief complaint, taking medical history and learning to communicate effectively with the patient. The clinic volunteer program is offered as an international elective by University of California schools and medical schools throughout the U.S. have participated in the program. Laura del Valle, MD, MPH, is the clinical director as well as an Assistant Clinical Professor with the Department of Family & Community Medicine at the University of California, San Francisco School of Medicine. The medical electives and residency rotation program require a 21 day minimum stay and consist of two components: clinical participation and Spanish study if needed. Also, nurse practitioners and physician assistants participating in the volunteer/study program have received as many as 60 CEUs for this course.

Placement opportunities for . . .	
People of only certain faiths?	No
Couples: both are health providers?	Yes
Couples: only one is a health provider?	Yes
Families with children?	Yes
Medical students?	Yes
Pre-medical or college students?	No
Other health professional students?	Yes
Doctors in training?	Yes
Health personnel who are US citizens?	Yes
Health personnel who are non-US citizens?	Yes
Health personnel with no prior experience in developing countries?	Yes
Health personnel who are not current members of your organization?	Yes

Organization/Service Specifics:		
Size of the Organization's Staff:		6-10
Number of providers sent or received/year:		11-20
Minimum term of assignment:		2 weeks
Maximum term of assignment:		2 years
Is funding available for travel?		No
Are room and board provided?		No
Is any other funding available?		No
Is training provided or available?		Yes
Is a language other than English required?	*1*	No

Health Professionals Placed:

Physicians:

All physician specialties

Allied Health Professionals:

All allied health professionals

Notes

1. Some spanish is very helpful.

Catholic Medical Mission Board, Inc.

Continents Served			
Africa ☑	Asia ☑	Europe ☐	The Americas ☑

Countries Served

Cameroon, China, Dominican Republic, Ecuador, El Salvador, Ghana, Guatemala, Guyana, Haiti, Honduras, Kenya, Malawi, Nicaragua, Papua-New Guinea, South Africa, Swaziland, Tanzania, Zambia

Address: **10 West 17th Street, New York, NY 10011-5765 U.S.A.**

Phone: **(212) 242-7757** FAX: **(212) 807-9161**

E-Mail: **info@cmmb.org** Web: **www.cmmb.org**

Mission: Since its founding in 1928, Catholic Medical Mission Board (CMMB) has addressed the dual burden of poverty and sickness. Through partnerships with other organizations, CMMB makes healthcare available to the world's needy through the provision of medical shipments, community healthcare training, programs for disease control and eradication, medical volunteer placements, and emergency assistance. All medical assistance is distributed without regard to creed, race, sex, or nationality. Volunteers can serve for short-term (1 week) assignment, or longer term (2 years) assignments. Spanish is especially helpful for volunteers travelling to Spanish speaking countries.

(continued)

Placement opportunities for . . .

People of only certain faiths? *1*	No
Couples: both are health providers?	Yes
Couples: only one is a health provider?	Yes
Families with children?	Yes
Medical students?	No
Pre-medical or college students?	No
Other health professional students?	No
Doctors in training?	Yes
Health personnel who are US citizens?	Yes
Health personnel who are non-US citizens? *2*	Yes
Health personnel with no prior experience in developing countries?	Yes
Health personnel who are not current members of your organization?	Yes

Organization/Service Specifics:

Size of the Organization's Staff:	21-50
Number of providers sent or received/year:	151-200
Minimum term of assignment: *4*	1 week
Maximum term of assignment:	2 years
Is funding available for travel?	Yes
Are room and board provided?	Yes
Is any other funding available?	
Is training provided or available?	
Is a language other than English required? *3*	Yes

Health Professionals Placed:

Physicians:

Physicians; Anesthesiologists; Dermatologists; Emergency Medicine Physicians; Family Practitioners; General Surgeons; Internal Medicine GPS & PCP; Neurologists; Neurosurgeons; OB/GYN; Ophthalmologists; Orthopedic Surgeons; Pediatricians; Plastic/Hand/Reconstructive Surgeons; Psychiatrists; Urologists

Allied Health Professionals:

Dental Hygienists; Dentists; Medical Technicians (lab, X-ray, etc); Nurses; Physical & Occupational Therapists; Physician Assistants

Notes

1. They accept all people who can work at a facility guided by Catholic teachings; *2.* Must be US or Candian licensed; *3.* Spanish is helpful for Latin American assignments, but not necessary; *4.* The length of assignments depend on the location.

Catholic Network of Volunteer Service

Address: **6930 Carroll Avenue, Suite 506, Takoma Park, MD 20912-4423 U.S.A.**

Phone: **(800) 543-5046** **(301) 270-0900** FAX: **(301) 270-0901**

E-Mail: **volunteer@cnvs.org** Web: **www.cnvs.org/**

Mission: Catholic Network of Volunteer Service (CNVS), a national association of faith-based volunteer programs, provides marketing, training, networking and technical assistance in order to help member programs accomplish their missions. CNVS promotes opportunities for men and women of all backgrounds and skills to respond to the Gospel through domestic and international volunteer service to people in need. Seeks students and physicians of all faiths and in a variety of fields for short- (2 weeks) to long-term stays in all four continents. Funding and room/board are available. Language restrictions vary depending on region.

Continents Served

Africa ✔ Asia ✔ Europe ✔ The Americas ✔

Countries Served

Argentina, Australia, Belgium, Belize, Bolivia, Brazil, Cambodia, Cameroon, Canada, Chile, China, Colombia, Congo, Costa Rica, Croatia, Cuba, Czech Republic, Dominican Republic, Ecuador, El Salvador, Ethiopia, France, Germany, Ghana, Guatemala, Guyana, Haiti, Honduras, Hungary, India, Indonesia, Ireland, Israel, Italy, Ivory Coast, Jamaica, Japan, Kenya, Korea, South, Laos, Liberia, Lithuania, Macedonia, Madagascar, Malawi, Mexico, Mozambique, Nepal, Netherlands, New Zealand, Nicaragua, Nigeria, Palestine, Panama, Papua-New Guinea, Paraguay, Peru, Philippines, Poland, Rwanda, Senegal, Sierra Leone, Slovakia, South Africa, Spain, Swaziland, Switzerland, Taiwan, Tanzania, Thailand, Uganda, United Kingdom, United States, Venezuela, Vietnam, Yugoslavia, former, Zambia, Zimbabwe

(continued)

Placement opportunities for . . .

People of only certain faiths?	No
Couples: both are health providers? *1*	Yes
Couples: only one is a health provider? *1*	Yes
Families with children?	Yes
Medical students?	Yes
Pre-medical or college students?	Yes
Other health professional students?	Yes
Doctors in training?	Yes
Health personnel who are US citizens?	Yes
Health personnel who are non-US citizens? *2*	Yes
Health personnel with no prior experience in developing countries?	Yes
Health personnel who are not current members of your organization?	Yes

Organization/Service Specifics:

Size of the Organization's Staff:	6-10
Number of providers sent or received/year:	
Minimum term of assignment:	2 weeks
Maximum term of assignment:	unlimited
Is funding available for travel?	Yes
Are room and board provided?	Yes
Is any other funding available? *3*	Yes
Is training provided or available?	Yes
Is a language other than English required?	Yes

Health Professionals Placed:

Physicians:

All physician specialties

Allied Health Professionals:

All allied health professionals

Notes

1. Certain programs can accommodate couples; *2.* This may be possible; *3.* There is sometimes a living stipend. Funding for travel is primarily at end of service.

CB International

Address: **1501 W. Mineral Ave., Littleton, CO 80120-5612 U.S.A.**

Phone: **(800) 487-4224** FAX: **(720) 283-9383**

E-Mail: **mob@cbi.org** Web: **www.cbi.org/**

Mission: In vital partnership with churches at home and abroad, the mission of CB International is to be a pioneering force in fulfilling Christ's commission to the final frontiers of the harvest. Volunteers are responsible for their own funding and can serve anywhere from 2 month assignments to life on the mission field.

Continents Served

Africa ☑ Asia ☑ Europe ☑ The Americas ☑

Countries Served

Angola	Argentina	Austria
Belgium	Belize	Bolivia
Cameroon	Central African Rep.	
Chile	Czech Republic	Ecuador
France	Germany	Ghana
Guinea	Hong Kong	Hungary
Indonesia	Ireland	Italy
Ivory Coast	Japan	Jordan
Kenya	Korea, South	Lebanon
Lithuania	Macau	Madagascar
Mali	Mongolia	Mozambique
Netherlands	Pakistan	Philippines
Poland	Portugal	Romania
Russia	Rwanda	Senegal
Singapore	Slovenia	Spain
Sudan	Taiwan	Thailand
Tibet	Uganda	Ukraine
United Kingdom		Uruguay
Venezuela	Zaire (DemRepCongo)	
Zambia		

Placement opportunities for . . .

People of only certain faiths? *1*	Yes
Couples: both are health providers?	Yes
Couples: only one is a health provider?	Yes
Families with children?	Yes
Medical students?	Yes
Pre-medical or college students?	Yes
Other health professional students?	Yes
Doctors in training?	Yes
Health personnel who are US citizens?	Yes
Health personnel who are non-US citizens?	No
Health personnel with no prior experience in developing countries?	Yes
Health personnel who are not current members of your organization?	Yes

Organization/Service Specifics:

Size of the Organization's Staff:	51-100
Number of providers sent or received/year:	>200
Minimum term of assignment:	2 month
Maximum term of assignment:	life
Is funding available for travel?	No
Are room and board provided?	No
Is any other funding available? *2*	No
Is training provided or available?	No
Is a language other than English required? *3*	Yes

(continued)

Health Professionals Placed:

Physicians:

Physicians; Anesthesiologists; Family Practitioners; General Surgeons; Internal Medicine GPS & PCP; OB/GYN; Pediatricians; Plastic/Hand/Reconstructive Surgeons

Allied Health Professionals:

Administrative Health Positions; Nurses; Pharmacists; Physical & Occupational Therapists; Psychologists; Public Health Specialists, Epidemiologists and Health Educators; Social Workers; Water/Sanitation Specialists

Notes

1. CBI personnel must be Evangelical Christians; *2.* All CBI personnel are responsible for raising their own financial support; *3.* Language requirements are dependent on the country of service.

CERT (Christian Emergency Relief Team) International

Address: **P.O. Box 1129, Crossville, TN 38557 U.S.A.**

Phone: **(931) 707-9328** FAX: **(931) 707-9406**

E-Mail: **george@certinternational.org** Web: **www.certinternational.org**

Mission: CERT International is a non-profit humanitarian organization based in Cumberland county with headquarters in Crossville, Tennessee. CERT provides short-term opportunities for volunteers from across the United States to become involved in humanitarian relief efforts in Africa, Europe, Asia, and the Americas. There are no language or religious restrictions, though the organization clearly follows a Christian mission.

Continents Served

Africa ☑ Asia ☑ Europe ☑ The Americas ☑

Countries Served

Afghanistan, Albania, Bosnia and Herzegovina, Bulgaria, China, Croatia, Dominican Republic, El Salvador, Ghana, Guatemala, Haiti, Honduras, India, Iraq, Malawi, Mexico, Mozambique, Nepal, Nicaragua, Papua New Guinea, Peru, Philippines, Romania, Russia, Swaziland, Thailand

Placement opportunities for . . .

People of only certain faiths?	No
Couples: both are health providers?	Yes
Couples: only one is a health provider?	Yes
Families with children?	Yes
Medical students?	Yes
Pre-medical or college students?	Yes
Other health professional students?	Yes
Doctors in training?	Yes
Health personnel who are US citizens?	Yes
Health personnel who are non-US citizens?	Yes
Health personnel with no prior experience in developing countries?	Yes
Health personnel who are not current members of your organization?	Yes

Organization/Service Specifics:

Size of the Organization's Staff:	0-5
Number of providers sent or received/year:	21-50
Minimum term of assignment:	2 weeks
Maximum term of assignment: *1*	1 year
Is funding available for travel?	No
Are room and board provided?	No
Is any other funding available?	No
Is training provided or available?	No
Is a language other than English required?	No

Health Professionals Placed:

Physicians:

Physicians; Emergency Medicine Physicians; Family Practitioners; General Surgeons; Internal Medicine GPS & PCP; Pediatricians

Allied Health Professionals:

Dental Hygienists; Dentists; Nurse Practitioners; Nurses; Physician Assistants; Water/Sanitation Specialists

Notes

1. Depends on the country and situation.

Chanet Community Organization

Address: **P.O. Box 1487, Mbale, Uganda**

Phone: **00 256 71 935168** FAX: **00 256 45 35750**

E-Mail: **ccomutufu@hotmail.com** Web: **www.cco.4mg.com**

Continents Served

Africa ☑ Asia ☐ Europe ☐ The Americas ☐

Countries Served

Mission: Chanet Community Organization works in Uganda to provide health care to disadvantaged communities. Volunteers will provide health care to needy people in the rural area Grassroot health clinic. There are high numbers of orphaned children with HIV/AIDS who need proper medical care. The majority of our patients are children below 10 years and elderly of low income.

(continued)

Placement opportunities for . . .		**Organization/Service Specifics:**	
People of only certain faiths?	No	Size of the Organization's Staff:	11-20
Couples: both are health providers?	No	Number of providers sent or received/year:	1-5
Couples: only one is a health provider?	No	Minimum term of assignment:	3 months
Families with children?	No	Maximum term of assignment:	6 months
Medical students?	Yes	Is funding available for travel?	No
Pre-medical or college students?	No	Are room and board provided?	No
Other health professional students?	Yes	Is any other funding available?	No
Doctors in training?	No	Is training provided or available?	No
Health personnel who are US citizens?	Yes	Is a language other than English required?	No
Health personnel who are non-US citizens?	Yes		
Health personnel with no prior experience in developing countries?	Yes		
Health personnel who are not current members of your organization?	Yes		

Health Professionals Placed:

Physicians:

Physicians; Family Practitioners; Internal Medicine GPS & PCP; Oral Surgeons; Pediatricians

Allied Health Professionals:

Dental Hygienists; Dentists; Medical Technicians (lab, X-ray, etc); Nurse Midwives; Nurse Practitioners; Nurses; Nutritionists & Dieticians; Paramedics; Pharmacists; Physical & Occupational Therapists; Physician Assistants; Public Health Specialists, Epidemiologists and Health Educators; Respiratory Therapists; Social Workers; Water/Sanitation Specialists

Notes

Child Family Health International

Address: **953 Mission Street, Suite 1104, San Francisco, CA 94103 U.S.A.**

Phone: **(415) 957-9000** FAX: **(415) 840-0486**

E-Mail: **students@cfhi.org** Web: **www.cfhi.org**

Continents Served

Africa ☐ Asia ☑ Europe ☐ The Americas ☑

Countries Served

Bolivia, Ecuador, India, Mexico, South Africa

Mission: Child Family Health International supports long-term health care projects and conducts educational programs in Asia and the Americas for medical residents, pre-medical, medical, nursing, public health, and alternative health students. Child Family Health International employs professionals that are local to program sites, whose assignments are short-term (4-8 weeks). There are no religious restrictions. Volunteers must provide their own funding, although room and board are both provided.

Placement opportunities for . . .		**Organization/Service Specifics:**	
People of only certain faiths?	No	Size of the Organization's Staff:	0-5
Couples: both are health providers?	No	Number of providers sent or received/year:	>200
Couples: only one is a health provider?	No	Minimum term of assignment:	4 weeks
Families with children?	No	Maximum term of assignment:	12 weeks
Medical students?	Yes	Is funding available for travel?	No
Pre-medical or college students?	Yes	Are room and board provided?	Yes
Other health professional students?	Yes	Is any other funding available?	Yes
Doctors in training?	Yes	Is training provided or available?	Yes
Health personnel who are US citizens?	Yes	Is a language other than English required? *1*	Yes
Health personnel who are non-US citizens?	Yes		
Health personnel with no prior experience in developing countries?	Yes		
Health personnel who are not current members of your organization?	Yes		

Health Professionals Placed:

Physicians:

Physicians; Family Practitioners; General Surgeons; Infectious Disease Spec.; Internal Medicine GPS & PCP; OB/GYN; Pediatricians; Plastic/Hand/Reconstructive Surgeons

Allied Health Professionals:

Public Health Specialists, Epidemiologists and Health Educators

Notes

1. One of the five Ecuador programs requires a minimal knowledge of Spanish.

Children's Cross Connection, International

Continents Served			
Africa ✔	Asia ☐	Europe ☐	The Americas ✔

Address: **220 Avon Drive, Fayetteville, GA 30215 U.S.A.**

Phone: **(770) 716-1926** FAX: **(770) 632-4009**

E-Mail: **Pam@cccinternational.org** Web: **www.cccinternational.org/index.html**

Countries Served

El Salvador, Ethiopia

Mission: Children's Cross Connection provides primary medical and dental care to rural areas of Ethiopia and El Salvador. We maintain mobile medical/dental teams as well as surgical support for longer term teaching projects within each country. Depending on need, volunteer doctors of all specialty areas are welcome. For each project we staff two teaching teams who rotate for one to two week tours every 6 months until the project can be maintained by the host country's doctors.

Placement opportunities for . . .

People of only certain faiths? *1*	Yes
Couples: both are health providers?	Yes
Couples: only one is a health provider?	No
Families with children?	No
Medical students? *2*	Yes
Pre-medical or college students?	Yes
Other health professional students?	Yes
Doctors in training?	Yes
Health personnel who are US citizens? *3*	Yes
Health personnel who are non-US citizens?	Yes
Health personnel with no prior experience in developing countries?	Yes
Health personnel who are not current members of your organization?	Yes

Organization/Service Specifics:

Size of the Organization's Staff:	6-10
Number of providers sent or received/year:	51-100
Minimum term of assignment:	1 week
Maximum term of assignment: *4*	2 weeks
Is funding available for travel?	No
Are room and board provided?	Yes
Is any other funding available?	No
Is training provided or available?	Yes
Is a language other than English required?	No

Health Professionals Placed:

Physicians:

All physician specialties

Allied Health Professionals:

All allied health professionals

Notes

1. Jewish or Christian; *2.* Students may observe medical procedures and act as support staff only; *3.* Must be accompanied by supervisory physician; *4.* Teaching teams up to 6 months.

Children's HeartLink

Continents Served			
Africa ✔	Asia ✔	Europe ✔	The Americas ✔

Address: **5075 Arcadia Ave. Minneapolis, MN 55436-2306 U.S.A.**

Phone: **(952) 928-4860 x-19** FAX: **(952) 928-4859**

E-Mail: **john@childrensheartlink.org** Web: **www.childrensheartlink.org**

Countries Served

China	Ecuador	Ethiopia
India	Israel	Kenya
Malaysia	USSR, former	

Mission: Children's HeartLink is an international medical charity dedicated to the treatment and prevention of heart disease in needy children. Children's HeartLink works in partnership with medical centers in emerging countries to promote sustainable and quality cardiovascular programs for indigent children.

Placement opportunities for . . .

People of only certain faiths?	No
Couples: both are health providers?	No
Couples: only one is a health provider?	No
Families with children?	No
Medical students?	No
Pre-medical or college students?	No
Other health professional students? *1*	Yes
Doctors in training?	No
Health personnel who are US citizens?	Yes
Health personnel who are non-US citizens?	Yes
Health personnel with no prior experience in developing countries?	Yes
Health personnel who are not current members of your organization?	Yes

Organization/Service Specifics:

Size of the Organization's Staff:	6-10
Number of providers sent or received/year:	51-100
Minimum term of assignment:	1 week
Maximum term of assignment:	3 months
Is funding available for travel?	Yes
Are room and board provided?	Yes
Is any other funding available?	No
Is training provided or available?	No
Is a language other than English required? *2*	Yes

(continued)

Health Professionals Placed:

Physicians:

Anesthesiologists; Cardiologists; General Surgeons; Infectious Disease Spec.

Allied Health Professionals:

Nurses

Notes

1. Public Health specialists;
2. Languages are preferred depending on the country.

Children's Medical Mission

Continents Served

Africa ☐ Asia ☑ Europe ☐ The Americas ☐

Countries Served

China

Address: **97 S. Professional Way, Payson, UT 84651 U.S.A.**

Phone: **(801) 465-4896** FAX: **(801) 465-4107**

E-Mail: **robclark@mstar.net** Web:

Mission: Children's Medical Mission provides short term training for physicians in developing countries to reduce maternal and newborn morbidity and mortality. There are no religious or language requirements and volunteers can serve for 1-3 week assignments. Training is available, but volunteers must provide their own funding for room and board and travel expenses.

Placement opportunities for . . .		**Organization/Service Specifics:**	
People of only certain faiths?	No	Size of the Organization's Staff:	0-5
Couples: both are health providers?	Yes	Number of providers sent or received/year:	11-20
Couples: only one is a health provider?	Yes	Minimum term of assignment:	1 weeks
Families with children?	Yes	Maximum term of assignment:	3 weeks
Medical students?	No	Is funding available for travel?	No
Pre-medical or college students?	No	Are room and board provided?	No
Other health professional students?	No	Is any other funding available?	No
Doctors in training?	Yes	Is training provided or available?	Yes
Health personnel who are US citizens?	Yes	Is a language other than English required?	No
Health personnel who are non-US citizens?	Yes		
Health personnel with no prior experience in developing countries?	Yes		
Health personnel who are not current members of your organization?	Yes		

Health Professionals Placed:

Physicians:

Physicians; Family Practitioners; OB/GYN; Pediatricians

Allied Health Professionals:

Nurses

Notes

Christian Dental Missions

Continents Served

Africa ☑ Asia ☑ Europe ☐ The Americas ☑

Countries Served

Bolivia	Ecuador	Haiti
Honduras	India	Korea, South
Mexico	Sierra Leone	Venezuela

Address: **64 Main Ave, Ocean Grove, NJ 07756 U.S.A.**

Phone: **(732) 774-8700** FAX: **(732) 774-8708**

E-Mail: **whildens@aol.com** Web:

Mission: The purpose of this organization shall be to promote, support and expand dental and health services to residents, missionaries, religious workers and all others in the mission fields of the United States and foreign countries by providing money, equipment, supplies, instruments, books and personnel, and in other ways helping those in need for the ultimate objective of advancing the Gospel of the Lord Jesus Christ throughout the world.

(continued)

Placement opportunities for . . .

People of only certain faiths? *1*	Yes
Couples: both are health providers?	Yes
Couples: only one is a health provider?	Yes
Families with children? *2*	Yes
Medical students?	No
Pre-medical or college students?	No
Other health professional students?	Yes
Doctors in training?	Yes
Health personnel who are US citizens?	Yes
Health personnel who are non-US citizens?	Yes
Health personnel with no prior experience in developing countries?	Yes
Health personnel who are not current members of your organization?	Yes

Organization/Service Specifics:

Size of the Organization's Staff:	0-5
Number of providers sent or received/year:	11-20
Minimum term of assignment:	1 week
Maximum term of assignment:	2 weeks
Is funding available for travel?	No
Are room and board provided?	Yes
Is any other funding available?	No
Is training provided or available?	No
Is a language other than English required?	No

Health Professionals Placed:

Physicians:

Allied Health Professionals:

Dental Hygienists; Dentists

Notes

1. Volunteers must be Protestant; *2.* Volunteers may bring teenaged children.

Christian Dental Society

Address: **PO Box 296, Sumner, IA 50674 U.S.A.**

Phone: **(800) 237-7368**
(563) 578-8887 FAX: **(800) 237-7368**

E-Mail: **twendel@christiandental.org** Web: **www.christiandental.org**

Mission: The Christian Dental Society is a fellowship and service organization that functions to provide oral health care to those in need. For over a quarter of a century, CDS has been a leader in dental missions worldwide. Traditionally, there have been far fewer dental mission volunteers compared to those involved in medical outreach programs. The need for short and long term dental outreach efforts continues into the new millenium. However, with the advances in portable equipment and increased exposure to potential volunteers, opportunities to relieve pain and suffering in the name of our Lord have rapidly expanded. The Christian Dental Society serves Christian dental efforts on an international basis. It cooperates with churches, volunteer agencies, and service organizations to provide volunteers, equipment, and supplies.

Continents Served

Africa ☑ Asia ☑ Europe ☑ The Americas ☑

Countries Served

Brazil, Cambodia, Cameroon, China, Colombia, Costa Rica, Dominican Republic, Ecuador, Guatemala, Haiti, Honduras, India, Jamaica, Laos, Mexico, Nepal, Nicaragua, Pakistan, Papua-New Guinea, Philippines, Singapore, Swaziland, United States, USSR, former, Vietnam, Zimbabwe

Placement opportunities for . . .

People of only certain faiths? *1*	Yes
Couples: both are health providers?	Yes
Couples: only one is a health provider?	Yes
Families with children?	Yes
Medical students?	Yes
Pre-medical or college students?	No
Other health professional students?	Yes
Doctors in training?	Yes
Health personnel who are US citizens?	Yes
Health personnel who are non-US citizens?	Yes
Health personnel with no prior experience in developing countries?	Yes
Health personnel who are not current members of your organization?	Yes

Organization/Service Specifics:

Size of the Organization's Staff:	0-5
Number of providers sent or received/year:	21-50
Minimum term of assignment:	1 week
Maximum term of assignment:	2 years
Is funding available for travel?	No
Are room and board provided?	No
Is any other funding available?	No
Is training provided or available?	Yes
Is a language other than English required?	No

Health Professionals Placed:

Physicians:

Oral Surgeons

Allied Health Professionals:

Dental Hygienists; Dentists

Notes

1. We seek dental professionals and students of Christian faith.

Christian Medical and Dental Associations- Global Health Outreach

Continents Served			
Africa ✔	Asia ☐	Europe ✔	The Americas ✔

Address: **PO Box 7500, Bristol, TN 37621 U.S.A.**

Phone: **(423) 844-1079, (423) 844-1000 or (888) 231-2637** FAX: **(423) 764-1417 (423) 844-1005**

E-Mail: **gho@cmdahome.org** Web: **www.cmdahome.org**

Countries Served

Afghanistan	Cameroon	China
Ecuador	El Salvador	Haiti
Honduras	Kenya	Maldova
Mexico	Nigeria	United States

Mission: The Christian Medical and Dental Associations (CMDA) are made up of the Christian Medical Association (CMA) and the Christian Dental Association (CDA). CMDA serves as a voice and ministry for Christian doctors. Founded in 1931, CMDA provides programs and services supporting its mission to "change hearts in healthcare" with a current membership of more than 17,800. CMDA promotes positions and addresses policies on healthcare issues; conducts overseas medical evangelism projects through its mission arm, Global Health Outreach; coordinates a network of Christian doctors for fellowship and professional growth; sponsors student ministries in medical and dental schools; distributes educational and inspirational resources; hosts marriage and family conferences; provides Third World missionary doctors with continuing education resources; and conducts academic exchange programs overseas.

Placement opportunities for . . .

People of only certain faiths? *1*	Yes
Couples: both are health providers?	Yes
Couples: only one is a health provider?	Yes
Families with children?	Yes
Medical students?	No
Pre-medical or college students?	No
Other health professional students?	No
Doctors in training?	Yes
Health personnel who are US citizens?	Yes
Health personnel who are non-US citizens?	Yes
Health personnel with no prior experience in developing countries?	Yes
Health personnel who are not current members of your organization?	Yes

Organization/Service Specifics:

Size of the Organization's Staff:	51-100
Number of providers sent or received/year:	>200
Minimum term of assignment:	1 week
Maximum term of assignment:	
Is funding available for travel?	No
Are room and board provided?	No
Is any other funding available?	No
Is training provided or available?	
Is a language other than English required?	No

Health Professionals Placed:

Physicians:

Not specified

Allied Health Professionals:

Not specified

Notes

1. Christian.

Christian Medical College (Vellore, India) Board

Continents Served			
Africa ☐	Asia ✔	Europe ☐	The Americas ☐

Address: **475 Riverside Drive, Ste 243, New York, NY 10115 U.S.A.**

Phone: **(212) 870-2640 (800) 875-6370** FAX: **(212) 870-2173**

E-Mail: **usaboard@vellorecmc.org** Web: **www.vellorecmc.org/index.html**

Countries Served

India

Mission: The Christian Medical College (CMC) in Vellore, India, is a major college and teaching hospital in South India which welcomes health professionals from around the world as volunteers. Volunteering needs vary with the needs of the hospital and college. CMC is especially interested in health care professionals who bring both a high level of expertise and a genuine desire to assist those less fortunate. As a major hospital and medical college, there are possibilities in all areas of health care. Volunteers are expected to pay for their costs including transportation to and from Vellore, lodging and living expenses (relatively inexpensive lodging is usually available on campus). The Vellore Board (NY) helps expedite the program for volunteers from North America by acting as a liason between the volunteer and CMC staff. Volunteers in the U.K. should contact the U.K. Friends of Vellore, while those in Australia can contact the Australian Friends of Vellore. Volunteers in other parts of the world can contact CMC/Vellore directly.

(continued)

Placement opportunities for . . .		Organization/Service Specifics:	
People of only certain faiths?	No	Size of the Organization's Staff:	6-10
Couples: both are health providers?	No	Number of providers sent or received/year:	6-10
Couples: only one is a health provider?	No	Minimum term of assignment:	2 weeks
Families with children?	No	Maximum term of assignment:	6 months
Medical students?	Yes	Is funding available for travel?	No
Pre-medical or college students?	No	Are room and board provided?	No
Other health professional students?	Yes	Is any other funding available?	No
Doctors in training?	Yes	Is training provided or available?	No
Health personnel who are US citizens?	Yes	Is a language other than English required?	No
Health personnel who are non-US citizens?	Yes		
Health personnel with no prior experience in developing countries?	Yes		
Health personnel who are not current members of your organization?	Yes		

Health Professionals Placed:

Notes

Physicians:

All physician specialties

Allied Health Professionals:

All allied health professionals

Christian Mission of Pignon Inc.

Address: **1200 Harpeth Lake Ct., Nashville, TN 37221 U.S.A.**

Phone: **(615) 646-5773** FAX: **(615) 646-5773**

E-Mail: **david.wilkins@pignon.org or CMPHaiti@aol.com** Web: **www.pignon.org**

Continents Served

Africa ☐ Asia ☐ Europe ☐ The Americas ☑

Countries Served

Haiti

Mission: The Comite de Bienfaisance de Pignon (CBP) is a non-governmental organization (NGO), officially recognized by the Republic of Haiti on September 6, 1984. The Christian Mission of Pignon, which was founded by Haitian-born and US trained surgeon Dr. Guy D. Theodore, carries out endeavors aimed at improving spiritual and socio-economic conditions for the population within its area. There is a preventive and curative medicine program run by the Hospital de Bienfaisance de Pignon, a full service hospital providing care and training, with its four satellite centers. Volunteers can serve from 1 week to 1 month. There are no language requirements and volunteers are responsible for their own funding.

Placement opportunities for . . .		Organization/Service Specifics:	
People of only certain faiths?	No	Size of the Organization's Staff:	0-5
Couples: both are health providers?	Yes	Number of providers sent or received/year:	21-50
Couples: only one is a health provider?	Yes	Minimum term of assignment:	1 week
Families with children?	No	Maximum term of assignment:	1 month
Medical students?	Yes	Is funding available for travel?	No
Pre-medical or college students?	Yes	Are room and board provided?	No
Other health professional students?	Yes	Is any other funding available?	No
Doctors in training?	Yes	Is training provided or available?	No
Health personnel who are US citizens?	Yes	Is a language other than English required?	No
Health personnel who are non-US citizens?	Yes		
Health personnel with no prior experience in developing countries?	Yes		
Health personnel who are not current members of your organization?	Yes		

Health Professionals Placed:

Notes

Physicians:

Physicians; Anesthesiologists; Cardiologists; Family Practitioners; General Surgeons; Hematologists; Oncologists; Infectious Disease Spec.; Internal Medicine GPS & PCP; OB/GYN; Ophthalmologists; Oral Surgeons; Optometrists; Orthopedic Surgeons; Pediatricians; Plastic/Hand/Reconstructive Surgeons; Pulmonary Specialists

Allied Health Professionals:

Administrative Health Positions; Dental Hygienists; Dentists; Medical Technicians (lab, X-ray, etc); Nurse Practitioners; Nurses; Pharmacists; Physical & Occupational Therapists; Public Health Specialists, Epidemiologists and Health Educators; Respiratory Therapists; Water/Sanitation Specialists

Christoffel-Blindenmission EV

Address: **Nibelungenstrasse 124 / D 64625 Bensheim, Hesse Germany**

Phone: **49 6251 131 182** FAX: **49 6251 131 270**

E-Mail: **Melanie.Raum@cbm-i.org** Web: **www.cbmi.org**

Mission: Since 1908 CBMI has been an independent interdenominational fellowship of committed professionals, dedicated to serving eye patients, blind and otherwise disabled people in the developing world, irrespective of nationality, race, sex, or religion. The work of CBMI centers around medical care—preventing and curing blindness—as well as the rehabilitation and training of disabled people and their integration into society. The main objective of the CBMI ophthalmologists, orthopedic surgeons, nurses, special teachers and rehabilitation experts is to equip and empower national specialists.

Continents Served

Africa ✔ Asia ✔ Europe ✔ The Americas ✔

Countries Served

Afghanistan, Argentina, Bangladesh, Belarus, Belize, Benin, Bhutan, Bolivia, Bosnia, Herzegovina, Botswana, Bulgaria, Burkina Faso, Burundi, Cambodia, Cameroon, Caroline Islands, Central African Rep., Chad, Chile, China, Congo, Costa Rica, Croatia, Cuba, Czech Republic, Djibouti, Dominican Republic, Ecuador, Egypt, El Salvador, Equatorial Guinea, Eritrea, Ethiopia, Fiji, Gabon, Gambia, Georgia, Germany, Ghana, Grenada, Guatemala, Guinea, Guinea-Bissau, Haiti, Honduras, India, Indonesia, Iran, Israel, Ivory Coast, Jamaica, Jordan, Kenya, Laos, Latvia, Lebanon, Lesotho, Liberia, Lithuania, Madagascar, Malawi, Malaysia, Mali, Mauritius, Mexico, Mongolia, Morocco, Namibia, Nepal, Nicaragua, Niger, Nigeria, Pakistan, Papua-New Guinea, Paraguay, Peru, Philippines, Poland, Russia, Rwanda, Samoa, Senegal, Sierra Leone, South Africa, Sri Lanka, Sudan, Swaziland, Syria, Tanzania, Thailand, Togo, Tonga, Trinidad and Tobago, Uganda, Ukraine, Uruguay, Vanuatu, Venezuela, Vietnam, Yemen, Zaire (DemRepCongo), Zambia, Zimbabwe

Placement opportunities for . . .

People of only certain faiths? *1*	Yes
Couples: both are health providers?	No
Couples: only one is a health provider?	Yes
Families with children?	Yes
Medical students?	No
Pre-medical or college students?	No
Other health professional students?	No
Doctors in training?	No
Health personnel who are US citizens?	Yes
Health personnel who are non-US citizens?	Yes
Health personnel with no prior experience in developing countries?	No
Health personnel who are not current members of your organization?	Yes

Organization/Service Specifics:

Size of the Organization's Staff:	101-150
Number of providers sent or received/year:	11-20
Minimum term of assignment:	2 years
Maximum term of assignment:	8 years
Is funding available for travel?	Yes
Are room and board provided?	Yes
Is any other funding available? *2*	Yes
Is training provided or available?	Yes
Is a language other than English required? *3*	Yes

Health Professionals Placed:

Physicians:

Ophthalmologists; Optometrists; Orthopedic Surgeons

Allied Health Professionals:

Nurses; Physical & Occupational Therapists

Notes

1. Volunteers must be Christian; *2.* Salary is based on German schemes; *3.* French for West Africa, Spanish for Latin America.

Church of the Nazarene World Mission Division

Address: **6401 The Paseo, Kansas City, MO 64131-1213 U.S.A.**

Phone: **(816) 333-7000, ext. 2350** FAX: **(816) 822-8296**

E-Mail: **nmi@nazarene.org** Web: **www.nazarene.org/**

Continents Served

Africa ✔ Asia ✔ Europe ✔ The Americas ✔

Countries Served

Australia, Brazil, India, Korea, South, Mexico, New Zealand, Papua-New Guinea, Philippines, Swaziland

Mission: The Church of the Nazarene offers many opportunities for volunteer ministries. In fact, the Church of the Nazarene is the second-largest of United States volunteer sending agencies. Thousands of people of all ages volunteer their time and talents for missions around the world. A main avenue of volunteer ministry through the Church of the Nazarene is the Nazarene Health Care Fellowship, through which health professionals serve in a specific site for one week to three years.

Placement opportunities for . . .	
People of only certain faiths? *1*	Yes
Couples: both are health providers?	Yes
Couples: only one is a health provider?	Yes
Families with children?	Yes
Medical students?	Yes
Pre-medical or college students?	No
Other health professional students?	Yes
Doctors in training?	Yes
Health personnel who are US citizens?	Yes
Health personnel who are non-US citizens?	Yes
Health personnel with no prior experience in developing countries?	Yes
Health personnel who are not current members of your organization?	Yes

Organization/Service Specifics:	
Size of the Organization's Staff:	>200
Number of providers sent or received/year:	1-5
Minimum term of assignment:	3 month
Maximum term of assignment:	4 year
Is funding available for travel?	Yes
Are room and board provided?	Yes
Is any other funding available? *2*	Yes
Is training provided or available?	No
Is a language other than English required?	No

Health Professionals Placed:

Physicians:

Physicians

Allied Health Professionals:

Administrative Health Positions; Nurses

Notes

1. Protestant; *2.* Negotiable.

Clinica Evangelica Morava Elective

Address: **203 West Bank St., Winston-Salem, NC 27101 U.S.A.**

Phone: **(336) 724-5786** FAX:

E-Mail: **rcamail@rca.org** Web:

Continents Served

Africa ☐ Asia ☐ Europe ☐ The Americas ✔

Countries Served

Honduras

Mission: Clinica Evangelica Morava serves Northeastern Honduras. Volunteers in most medical fields are needed. Volunteers staying several months may be able to receive a stipend. Urgently needed volunteers may be accepted without Spanish language proficiency. The need is greatest for Family Practitioners, General Surgeons, OB/GYN, Ophthalmologists, Pediatricians and Water Specialist.

Placement opportunities for . . .	
People of only certain faiths? *1*	Yes
Couples: both are health providers?	Yes
Couples: only one is a health provider?	No
Families with children?	No
Medical students?	No
Pre-medical or college students?	No
Other health professional students?	No
Doctors in training?	Yes
Health personnel who are US citizens?	Yes
Health personnel who are non-US citizens?	Yes
Health personnel with no prior experience in developing countries? *3*	Yes
Health personnel who are not current members of your organization?	Yes

Organization/Service Specifics:	
Size of the Organization's Staff:	0-5
Number of providers sent or received/year:	1-5
Minimum term of assignment:	2 weeks
Maximum term of assignment:	6 months
Is funding available for travel?	No
Are room and board provided?	No
Is any other funding available?	No
Is training provided or available?	No
Is a language other than English required? *2*	Yes

(continued)

Health Professionals Placed:

Physicians:

Physicians; Anesthesiologists; Dermatologists; Emergency Medicine Physicians; Family Practitioners; General Surgeons; Infectious Disease Spec.; Internal Medicine GPS & PCP

Allied Health Professionals:

Notes

1. Christian or sympathetic to Christian outreach programs; *2.* Spanish; *3.* Experience preferred.

Clínica Maxena

Continents Served

Africa ☐ Asia ☐ Europe ☐ The Americas ☑

Countries Served

Guatemala India Russia

Address: **Santo Tomas La Union Suchitepequez, 10017 Guatemala, C.A.**

Phone: **(502) 872-8107** FAX: **(502) 872-8107**

E-Mail: **cm10017@intelnet.net.gt** Web:

Mission: Clínica Maxena serves a parish covering a large mountainous area of Solola and the indiginous Mayans. We struggle at times to maintain funding for the clinic and we appreciate hardworking, conscientious, respectful volunteers who want to work hard and contribute. We cannot accommodate guests of volunteers. Greatest needs are for dental/oral specialists, radiologists and radiology techs, and medical support.

Placement opportunities for . . .		Organization/Service Specifics:	
People of only certain faiths? *1*	Yes	Size of the Organization's Staff:	6-10
Couples: both are health providers?	Yes	Number of providers sent or received/year:	6-10
Couples: only one is a health provider?	No	Minimum term of assignment:	1 month
Families with children?	No	Maximum term of assignment:	1 year
Medical students?	No	Is funding available for travel?	No
Pre-medical or college students?	No	Are room and board provided?	No
Other health professional students?	No	Is any other funding available?	No
Doctors in training?	No	Is training provided or available?	No
Health personnel who are US citizens?	Yes	Is a language other than English required? *2*	Yes
Health personnel who are non-US citizens?	Yes		
Health personnel with no prior experience in developing countries?	Yes		
Health personnel who are not current members of your organization?	Yes		

Health Professionals Placed:

Physicians:

Physicians; Dermatologists; Emergency Medicine Physicians; Endocrinologists; Family Practitioners; Infectious Disease Spec.; Internal Medicine GPS & PCP; OB/GYN; Ophthalmologists; Oral Surgeons; Orthopedic Surgeons; Pediatricians; Pulmonary Specialists; Radiologists

Allied Health Professionals:

Dentists; Medical Technicians (lab, X-ray, etc); Nurse Practitioners; Nurses; Nutritionists & Dieticians; Physician Assistants; Public Health Specialists, Epidemiologists and Health Educators; Social Workers; Water/Sanitation Specialists

Notes

1. Christian; *2.* Spanish.

College of Medicine, Malawi

Continents Served

Africa ☑ Asia ☐ Europe ☐ The Americas ☐

Countries Served

Malawi

Address: **Private Bag 360 Chichiri, Blanty RE3, Malawi**

Phone: **+265 (0) 1 677 245** FAX: **674700673148 or +265 (0) 1 674 700**

E-Mail: **Principal@medcol.mw** Web: **www.medcol.mw/**

Mission: College of Medicine aims to provide training to Malawian doctors, to cater to the specific health needs of Malawi, and to conduct research of the highest quality to address the health needs of Malawi. Health care personnel, physicians, medical students, and a limited number of residents are offered the opportunity for 8-week to 2-year stays in Malawi, where room and board and training are provided.

(continued)

Placement opportunities for . . .

People of only certain faiths?	No
Couples: both are health providers?	Yes
Couples: only one is a health provider?	Yes
Families with children?	Yes
Medical students?	Yes
Pre-medical or college students?	
Other health professional students?	No
Doctors in training? *1*	Yes
Health personnel who are US citizens?	Yes
Health personnel who are non-US citizens?	Yes
Health personnel with no prior experience in developing countries?	Yes
Health personnel who are not current members of your organization?	Yes

Organization/Service Specifics:

Size of the Organization's Staff:	51-100
Number of providers sent or received/year:	unlimited
Minimum term of assignment:	8 weeks
Maximum term of assignment:	2 years
Is funding available for travel?	No
Are room and board provided?	Yes
Is any other funding available?	No
Is training provided or available?	Yes
Is a language other than English required?	No

Health Professionals Placed:

Physicians:

Physicians; Anesthesiologists; Cardiologists; Dermatologists; Emergency Medicine Physicians; Endocrinologists; Family Practitioners; Gastroenterologists; General Surgeons; Hematologists; Oncologists; Infectious Disease Spec.; Internal Medicine GPS & PCP; Nephrologists; Neurologists; Neurosurgeons; OB/GYN; Ophthalmologists; Oral Surgeons; Orthopedic Surgeons; Otolaryngologists; Pathologists; Pediatricians; Plastic/Hand/Reconstructive Surgeons; Psychiatrists; Pulmonary Specialists; Radiologists; Urologists

Allied Health Professionals:

Administrative Health Positions; Dentists; Medical Technicians (lab, X-ray, etc); Nutritionists & Dieticians; Paramedics; Psychologists; Public Health Specialists, Epidemiologists and Health Educators

Notes

1. Space for doctors in training is limited.

Comitato Collaborazione Medica (Doctors for Developing Countries)

Continents Served

Africa ☑ Asia ☐ Europe ☐ The Americas ☑

Countries Served

Burundi, Guatemala, Kenya, Sudan, Uganda

Address: **Corso Giovanni Lanza, 100 Torino, 10133 Italy**

Phone: **(011) 660-2793** FAX: **(011) 383-9455**

E-Mail: **ccm@comitato medico.191.it** Web: **www.ccm-italia.org/**

Mission: The CCM, a non-governmental organization (NGO), was formed in Turin, Italy, in 1968 with the purpose of promoting international aid by the assistance of civil volunteers to health programs. By its programs, the CCM intends to promote, besides the development of curative medicine, the implementation of Primary Health Care and Expanded Programs of Immunization advocated by WHO and accepted by Developing Countries. A special effort is made to train local personnel for health care and health education, in order to assure the autonomy of newly-established services. CCM has short term (3 month) and longer term (2 years) trips. French is a required language for some placements but there are no religious requirements.

Placement opportunities for . . .

People of only certain faiths?	No
Couples: both are health providers?	Yes
Couples: only one is a health provider?	Yes
Families with children?	Yes
Medical students?	No
Pre-medical or college students?	No
Other health professional students?	Yes
Doctors in training?	Yes
Health personnel who are US citizens?	No
Health personnel who are non-US citizens?	Yes
Health personnel with no prior experience in developing countries?	No
Health personnel who are not current members of your organization?	Yes

Organization/Service Specifics:

Size of the Organization's Staff:	0-5
Number of providers sent or received/year:	6-10
Minimum term of assignment:	3 month
Maximum term of assignment:	2 years
Is funding available for travel?	Yes
Are room and board provided?	Yes
Is any other funding available? *1*	Yes
Is training provided or available?	No
Is a language other than English required? *2*	Yes

Health Professionals Placed:

Physicians:

General Surgeons; Internal Medicine GPS & PCP

Allied Health Professionals:

Administrative Health Positions; Nurse Midwives

Notes

1. Other funding depends on the length of the misson period;
2. French may be required for some assignments.

Commonwealth Health Center

Address: **P.O. Box 500-409 CK Saipan, MP 96950-0409 U.S.A.**

Phone: **(670) 236-8206 or (670) 234-8950 x-2702/03** FAX: **(670) 236-8638 (670) 234-8930**

E-Mail: **bjohnson@gtepacifica.net** Web: **www.dphsaipan.com/**

Continents Served
Africa ☐ Asia ☑ Europe ☐ The Americas ☐

Countries Served
Northern Mariana Isl.

Mission: The Commonwealth Health Center is the only island hospital of the Northern Mariana Islands. The general mission of the facility is to provide the best possible quality medical care, in a respectful and caring manner, to all NMI residents, guest workers, and visitors. Volunteers can serve for short-term (1 week) to longer term (1 year) assignments. There are no religious or language requirements.

Placement opportunities for . . .		Organization/Service Specifics:	
People of only certain faiths?	No	Size of the Organization's Staff:	21-50
Couples: both are health providers?	Yes	Number of providers sent or received/year:	6-10
Couples: only one is a health provider?	Yes	Minimum term of assignment:	1 week
Families with children?	Yes	Maximum term of assignment:	1 year
Medical students?	No	Is funding available for travel?	Yes
Pre-medical or college students?	No	Are room and board provided?	Yes
Other health professional students?	Yes	Is any other funding available?	No
Doctors in training?	Yes	Is training provided or available?	Yes
Health personnel who are US citizens?	Yes	Is a language other than English required?	No
Health personnel who are non-US citizens?	Yes		
Health personnel with no prior experience in developing countries?	Yes		
Health personnel who are not current members of your organization?	Yes		

Health Professionals Placed: **Notes**

Physicians:

Physicians; Anesthesiologists; Cardiologists; Dermatologists; Emergency Medicine Physicians; Gastroenterologists; General Surgeons; Infectious Disease Spec.; Internal Medicine GPS & PCP; Nephrologists; OB/GYN; Orthopedic Surgeons; Otolaryngologists; Pathologists; Pediatricians; Psychiatrists; Radiologists

Allied Health Professionals:

Dentists; Medical Technicians (lab, X-ray, etc); Nurse Midwives; Nurse Practitioners; Nutritionists & Dieticians; Pharmacists; Physical & Occupational Therapists; Physician Assistants; Respiratory Therapists

---

Community of Caring

Address: **245 East 8th St, Erie, PA 16503 U.S.A.**

Phone: **(814) 456-6661** FAX: **(814) 459-5864**

E-Mail: **caring@velocity.net** Web:

Continents Served
Africa ☑ Asia ☐ Europe ☐ The Americas ☑

Countries Served
Colombia, Cuba, Dominican Republic, Haiti, Ivory Coast, Liberia, Sierra Leone, Zaire (DemRepCongo), Zambia

Mission: The mission of the Community of Caring is to help impoverished people throughout the world to meet their unmet needs, both physical (food, clothing, and shelter) and spiritual, so far as resources permit. This is to be done in a caring and compassionate way, reflecting the love of Christ, so as to preserve the dignity of the individual. Family practitioners are particularly needed for 1-3 week assignments. While there are no religious requirements, most volunteers have been Christian.

Placement opportunities for . . .		Organization/Service Specifics:	
People of only certain faiths? *1*	No	Size of the Organization's Staff:	11-20
Couples: both are health providers?	Yes	Number of providers sent or received/year:	11-20
Couples: only one is a health provider?	Yes	Minimum term of assignment:	1 weeks
Families with children?	Yes	Maximum term of assignment: *3*	3 weeks
Medical students?	Yes	Is funding available for travel?	No
Pre-medical or college students?	Yes	Are room and board provided?	Yes
Other health professional students?	Yes	Is any other funding available?	No
Doctors in training?	Yes	Is training provided or available?	Yes
Health personnel who are US citizens?	Yes	Is a language other than English required? *2*	No
Health personnel who are non-US citizens?	Yes		
Health personnel with no prior experience in developing countries?	Yes		
Health personnel who are not current members of your organization?	Yes		

(continued)

Health Professionals Placed:

Physicians:

Physicians; Family Practitioners

Allied Health Professionals:

Nurse Midwives; Physician Assistants; Prosthetists; Psychologists; Water/Sanitation Specialists

Notes

1. Volunteers have been predominantly Christian, but they are open to non-Christians as well; *2.* French and Spanish are desirable for some assignments; *3.* Longer term assignments can be arranged.

Complete Basic Health 2000

Continents Served			
Africa ☑	Asia ☐	Europe ☐	The Americas ☐

Address: **15401 Suffolk Lane, Chagrin Falls, OH 44022 U.S.A.**

Phone: **(216) 541-3600**
(888) 505-6566

FAX: **(216) 541-5528**

E-Mail: **etuffuor@aol.com**

Web: **ghanacare.org**

Countries Served

Ghana

Mission: The mission of Complete Basic Health 2000 is to promote goodwill and understanding among people through exchange of medical knowledge and to provide medical services to the needy. Physicians can travel to Ghana for a minimum of 1 month. There are no language or religious requirements. Funding is provided for room and board. Additional funding is available for longer than 1 year terms.

Placement opportunities for . . .	
People of only certain faiths?	No
Couples: both are health providers?	Yes
Couples: only one is a health provider?	Yes
Families with children?	Yes
Medical students?	Yes
Pre-medical or college students?	Yes
Other health professional students?	Yes
Doctors in training?	Yes
Health personnel who are US citizens?	Yes
Health personnel who are non-US citizens?	Yes
Health personnel with no prior experience in developing countries?	Yes
Health personnel who are not current members of your organization?	Yes

Organization/Service Specifics:	
Size of the Organization's Staff:	0-5
Number of providers sent or received/year:	6-10
Minimum term of assignment:	1 month
Maximum term of assignment:	no limit
Is funding available for travel?	No
Are room and board provided?	Yes
Is any other funding available? *1*	Yes
Is training provided or available?	No
Is a language other than English required?	No

Health Professionals Placed:

Physicians:

Physicians; Emergency Medicine Physicians; Gastroenterologists; General Surgeons; Internal Medicine GPS & PCP; OB/GYN; Orthopedic Surgeons; Urologists

Allied Health Professionals:

Medical Technicians (lab, X-ray, etc); Physical & Occupational Therapists

Notes

1. Additional funding is available if longer than a 1-year term.

CONCERN

Continents Served			
Africa ☑	Asia ☑	Europe ☐	The Americas ☐

Address: **52-55 Lower Camden Street, Dublin 2, Ireland**

Phone: **01 417 7700 or 7706 (J. Jennings)**

FAX: **01 475 7362**

E-Mail: **joe.jennings@concern.net**

Web: **www.concern.ie**

Countries Served

Afghanistan	Angola	Bangladesh
Burundi	Cambodia	Dominica
Eritrea	Ethiopia	Haiti
India	Kenya	Korea, North
Laos	Liberia	Malawi
Montserrat	Mozambique	Niger
Pakistan	Rwanda	Sierra Leone
Somalia	St. Kitts	Sudan
Tanzania	Timor Leste	Uganda
Zaire (DemRepCongo)		Zambia

Mission: CONCERN is a voluntary non-governmental organization devoted to the relief, assistance and advancement of peoples in need in less developed areas of the world. CONCERN directs its resources towards people who live in extreme or absolute poverty. Our integrated program strategy towards poverty elimination is carried out in three key areas: emergency response, development work, and advocacy & development education. Assignments are 2 years long. Funding for travel and room and board, as well as a monthly allowance are provided. French or Portuguese may be required for some assignments. *(continued)*

Placement opportunities for . . .		Organization/Service Specifics:	
People of only certain faiths?	No	Size of the Organization's Staff:	
Couples: both are health providers?	Yes	Number of providers sent or received/year:	
Couples: only one is a health provider?	Yes	Minimum term of assignment:	2 years
Families with children?	Yes	Maximum term of assignment:	2 years
Medical students?	No	Is funding available for travel?	Yes
Pre-medical or college students?	No	Are room and board provided?	Yes
Other health professional students?	No	Is any other funding available? *1*	Yes
Doctors in training?	No	Is training provided or available?	Yes
Health personnel who are US citizens?	Yes	Is a language other than English required? *2*	Yes
Health personnel who are non-US citizens?	Yes		
Health personnel with no prior experience in developing countries?	No		
Health personnel who are not current members of your organization?	Yes		

Health Professionals Placed:

Physicians:

Internal Medicine GPS & PCP

Allied Health Professionals:

Nurse Midwives; Nutritionists & Dieticians; Public Health Specialists, Epidemiologists and Health Educators; Social Workers

Notes

1. Volunteers receive a monthly allowance; *2.* French or Portuguese may be required for some assignments.

CONCERN America

Address: **P.O. Box 1790, Santa Ana, CA 92702 U.S.A.**

Phone: **(714) 953-8575 or (800) 266-2376** FAX: **(714) 953-1242**

E-Mail: **concamerinc@earthlink.net** Web: **www.concernamerica.org**

Continents Served

Africa ☑ Asia ☐ Europe ☐ The Americas ☑

Countries Served

El Salvador, Guatemala, Guinea, Honduras, Mexico, Mozambique, Nicaragua

Mission: CONCERN America is an international development and refugee aid organization, incorporated as an independent nonprofit in California. Through the work of volunteers, who are professionals in the fields of health, public health, nutrition, health education, adult literacy, sanitation, agroforestry, appropriate technology, and community organization, CONCERN America assists impoverished communities and refugees in developing countries in their efforts to improve their living conditions. CONCERN America programs emphasize the training of community members in order to impart skills and knowledge which remain with the community long after the volunteer is gone.

Placement opportunities for . . .		Organization/Service Specifics:	
People of only certain faiths?	No	Size of the Organization's Staff:	6-10
Couples: both are health providers?	Yes	Number of providers sent or received/year:	>200
Couples: only one is a health provider?	Yes	Minimum term of assignment:	2 years
Families with children?	Yes	Maximum term of assignment:	no limit
Medical students?	No	Is funding available for travel?	Yes
Pre-medical or college students?	No	Are room and board provided?	Yes
Other health professional students?	No	Is any other funding available? *1*	Yes
Doctors in training?	No	Is training provided or available?	Yes
Health personnel who are US citizens?	Yes	Is a language other than English required? *2*	Yes
Health personnel who are non-US citizens?	Yes		
Health personnel with no prior experience in developing countries?	Yes		
Health personnel who are not current members of your organization?	Yes		

Health Professionals Placed:

Physicians:

Physicians; Family Practitioners; Internal Medicine GPS & PCP; OB/GYN; Pediatricians

Allied Health Professionals:

Nurse Midwives; Nurse Practitioners; Nurses; Nutritionists & Dieticians; Physician Assistants; Public Health Specialists, Epidemiologists and Health Educators

Notes

1. Stipend of $250 per month plus insurance and registration allowance; *2.* Either Spanish or Portuguese is required depending on the assignment.

Cross-Cultural Solutions

Continents Served			
Africa ✔	Asia ✔	Europe ✔	The Americas ✔

Countries Served

Brazil	China	Costa Rica
Ghana	Guatemala	India
Peru	Russia	Tanzania
Thailand		

Address: **2 Clinton Place, New Rochelle, NY 10801 U.S.A.**

Phone: **(800) 380-4777** **(914) 632-0022** FAX: **(914) 632-8494**

E-Mail: **info@crossculturalsolutions.org** Web: **www.crossculturalsolutions.org/**

Mission: Cross-Cultural Solutions is a nonprofit, public benefit organization that employs volunteer humanitarian action to empower local communities, foster cultural sensitivity and understanding, and contribute grassroots solutions to the global challenge of providing health care and education and promoting social development. It places volunteers for short (1-2 weeks) to long-term (6 months or more) stays in countries around the world. There are no religious or language restrictions. Funding is not provided. The *New York Times* called it "something akin to a mini-stint in the Peace Corps."

Placement opportunities for . . .	
People of only certain faiths?	No
Couples: both are health providers?	Yes
Couples: only one is a health provider?	Yes
Families with children?	Yes
Medical students?	Yes
Pre-medical or college students?	Yes
Other health professional students?	Yes
Doctors in training?	Yes
Health personnel who are US citizens?	Yes
Health personnel who are non-US citizens?	Yes
Health personnel with no prior experience in developing countries?	Yes
Health personnel who are not current members of your organization?	Yes

Organization/Service Specifics:	
Size of the Organization's Staff:	51-100
Number of providers sent or received/year:	101-150
Minimum term of assignment:	3 weeks
Maximum term of assignment:	6 months
Is funding available for travel?	No
Are room and board provided? *1*	No
Is any other funding available?	No
Is training provided or available?	No
Is a language other than English required? *2*	No

Health Professionals Placed:

Physicians:

Not specified

Allied Health Professionals:

Not specified

Notes

1. Live and work with other volunteers as a community in CCS housing (food also part of the package); *2.* Spanish is helpful in Peru but not required. Language training in other countries is provided.

CrossWorld

Continents Served			
Africa ✔	Asia ✔	Europe ☐	The Americas ✔

Countries Served

Brazil	Haiti	Indonesia
Mexico	Zaire (DemRepCongo)	

Address: **306 Bala Avenue, P.O. Box 306, Bala Cynwyd, PA 19004 U.S.A.**

Phone: **(610) 667-7660** FAX: **(610) 660-9068**

E-Mail: **info@crossworld.org** Web: **www.crossworld.org/**

Mission: Missionary organizations consider medical work important because it provides people with an opportunity to have both their physical and spiritual needs met. Missions are not simply charitable institutions concerned only with social privations of people. UFM International's commission puts the priority on proclamation of the Gospel of Jesus Christ, in consideration of one's eternal welfare and salvation. We do, however, care about the whole person and seek also to help them physically. Evangelical Protestant volunteers can serve for a minimum of 3 months and expenses are paid through individual fundraising. Haitian Creole, French, or Indonesian are required depending on the country of service.

(continued)

Placement opportunities for . . .		**Organization/Service Specifics:**	
People of only certain faiths? *1*	Yes	Size of the Organization's Staff:	>200
Couples: both are health providers?	Yes	Number of providers sent or received/year:	6-10
Couples: only one is a health provider?	Yes	Minimum term of assignment:	2 weeks
Families with children?	Yes	Maximum term of assignment:	life
Medical students?	Yes	Is funding available for travel?	No
Pre-medical or college students?		Are room and board provided?	No
Other health professional students?	Yes	Is any other funding available? *2*	No
Doctors in training?	Yes	Is training provided or available?	Yes
Health personnel who are US citizens?	Yes	Is a language other than English required? *3*	Yes
Health personnel who are non-US citizens?	No		
Health personnel with no prior experience in developing countries?	Yes		
Health personnel who are not current members of your organization?	Yes		

Health Professionals Placed:

Physicians:

Physicians; Anesthesiologists; Family Practitioners; General Surgeons; Internal Medicine GPS & PCP; OB/GYN; Pediatricians

Allied Health Professionals:

Dentists; Nurse Midwives; Pharmacists; Water/Sanitation Specialists

Notes

1. Volunteers must be Evangelical Protestant; *2.* Faculty are funded by churches, family, and friends; *3.* Language requirements depend on place of service.

Crudem Foundation

Address: **9043 Ladue Road, St. Louis, MO 63124-1901 U.S.A.**

Phone: **(413) 596-2692** FAX:

E-Mail: **lppjs@aol.com** Web:

Continents Served

Africa ☐ Asia ☐ Europe ☐ The Americas ☑

Countries Served

Haiti

Mission: The Crudem Foundation is a tax exempt public charity whoe purpose is to support Project Crudem in Milot, Haiti. We support a sixty-four bed full service general hospital there. It has a permanent staff of six physicians and one dentist. This care is supplemented by visits of short term volunteer medical teams in practically every specialty, including open heart surgery. In 2000, we had 138 volunteers. Thirty thousand patients were treated at the hospital. A Nutrition Center is also present on the hospital campus, which provides two free meals daily to up to eighty malnourished preschool children. Volunteers can serve for short term (1 week) to longer term (1 year) assignments. The Crudem Foundation has no religious or language requirements.

Placement opportunities for . . .		**Organization/Service Specifics:**	
People of only certain faiths?	No	Size of the Organization's Staff:	0-5
Couples: both are health providers?	Yes	Number of providers sent or received/year:	151-200
Couples: only one is a health provider?	Yes	Minimum term of assignment:	1 week
Families with children?	No	Maximum term of assignment: *1*	1 year
Medical students?	No	Is funding available for travel?	No
Pre-medical or college students?	No	Are room and board provided?	Yes
Other health professional students?	Yes	Is any other funding available?	No
Doctors in training?	Yes	Is training provided or available?	No
Health personnel who are US citizens?	Yes	Is a language other than English required?	No
Health personnel who are non-US citizens?	Yes		
Health personnel with no prior experience in developing countries?	Yes		
Health personnel who are not current members of your organization?	Yes		

Health Professionals Placed:

Physicians:

Physicians; Anesthesiologists; Cardiologists; Family Practitioners; General Surgeons; Hematologists; Oncologists; Infectious Disease Spec.; Internal Medicine GPS & PCP; Neurologists; OB/GYN; Ophthalmologists; Optometrists; Orthopedic Surgeons; Otolaryngologists; Pediatricians; Plastic/Hand/Reconstructive Surgeons; Urologists

Allied Health Professionals:

Medical Technicians (lab, X-ray, etc); Nurses; Nutritionists & Dieticians; Pharmacists; Physical & Occupational Therapists; Physician Assistants; Public Health Specialists, Epidemiologists and Health Educators

Notes

1. Trips generally 1-3 weeks.

Curamericas

Address: **224 East Martin Street, Raleigh, NC 27601 U.S.A.**
Phone: **(919) 821-8000** FAX: **(919) 821-8087**
E-Mail: **twolf@curamericas.org** Web: **www.curamericas.org**

Continents Served
Africa ☐ Asia ☐ Europe ☐ The Americas ☑

Countries Served
Bolivia Guatemala Haiti Mexico

Mission: Moved by our faith, we are committed to the measurable improvement of health and the prevention of unnecessary suffering, sickness, and death. We bring hope through health, working through self-sustaining local partnerships in communities lacking access to basic services.

Placement opportunities for . . .		Organization/Service Specifics:	
People of only certain faiths?	No	Size of the Organization's Staff:	6-10
Couples: both are health providers?	Yes	Number of providers sent or received/year:	151-200
Couples: only one is a health provider?	Yes	Minimum term of assignment: *1*	2 weeks
Families with children?	No	Maximum term of assignment: *2*	1 years
Medical students?	No	Is funding available for travel?	No
Pre-medical or college students?	No	Are room and board provided? *3*	No
Other health professional students?	No	Is any other funding available?	No
Doctors in training?	Yes	Is training provided or available?	Yes
Health personnel who are US citizens?	Yes	Is a language other than English required?	No
Health personnel who are non-US citizens?	No		
Health personnel with no prior experience in developing countries?	Yes		
Health personnel who are not current members of your organization?	No		

Health Professionals Placed:

Physicians:

Physicians; Anesthesiologists; Dermatologists; Emergency Medicine Physicians; Family Practitioners; Gastroenterologists; General Surgeons; Internal Medicine GPS & PCP; Neurologists; OB/GYN; Ophthalmologists; Optometrists; Orthopedic Surgeons; Pediatricians; Psychiatrists; Pulmonary Specialists

Allied Health Professionals:

Dentists; Medical Technicians (lab, X-ray, etc); Nurse Midwives; Nurse Practitioners; Nurses; Pharmacists; Physical & Occupational Therapists; Physician Assistants; Prosthetists; Psychologists; Public Health Specialists, Epidemiologists and Health Educators; Respiratory Therapists

Notes

1. 2 weeks for medical teams and 3 months for individual health volunteer; *2.* 2 weeks for medical teams and 1 year for individual health volunteer; *3.* Room and board are included in the flat rate.

Dental Health International

Address: **847 South Milledge Avenue, Athens, GA 30605-1331 U.S.A.**
Phone: **(706) 546-1716** FAX: **(706) 546-1715**
E-Mail: **bsdds@earthlink.net** Web:

Continents Served
Africa ☑ Asia ☑ Europe ☐ The Americas ☐

Countries Served
Bhutan Cameroon Cook Islands
Lesotho Rwanda Vietnam

Mission: The mission of Dental Health International is to provide dental equipment for remote rural areas of developing countries both portable and fixed, to provide dentists and dental lab personnel in the installation and teaching of operation of the equipment in those areas, and to provide teaching in the surrounding school systems as to the benefits of dentistry. There is a three month commitment for volunteers. Room and board are provided. There are no language or religious requirements.

Placement opportunities for . . .		Organization/Service Specifics:	
People of only certain faiths?	No	Size of the Organization's Staff:	0-5
Couples: both are health providers?	Yes	Number of providers sent or received/year:	
Couples: only one is a health provider?	No	Minimum term of assignment:	3 month
Families with children?	No	Maximum term of assignment:	more
Medical students?	No	Is funding available for travel?	No
Pre-medical or college students?	No	Are room and board provided?	Yes
Other health professional students?	No	Is any other funding available?	No
Doctors in training?	No	Is training provided or available?	Yes
Health personnel who are US citizens?	Yes	Is a language other than English required?	No
Health personnel who are non-US citizens?	No		
Health personnel with no prior experience in developing countries?	Yes		
Health personnel who are not current members of your organization?	Yes		

(continued)

Health Professionals Placed:

Physicians:

Oral Surgeons

Allied Health Professionals:

Dentists; Dental Technicians

Notes

DePauw University Winter Term in Service

Address: **The Hartman Center 500 E. Seminary St., Greencastle, IN 46135 U.S.A.**

Phone: **(765) 658-4355** **(765) 658-8000** FAX: **(765) 658-4868**

E-Mail: **winterterm@depauw.edu** Web: **www.depauw.edu/admin/winterterm/wtis.asp**

Continents Served

Africa ☑ Asia ☑ Europe ☐ The Americas ☑

Countries Served

Argentina	Bangladesh	Bolivia
Costa Rica	Dominican Republic	
Ecuador	El Salvador	Ghana
Guatemala	Haiti	Honduras
Jamaica	Kenya	Mexico
Nicaragua	Nigeria	Paraguay
Philippines	United States	

Mission: The mission of the Winter Term in Service Program is to provide students, faculty members, and professionals with an opportunity to serve others in need while increasing students' awareness and understanding of the interconnectedness of diverse communities through immersion in another culture and critical reflection on their values and experiences. Room and board are provided, but volunteers must provide the rest of the funding. Trips last between 1-3 weeks.

Placement opportunities for . . .

People of only certain faiths?	No
Couples: both are health providers?	Yes
Couples: only one is a health provider?	Yes
Families with children?	No
Medical students?	No
Pre-medical or college students?	No
Other health professional students?	No
Doctors in training?	Yes
Health personnel who are US citizens?	Yes
Health personnel who are non-US citizens?	Yes
Health personnel with no prior experience in developing countries?	Yes
Health personnel who are not current members of your organization?	Yes

Organization/Service Specifics:

Size of the Organization's Staff:	6-10
Number of providers sent or received/year:	11-20
Minimum term of assignment:	1 week
Maximum term of assignment:	3 weeks
Is funding available for travel?	No
Are room and board provided?	Yes
Is any other funding available?	No
Is training provided or available?	No
Is a language other than English required?	No

Health Professionals Placed:

Physicians:

Physicians; Dermatologists; Emergency Medicine Physicians; Family Practitioners; Infectious Disease Spec.; Internal Medicine GPS & PCP; OB/GYN; Optometrists; Pathologists; Pediatricians; Psychiatrists; Pulmonary Specialists; Radiologists; Urologists

Allied Health Professionals:

Dental Hygienists; Dentists; Nurse Midwives; Nurse Practitioners; Nurses; Nutritionists & Dieticians; Paramedics; Pharmacists; Physical & Occupational Therapists; Physician Assistants; Psychologists; Public Health Specialists, Epidemiologists and Health Educators; Respiratory Therapists; Social Workers; Water/Sanitation Specialists

Notes

DoCare International, Inc.

Address: **430 King Avenue, East Dundee, Il 60118 U.S.A.**

Phone: **(847) 836-8022** FAX:

E-Mail: Web: **www.docareintl.org**

Continents Served

Africa ☐ Asia ☐ Europe ☐ The Americas ☑

Countries Served

Ecuador	El Salvador	Guatemala
Mexico	Peru	

Mission: DoCare International has been bringing needed health-care service to primitive and isolated people in the remote areas of the western hemisphere for over 40 years. While DoCare consists of mostly osteopathic physicians, its members also include allopathic physicians, nurses, dentists, veterinarians, pharmacists, optometrists, podiatrists, physician assistants, and interested lay people who contribute special skills. DoCare prefers to have the help of local physicians when possible, and will continue to provide aid until the local medical services are adequate. There are no religious or language requirements, although Spanish is helpful. Interested personnel must first become members of DoCare to become involved with medical service.

Placement opportunities for . . .

People of only certain faiths?	No
Couples: both are health providers?	Yes
Couples: only one is a health provider?	Yes
Families with children?	Yes
Medical students?	Yes
Pre-medical or college students?	Yes
Other health professional students?	Yes
Doctors in training?	Yes
Health personnel who are US citizens?	Yes
Health personnel who are non-US citizens?	No
Health personnel with no prior experience in developing countries?	Yes
Health personnel who are not current members of your organization?	No

Organization/Service Specifics:

Size of the Organization's Staff:	0-5
Number of providers sent or received/year:	>200
Minimum term of assignment:	1 week
Maximum term of assignment:	2 weeks
Is funding available for travel?	No
Are room and board provided?	No
Is any other funding available?	No
Is training provided or available?	
Is a language other than English required? *1*	No

Health Professionals Placed:

Physicians:

Physicians; Cardiologists; Dermatologists; Emergency Medicine Physicians; Family Practitioners; Gastroenterologists; General Surgeons; Infectious Disease Spec.; OB/GYN; Ophthalmologists; Oral Surgeons; Optometrists; Orthopedic Surgeons; Otolaryngologists; Pediatricians; Psychiatrists; Urologists

Allied Health Professionals:

Dentists; Nurse Midwives; Nurse Practitioners; Nurses; Paramedics; Pharmacists; Physical & Occupational Therapists; Physician Assistants; Podiatrists; Public Health Specialists, Epidemiologists and Health Educators

Notes

1. Spanish is not required, but it is helpful.

Doctors for Global Health

Address: **P.O. Box 1761, Decatur, GA 30031 U.S.A.**

Phone: **(979) 774-4079** FAX: **(404) 377-3566**

E-Mail: **development@dghonline.org & dghinfo@dghonline.org** Web: **www.dghonline.org**

Continents Served

Africa ☑ Asia ☐ Europe ☐ The Americas ☑

Countries Served

Argentina	El Salvador	Guatemala
Mexico	Nicaragua	Uganda

Mission: The Doctors for Global Health mission is "to improve health and foster other human rights with those most in need by accompanying communities, while educating and inspiring others to action." The organization works to improve accessibility to health, education, art and other human rights throughout the world. Health care providers are encouraged to go overseas to Spanish speaking countries, and help accomplish their mission.

(continued)

Placement opportunities for . . .

People of only certain faiths?	No
Couples: both are health providers?	Yes
Couples: only one is a health provider?	Yes
Families with children? *1*	No
Medical students?	Yes
Pre-medical or college students?	Yes
Other health professional students?	Yes
Doctors in training?	Yes
Health personnel who are US citizens?	Yes
Health personnel who are non-US citizens?	Yes
Health personnel with no prior experience in developing countries?	Yes
Health personnel who are not current members of your organization?	Yes

Organization/Service Specifics:

Size of the Organization's Staff:	0-5
Number of providers sent or received/year:	>200
Minimum term of assignment:	6 weeks
Maximum term of assignment:	
Is funding available for travel?	No
Are room and board provided?	No
Is any other funding available?	No
Is training provided or available?	No
Is a language other than English required? *2*	Yes

Health Professionals Placed:

Physicians:

Physicians; Emergency Medicine Physicians; Endocrinologists; Family Practitioners; Infectious Disease Spec.; Internal Medicine GPS & PCP; Nephrologists; OB/GYN; Pediatricians

Allied Health Professionals:

Administrative Health Positions; Dental Hygienists; Dentists; Nurse Midwives; Nurse Practitioners; Nurses; Physician Assistants; Psychologists; Public Health Specialists, Epidemiologists and Health Educators; Social Workers; Water/Sanitation Specialists

Notes

1. Do not usually send families with children; *2.* All sites require Spanish, except Uganda, where English is required.

Doctors of the World

Address: **375 W. Broadway, 4th Floor, New York, NY 10012 U.S.A.**

Phone: **(212) 226-9890 or (888) 817-HELP** FAX: **(212) 226-7026**

E-Mail: **info@dowusa.org** Web: **www.doctorsoftheworld.org**

Mission: Doctors of the World is dedicated to improving the health and relieving the suffering of vulnerable populations in the United States and abroad; committed to developing approaches to the delivery of medical care and public health that enhances respect for human dignity; committed to exposing and bearing witness to human rights violations where health is at stake; dedicated to fulfilling the ideals of medicine by encouraging health professionals to provide voluntary services to underserved populations.

Continents Served

Africa ✔ Asia ✔ Europe ✔ The Americas ✔

Countries Served

Afghanistan	Brazil	Cambodia
Canada	El Salvador	Ethiopia
France	Guatemala	Haiti
India	Indonesia	Iran
Kenya	Kosovo	Liberia
Maldova	Mexico	Mozambique
Romania	Russia	South Africa
Sri Lanka	Tanzania	Thailand
United States	Vietnam	
Yugoslavia, former		

Placement opportunities for . . .

People of only certain faiths?	No
Couples: both are health providers?	Yes
Couples: only one is a health provider?	Yes
Families with children?	Yes
Medical students?	No
Pre-medical or college students?	No
Other health professional students?	No
Doctors in training?	No
Health personnel who are US citizens?	Yes
Health personnel who are non-US citizens?	Yes
Health personnel with no prior experience in developing countries?	No
Health personnel who are not current members of your organization?	Yes

Organization/Service Specifics:

Size of the Organization's Staff:	21-50
Number of providers sent or received/year:	51-100
Minimum term of assignment:	1 month
Maximum term of assignment:	3 years
Is funding available for travel?	Yes
Are room and board provided?	Yes
Is any other funding available? *1*	Yes
Is training provided or available?	No
Is a language other than English required? *2*	Yes

(continued)

Health Professionals Placed:

Physicians:

Physicians; Emergency Medicine Physicians; Family Practitioners; Infectious Disease Spec.; Internal Medicine GPS & PCP; OB/GYN; Ophthalmologists; Pediatricians; Psychiatrists; Pulmonary Specialists

Allied Health Professionals:

Administrative Health Positions; Nurse Midwives; Nurse Practitioners; Nurses; Physician Assistants; Public Health Specialists, Epidemiologists and Health Educators

Notes

1. Additional funding depends on the position; *2.* Language requirements depend on the country of service.

Duke University Medical Center, Division of Infectious Diseases and Int'l Health

Continents Served

Africa ☑ Asia ☑ Europe ☐ The Americas ☑

Countries Served

Australia, Brazil, China, Kenya, New Zealand, Taiwan, Tanzania, Thailand

Address: **Box 3867, Duke University Medical Center, Durham, NC 27710 U.S.A.**

Phone: **(919) 684-2660** FAX: **(919) 684-8902**

E-Mail: **hamil008@mc.duke.edu** Web: **http://medicine.duke.edu/modules/fellowship/index**

Mission: The Division of Infectious Diseases and International Health at Duke University Medical Center is an academic unit specializing in the diagosis, treatment, and clinical and laboratory investigation of infections. Division activities emphasize three main areas: clinical care of inpatients and outpatients, training of students and postgraduates, and basic and applied research. Duke University medical school students and residents are accepted for placement each year.

Placement opportunities for . . .	
People of only certain faiths?	No
Couples: both are health providers?	No
Couples: only one is a health provider?	No
Families with children?	No
Medical students? *1*	Yes
Pre-medical or college students?	No
Other health professional students?	No
Doctors in training? *2*	Yes
Health personnel who are US citizens?	No
Health personnel who are non-US citizens?	No
Health personnel with no prior experience in developing countries?	No
Health personnel who are not current members of your organization?	No

Organization/Service Specifics:	
Size of the Organization's Staff:	21-50
Number of providers sent or received/year:	6-10
Minimum term of assignment:	1 month
Maximum term of assignment:	1 year
Is funding available for travel? *3*	Yes
Are room and board provided?	No
Is any other funding available?	No
Is training provided or available?	No
Is a language other than English required? *4*	No

Health Professionals Placed:

Physicians:

Medical students and residents only

Allied Health Professionals:

Notes

1. Duke Medical Students only; *2.* Duke residents and fellows only; *3.* Travel funding is for Duke residents only; *4.* Swahili is desirable, but not required, if going to Kenya or Tanzania.

Edmundite Missions Corps

Continents Served

Africa ☐ Asia ☐ Europe ☐ The Americas ☑

Countries Served

United States

Address: **1428 Broad St., Selma, AL 36701 U.S.A.**

Phone: **(334) 872-2359** FAX: **(334) 875-8189**

E-Mail: **information@edmunditemissions.org** Web: **www.edmunditemissions.org**

Mission: The Edmundite Missions Corps (EMC) is a service-learning program for those who wish to assist economically disadvantaged African-American communities in central Alabama. The Missions support health clinics and provide home health care services in several rural Alabama locations. EMC members volunteer to work directly with the poor and express their faith.

(continued)

Placement opportunities for . . .

People of only certain faiths? *1*	Yes
Couples: both are health providers?	Yes
Couples: only one is a health provider?	Yes
Families with children?	Yes
Medical students?	Yes
Pre-medical or college students?	Yes
Other health professional students?	Yes
Doctors in training?	Yes
Health personnel who are US citizens?	Yes
Health personnel who are non-US citizens?	Yes
Health personnel with no prior experience in developing countries?	Yes
Health personnel who are not current members of your organization?	Yes

Organization/Service Specifics:

Size of the Organization's Staff:	6-10
Number of providers sent or received/year:	21-50
Minimum term of assignment: *2*	1 week
Maximum term of assignment: *2*	2 years
Is funding available for travel?	Yes
Are room and board provided?	Yes
Is any other funding available?	
Is training provided or available?	
Is a language other than English required?	No

Health Professionals Placed:

Physicians:

Not specified

Allied Health Professionals:

Not specified

Notes

1. Christian; *2.* Usually 10 months.

Edward A. Ulzen Memorial Foundation (EAUMF)

Continents Served

Africa ☑ Asia ☐ Europe ☐ The Americas ☐

Countries Served

Ghana

Address: **P.M.B. 214 / 400-740 Greenville Blvd S. E., Greenville, NC 27858 U.S.A.**

Phone: **(252) 412-0415** FAX: **(252) 561-7312**

E-Mail: **medicalvolunteer@elwininternational.com** Web: **elwininternational.com/healthcare_volunteer.html**

Mission: The Edward A. Ulzen Memorial Foundation (EAUMF) is named for a well-known educator and international public servant from Elmina who served Africa during his professional life and died in October 1999. His professional career spanned more than four decades. He was a pillar in the field of adult education and literacy. He was also involved in public health education and was a renowned univeristy administrator. The foundation was established to provide opportunities in higher education for youth from Elmina and the surrounding district. It also exists to promote primary care and public health initiatives in the KEEA district. The EAUMF also operates the Elmina-Java Museum dedicated to archiving Elmina's history for posterity.

Placement opportunities for . . .

People of only certain faiths?	No
Couples: both are health providers?	
Couples: only one is a health provider?	
Families with children?	
Medical students?	
Pre-medical or college students?	
Other health professional students?	Yes
Doctors in training?	Yes
Health personnel who are US citizens?	Yes
Health personnel who are non-US citizens?	
Health personnel with no prior experience in developing countries?	
Health personnel who are not current members of your organization?	Yes

Organization/Service Specifics:

Size of the Organization's Staff:	
Number of providers sent or received/year:	
Minimum term of assignment:	2 weeks
Maximum term of assignment:	3 months
Is funding available for travel?	
Are room and board provided?	
Is any other funding available?	
Is training provided or available?	
Is a language other than English required?	No

Health Professionals Placed:

Physicians:

Family Practitioners; Internal Medicine GPS & PCP

Allied Health Professionals:

Dental Hygienists; Dentists; Nurses; Physician Assistants

Notes

Emergency International, Inc.

Address: **1722 Thames St., Baltimore, MD 21231 U.S.A.**
Phone: **(410) 955-2280** FAX: **(410) 614-7298**
E-Mail: **ggreen@jhmi.edu** Web:

Continents Served
Africa ☐ Asia ☑ Europe ☐ The Americas ☑

Countries Served
China Guatemala Nicaragua Panama

Mission: Emergency International is dedicated to improving the quality of emergency medical care worldwide. Emergency International is involved with leadership development, physician, nurse and pre-hospital provider training, and medical equipment and supply donation. Membership is open to all interested individuals, including: physicians, nurses, pre-hospital care providers, other medical professionals, administrators, public health officials, and the public. Funding is not provided. There are no religious or language requirements, but language skills are beneficial.

Placement opportunities for . . .

People of only certain faiths?	No
Couples: both are health providers?	Yes
Couples: only one is a health provider?	No
Families with children?	No
Medical students?	Yes
Pre-medical or college students?	No
Other health professional students?	Yes
Doctors in training?	Yes
Health personnel who are US citizens?	Yes
Health personnel who are non-US citizens?	Yes
Health personnel with no prior experience in developing countries?	Yes
Health personnel who are not current members of your organization?	Yes

Organization/Service Specifics:

Size of the Organization's Staff:	*1*	0-5
Number of providers sent or received/year:		11-20
Minimum term of assignment:		1 week
Maximum term of assignment:		
Is funding available for travel?	*2*	No
Are room and board provided?		No
Is any other funding available?		No
Is training provided or available?		Yes
Is a language other than English required?	*3*	No

Health Professionals Placed:

Physicians:

Physicians; Emergency Medicine Physicians

Allied Health Professionals:

Notes

1. EI is in a state of administrative reorganization but will soon resume services. Please contact Dr Gary Green (president) for more information - 2/06; *2.* Funding is sometimes available; *3.* No language is required, but language skills are useful.

Esperanca, Inc.

Address: **1911 West Earll Drive, Phoenix, AZ 85015-6095 U.S.A.**
Phone: **(602) 252-7772** FAX: **(602) 340-9197**
(888) 701-5150
E-Mail: **info@esperanca.org** Web: **www.esperanca.org/**

Continents Served
Africa ☑ Asia ☐ Europe ☐ The Americas ☑

Countries Served
Bolivia Mozambique Nicaragua
United States

Mission: Esperanca is Saving Children's Lives Now because every child deserves a healthy life. Hence we seek to nurture the seeds of self-reliance in health through prevention, training, and treatment in areas of greatest need throughout the world. Volunteers can serve for 1- to 3-week assignments, and while there are no language requirements, knowledge of Portuguese and Spanish is helpful.

Placement opportunities for . . .

People of only certain faiths?	No
Couples: both are health providers?	Yes
Couples: only one is a health provider?	No
Families with children?	No
Medical students?	No
Pre-medical or college students?	No
Other health professional students?	Yes
Doctors in training?	No
Health personnel who are US citizens?	Yes
Health personnel who are non-US citizens?	Yes
Health personnel with no prior experience in developing countries?	Yes
Health personnel who are not current members of your organization?	Yes

Organization/Service Specifics:

Size of the Organization's Staff:		11-20
Number of providers sent or received/year:		11-20
Minimum term of assignment:		1 weeks
Maximum term of assignment:		3 weeks
Is funding available for travel?		No
Are room and board provided?		Yes
Is any other funding available?		No
Is training provided or available?		No
Is a language other than English required?	*1*	No

(continued)

Health Professionals Placed:

Physicians:

Anesthesiologists; General Surgeons; Orthopedic Surgeons; Plastic/Hand/Reconstructive Surgeons

Allied Health Professionals:

Nurse Practitioners; Nurses

Notes

1. No language requirements, but Portuguese and Spanish are desirable for some assignments.

Evangelical Alliance Mission (TEAM World)

Address: **P.O. Box 969, Wheaton, IL 60189-0969 U.S.A.**

Phone: **(630) 653-5300** FAX: **(630) 653-1826**
(800) 343-3144

E-Mail: **team@teamworld.org** Web: **www.teamworld.org**

Continents Served

Africa ☑ Asia ☑ Europe ☐ The Americas ☐

Countries Served

Chad, Indonesia, South Africa, Zimbabwe

Mission: TEAM seeks to spread the word of God to areas of the world in need. Starting new churches that in turn start more new churches is the key to our mission's success. We have hundreds of people called by God and strategically placed around the world trained for our mission. Many men and women will never understand the love of Jesus until they experience His healing through the hands of our health care volunteers.

Placement opportunities for . . .	
People of only certain faiths? *1*	Yes
Couples: both are health providers?	Yes
Couples: only one is a health provider?	Yes
Families with children?	Yes
Medical students?	Yes
Pre-medical or college students?	No
Other health professional students?	Yes
Doctors in training?	No
Health personnel who are US citizens?	Yes
Health personnel who are non-US citizens?	Yes
Health personnel with no prior experience in developing countries?	Yes
Health personnel who are not current members of your organization?	Yes

Organization/Service Specifics:	
Size of the Organization's Staff:	151-200
Number of providers sent or received/year:	21-50
Minimum term of assignment:	2 weeks
Maximum term of assignment:	none
Is funding available for travel?	No
Are room and board provided?	No
Is any other funding available?	No
Is training provided or available?	Yes
Is a language other than English required? *2*	No

Health Professionals Placed: *3*

Physicians:

Physicians; Anesthesiologists; Cardiologists; Dermatologists; Family Practitioners; General Surgeons; Infectious Disease Spec.; Neurologists; Ophthalmologists; Pathologists; Pediatricians; Psychiatrists; Radiologists; Urologists

Allied Health Professionals:

Administrative Health Positions; Dental Hygienists; Dentists; Medical Technicians (lab, X-ray, etc); Nurse Midwives; Nurse Practitioners; Nurses; Nutritionists & Dieticians; Physical & Occupational Therapists; Public Health Specialists, Epidemiologists and Health Educators; Social Workers; Water/Sanitation Specialists

Notes

1. Born-again christians with recommendation from pastor; *2.* Sometimes; TEAM provides language training; *3.* Other specialties often needed as well.

Evangelical Free Church of America Mission

Address: **901 E 78th St., Minneapolis, MN 55420-1300 U.S.A.**

Phone: **(800) 745-2202** FAX: **(952) 853-8474**
(952) 854-1300

E-Mail: **efcm@efca.org or tcairns@efca.org** Web: **www.efca.org**

Continents Served

Africa ☑ Asia ☑ Europe ☑ The Americas ☑

Countries Served

Central African Rep., China, Congo, Hong Kong, Macau, Tanzania, Tibet

Mission: To gain insight into a wide variety of cross-cultural ministries and seek an answer to the question "Has God called me and gifted me to serve as a cross-cultural missionary?" To provide meaningful help for our career missionaries. To become a well informed promoter of missions in the local church at home. Medical service opportunities are available, among a host of other evangelical opportunities. Missionaries can serve for short term assignments or can commit their lives to overseas work. Volunteers must be Evangelical Christians.

(continued)

Placement opportunities for . . .

People of only certain faiths? *1*	Yes
Couples: both are health providers?	Yes
Couples: only one is a health provider?	Yes
Families with children?	Yes
Medical students?	Yes
Pre-medical or college students?	Yes
Other health professional students?	Yes
Doctors in training?	Yes
Health personnel who are US citizens?	Yes
Health personnel who are non-US citizens?	Yes
Health personnel with no prior experience in developing countries?	Yes
Health personnel who are not current members of your organization?	No

Organization/Service Specifics:

Size of the Organization's Staff:	>200
Number of providers sent or received/year:	101-150
Minimum term of assignment:	3 weeks
Maximum term of assignment:	life
Is funding available for travel?	No
Are room and board provided?	Yes
Is any other funding available?	No
Is training provided or available?	No
Is a language other than English required? *2*	Yes

Health Professionals Placed:

Physicians:

Physicians; Family Practitioners; General Surgeons; Pediatricians

Allied Health Professionals:

Medical Technicians (lab, X-ray, etc); Nurses

Notes

1. Volunteers must be Evangelical Christians; *2.* There may be language requirements for longer missions.

Evangelical Lutheran Church in America

Address: **Division for Global Mission**
8765 West Higgins Rd., Chicago, IL 60631-4177
U.S.A.

Phone: **(773) 380-2648 or (800) 638-3522 x2648** FAX: **(773) 380-2410**

E-Mail: **dgmserve@elca.org** Web: **www.elca.org/globalmission/**

Continents Served

Africa ☑ Asia ☑ Europe ☐ The Americas ☐

Countries Served

Bangladesh; Cameroon; Central African Rep.; India; Liberia; Madagascar; Malawi; Namibia; Nepal; Papua-New Guinea; Senegal; South Africa; Tanzania

Mission: The Evangelical Lutheran Church in America is a 5.1 million member church that also works in the context of the global church. Many global mission service opportunities are available through us as we faithfully serve our God and church in mission. Missionaries can serve for short term (2 month) to longer term (2 year) assignments. There are medical placements for a variety of health care professionals. Volunteers must be Christian. Room, but not board, is provided. The volunteer is responsible for all other funding.

Placement opportunities for . . .

People of only certain faiths? *1*	Yes
Couples: both are health providers?	Yes
Couples: only one is a health provider?	Yes
Families with children?	No
Medical students?	Yes
Pre-medical or college students?	
Other health professional students?	No
Doctors in training?	Yes
Health personnel who are US citizens?	Yes
Health personnel who are non-US citizens?	No
Health personnel with no prior experience in developing countries?	Yes
Health personnel who are not current members of your organization?	Yes

Organization/Service Specifics:

Size of the Organization's Staff:	21-50
Number of providers sent or received/year:	101-150
Minimum term of assignment:	2 months
Maximum term of assignment:	2 years
Is funding available for travel?	No
Are room and board provided? *2*	No
Is any other funding available?	No
Is training provided or available?	Yes
Is a language other than English required?	No

Health Professionals Placed:

Physicians:

Physicians; Cardiologists; Family Practitioners; General Surgeons; Infectious Disease Spec.; Internal Medicine GPS & PCP; OB/GYN; Ophthalmologists; Oral Surgeons; Orthopedic Surgeons; Pathologists; Pediatricians; Plastic/Hand/Reconstructive Surgeons

Allied Health Professionals:

Dentists; Medical Technicians (lab, X-ray, etc); Nurse Midwives; Nurses; Physical & Occupational Therapists

Notes

1. Volunteers must be Christian; *2.* Room, but not board, is provided.

Father Carr's Place 2B

Continents Served			
Africa ☐	Asia ☐	Europe ☐	The Americas ☑

Countries Served
United States

Address: **1965 Oshkosh Ave., Oshkosh, WI 54901 U.S.A.**

Phone: **(920) 231-2378** FAX: **(920) 231-2502**

E-Mail: Web:

Mission: Father Carr's Place 2B is a free walk-in clinic fully volunteer-staffed in Oshkosh, Wisconsin. We are dedicated to providing quality health care. Human caring and compassion are our specialty. Comprehensive health care, full service clinic to uninsured and underinsured, AIDS testing/screening available. Volunteers can serve a minimum of 6 months and there is no maximum period of service. Room and board are provided, but other funding is not available.

Placement opportunities for . . .		Organization/Service Specifics:	
People of only certain faiths?	No	Size of the Organization's Staff:	11-20
Couples: both are health providers?	Yes	Number of providers sent or received/year:	
Couples: only one is a health provider?	Yes	Minimum term of assignment:	6 month
Families with children?	Yes	Maximum term of assignment:	life
Medical students?	Yes	Is funding available for travel?	No
Pre-medical or college students?	Yes	Are room and board provided?	Yes
Other health professional students?	Yes	Is any other funding available?	No
Doctors in training?	Yes	Is training provided or available?	No
Health personnel who are US citizens?	Yes	Is a language other than English required?	No

Health personnel who are non-US citizens?	No
Health personnel with no prior experience in developing countries?	Yes
Health personnel who are not current members of your organization?	Yes

Health Professionals Placed:

Physicians:

Physicians; Family Practitioners

Allied Health Professionals:

Dentists; Nurses

Notes

Feed the Children

Continents Served			
Africa ☐	Asia ☑	Europe ☑	The Americas ☑

Countries Served

Guatemala	Mexico	Moldova
Nicaragua	Romania	Thailand

Address: **333 North Meridian, Oklahoma City, OK 73107-6568 U.S.A.**

Phone: **(800) 627-4556** **(405) 942-0228** FAX: **(405) 945-4177**

E-Mail: **ftc@feedthechildren.org** Web: **www.feedthechildren.org**

Mission: Feed the Children is a Christian, international, nonprofit relief organization that delivers food, medicine, clothing and other necessities to children and families who lack these essentials due to famine, war, poverty or natural disaster. The Medical Team is made up of volunteer doctors, nurses, dentists, optometrists and laypersons who reach out to minister to the physical and spiritual needs of children and families in developing countries. Led by Dr. Larry Biehle, four mission trips are scheduled each year.

Placement opportunities for . . .		Organization/Service Specifics:	
People of only certain faiths?	No	Size of the Organization's Staff:	151-200
Couples: both are health providers?	Yes	Number of providers sent or received/year:	21-50
Couples: only one is a health provider?	No	Minimum term of assignment:	10 days
Families with children?	No	Maximum term of assignment:	2 weeks
Medical students?	No	Is funding available for travel?	No
Pre-medical or college students?	No	Are room and board provided?	No
Other health professional students?	Yes	Is any other funding available?	No
Doctors in training?	No	Is training provided or available?	No
Health personnel who are US citizens?	Yes	Is a language other than English required?	No

Health personnel who are non-US citizens?	Yes
Health personnel with no prior experience in developing countries?	Yes
Health personnel who are not current members of your organization?	Yes

(continued)

Health Professionals Placed:

Physicians:

Physicians; Optometrists

Allied Health Professionals:

Dentists; Nurse Practitioners; Nurses; Pharmacists; Physician Assistants

Notes

Fellowship of Associates of Medical Evangelism

Address: **4545 Southeastern Avenue**
P.O. Box 33548, Indianapolis, IN 46203 U.S.A.

Phone: **(317) 358-2480** FAX: **(317) 358-2483**

E-Mail: **medicalmissions@fameworld.org** Web: **www.fameworld.org/**

Mission: FAME is dedicated to bringing help and hope to people in underdeveloped nations through medical evangelism with special concern for those untouched by the Gospel of Christ. FAME works to provide medical facilities, medicines, and medical equipment, as well as mobilizing medical personnel and evangelistic teams to the poorest of the poor around the world. Christian volunteers can serve for 1- to 4-week terms. Funding is not provided, although room and board will be arranged by FAME.

Continents Served

Africa ☑ Asia ☑ Europe ☑ The Americas ☑

Countries Served

Central African Rep.; China; Dominican Republic; Ghana; Haiti; Honduras; India; Jamaica; Korea, South; Kosovo; Mexico; Nigeria; Panama; Philippines; Tanzania; Thailand; Zimbabwe

Placement opportunities for . . .

People of only certain faiths? *1*	No
Couples: both are health providers?	Yes
Couples: only one is a health provider?	Yes
Families with children?	Yes
Medical students?	Yes
Pre-medical or college students?	Yes
Other health professional students?	Yes
Doctors in training?	Yes
Health personnel who are US citizens?	Yes
Health personnel who are non-US citizens?	No
Health personnel with no prior experience in developing countries?	Yes
Health personnel who are not current members of your organization?	No

Organization/Service Specifics:

Size of the Organization's Staff:	6-10
Number of providers sent or received/year:	51-100
Minimum term of assignment:	1 week
Maximum term of assignment:	4 weeks
Is funding available for travel?	No
Are room and board provided?	No
Is any other funding available?	No
Is training provided or available?	Yes
Is a language other than English required?	No

Health Professionals Placed:

Physicians:

Physicians; Emergency Medicine Physicians; Family Practitioners; General Surgeons; Nephrologists; OB/GYN

Allied Health Professionals:

Nurse Practitioners; Nurses; Paramedics; Pharmacists; Physician Assistants

Notes

1. Volunteers must be Christian.

Filipino-American Medical Inc.

Address: **P.O. Box 161, New York, NY 10101-0161 U.S.A.**

Phone: **(212) 582-3304** FAX:

E-Mail: **mperlas@att.net** Web: **www.ifami.org/index.htm**

Continents Served

Africa ☐ Asia ☑ Europe ☐ The Americas ☐

Countries Served

Philippines

Mission: Filipino-American Medical Inc. brings American and Filipino American health professionals to the Philippines to serve poor people in need. Medical & Surgical Missions are usually held in the last two weeks of February and are coordinated with local non-government organizations and non-profit foundations at a designated charity hospital. These hospitals are normally equipped with basic operating room equipment The FAMI mission volunteer process is a combination of invitations sent to essential medical professionals, FAMI board members and an open lottery.

(continued)

Placement opportunities for . . .	
People of only certain faiths?	No
Couples: both are health providers?	Yes
Couples: only one is a health provider?	Yes
Families with children?	No
Medical students?	No
Pre-medical or college students?	No
Other health professional students?	Yes
Doctors in training?	No
Health personnel who are US citizens?	Yes
Health personnel who are non-US citizens? *1*	Yes
Health personnel with no prior experience in developing countries?	Yes
Health personnel who are not current members of your organization?	Yes

Organization/Service Specifics:	
Size of the Organization's Staff:	11-20
Number of providers sent or received/year:	21-50
Minimum term of assignment:	1 week
Maximum term of assignment:	1 week
Is funding available for travel?	No
Are room and board provided?	Yes
Is any other funding available?	No
Is training provided or available?	No
Is a language other than English required?	No

Health Professionals Placed:

Physicians:

Physicians; Anesthesiologists; Cardiologists; Family Practitioners; General Surgeons; Internal Medicine GPS & PCP; Pediatricians; Plastic/Hand/Reconstructive Surgeons

Allied Health Professionals:

Nurse Practitioners; Nurses; Pharmacists; Physician Assistants

Notes

1. Phillipines.

Florida Association of Voluntary Agencies for Caribbean Action, Inc. (FAVACA)

Continents Served

Africa ☐ Asia ☐ Europe ☐ The Americas ☑

Countries Served

Barbados, Belize, Costa Rica, Dominican Republic, El Salvador, Guatemala, Guyana, Haiti, Honduras, Jamaica, Nicaragua, Panama, St. Lucia, Trinidad and Tobago

Address: **1310 N. Paul Russell Rd., Tallahassee, FL 32301 U.S.A.**

Phone: **(850) 410-3100** FAX: **(850) 922-4849**

E-Mail: **favaca@favaca.org** Web: **www.favaca.org**

Mission: The Florida Association of Voluntary Agencies for Caribbean Action, Inc. (FAVACA), is a private, not for profit organization formed in 1981. A state appropriation provides a funding base for an estimated 150 volunteer missions to Central America and the Caribbean this year. Florida's International Volunteer Corps is a one of a kind development partnership between Floridians and our Caribbean neighbors. It is volunteers providing on-site, overseas technical assistance and training in health, agriculture, social services, and education towards projects that create jobs, increase productivity, promote self-sufficiency, and improve living conditions. We cover the expenses of Corps volunteers who donate their time and skills on short-term technical assistance missions to help Florida's neighbors help themselves.

Placement opportunities for . . .	
People of only certain faiths?	
Couples: both are health providers?	No
Couples: only one is a health provider?	No
Families with children?	No
Medical students?	No
Pre-medical or college students?	No
Other health professional students?	No
Doctors in training?	No
Health personnel who are US citizens?	Yes
Health personnel who are non-US citizens?	No
Health personnel with no prior experience in developing countries?	No
Health personnel who are not current members of your organization?	No

Organization/Service Specifics:	
Size of the Organization's Staff:	6-10
Number of providers sent or received/year:	6-10
Minimum term of assignment:	1 week
Maximum term of assignment:	4 weeks
Is funding available for travel?	Yes
Are room and board provided?	Yes
Is any other funding available?	No
Is training provided or available?	No
Is a language other than English required? *1*	Yes

Health Professionals Placed:

Physicians:

Not specified

Allied Health Professionals:

Not specified

Notes

1. French, Spanish, or Creole may be required depending on the location.

Flying Doctors of America

Continents Served			
Africa ✔	Asia ✔	Europe ☐	The Americas ✔

Countries Served

Belize	Bolivia	China
Dominican Republic		Guatemala
India	Jamaica	Macau
Mexico	Mongolia	Peru
Tibet		

Address: **15 Medical Drive, Cartersville, GA 30121 U.S.A.**

Phone: **(404) 815-7044** **(770) 386-5221** FAX: **(404) 892-6672**

E-Mail: **fdoamerica@aol.com or pittsman54@aol.com** Web: **www.fdoamerica.org**

Mission: For more than a decade, Flying Doctors of America has been bringing together physicians, dentists, nurses, chiropractors, other health professionals and non-medical support volunteers to care for people who otherwise would never receive professional medical care. We operate under the "Mother Teresa Principle," focusing on the poorest of the poor who live in conditions that are difficult for most Americans to imagine. Knowing that someone cares renews hope for these people who live in an otherwise hopeless situation. Flying Doctors of America was founded by Allan Gathercoal in 1990 with $700, a wing and a prayer. Today it's an established non-profit, non-sectarian organization. In the past 12 years the organization has flown more than 100 missions and provided free medical care to over 85,000 children, women and men. Among the areas served are Mexico, South and Central America, the Dominican Republic, Jamaica, India, Africa, Mongolia, and Thailand.

Placement opportunities for . . .	
People of only certain faiths?	No
Couples: both are health providers?	
Couples: only one is a health provider?	
Families with children?	No
Medical students?	No
Pre-medical or college students?	No
Other health professional students?	Yes
Doctors in training?	No
Health personnel who are US citizens?	Yes
Health personnel who are non-US citizens?	No
Health personnel with no prior experience in developing countries?	Yes
Health personnel who are not current members of your organization?	Yes

Organization/Service Specifics:	
Size of the Organization's Staff:	6-10
Number of providers sent or received/year:	21-50
Minimum term of assignment:	3 days
Maximum term of assignment:	2 weeks
Is funding available for travel?	No
Are room and board provided?	No
Is any other funding available?	No
Is training provided or available?	No
Is a language other than English required? *1*	No

Health Professionals Placed: *2*

Physicians:

Physicians

Allied Health Professionals:

Dentists; Nurses

Notes

1. Spanish helpful; *2.* Medical support team depending on trip.

Flying Samaritans

Continents Served			
Africa ☐	Asia ☐	Europe ☐	The Americas ✔

Countries Served

Address: **1203 E. Meda Ave., Glendora, CA 91741 U.S.A.**

Phone: **(800) 775-9018** FAX:

E-Mail: **OCsams@flyingsamaritans.org** Web: **www.flyingsamaritans.org/index.html**

Mission: The Flying Sams, as we are often called, have four basic missions—primary care, specialty care, education and emergency care. In our primary care role, the Sams fly (and drive) to clinics where they provide non-emergency services, such as family medicine, optometry, audiology, dentistry and dental hygiene, and preventative health care. Most patients are the 60% of the Mexican population who are not eligible for Mexican Social Security medical care. Unless the Sams are working with Mexican doctors, they can only practice in areas where there are no doctors. Our physicians usually perform surgery only when another doctor is present to provide follow-up care. The second mission, specialty care, is a cooperative effort with Buen Pastor Hospital in San Quintin where follow-up care is available that many clinics cannot provide. Our third mission is education in the training of pasantes, medical and dental graduates interested in additional education. Lastly, to meet medical emergencies, our professionals assist with disasters and critical medical patients.

(continued)

Placement opportunities for . . .

People of only certain faiths?	No
Couples: both are health providers?	Yes
Couples: only one is a health provider?	No
Families with children?	No
Medical students?	No
Pre-medical or college students?	No
Other health professional students?	Yes
Doctors in training?	Yes
Health personnel who are US citizens?	Yes
Health personnel who are non-US citizens?	No
Health personnel with no prior experience in developing countries?	Yes
Health personnel who are not current members of your organization?	Yes

Organization/Service Specifics:

Size of the Organization's Staff:	51-100
Number of providers sent or received/year:	21-50
Minimum term of assignment:	1 wknd/month
Maximum term of assignment:	1 wknd/month
Is funding available for travel?	No
Are room and board provided?	No
Is any other funding available?	No
Is training provided or available?	No
Is a language other than English required? *1*	No

Health Professionals Placed:

Physicians:

Physicians; Emergency Medicine Physicians; Family Practitioners; General Surgeons; Optometrists

Allied Health Professionals:

Dental Hygienists; Dentists; Nurse Practitioners; Nurses; Pharmacists; Physician Assistants; Public Health Specialists, Epidemiologists and Health Educators

Notes

1. Spanish is helpful.

FOCUS Inc.

Address: **1855 W. Taylor St., Chicago, IL 60612 U.S.A.**

Phone: **(312) 996-7445** FAX: **(312) 413-4916**

E-Mail: **marimill@uic.edu** Web: **www.focuseye.org**

Continents Served

Africa ☑ Asia ☐ Europe ☐ The Americas ☐

Countries Served

Nigeria

Mission: FOCUS provides vital medical, surgical opthalmic services and support in areas of extreme need by recruiting volunteer physicians, collecting donated medical supplies, and raising money to fund its work. For the past 25 years, FOCUS has concentrated its efforts in a remote area of Nigeria. Recognized by the Chicago Opthalmological Society, FOCUS is headquartered at the University of Illinois School of Opthalmology.

Placement opportunities for . . .

People of only certain faiths?	No
Couples: both are health providers?	Yes
Couples: only one is a health provider?	Yes
Families with children? *1*	No
Medical students?	No
Pre-medical or college students?	No
Other health professional students?	No
Doctors in training?	No
Health personnel who are US citizens?	Yes
Health personnel who are non-US citizens?	Yes
Health personnel with no prior experience in developing countries?	Yes
Health personnel who are not current members of your organization?	Yes

Organization/Service Specifics:

Size of the Organization's Staff:	0-5
Number of providers sent or received/year:	101-150
Minimum term of assignment:	1 weeks
Maximum term of assignment:	3 weeks
Is funding available for travel?	No
Are room and board provided?	Yes
Is any other funding available?	No
Is training provided or available?	No
Is a language other than English required?	No

Health Professionals Placed:

Physicians:

Physicians; Ophthalmologists

Allied Health Professionals:

Notes

1. No placements for families with children under 18.

(continued)

Foundation for International Medical Relief of Children

Continents Served
Africa ☑ Asia ☑ Europe ☐ The Americas ☑

Countries Served
Costa Rica, Ethiopia, India

Address: **1711 Massachusetts Ave., NW Suite 526, Washington, DC 20036 U.S.A.**

Phone: **(888) 211-8575** FAX: **(888) 735-6530**

E-Mail: **info@fimrc.org** Web: **www.fimrc.org/**

Mission: Foundation for International Medical Relief of Children is dedicated to improving children's lives around the world by providing children with the most basic of medical needs. At each mission location, FIMRC runs a clinic where patients receive care. Doctors and nurses who travel to these missions will treat children with acute health issues, conduct "well child visits," and provide prenatal care. Health care workers may also be asked to travel into the community to provide care when needed. FIMRC maintains clinics with basic medical supplies and charting systems. In addition to doctors and nurses, FIMRC also welcomes medical students, public health students, and undergraduate volunteers.

Placement opportunities for . . .

People of only certain faiths?	No
Couples: both are health providers?	Yes
Couples: only one is a health provider?	Yes
Families with children?	Yes
Medical students?	Yes
Pre-medical or college students?	Yes
Other health professional students?	Yes
Doctors in training?	No
Health personnel who are US citizens?	Yes
Health personnel who are non-US citizens?	Yes
Health personnel with no prior experience in developing countries?	Yes
Health personnel who are not current members of your organization?	Yes

Organization/Service Specifics:

Size of the Organization's Staff:	>200
Number of providers sent or received/year:	51-100
Minimum term of assignment:	1 week
Maximum term of assignment:	none
Is funding available for travel? *1*	No
Are room and board provided?	Yes
Is any other funding available?	No
Is training provided or available?	Yes
Is a language other than English required? *2*	No

Health Professionals Placed:

Physicians:

Not specified

Allied Health Professionals:

Not specified

Notes

1. Only if greater than 3-month volunteer; *2.* Other languages always helpful.

Foundation Human Nature (MeHiPro)

Continents Served
Africa ☑ Asia ☐ Europe ☐ The Americas ☑

Countries Served
Ecuador, Ghana

Address: **1823 Westridge Road, Los Angeles, CA 90049 U.S.A.**

Phone: **(919) 949-0459** FAX:

E-Mail: **info@fhnusa.org or jessica@fhnusa.org** Web: **www.f-h-n.org/**

Mission: As a branch of FHN International, FHN USA raises awareness of FHN's programs, solicits financial and technical support, and recruits volunteers. Our current projects focus on supporting the operation of much-needed medical clinics in Ecuador and Ghana. In addition to helping manage these clinics, FHN works to develop sustainable and locally appropriate approaches to healthcare that include related programs in education, economic alternatives and environmental health.

(continued)

Placement opportunities for . . .

People of only certain faiths?	No
Couples: both are health providers?	No
Couples: only one is a health provider?	No
Families with children?	No
Medical students?	Yes
Pre-medical or college students?	Yes
Other health professional students?	Yes
Doctors in training? *1*	Yes
Health personnel who are US citizens?	Yes
Health personnel who are non-US citizens?	Yes
Health personnel with no prior experience in developing countries?	Yes
Health personnel who are not current members of your organization?	Yes

Organization/Service Specifics:

Size of the Organization's Staff:	6-10
Number of providers sent or received/year:	21-50
Minimum term of assignment:	3 months
Maximum term of assignment:	6 months
Is funding available for travel?	No
Are room and board provided?	No
Is any other funding available?	No
Is training provided or available?	No
Is a language other than English required? *2*	Yes

Health Professionals Placed:

Physicians:

All physician specialties

Allied Health Professionals:

All allied health professionals

Notes

1. Note that many projects have minimum time commitments;
2. Spanish.

Foundation of Compassionate American Samaritans

Address: **P.O. Box 428760, Cincinnati, OH 45242-8760 U.S.A.**

Phone: **(513) 621-5300** FAX: **(513) 621-5307**

E-Mail: **focas@focas-us.org** Web: **focas-us.org**

Continents Served

Africa ☐ Asia ☐ Europe ☐ The Americas ☑

Countries Served

Haiti

Mission: Foundation of Compassionate American Samaritans (FOCAS) is a Christian organization dedicated to helping the desperately poor in remote areas of Haiti to meet their basic physical and spiritual needs—including elementary and vocational education, food security, and medical care. FOCAS' Child Survival project in Haiti aims at bringing about behavioral changes among a marginalized population of 77,000 from two rural districts, to reduce mortality and morbidity of infants, children, and women. This four-year project was launched in Haiti in 1997, with USAID central grants. Andcan Rural Health Care (ARHC) is the mentoring organization for FOCAS, to transfer technology and lessons learned from the ARHC experience in Bolivia to the FOCAS Child Survival project in Haiti. Placements are made on a short (2 weeks) and longer term (2 years) basis; health care providers must know Creole/French.

Placement opportunities for . . .

People of only certain faiths? *1*	Yes
Couples: both are health providers?	Yes
Couples: only one is a health provider?	Yes
Families with children?	No
Medical students?	Yes
Pre-medical or college students?	Yes
Other health professional students?	Yes
Doctors in training?	No
Health personnel who are US citizens?	Yes
Health personnel who are non-US citizens?	Yes
Health personnel with no prior experience in developing countries?	No
Health personnel who are not current members of your organization?	Yes

Organization/Service Specifics:

Size of the Organization's Staff:	0-5
Number of providers sent or received/year:	>200
Minimum term of assignment:	10 days
Maximum term of assignment:	2 years
Is funding available for travel?	No
Are room and board provided?	No
Is any other funding available? *2*	Yes
Is training provided or available?	Yes
Is a language other than English required? *3*	No

Health Professionals Placed:

Physicians:

Physicians; Internal Medicine GPS & PCP; OB/GYN; Pediatricians

Allied Health Professionals:

Dental Hygienists; Dentists; Nurse Midwives; Nurses; Nutritionists & Dieticians; Public Health Specialists, Epidemiologists and Health Educators; Respiratory Therapists; Social Workers; Water/Sanitation Specialists

Notes

1. Volunteers must be Christian;
2. Limited subsidy may be provided by organization;
3. Haitian Creole and/or French.

Foundation of International Education in Neurological Surgery (FIENS)

Continents Served			
Africa ✔	Asia ✔	Europe ☐	The Americas ✔

Countries Served

Belize	Ecuador	Ghana
Guatemala	Honduras	India
Indonesia	Kenya	Nepal
Peru	Philippines	Taiwan
Thailand	Zimbabwe	

Address: **University of Wisconsin, H4/ 338, 600 Highland Ave, Madison, WI 53792 U.S.A.**

Phone: **(608) 224-1036** FAX: **(608) 224-1036**

E-Mail: **dempsey@neurosurg.wisc.edu** Web: **www.fiens.org**

Mission: The Foundation for International Education in Neurological Surgery (FIENS) seeks to promote education and development of neurosurgery in the areas of Africa, Asia, and the Americas. The activities of FIENS are implemented primarily through the recruitment and coordination of those who are willing to serve as volunteers in the projects and areas that they support. Although the focus is primarily towards neurosurgeons, persons from related disciplines as well as residents are welcome for areas of specific need. Stays are typically 4 weeks to 6 months.

Placement opportunities for . . .	
People of only certain faiths?	No
Couples: both are health providers?	No
Couples: only one is a health provider?	No
Families with children?	No
Medical students?	No
Pre-medical or college students?	No
Other health professional students?	No
Doctors in training?	No
Health personnel who are US citizens?	Yes
Health personnel who are non-US citizens?	Yes
Health personnel with no prior experience in developing countries?	Yes
Health personnel who are not current members of your organization?	Yes

Organization/Service Specifics:	
Size of the Organization's Staff:	0-5
Number of providers sent or received/year:	6-10
Minimum term of assignment:	4 weeks
Maximum term of assignment:	6 months
Is funding available for travel? *1*	Yes
Are room and board provided?	Yes
Is any other funding available?	No
Is training provided or available?	No
Is a language other than English required?	No

Health Professionals Placed:

Physicians:

Neurosurgeons

Allied Health Professionals:

Notes

1. For those volunteers who spend a minimum of four weeks in the host country, FIENS will provide round trip economy air fare and a small discretionary fund to be used in support of local activities as the volunteer sees fit.

Friends Lugulu Hospital

Continents Served			
Africa ✔	Asia ☐	Europe ☐	The Americas ☐

Countries Served

Kenya

Address: **P.O. Box 43, Webuye, Kenya**

Phone: **(003) 374-1114** FAX: **(003) 374-1513**

E-Mail: Web:

Mission: Friends Lugulu Hospital is a 110 bed Quaker-affiliated hospital located in a densely populated rural area of western Kenya. Friends Lugulu Hospital's stated intent is, "to help build the Kingdom of God by reaching out with healing to the poor and suffering of western Kenya, and by demonstrating, in a tangible way through its health care provision, the love and compassion of Christ." Hospital services have been developed since 1977. Lugulu also provides health care services to outlying areas through a series of health clinics and dispensaries. Both at Lugulu and in the major satellite clinics, a full range of services are rendered, including inpatient and outpatient care; pre-natal care; family planning services; and child immunizations.

(continued)

Placement opportunities for . . .	
People of only certain faiths?	No
Couples: both are health providers?	Yes
Couples: only one is a health provider?	Yes
Families with children?	Yes
Medical students?	Yes
Pre-medical or college students?	No
Other health professional students?	No
Doctors in training?	No
Health personnel who are US citizens?	Yes
Health personnel who are non-US citizens?	Yes
Health personnel with no prior experience in developing countries?	Yes
Health personnel who are not current members of your organization?	Yes

Organization/Service Specifics:	
Size of the Organization's Staff:	101-150
Number of providers sent or received/year:	1-5
Minimum term of assignment:	3 months
Maximum term of assignment:	3 years
Is funding available for travel?	No
Are room and board provided?	Yes
Is any other funding available?	No
Is training provided or available?	No
Is a language other than English required?	No

Health Professionals Placed:

Physicians:

Physicians; Pediatricians; Plastic/Hand/Reconstructive Surgeons

Allied Health Professionals:

Notes

Friends Without a Border

Continents Served

Africa ☐ Asia ☑ Europe ☐ The Americas ☐

Countries Served

Address: **1123 Broadway, Suite 1210, New York, NY 10010 U.S.A.**

Phone: **(212) 691-0909** FAX: **(212) 337-8052**

E-Mail: **fwab@fwab.org** Web: **www.fwab.org**

Mission: Friends Without a Border (Friends) is a not-for-profit organization which funds and operates Angkor Hospital for Children (AHC) in Siem Reap, Cambodia. Friends and AHC are dedicated to improving the health and future of Cambodia's children by providing pediatric medical care and medical education. AHC is centrally located in Siem Reap City in Cambodia (population 90,000) and serves the entire province of Siem Reap (population 700,000). The hospital treats children ranging in age from newborn to 15 years. Staffed by an international team of health care professionals, AHC currently offers outpatient and inpatient services, basic surgery, 24-hour emergency service, dental care and pediatric medical training for Cambodian doctors and nurses.

Placement opportunities for . . .	
People of only certain faiths?	No
Couples: both are health providers?	Yes
Couples: only one is a health provider?	No
Families with children?	No
Medical students?	Yes
Pre-medical or college students?	Yes
Other health professional students?	Yes
Doctors in training?	
Health personnel who are US citizens?	
Health personnel who are non-US citizens?	
Health personnel with no prior experience in developing countries?	
Health personnel who are not current members of your organization?	

Organization/Service Specifics:		
Size of the Organization's Staff:	*1*	101-150
Number of providers sent or received/year:		51-100
Minimum term of assignment:	*2*	none
Maximum term of assignment:		none
Is funding available for travel?	*3*	No
Are room and board provided?		Yes
Is any other funding available?	*4*	Yes
Is training provided or available?		Yes
Is a language other than English required?	*5*	No

Health Professionals Placed:

Physicians:

All physician specialties

Allied Health Professionals:

All allied health professionals

Notes

1. Represents staff in Cambodia; *2.* No min or maximum although 6 months-1 year is usual time period; *3.* Org. pays a small stipend that varies depending on experience of volunteer; *4.* Org. may pay for long-term volunteers (>6 months); *5.* French is helpful.

General Baptist International

Address: **100 Stinson Dr., Poplar Bluff, MO 63901 U.S.A.**

Phone: **(573) 785-7746** FAX: **(573) 785-0564**

E-Mail: **imdir@generalbaptist.com** Web: **generalbaptist.com**

Continents Served

Africa ☐ Asia ☑ Europe ☐ The Americas ☑

Countries Served

Guam, Honduras, India, Jamaica, Mexico, Northern Mariana Isl., Philippines

Mission: General Baptist International is a Christian missionary that provides humanitarian service to the indigent and sick in the Philippines and Honduras. It provides room and board for short-term assignments (1-2 weeks). Its purpose is to help the poor through the sharing of faith and discipling of people.

Placement opportunities for . . .	
People of only certain faiths?	No
Couples: both are health providers?	Yes
Couples: only one is a health provider?	Yes
Families with children?	Yes
Medical students?	Yes
Pre-medical or college students?	Yes
Other health professional students?	Yes
Doctors in training?	Yes
Health personnel who are US citizens?	Yes
Health personnel who are non-US citizens?	Yes
Health personnel with no prior experience in developing countries?	No
Health personnel who are not current members of your organization?	Yes

Organization/Service Specifics:	
Size of the Organization's Staff:	0-5
Number of providers sent or received/year:	>200
Minimum term of assignment:	1 week
Maximum term of assignment:	3 months
Is funding available for travel?	No
Are room and board provided?	Yes
Is any other funding available?	No
Is training provided or available?	No
Is a language other than English required?	No

Health Professionals Placed:

Physicians:

Physicians

Allied Health Professionals:

Notes

General Board of Global Ministries/ The United Methodist Church

Address: **475 Riverside Dr., Room 330, New York, NY 10115 U.S.A.**

Phone: **(212) 870-3660** **(800) 862-4246** FAX: **(212) 870-3624**

E-Mail: **voluntrs@gbgm-umc.org** Web: **http://gbgm-umc.org/vim**

Continents Served

Africa ☑ Asia ☑ Europe ☑ The Americas ☑

Countries Served

Afghanistan, Algeria, Angola, Armenia, Bolivia, Bosnia, Herzegovina, Botswana, Brazil, Cambodia, Chile, China, Congo, Costa Rica, Cuba, Dominican Republic, El Salvador, Estonia, Georgia, Ghana, Guatemala, Haiti, Honduras, India, Indonesia, Israel, Italy, Ivory Coast, Jamaica, Japan, Kenya, Laos, Liberia, Mexico, Mozambique, Nepal, Nicaragua, Nigeria, Pakistan, Palestine, Panama, Papua-New Guinea, Peru, Philippines, Puerto Rico, Rwanda, Senegal, Sierra Leone, South Africa, Swaziland, Taiwan, Thailand, Uganda, Ukraine, United Kingdom, United States, Uruguay, Venezuela, Vietnam, Yugoslavia, former, Zambia, Zimbabwe

Mission: The four goals of the General Board of Global Ministries are:

1. Witness to the Gospel for Initial decision to follow Jesus Christ—We will proclaim and live the Gospel of Jesus and similarly, challenge others to discipleship and through Christian communities.
2. Strengthen, develop and renew Christian congregations and communities.
3. Alleviate human suffering—we will help to initiate, strengthen and support ministries to the spiritual, physical, emotional and social needs of people.
4. Seek justice, freedom and peace—we will participate with people oppressed by unjust economic, political and social systems in programs that seek to build just, free and peaceful societies.

Volunteers can serve for 2 year terms, language training is provided, as well as all funding and room and board.

(continued)

Placement opportunities for . . .		Organization/Service Specifics:	
People of only certain faiths? *1*	Yes	Size of the Organization's Staff:	>200
Couples: both are health providers?	Yes	Number of providers sent or received/year:	>200
Couples: only one is a health provider?	Yes	Minimum term of assignment:	1 week
Families with children?	Yes	Maximum term of assignment:	2 years
Medical students?	Yes	Is funding available for travel? *2*	No
Pre-medical or college students?	Yes	Are room and board provided?	No
Other health professional students?	Yes	Is any other funding available?	No
Doctors in training?	Yes	Is training provided or available?	Yes
Health personnel who are US citizens?	Yes	Is a language other than English required? *3*	Yes
Health personnel who are non-US citizens?	Yes		
Health personnel with no prior experience in developing countries?	Yes		
Health personnel who are not current members of your organization?	Yes		

Health Professionals Placed:

Physicians:

Physicians; Cardiologists; Dermatologists; Emergency Medicine Physicians; Family Practitioners; General Surgeons; Internal Medicine GPS & PCP; Neurologists; OB/GYN; Ophthalmologists; Oral Surgeons; Optometrists; Orthopedic Surgeons; Pediatricians

Allied Health Professionals:

Administrative Health Positions; Dental Hygienists; Dentists; Nurse Practitioners; Nurses; Nutritionists & Dieticians; Social Workers

Notes

1. Volunteers must be Christian; *2.* Volunteers raise their own fund ahead of time; *3.* Language training is provided.

General Dept. of World Missions, The Wesleyan Church

Continents Served

Africa ☑ Asia ☐ Europe ☑ The Americas ☑

Countries Served

Haiti Kosovo Russia Zambia

Address: **P.O. Box 50434, Indianapolis, IN 46250-0434 U.S.A.**

Phone: **(317) 774-7950 or (800) 707-7715 or (317) 570-5170** FAX: **(317) 774-7958**

E-Mail: **globalpartners@wesleyan.org** Web: **www.wesleyan.org**

Mission: Wesleyan World Missions exists to exalt Jesus Christ by calling Wesleyans to evangelism, church planting, leadership development, and ministries of compassion for establishing a flourishing international church. Volunteers can serve from 1 year to life. There are no language requirements, and while funding is not directly available, the Wesleyan Church will help volunteers raise monetary support.

Placement opportunities for . . .		Organization/Service Specifics:	
People of only certain faiths? *1*	Yes	Size of the Organization's Staff:	151-200
Couples: both are health providers?	Yes	Number of providers sent or received/year:	
Couples: only one is a health provider?	Yes	Minimum term of assignment:	1 year
Families with children?	Yes	Maximum term of assignment:	100 years
Medical students?	No	Is funding available for travel?	No
Pre-medical or college students?	No	Are room and board provided?	No
Other health professional students?	No	Is any other funding available? *2*	No
Doctors in training?	No	Is training provided or available?	Yes
Health personnel who are US citizens?	Yes	Is a language other than English required?	No
Health personnel who are non-US citizens?	No		
Health personnel with no prior experience in developing countries?	No		
Health personnel who are not current members of your organization?	Yes		

Health Professionals Placed:

Physicians:

Physicians

Allied Health Professionals:

Nurses; Physician Assistants

Notes

1. Volunteers must be Protestant Christians; *2.* We help volunteers raise monetary support.

Global Operations & Development

Address: **8332 Commonwealth Ave, Buena Park, CA 90621 U.S.A.**

Phone: **(714) 523-4454** FAX: **(714) 523-4474**

E-Mail: **global@godaid.com** Web: **www.godaid.com**

Mission: Global Operations & Development (GO&D) seeks to improve the physical, spiritual, and emotional well being of the world's neediest children. It provides medical care and supplies to areas in all parts of the world. For example, in Siberia, Russia, GO&D helped to construct, equip, and supply the Mount Olive Medical Clinic in the Buryatia Republic. GO&D seeks health care practitioners of the Catholic or Protestant faith for shorter (2 week) to longer (3 years) term stays. There are no language requirements. Room, board, and funding, but not training, are provided.

Continents Served

Africa ✔ Asia ✔ Europe ✔ The Americas ✔

Countries Served

Austria, Bosnia and Herzegovina, China, Cuba, El Salvador, Honduras, Iraq, Kenya, Korea, North, Nepal, Nigeria, Peru, Philippines, Romania, Russia, Serbia and Montenegro, Tajikistan, Tanzania, Uganda, Vietnam

Placement opportunities for . . .

People of only certain faiths? *1*	Yes
Couples: both are health providers?	Yes
Couples: only one is a health provider?	Yes
Families with children?	Yes
Medical students?	Yes
Pre-medical or college students?	Yes
Other health professional students?	Yes
Doctors in training?	Yes
Health personnel who are US citizens?	Yes
Health personnel who are non-US citizens?	Yes
Health personnel with no prior experience in developing countries?	Yes
Health personnel who are not current members of your organization?	Yes

Organization/Service Specifics:

Size of the Organization's Staff:	51-100
Number of providers sent or received/year:	6-10
Minimum term of assignment:	2 weeks
Maximum term of assignment:	3 years
Is funding available for travel?	No
Are room and board provided?	Yes
Is any other funding available? *2*	Yes
Is training provided or available?	
Is a language other than English required?	No

Health Professionals Placed:

Physicians:

Physicians; Family Practitioners; Internal Medicine GPS & PCP

Allied Health Professionals:

Administrative Health Positions; Nurses; Public Health Specialists, Epidemiologists and Health Educators

Notes

1. Volunteers must be Catholic or Protestant; *2.* Project funds are available, but in terms of travel expenses, participants must raise own support.

Global Outreach International

Address: **P.O. Box 1, Tupelo, MS 38802 U.S.A.**

Phone: **(662) 842-4615** FAX: **(662) 842-4620**

E-Mail: **go@globaloutreach.org** Web: **www.globaloutreach.org**

Mission: Our mission is to partner with churches to carry out the Great Commission by providing opportunities in a ministry-evangelism based mission endeavor. Medical assignments can be as short as 1 week and there is no maximum term. Volunteers must be Protestant Christians and must provide their own funding for travel and room and board. There are no language requirements.

Continents Served

Africa ✔ Asia ✔ Europe ✔ The Americas ✔

Countries Served

Belize, Brazil, Chile, China, Costa Rica, Ecuador, Guyana, Haiti, Honduras, India, Israel, Kenya, Mexico, Philippines, Poland, Romania, Russia, Uganda

(continued)

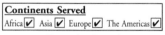

Placement opportunities for . . .

People of only certain faiths? *1*	Yes
Couples: both are health providers?	Yes
Couples: only one is a health provider?	Yes
Families with children?	Yes
Medical students?	Yes
Pre-medical or college students?	Yes
Other health professional students?	Yes
Doctors in training?	Yes
Health personnel who are US citizens?	Yes
Health personnel who are non-US citizens?	No
Health personnel with no prior experience in developing countries?	Yes
Health personnel who are not current members of your organization?	Yes

Organization/Service Specifics:

Size of the Organization's Staff:	101-150
Number of providers sent or received/year:	6-10
Minimum term of assignment:	1 week
Maximum term of assignment:	no limit
Is funding available for travel?	No
Are room and board provided?	No
Is any other funding available?	No
Is training provided or available?	Yes
Is a language other than English required?	No

Health Professionals Placed:

Physicians:

Physicians; Family Practitioners

Allied Health Professionals:

Dentists; Nurse Midwives; Nurse Practitioners; Nurses; Paramedics; Water/Sanitation Specialists

Notes

1. Protestant, non-denominational Christian.

Global Service Corps/Earth Island Institute

Continents Served

Africa ☑ Asia ☑ Europe ☐ The Americas ☑

Countries Served

Tanzania Thailand

Address: **300 Broadway, Suite 28, San Francisco, CA 94133-3312 U.S.A.**

Phone: **(415) 788-3666 Ext. 128** FAX: **(415) 788-7324**

E-Mail: **gsc@earthisland.org** Web: **www.globalservicecorps.org**

Mission: Global Service Corps (GSC) provides opportunities for physicians, health administrators, and public health workers to serve abroad and help underserved people. GSC provides cross-cultural learning and community service adventures for adults in Tanzania and Thailand for a fee. Short-term (2-4 weeks), long-term (2-6 months), and student internship programs for pre-med and medical students are available. Volunteers live and work in a developing country alongside local people. There are no language or religious restrictions.

Placement opportunities for . . .

People of only certain faiths?	No
Couples: both are health providers?	Yes
Couples: only one is a health provider?	Yes
Families with children?	Yes
Medical students?	Yes
Pre-medical or college students?	Yes
Other health professional students?	Yes
Doctors in training?	Yes
Health personnel who are US citizens?	Yes
Health personnel who are non-US citizens?	Yes
Health personnel with no prior experience in developing countries?	Yes
Health personnel who are not current members of your organization?	Yes

Organization/Service Specifics:

Size of the Organization's Staff:	0-5
Number of providers sent or received/year:	>200
Minimum term of assignment:	2 weeks
Maximum term of assignment:	1 year
Is funding available for travel?	No
Are room and board provided?	Yes
Is any other funding available?	No
Is training provided or available?	Yes
Is a language other than English required?	No

Health Professionals Placed:

Physicians:

Physicians

Allied Health Professionals:

Administrative Health Positions; Public Health Specialists, Epidemiologists and Health Educators

Notes

Global Volunteers

Continents Served			
Africa ✔	Asia ✔	Europe ✔	The Americas ✔

Address: **375 E. Little Canada Road, St. Paul, MN 55117 U.S.A.**
Phone: **(651) 407-6100**
(800) 487-1074
FAX: **(651) 482-0915**
E-Mail: **email@globalvolunteers.org**
Web: **www.globalvolunteers.org**

Countries Served

Cook Islands	Costa Rica	Ecuador
Ghana	Greece	Jamaica
Romania	Tanzania	

Mission: As a non-governmental organization (NGO) in special consultative status with the United Nations, Global Volunteers mobilizes some 150 service-learning teams year-around to work in 18 countries on six continents. Global Volunteers continues to provide health care assistance in more than a third of those countries. Because the access to medical services in developing communities is often limited, health-care volunteers are needed to provide a variety of services both in the clinics and surrounding areas.

Placement opportunities for . . .		Organization/Service Specifics:	
People of only certain faiths?	No	Size of the Organization's Staff:	21-50
Couples: both are health providers?	Yes	Number of providers sent or received/year:	51-100
Couples: only one is a health provider?	Yes	Minimum term of assignment:	2 weeks
Families with children?	No	Maximum term of assignment:	3 weeks
Medical students?	Yes	Is funding available for travel?	No
Pre-medical or college students?	Yes	Are room and board provided?	No
Other health professional students?	Yes	Is any other funding available?	No
Doctors in training?	Yes	Is training provided or available?	No
Health personnel who are US citizens?	Yes	Is a language other than English required?	No
Health personnel who are non-US citizens?	Yes		
Health personnel with no prior experience in developing countries?	Yes		
Health personnel who are not current members of your organization?	Yes		

Health Professionals Placed:

Physicians:

All physician specialties

Allied Health Professionals:

All allied health professionals

Notes

Grace Ministries International

Continents Served			
Africa ✔	Asia ✔	Europe ☐	The Americas ✔

Address: **2125 Martindale Ave. SW, Grand Rapids, MI 49509 U.S.A.**
Phone: **(616) 241-5666**
FAX: **(616) 241-2542**
E-Mail: **gmi@gracem.org**
Web: **www.gracem.org**

Countries Served

Congo Tanzania

Mission: Grace Ministries International is an evangelical mission agency with the goal of bringing people to experience salvation in the Lord Jesus Christ and incorporating them into strong, self-sustaining churches. Depending on the particular needs of the host countries, GMI will also be involved in medical work, educational ministries, and community development. Volunteers are needed to support ongoing mission work.

Placement opportunities for . . .		Organization/Service Specifics:	
People of only certain faiths? *1*	No	Size of the Organization's Staff:	51-100
Couples: both are health providers?	Yes	Number of providers sent or received/year:	6-10
Couples: only one is a health provider?	Yes	Minimum term of assignment:	2 weeks
Families with children?	Yes	Maximum term of assignment:	4 weeks
Medical students?	No	Is funding available for travel?	No
Pre-medical or college students?	No	Are room and board provided?	Yes
Other health professional students?	Yes	Is any other funding available?	Yes
Doctors in training?	No	Is training provided or available?	Yes
Health personnel who are US citizens?	Yes	Is a language other than English required? *2*	No
Health personnel who are non-US citizens?	Yes		
Health personnel with no prior experience in developing countries?	Yes		
Health personnel who are not current members of your organization?	Yes		

(continued)

Health Professionals Placed:

Physicians:

Physicians; Anesthesiologists; Family Practitioners; General Surgeons; Hematologists; Oncologists; Infectious Disease Spec.; OB/GYN; Ophthalmologists; Optometrists; Orthopedic Surgeons; Pediatricians; Urologists

Allied Health Professionals:

Administrative Health Positions; Dentists; Physician Assistants

Notes

1. Prefer Protestants; *2.* French training available.

Grokha Association of Social Health

Address: **G.P.O.8975, E.P.C.2446, Kathmandu, Nepal**

Phone: **0977-1-2122028** FAX:

E-Mail: **bless_smn@yahoo.com** Web: **www.geocities.com/gash_nepal**

Continents Served

Africa ☐ Asia ☑ Europe ☐ The Americas ☐

Countries Served

Nepal

Mission: Grokha Association of Social Health established to serve the health needs of the rural area of Nepal, especially the area of the rural district Gorkha. The goal is to gradually provide specific health services to all of Nepal's rural communities. Most rural community members believe that diseases are caused by the anger of many types of Gods. They do not know the scientific causes (bacteria, virus, etc). The government health sector provides care to the fortunate members of urban society but this is not as true in the rural communities. GASH hopes to spread awareness to the rural areas of Nepal and provide the specific health services they so badly need.

Placement opportunities for . . .	
People of only certain faiths?	No
Couples: both are health providers?	Yes
Couples: only one is a health provider?	No
Families with children?	No
Medical students?	No
Pre-medical or college students?	No
Other health professional students?	Yes
Doctors in training?	No
Health personnel who are US citizens?	Yes
Health personnel who are non-US citizens?	Yes
Health personnel with no prior experience in developing countries?	Yes
Health personnel who are not current members of your organization?	Yes

Organization/Service Specifics:	
Size of the Organization's Staff:	6-10
Number of providers sent or received/year:	1-5
Minimum term of assignment:	1 month
Maximum term of assignment:	3 months
Is funding available for travel?	No
Are room and board provided?	No
Is any other funding available?	No
Is training provided or available?	No
Is a language other than English required?	No

Health Professionals Placed: *1*

Physicians:

Physicians; Family Practitioners; Infectious Disease Spec.; Internal Medicine GPS & PCP; Pediatricians; Urologists

Allied Health Professionals:

Dental Hygienists; Dentists; Medical Technicians (lab, X-ray, etc); Nurse Midwives; Nurse Practitioners; Nurses; Paramedics; Pharmacists; Physical & Occupational Therapists; Physician Assistants; Public Health Specialists, Epidemiologists and Health Educators; Water/Sanitation Specialists

Notes

1. Other specialty areas may be requested according to community needs.

Guinea Development Foundation, Inc.

Address: **140 West End Ave., Suite 17G, New York, NY 10023 U.S.A.**

Phone: **(212) 874-2911** FAX: **(212) 496-9549**

E-Mail: **GDF@guineadev.org** Web: **www.guineadev.org/**

Continents Served

Africa ☑ Asia ☐ Europe ☐ The Americas ☐

Countries Served

Guinea

Mission: To improve the overall health of the citizens of the Republic of Guinea. The Foundation is particularly concerned with reducing the rates of infant and maternal mortality, with reducing morbidity resulting from the nation's high incidence of malaria, reducing the impact of childhood diseases, and treating patients affected by diarrhoeal and respiratory illnesses. The program for action includes: training doctors, nurses, nurse aides and village health workers; training public health workers in preventive health care education for the rural population; establishing fully operational health centers in areas of pressing need; promoting modern medical standards and integrating them with traditional healing practices; implementing effective and culturally acceptable family planning techniques; educating people in the prevention of AIDS; spreading the knowledge and practice of environmental responsibility: concerning pollution, recycling, energy conservation, etc.

Placement opportunities for . . .	
People of only certain faiths?	No
Couples: both are health providers?	Yes
Couples: only one is a health provider?	Yes
Families with children?	No
Medical students?	Yes
Pre-medical or college students?	Yes
Other health professional students?	Yes
Doctors in training?	Yes
Health personnel who are US citizens?	Yes
Health personnel who are non-US citizens?	Yes
Health personnel with no prior experience in developing countries?	Yes
Health personnel who are not current members of your organization?	Yes

Organization/Service Specifics:	
Size of the Organization's Staff:	0-5
Number of providers sent or received/year:	11-20
Minimum term of assignment:	6 months
Maximum term of assignment:	3 years
Is funding available for travel?	Yes
Are room and board provided?	Yes
Is any other funding available? *1*	Yes
Is training provided or available?	Yes
Is a language other than English required? *2*	Yes

Health Professionals Placed:

Physicians:

Physicians; Anesthesiologists; Cardiologists; Dermatologists; Emergency Medicine Physicians; Endocrinologists; Family Practitioners; Gastroenterologists; General Surgeons; Hematologists; Oncologists; Infectious Disease Spec.; Internal Medicine GPS & PCP; Nephrologists; Neurologists; Neurosurgeons; OB/GYN; Ophthalmologists; Oral Surgeons; Optometrists; Orthopedic Surgeons; Otolaryngologists; Pediatricians; Plastic/Hand/Reconstructive Surgeons; Pulmonary Specialists; Radiologists; Urologists

Allied Health Professionals:

Dental Hygienists; Dentists; Medical Technicians (lab, X-ray, etc); Nurse Midwives; Nurse Practitioners; Nurses; Nutritionists & Dieticians; Paramedics; Pharmacists; Physical & Occupational Therapists; Physician Assistants; Podiatrists; Prosthetists; Psychologists; Public Health Specialists, Epidemiologists and Health Educators; Respiratory Therapists; Social Workers; Water/Sanitation Specialists

Notes

1. Stipends are available for foreign medical doctors;
2. French is required.

Haitian Health Foundation, Inc.

Address: **97 Sherman Street, Norwich, CT 06360 U.S.A.**

Phone: **(860) 886-4357** FAX: **(860) 859-9887**

E-Mail: **HHF@Haitianhealthfoundation.org** Web: **www.haitianhealthfoundation.org/**

Continents Served

Africa ☐ Asia ☐ Europe ☐ The Americas ☑

Countries Served

Haiti

Mission: The mission of the Haitian Health Foundation is to improve the health and well being of the poor, the sick, and the infirm of the greater Jeremie area. This is accomplished through a secondary care outpatient clinic, a public health outreach program, nutritional rehabilitation services, safe motherhood services, community development programs, self-help programs which advance family and community self-sufficiency, responding to emergencies and crises with humanitarian relief, and programs to facilitate the exchange of knowledge and expertise between Haitians and the international community. Volunteers can serve for 2 week to 6 month terms. Knowledge of French or Creole is required.

(continued)

Placement opportunities for . . .		Organization/Service Specifics:		
People of only certain faiths?	No	Size of the Organization's Staff:		11-20
Couples: both are health providers?	Yes	Number of providers sent or received/year:		51-100
Couples: only one is a health provider?	Yes	Minimum term of assignment:		2 weeks
Families with children?		Maximum term of assignment:		6 months
Medical students?	Yes	Is funding available for travel?		No
Pre-medical or college students?	No	Are room and board provided?		No
Other health professional students?	Yes	Is any other funding available?		No
Doctors in training?	Yes	Is training provided or available?		No
Health personnel who are US citizens?	Yes	Is a language other than English required?	*1*	Yes
Health personnel who are non-US citizens?	Yes			
Health personnel with no prior experience in developing countries?	Yes			
Health personnel who are not current members of your organization?	Yes			

Health Professionals Placed:

Physicians:

Physicians; Dermatologists; Family Practitioners; Gastroenterologists; Infectious Disease Spec.; Internal Medicine GPS & PCP; OB/GYN; Ophthalmologists; Oral Surgeons; Optometrists; Otolaryngologists; Pathologists; Pediatricians; Radiologists

Allied Health Professionals:

Dental Hygienists; Dentists; Medical Technicians (lab, X-ray, etc); Nurse Practitioners; Nurses; Nutritionists & Dieticians; Pharmacists; Physical & Occupational Therapists; Physician Assistants; Public Health Specialists, Epidemiologists and Health Educators

Notes

1. French or Creole is required.

Hands Together, Inc.

Address: **PO Box 80985, Springfield, MA 01138 U.S.A.**

Phone: **(413) 731-7716** FAX: **(413) 731-6405**

E-Mail: **handstog@aol.com** Web: **www.handstogether.org**

Continents Served

Africa ☐ Asia ☐ Europe ☐ The Americas ☑

Countries Served

Haiti

Mission: Hands Together is a non-profit organization devoted to educating, inspiring, and encouraging people to understand and respond to the needs of all people, especially the poor and disadvantaged. Our mission, as we strive to build a more compassionate and human world, proceeds from the belief that all people are members of one equal, interconnected family under a loving God. Volunteers can serve for 1 week to 6 month terms. While room and board are provided, volunteers are responsible for other funding.

Placement opportunities for . . .			Organization/Service Specifics:		
People of only certain faiths?		No	Size of the Organization's Staff:		0-5
Couples: both are health providers?		Yes	Number of providers sent or received/year:		>200
Couples: only one is a health provider?		Yes	Minimum term of assignment:		1 weeks
Families with children?		No	Maximum term of assignment:		6 months
Medical students?		Yes	Is funding available for travel?		No
Pre-medical or college students?	*1*	Yes	Are room and board provided?		Yes
Other health professional students?		Yes	Is any other funding available?		No
Doctors in training?		Yes	Is training provided or available?		Yes
Health personnel who are US citizens?		Yes	Is a language other than English required?	*2*	No
Health personnel who are non-US citizens?		Yes			
Health personnel with no prior experience in developing countries?		Yes			
Health personnel who are not current members of your organization?		Yes			

Health Professionals Placed:

Physicians:

Physicians; Family Practitioners; General Surgeons; Infectious Disease Spec.; Internal Medicine GPS & PCP; OB/GYN; Oral Surgeons; Pediatricians; Plastic/Hand/Reconstructive Surgeons

Allied Health Professionals:

Dentists; Nurse Midwives; Nurse Practitioners; Nurses; Public Health Specialists, Epidemiologists and Health Educators; Water/Sanitation Specialists

Notes

1. If they have a health background; *2.* French is helpful.

Harlem Hospital, Plastic Surgery Program Rm. 11101

Address: **506 Lenox Avenue, New York, NY 10037 U.S.A.**
Phone: **(212) 939-3538** FAX: **(212) 939-3599**
E-Mail: **fao1@columbia.edu** Web:

Continents Served
Africa ☑ Asia ☐ Europe ☐ The Americas ☑

Countries Served
Haiti Nigeria

Mission: Harlem Hospital, in New York City, places plastic surgeons in Haiti and potentially in a pending program located in Africa. As of 4/04, this group only sends plastic surgeons from Harlem Hospital, though the group director, Dr Ofodile, states they may be open to others joining them in the future.

Placement opportunities for . . .		Organization/Service Specifics:	
People of only certain faiths?	No	Size of the Organization's Staff:	0-5
Couples: both are health providers?	Yes	Number of providers sent or received/year:	1-5
Couples: only one is a health provider?	No	Minimum term of assignment:	1 week
Families with children?	No	Maximum term of assignment:	
Medical students?	No	Is funding available for travel?	Yes
Pre-medical or college students?	No	Are room and board provided?	Yes
Other health professional students?	No	Is any other funding available?	No
Doctors in training?	No	Is training provided or available?	Yes
Health personnel who are US citizens?	Yes	Is a language other than English required?	No
Health personnel who are non-US citizens?	No		
Health personnel with no prior experience in developing countries?	Yes		
Health personnel who are not current members of your organization?	Yes		

Health Professionals Placed:

Physicians:

Physicians; Plastic/Hand/Reconstructive Surgeons

Allied Health Professionals:

Notes

HBS Foundation, Inc. / Hopital Bon Samaritain

Address: **P.O. Box 1290, Lake Worth, FL 33460 U.S.A.**
Phone: **(561) 533-0883** FAX: **(561) 533-0884**
E-Mail: **hbsfl@bellsouth.net** Web: **www.hbslimbe.org/**

Continents Served
Africa ☐ Asia ☐ Europe ☐ The Americas ☑

Countries Served
Haiti

Mission:

Placement opportunities for . . .		Organization/Service Specifics:	
People of only certain faiths?	No	Size of the Organization's Staff:	0-5
Couples: both are health providers?	Yes	Number of providers sent or received/year:	21-50
Couples: only one is a health provider?	Yes	Minimum term of assignment:	none
Families with children?	Yes	Maximum term of assignment:	none
Medical students?	Yes	Is funding available for travel?	No
Pre-medical or college students?	Yes	Are room and board provided?	Yes
Other health professional students?	Yes	Is any other funding available?	No
Doctors in training?	Yes	Is training provided or available?	Yes
Health personnel who are US citizens?	Yes	Is a language other than English required? *2*	No
Health personnel who are non-US citizens?	Yes		
Health personnel with no prior experience in developing countries? *1*	Yes		
Health personnel who are not current members of your organization?	Yes		

Health Professionals Placed: *3*

Physicians:

Physicians; Anesthesiologists; Dermatologists; Family Practitioners; General Surgeons; Infectious Disease Spec.; OB/GYN; Orthopedic Surgeons

Allied Health Professionals:

Administrative Health Positions; Medical Technicians (lab, X-ray, etc); Nurse Midwives; Nurse Practitioners; Nurses; Nutritionists & Dieticians; Physical & Occupational Therapists; Physician Assistants; Public Health Specialists, Epidemiologists and Health Educators; Social Workers; Water/Sanitation Specialists

Notes

1. Experience helpful; *2.* French helpful; *3.* Other specialties welcome.

Healing the Children Northeast, Inc.

Address: **219 Kent Rd., Suite 20, PO Box 129, New Milford, CT 06776 U.S.A.**

Phone: **(860) 355-1828** FAX: **(860) 350-6634**

E-Mail: **Info@htcne.org** Web: **www.htcne.org**

Continents Served

Africa ☑ Asia ☑ Europe ☑ The Americas ☑

Countries Served

Bangladesh	Belize	Bolivia
Brazil	China	Colombia
Dominican Republic		Ecuador
Egypt	El Salvador	Ethiopia
Guatemala	India	Jamaica
Kenya	Korea, South	
Nicaragua	Romania	Russia
Venezuela	Vietnam	

Mission: Healing the Children is a non-profit, non-partisan, volunteer organization whose main purpose is to secure and make available medical treatment for children from the United States and around the world. Healing the Children also brings children to the United States. Funding is not available for travel in all cases, although room and board are provided. Service terms last between 1 week and 2 weeks. There are no language requirements for volunteers, although foreign languages are helpful for some assignments.

Placement opportunities for . . .

People of only certain faiths?	No
Couples: both are health providers?	Yes
Couples: only one is a health provider?	No
Families with children?	No
Medical students?	No
Pre-medical or college students?	No
Other health professional students?	Yes
Doctors in training?	Yes
Health personnel who are US citizens?	Yes
Health personnel who are non-US citizens?	Yes
Health personnel with no prior experience in developing countries?	Yes
Health personnel who are not current members of your organization?	Yes

Organization/Service Specifics:

Size of the Organization's Staff:	6-10
Number of providers sent or received/year:	>200
Minimum term of assignment:	1 week
Maximum term of assignment:	2 weeks
Is funding available for travel? *1*	No
Are room and board provided?	Yes
Is any other funding available?	Yes
Is training provided or available?	Yes
Is a language other than English required? *2*	No

Health Professionals Placed:

Physicians:

Physicians; Anesthesiologists; Cardiologists; Emergency Medicine Physicians; Endocrinologists; Family Practitioners; Gastroenterologists; General Surgeons; Internal Medicine GPS & PCP; Neurologists; Neurosurgeons; OB/GYN; Ophthalmologists; Oral Surgeons; Optometrists; Orthopedic Surgeons; Otolaryngologists; Pediatricians; Plastic/Hand/Reconstructive Surgeons; Pulmonary Specialists; Radiologists; Urologists

Allied Health Professionals:

Administrative Health Positions; Dental Hygienists; Dentists; Nurse Practitioners; Nurses; Physical & Occupational Therapists; Physician Assistants; Respiratory Therapists; Social Workers

Notes

1. Grants for travel depend on the time and place of service; *2.* No language requirements, but foreign languages would be helpful for some assignments.

Health Alliance International

Address: **1107 NE 45th St., Suite 427, Seattle, WA 98105 U.S.A.**

Phone: **(206) 543-8382** FAX: **(206) 685-4184**

E-Mail: **hai@u.washington.edu** Web: **http://depts.washington.edu/haiuw/**

Continents Served

Africa ☑ Asia ☐ Europe ☐ The Americas ☐

Countries Served

East Timor Mozambique

Mission: Health Alliance Internatinoal is a non-profit organization associated with the University of Washington School of Public Health and Community Medicine. HAI provides technical and material assistance to government and community institutions to evaluate, strengthen, and sustain effective health services, as well as focus on changing the inequitable conditions that contribute to poor health. A principal goal of HAI is to enable university and community-based practitioners to develop public health service projects.

(continued)

Placement opportunities for . . .		**Organization/Service Specifics:**	
People of only certain faiths?	No	Size of the Organization's Staff:	11-20
Couples: both are health providers?	Yes	Number of providers sent or received/year:	1-5
Couples: only one is a health provider?	Yes	Minimum term of assignment:	2 months
Families with children?	Yes	Maximum term of assignment:	3 years
Medical students?	Yes	Is funding available for travel?	Yes
Pre-medical or college students?	No	Are room and board provided?	Yes
Other health professional students?	Yes	Is any other funding available? *1*	Yes
Doctors in training?	Yes	Is training provided or available?	No
Health personnel who are US citizens?	Yes	Is a language other than English required? *2*	Yes

Health personnel who are non-US citizens?	Yes
Health personnel with no prior experience in developing countries?	No
Health personnel who are not current members of your organization?	Yes

Health Professionals Placed:

Physicians:

Physicians

Allied Health Professionals:

Administrative Health Positions; Nurses; Public Health Specialists, Epidemiologists and Health Educators

Notes

1. Some salaried positions are available; *2.* Portuguese is required for some placements.

Health and Child Survival Fellows Program

Address: **P.O. Box 2216, Baltimore, MD 21203-2216 U.S.A.**

Phone: **(410) 659-4108** FAX: **(410) 659-4118**

E-Mail: **pseaton@jhsph.edu** Web: **jhuhcsfp.org**

Mission: The Institute for International Programs, John Hopkins Bloomberg School of Public Health, serves as National Secretariat for the Health and Child Survival Fellows Program (HCSFP). With its objective being the establishment and fostering of a cadre of field-experienced technical experts in child survival and international health, the National Secretariat identifies, places, supports and supervises junior, mid-level and senior experts in assignments in the broad fields of child survival and international health. These assignments contribute to health and child survival programs in developing countries, as well as to the career development and commitment of the experts themselves. No opportunities for health care services are offered. Candidate must have a masters degree in a health-related field and an interest in a career in international health and child survival.

Continents Served

Africa ☑ Asia ☑ Europe ☑ The Americas ☑

Countries Served

Angola	Bangladesh	Barbados
Brazil	Cambodia	Egypt
Ghana	Guyana	Honduras
India	Indonesia	Jamaica
Kenya	Mozambique	Nepal
Nicaragua	Nigeria	Thailand
Uganda	United States	USSR, former
Zambia		

Placement opportunities for . . .		**Organization/Service Specifics:**	
People of only certain faiths?	No	Size of the Organization's Staff:	0-5
Couples: both are health providers?	Yes	Number of providers sent or received/year:	21-50
Couples: only one is a health provider?	Yes	Minimum term of assignment:	2 years
Families with children?	Yes	Maximum term of assignment:	4 years
Medical students?	No	Is funding available for travel?	Yes
Pre-medical or college students?	No	Are room and board provided?	Yes
Other health professional students?	Yes	Is any other funding available? *1*	Yes
Doctors in training?	No	Is training provided or available?	Yes
Health personnel who are US citizens?	Yes	Is a language other than English required?	No

Health personnel who are non-US citizens?	No
Health personnel with no prior experience in developing countries?	Yes
Health personnel who are not current members of your organization?	Yes

Health Professionals Placed:

Physicians:

Physicians; Infectious Disease Spec.; Internal Medicine GPS & PCP; OB/GYN; Pediatricians

Allied Health Professionals:

Administrative Health Positions; Nurse Midwives; Nurse Practitioners; Nurses; Nutritionists & Dieticians; Pharmacists; Public Health Specialists, Epidemiologists and Health Educators; Water/Sanitation Specialists

Notes

1. Both salary and benefits are provided.

Health Teams International

Address: **10056 Applegate Lane, Brighton, MI 48114 U.S.A.**

Phone: **(810) 229-9247** FAX: **(810) 229-4336**

E-Mail: **ddchar@ismi.net** Web:

Mission: We are an ecumenical missionary organization. Our purpose is to assist in the evangelization of the unreached groups of the world through the ministrations of short term Chirsitian health care teams. Volunteers can travel on 1-3 week missions. There is funding available for travel, but room and board are not provided. Volunteers must be Catholic or Protestant.

Continents Served

Africa ✔ Asia ✔ Europe ✔ The Americas ✔

Countries Served *2*

Brazil	Burkina Faso	Cambodia
Cameroon	Central African Rep.	
Ghana	Guatemala	Honduras
India	Indonesia	Madagascar
Mexico	Mozambique	Nepal
Sierra Leone	Sri Lanka	Thailand
USSR, former		

Placement opportunities for . . .

People of only certain faiths? *1*	Yes
Couples: both are health providers?	Yes
Couples: only one is a health provider?	Yes
Families with children?	Yes
Medical students?	Yes
Pre-medical or college students?	Yes
Other health professional students?	Yes
Doctors in training?	Yes
Health personnel who are US citizens?	Yes
Health personnel who are non-US citizens?	Yes
Health personnel with no prior experience in developing countries?	Yes
Health personnel who are not current members of your organization?	Yes

Organization/Service Specifics:

Size of the Organization's Staff:	0-5
Number of providers sent or received/year:	51-100
Minimum term of assignment:	1 week
Maximum term of assignment:	3 weeks
Is funding available for travel?	Yes
Are room and board provided?	No
Is any other funding available?	No
Is training provided or available?	Yes
Is a language other than English required?	No

Health Professionals Placed:

Physicians:

Physicians; Anesthesiologists; Cardiologists; Dermatologists; Emergency Medicine Physicians; Endocrinologists; Family Practitioners; Gastroenterologists; General Surgeons; Hematologists; Oncologists; Infectious Disease Spec.; Internal Medicine GPS & PCP; Nephrologists; Neurologists; Neurosurgeons; OB/GYN; Ophthalmologists; Oral Surgeons; Optometrists; Orthopedic Surgeons; Otolaryngologists; Pathologists; Pediatricians; Plastic/Hand/Reconstructive Surgeons; Psychiatrists; Pulmonary Specialists; Radiologists; Urologists

Allied Health Professionals:

Administrative Health Positions; Dental Hygienists; Dentists; Medical Technicians (lab, X-ray, etc); Nurse Midwives; Nurse Practitioners; Nurses; Nutritionists & Dieticians; Paramedics; Pharmacists; Physical & Occupational Therapists; Physician Assistants; Podiatrists; Prosthetists; Psychologists; Public Health Specialists, Epidemiologists and Health Educators; Respiratory Therapists; Social Workers; Water/Sanitation Specialists

Notes

1. Volunteers must be Catholic or Protestant. *2.* Organization serves 52 countries as of 2/05-specific countries beyond those listed are unavailable. Please contact organization for details.

Health Volunteers Overseas

Address: **1900 L Street, NW, Washington, DC 20036 U.S.A.**

Phone: **(202) 296-0928** FAX: **(202) 296-8018**

E-Mail: **info@hvousa.org** Web: **www.hvousa.org/**

Mission: Most developing countries lack the trained health professionals necessary to provide appropriate care. They also lack the financial resources to provide adequate training. HVO, a private nonprofit organization, is dedicated to making this training and education available. HVO volunteers train more than 750 health care providers each year. Since 1986, over 3000 volunteers have served with HVO. Volunteers can serve for short term (2 weeks) to longer term (1 year) assignments. Funding is occasionally available, and while there is no formal training, there is an orientation period.

Continents Served

Africa ✔ Asia ✔ Europe ✔ The Americas ✔

Countries Served

Belize	Bhutan	Brazil
Cambodia	Costa Rica	Ethiopia
Guyana	Haiti	Honduras
India	Kenya	Nepal
Nicaragua	Peru	Philippines
South Africa	St. Lucia	Suriname
Tanzania	Trinidad and Tobago	
Uganda	Vietnam	

(continued)

Placement opportunities for . . .

People of only certain faiths?	No
Couples: both are health providers?	Yes
Couples: only one is a health provider?	Yes
Families with children?	Yes
Medical students?	No
Pre-medical or college students?	No
Other health professional students?	Yes
Doctors in training?	Yes
Health personnel who are US citizens?	Yes
Health personnel who are non-US citizens?	Yes
Health personnel with no prior experience in developing countries?	Yes
Health personnel who are not current members of your organization?	Yes

Organization/Service Specifics:

Size of the Organization's Staff:	6-10
Number of providers sent or received/year:	>200
Minimum term of assignment:	2 weeks
Maximum term of assignment:	1 year
Is funding available for travel?	Yes
Are room and board provided?	Yes
Is any other funding available? *1*	Yes
Is training provided or available? *2*	No
Is a language other than English required?	No

Health Professionals Placed:

Physicians:

Anesthesiologists; Dermatologists; General Surgeons; Internal Medicine GPS & PCP; Oral Surgeons; Orthopedic Surgeons; Pediatricians; Plastic/Hand/Reconstructive Surgeons

Allied Health Professionals:

Dentists; Nurses; Physical & Occupational Therapists

Notes

1. Funding for travel and room and board are occasionally provided; *2.* Orientation, not training, is provided.

Helen Keller International

Address: **352 Park Avenue South, 12th Floor, New York, NY 10010 U.S.A.**

Phone: **(877) 535-5374**
(212) 532-0544 FAX: **(212) 791-7590**

E-Mail: **info@hkworld.org** Web: **www.hki.org**

Mission: Helen Keller International prevents blindness, restores sight, and provides rehabilitation sources to blind people. We save the sight and lives of the most vulnerable people in the human family. There are no language requirements and funding is not available.

Continents Served

Africa ✔ Asia ✔ Europe ✔ The Americas ✔

Countries Served

Bangladesh	Burkina Faso	Cambodia
Cameroon	China	France
Guinea	Indonesia	Ivory Coast
Mali	Morocco	Mozambique
Myanmar (Burma)		Nepal
Niger	Nigeria	Philippines
South Africa	Tanzania	Vietnam

Placement opportunities for . . .

People of only certain faiths?	No
Couples: both are health providers?	Yes
Couples: only one is a health provider?	Yes
Families with children?	Yes
Medical students?	Yes
Pre-medical or college students?	No
Other health professional students?	Yes
Doctors in training?	Yes
Health personnel who are US citizens?	Yes
Health personnel who are non-US citizens?	Yes
Health personnel with no prior experience in developing countries?	Yes
Health personnel who are not current members of your organization?	Yes

Organization/Service Specifics:

Size of the Organization's Staff:	>200
Number of providers sent or received/year:	>200
Minimum term of assignment:	
Maximum term of assignment:	
Is funding available for travel?	No
Are room and board provided?	No
Is any other funding available?	No
Is training provided or available?	No
Is a language other than English required? *1*	No

Health Professionals Placed:

Physicians:

Ophthalmologists; Optometrists

Allied Health Professionals:

Notes

1. Other languages are useful, but not required.

Helping Hands Health Education

Continents Served			
Africa ☐	Asia ☑	Europe ☐	The Americas ☐

Address: **948 Pearl Street, Boulder, CO 80302 U.S.A.**

Phone: **(303) 448-1811**
(888) 241-0710
FAX: **(303) 440-7328**

E-Mail: **helpinghands@sannr.com** Web: **www.helpinghandsusa.org/**

Countries Served
Nepal Vietnam

Mission: Helping Hands Health Education is a non-profit organization aimed at bringing low cost quality medical care to people in rural villages of Nepal through the help of Western medical and non-medical volunteers. It provides volunteering opportunities for medical professionals, medical students and nonmedical volunteers to serve in Nepal. Along with two permanent clinics in the capital city of Kathmandu, Helping Hands has formed a permanent clinic in the eastern village of Khandbar. Medical volunteers get opportunities to work in these permanent clinics as well as in the mobile health camps that are organized through the year.

Placement opportunities for . . .		Organization/Service Specifics:	
People of only certain faiths?	No	Size of the Organization's Staff:	0-5
Couples: both are health providers?	Yes	Number of providers sent or received/year:	21-50
Couples: only one is a health provider?	Yes	Minimum term of assignment:	2 weeks
Families with children?	No	Maximum term of assignment:	2 months
Medical students?	Yes	Is funding available for travel?	No
Pre-medical or college students?	Yes	Are room and board provided?	No
Other health professional students?	Yes	Is any other funding available?	No
Doctors in training?	Yes	Is training provided or available?	Yes
Health personnel who are US citizens?	Yes	Is a language other than English required?	No

Health personnel who are non-US citizens?	Yes
Health personnel with no prior experience in developing countries?	Yes
Health personnel who are not current members of your organization?	Yes

Health Professionals Placed: **Notes**

Physicians:

Physicians; General Surgeons; Internal Medicine GPS & PCP; OB/GYN; Ophthalmologists; Pediatricians

Allied Health Professionals:

Dentists; Nurses; Water/Sanitation Specialists

HELPS International

Continents Served			
Africa ☐	Asia ☐	Europe ☐	The Americas ☑

Address: **15301 Dallas Pkwy #200, Addison, TX 75001 U.S.A.**

Phone: **(972) 386-2901 or**
(800) 41-HELPS
FAX: **(972) 386-4294**

Countries Served
Guatemala

E-Mail: **info@helpsinternational.com** Web: **helpsintl.org**

Mission: HELPS International is a non-denominational Christian organization that provides assistance to the people of rural Guatemala through the personal interaction and efforts of volunteers dedicated to service to others. In cooperation with government authorities and with local support, HELPS develops enduring programs in medical care, health promotion, construction, infrastructure, education, and economic development. Trips to Guatelmala last for 10 days, and volunteers are required to come up with their own funding.

Placement opportunities for . . .		Organization/Service Specifics:	
People of only certain faiths? *1*	No	Size of the Organization's Staff:	6-10
Couples: both are health providers?	Yes	Number of providers sent or received/year:	>200
Couples: only one is a health provider?	Yes	Minimum term of assignment:	10 days
Families with children?	No	Maximum term of assignment:	10 days
Medical students?	Yes	Is funding available for travel?	No
Pre-medical or college students?	No	Are room and board provided?	No
Other health professional students?	Yes	Is any other funding available? *2*	No
Doctors in training?	Yes	Is training provided or available?	No
Health personnel who are US citizens?	Yes	Is a language other than English required?	No

Health personnel who are non-US citizens?	Yes
Health personnel with no prior experience in developing countries?	Yes
Health personnel who are not current members of your organization?	Yes

(continued)

Health Professionals Placed:

Physicians:

Physicians; Anesthesiologists; Dermatologists; Emergency Medicine Physicians; Family Practitioners; General Surgeons; Infectious Disease Spec.; Internal Medicine GPS & PCP; OB/GYN; Ophthalmologists; Oral Surgeons; Pediatricians; Plastic/Hand/Reconstructive Surgeons; Radiologists; Urologists

Allied Health Professionals:

Dental Hygienists; Dentists; Nurse Practitioners; Nurses; Physician Assistants

Notes

1. All faiths are welcome; *2.* Each person is responsible for raising $1400.

Hillside Healthcare Center

Continents Served

Africa ☐ Asia ☐ Europe ☐ The Americas ☑

Countries Served

Belize

Address: **P.O. Box 27, Punta Gorda, Toledo District, Belize, C.A.**

Phone: **011 501-722-2312** FAX:

E-Mail: **doctor@hillsidebelize.net** Web: **www.hillsidebelize.net/**

Mission: Hillside Healthcare Center is a non-profit agency providing free care to the people of the Toledo District in Southern Belize. HHC center is staffed by nurses and physicians who work together with medical professionals taking part in a cross cultural training program in primary care medicine. Medical students, physician assistant students, and residents may come to provide quality medical care in a cross cultural setting. HHC has a close affiliation with the Department of Family and Community Medicine at the Medical College of Wisconsin who participated in the design and planning of the program. HHC also welcomes volunteer health care workers including physician specialists who wish to offer their service. Nurses, physical and occupational therapists, pharmacists, and dental teams are also encouraged to contact us about volunteering in the clinic.

Placement opportunities for . . .	
People of only certain faiths?	No
Couples: both are health providers?	Yes
Couples: only one is a health provider?	No
Families with children?	No
Medical students?	Yes
Pre-medical or college students?	No
Other health professional students?	Yes
Doctors in training?	Yes
Health personnel who are US citizens?	Yes
Health personnel who are non-US citizens?	Yes
Health personnel with no prior experience in developing countries?	Yes
Health personnel who are not current members of your organization?	Yes

Organization/Service Specifics:		
Size of the Organization's Staff:		0-5
Number of providers sent or received/year:		6-10
Minimum term of assignment:		1 week
Maximum term of assignment:	*1*	years
Is funding available for travel?		No
Are room and board provided?		No
Is any other funding available?	*1*	Yes
Is training provided or available?		Yes
Is a language other than English required?		No

Health Professionals Placed:

Physicians:

Physicians; Dermatologists; General Surgeons; OB/GYN; Ophthalmologists; Oral Surgeons; Optometrists; Pediatricians

Allied Health Professionals:

Dentists; Nurse Practitioners; Nurses; Pharmacists; Physical & Occupational Therapists; Physician Assistants; Podiatrists

Notes

1. Long-term volunteers stay 1 year or more and qualify for aid.

Himalayan Health Exchange

Continents Served
Africa ☐ Asia ☑ Europe ☐ The Americas ☐

Countries Served
India

Address: **P.O. Box 610, Decatur, GA 30031-0610 U.S.A.**

Phone: **(404) 929-9399** FAX: **(404) 929-9321**

E-Mail: **info@himalayanihealth.com** Web: **www.himalayanhealth.com/**

Mission: Himalayan Health Exchange is a humanitarian service and educational program bringing together health care professionals who give of their time, talent and resources to provide care to the underserved populations in select, remote ares of Indo-Tibetan Borderlands and North Indian Himalayas. Each trip combines service and adventure, with team members providing care while also experiencing the land, its natural environment, people and culture.

Placement opportunities for . . .		Organization/Service Specifics:	
People of only certain faiths?	No	Size of the Organization's Staff:	6-10
Couples: both are health providers?	Yes	Number of providers sent or received/year:	151-200
Couples: only one is a health provider?	Yes	Minimum term of assignment:	2 weeks
Families with children?	No	Maximum term of assignment:	6 weeks
Medical students? *1*	Yes	Is funding available for travel?	No
Pre-medical or college students?	Yes	Are room and board provided? *2*	Yes
Other health professional students?	Yes	Is any other funding available? *3*	Yes
Doctors in training?	Yes	Is training provided or available?	No
Health personnel who are US citizens?	Yes	Is a language other than English required?	No
Health personnel who are non-US citizens?	Yes		
Health personnel with no prior experience in developing countries?	Yes		
Health personnel who are not current members of your organization?	Yes		

Health Professionals Placed:

Physicians:

Family Practitioners; Internal Medicine GPS & PCP; OB/GYN; Optometrists; Pediatricians

Allied Health Professionals:

Dentists; Nurses

Notes

1. Faculty physicians and residents also; *2.* Accommodations may include hotels, guest houses, lodges or tents; *3.* Past participants have been able to receive funds through their schools, hospitals or civic organizations.

Himalayan HealthCare Inc.

Continents Served
Africa ☐ Asia ☑ Europe ☐ The Americas ☐

Countries Served
Nepal

Address: **PO Box 737, Planetarium Station, New York, NY 10024 U.S.A.**

Phone: **(212) 829-8691** FAX: **(212) 225-3999**

E-Mail: **info@himalayan-healthcare.org** Web: **www.himalayan-healthcare.org/**

Mission: Himlayan HealthCare Inc. was established to address the health crisis in rural Nepal. The primary objectives of the organization are to provide immediate medical treatment to people living in remote mountain villages and to improve the general health conditions of the rural population of Nepal who do not have access to health care at times of critical need. Nepali medical professionals sustain Himalayan HealthCare's community development programs. The organization also arranges for groups of foreign physicians and health workers to participate in medical treks to supplement the efforts of our Nepalese medical staff.

Placement opportunities for . . .		Organization/Service Specifics:	
People of only certain faiths?	No	Size of the Organization's Staff:	21-50
Couples: both are health providers?	Yes	Number of providers sent or received/year:	21-50
Couples: only one is a health provider?	No	Minimum term of assignment:	3 weeks
Families with children?	No	Maximum term of assignment:	3 weeks
Medical students?	No	Is funding available for travel?	No
Pre-medical or college students?	No	Are room and board provided?	No
Other health professional students?	No	Is any other funding available?	No
Doctors in training?	Yes	Is training provided or available?	No
Health personnel who are US citizens?	Yes	Is a language other than English required?	No
Health personnel who are non-US citizens?	Yes		
Health personnel with no prior experience in developing countries?	Yes		
Health personnel who are not current members of your organization?	Yes		

(continued)

Health Professionals Placed:

Notes

Physicians:

Physicians; Cardiologists; Dermatologists; Family Practitioners; Gastroenterologists; Hematologists; Oncologists; Infectious Disease Spec.; Internal Medicine GPS & PCP; Nephrologists; OB/GYN; Oral Surgeons; Pediatricians; Psychiatrists; Pulmonary Specialists

Allied Health Professionals:

Dentists; Nurse Midwives; Nurse Practitioners; Nurses; Public Health Specialists, Epidemiologists and Health Educators

---

Honduras Outreach, Inc.

Address: **150 East Ponce de Leon Ave., Suite 100, Decatur, GA 30030 U.S.A.**

Phone: **(404) 378-0919** FAX: **(404) 378-8429**

E-Mail: **askhoi@hoi.org** Web: **www.hoi.org/**

Continents Served

Africa ☐ Asia ☐ Europe ☐ The Americas ☑

Countries Served

Honduras

Mission: Honduras Outreach, Inc. is a transdenomenational mission program dedicated to improving lives of residents of and visitors in Olancho. Through short-term missions working continuously on long-term projects, Hondurans and North Americans minister to each other and share the love of Jesus Christ. The Ministry of Health has assigned Honduras Outreach 38 villages representing over 35,000 people. HOI operates four medical clinics with Honduran medical staff and also has a large clinic on the Ranch. These clinics provide vaccinations, dental work, public health information, and many other basic health needs for thousands of Hondurans.

Placement opportunities for . . .

People of only certain faiths?	No
Couples: both are health providers?	Yes
Couples: only one is a health provider?	Yes
Families with children?	No
Medical students?	Yes
Pre-medical or college students?	Yes
Other health professional students?	Yes
Doctors in training?	Yes
Health personnel who are US citizens?	Yes
Health personnel who are non-US citizens?	Yes
Health personnel with no prior experience in developing countries?	Yes
Health personnel who are not current members of your organization?	Yes

Organization/Service Specifics:

Size of the Organization's Staff:	6-10
Number of providers sent or received/year:	21-50
Minimum term of assignment:	1 week
Maximum term of assignment:	2 weeks
Is funding available for travel?	No
Are room and board provided?	No
Is any other funding available?	No
Is training provided or available?	Yes
Is a language other than English required? *1*	No

Health Professionals Placed:

Physicians:

Physicians; Cardiologists; Dermatologists; Emergency Medicine Physicians; Endocrinologists; Family Practitioners; General Surgeons; Infectious Disease Spec.; Internal Medicine GPS & PCP; Nephrologists; Neurologists; OB/GYN; Ophthalmologists; Oral Surgeons; Orthopedic Surgeons; Pediatricians; Plastic/Hand/Reconstructive Surgeons; Radiologists

Allied Health Professionals:

Dental Hygienists; Dentists; Medical Technicians (lab, X-ray, etc); Nurse Midwives; Nurse Practitioners; Nurses; Nutritionists & Dieticians; Pharmacists; Physical & Occupational Therapists; Physician Assistants; Public Health Specialists, Epidemiologists and Health Educators; Social Workers; Water/Sanitation Specialists

Notes

1. Spanish preferable.

Hope Alliance

Continents Served			
Africa ✔	Asia ☐	Europe ☐	The Americas ✔

Countries Served

Cambodia	Ghana	Guatemala
Haiti	Peru	Philippines
United States	Vanuatu	

Address: **980 South 700 West, Suite 11, Salt Lake City, UT 84104 U.S.A.**

Phone: **(801) 952-0400** FAX: **(801) 952-0401**

E-Mail: **info@hopealliance.com** Web: **www.hopealliance.com**

Mission: The Hope Alliance is a secular organization connecting people and resources to humanitarian needs in areas of Africa and the Americas. This is accomplished by delivering projects which provide (1) short-term relief to communities in emergency crisis or natural disaster situations, and/or (2) long-term capital commitments to specific communities that meaningfully add value to the overall quality of life. The Hope Alliance provides funding, room/board, and training to physicians for short- and long-term stays in underserved regions of the United States, Ghana, Cambodia, Vanuatu, Peru, and Haiti.

Placement opportunities for . . .	
People of only certain faiths?	No
Couples: both are health providers?	Yes
Couples: only one is a health provider?	Yes
Families with children? *1*	No
Medical students?	Yes
Pre-medical or college students? *1*	Yes
Other health professional students?	Yes
Doctors in training?	Yes
Health personnel who are US citizens?	Yes
Health personnel who are non-US citizens?	Yes
Health personnel with no prior experience in developing countries?	Yes
Health personnel who are not current members of your organization?	Yes

Organization/Service Specifics:	
Size of the Organization's Staff:	0-5
Number of providers sent or received/year:	21-50
Minimum term of assignment:	1 week
Maximum term of assignment:	no max
Is funding available for travel?	Yes
Are room and board provided?	Yes
Is any other funding available?	Yes
Is training provided or available?	Yes
Is a language other than English required? *2*	No

Health Professionals Placed:

Physicians:

Physicians; Anesthesiologists; Cardiologists; Dermatologists; Emergency Medicine Physicians; Endocrinologists; Family Practitioners; Gastroenterologists; General Surgeons; Hematologists; Oncologists; Infectious Disease Spec.; Internal Medicine GPS & PCP; Nephrologists; Neurologists; Neurosurgeons; OB/GYN; Ophthalmologists; Oral Surgeons; Optometrists; Orthopedic Surgeons; Otolaryngologists; Pathologists; Pediatricians; Plastic/Hand/Reconstructive Surgeons; Psychiatrists; Pulmonary Specialists; Radiologists; Urologists

Allied Health Professionals:

Administrative Health Positions; Dental Hygienists; Dentists; Medical Technicians (lab, X-ray, etc); Nurse Midwives; Nurse Practitioners; Nurses; Nutritionists & Dieticians; Paramedics; Pharmacists; Physical & Occupational Therapists; Physician Assistants; Podiatrists; Prosthetists; Psychologists; Public Health Specialists, Epidemiologists and Health Educators; Respiratory Therapists; Social Workers; Water/Sanitation Specialists

Notes

1. Children must be over 16;
2. Spanish and Creole are helpful.

Hope Worldwide

Continents Served			
Africa ✔	Asia ✔	Europe ✔	The Americas ✔

Countries Served

Brazil	Cambodia	Colombia
Guatemala	Honduras	India
Indonesia	Ivory Coast	Jamaica
Malaysia	Mali	Mexico
Papua-New Guinea		Philippines
Russia	Senegal	Somalia
South Africa	United States	
Zaire (DemRepCongo)		

Address: **353 W. Lancaster Ave., Suite 200, Wayne, PA 19087 U.S.A.**

Phone: **(610) 254-8800** FAX: **(610) 254-8989**

E-Mail: **webmaster@hopeww.org** Web: **www.hopeww.org**

Mission: A US-based charity with projects in 106 cities in all parts of the world, Hope Worldwide is dedicated to helping the poor and sick, focusing on health, education, children, seniors, and global outreach. This Christian charity seeks a variety of different types of physicians, nurses, other health care professionals, and medical/health professional students, either with or without prior international health experience, for short to long (2 weeks to 5 years) term stays. Participants must be a part of the Christian faith; there are no language restrictions. Funding is available for travel, room/board, as well as other expenses, and salaries can be arranged for longer-term stays.

(continued)

Placement opportunities for . . .		**Organization/Service Specifics:**	
People of only certain faiths? *1*	Yes	Size of the Organization's Staff:	>200
Couples: both are health providers?	Yes	Number of providers sent or received/year:	>200
Couples: only one is a health provider?	Yes	Minimum term of assignment:	2 weeks
Families with children?	Yes	Maximum term of assignment:	5 years
Medical students?	Yes	Is funding available for travel?	Yes
Pre-medical or college students?		Are room and board provided?	Yes
Other health professional students?	Yes	Is any other funding available? *2*	Yes
Doctors in training?	Yes	Is training provided or available?	Yes
Health personnel who are US citizens?	Yes	Is a language other than English required?	No
Health personnel who are non-US citizens?	Yes		
Health personnel with no prior experience in developing countries?	Yes		
Health personnel who are not current members of your organization?	Yes		

Health Professionals Placed:

Physicians:

Physicians; Anesthesiologists; Cardiologists; Emergency Medicine Physicians; Endocrinologists; Family Practitioners; General Surgeons; Hematologists; Oncologists; Infectious Disease Spec.; Internal Medicine GPS & PCP; Nephrologists; Neurologists; OB/GYN; Ophthalmologists; Optometrists; Orthopedic Surgeons; Pathologists; Pediatricians; Plastic/Hand/Reconstructive Surgeons; Psychiatrists; Pulmonary Specialists; Radiologists; Urologists

Allied Health Professionals:

Administrative Health Positions; Dental Hygienists; Dentists; Medical Technicians (lab, X-ray, etc); Nurse Practitioners; Nurses; Nutritionists & Dieticians; Paramedics; Pharmacists; Podiatrists; Prosthetists; Public Health Specialists, Epidemiologists and Health Educators; Respiratory Therapists; Social Workers

Notes

1. Christian; *2.* Salary is available for longer appointments.

Hospital Albert Schweitzer

Continents Served

Africa ☐ Asia ☐ Europe ☐ The Americas ☑

Countries Served

Haiti

Address: **1360 Whitfield Avenue, Sarasota, FL 34243 U.S.A.**

Phone: **(941) 752-1525** FAX: **(941) 752-0755**

E-Mail: **hertha@hashaiti.org** Web: **www.hashaiti.org**

Mission: The mission of Hopital Albert Schweitzer is to collaborate with the people in its district of the Artibonite Valley of Haiti as they strive to improve their health and quality of life. Room and board are provided, although volunteers are responsible for other funding. Volunteers can serve for short-term (2 weeks) to longer term (5 years) assignments. While other languages are not absolutely required, French and Creole are helpful.

Placement opportunities for . . .		**Organization/Service Specifics:**	
People of only certain faiths?	No	Size of the Organization's Staff:	>200
Couples: both are health providers?	Yes	Number of providers sent or received/year:	>200
Couples: only one is a health provider?	Yes	Minimum term of assignment:	2 weeks
Families with children?	Yes	Maximum term of assignment:	5 years
Medical students?	No	Is funding available for travel? *1*	Yes
Pre-medical or college students?	No	Are room and board provided?	Yes
Other health professional students?	Yes	Is any other funding available?	No
Doctors in training?	Yes	Is training provided or available?	Yes
Health personnel who are US citizens?	Yes	Is a language other than English required? *2*	Yes
Health personnel who are non-US citizens?	Yes		
Health personnel with no prior experience in developing countries?	Yes		
Health personnel who are not current members of your organization?	Yes		

Health Professionals Placed:

Physicians:

Anesthesiologists; Emergency Medicine Physicians; Family Practitioners; General Surgeons; Internal Medicine GPS & PCP; OB/GYN; Ophthalmologists; Orthopedic Surgeons; Pediatricians; Plastic/Hand/Reconstructive Surgeons; Pulmonary Specialists; Radiologists; Urologists

Allied Health Professionals:

Administrative Health Positions; Dentists; Medical Technicians (lab, X-ray, etc); Physical & Occupational Therapists; Public Health Specialists, Epidemiologists and Health Educators; Water/Sanitation Specialists

Notes

1. Travel expenses are provided for doctors who plan to spend more than 2 years at the hospital; *2.* French and Creole are helpful.

Indochina Surgical Educational Exchange

Continents Served
Africa ☐ Asia ☑ Europe ☐ The Americas ☐

Countries Served
Myanmar (Burma)

Address: **Massachusetts General Hospital, ACC #453, Boston, MA 02114 U.S.A.**

Phone: **(508) 653-1395** FAX: **(508) 653-4017**

E-Mail: **jdc500@aol.com** Web:

Mission: Originally the IndoChina Surgical Education Exchange sent teams of 2 or 3 surgeons to Vietnam. Now, they mostly sponsor Vietnamese doctors to study in the United States for 6 months at a time in accordance with the Vietnamese needs. Volunteers can serve for 2-4 weeks. While room and board are provided, volunteers must provide their own funding.

Placement opportunities for . . .		Organization/Service Specifics:	
People of only certain faiths?	No	Size of the Organization's Staff:	0-5
Couples: both are health providers?	No	Number of providers sent or received/year:	1-5
Couples: only one is a health provider?	No	Minimum term of assignment:	2 weeks
Families with children?	No	Maximum term of assignment:	4 weeks
Medical students?	No	Is funding available for travel?	No
Pre-medical or college students?	No	Are room and board provided?	Yes
Other health professional students?	No	Is any other funding available?	No
Doctors in training?	No	Is training provided or available?	No
Health personnel who are US citizens?	Yes	Is a language other than English required?	No

Health personnel who are non-US citizens?	Yes
Health personnel with no prior experience in developing countries?	Yes
Health personnel who are not current members of your organization?	Yes

Health Professionals Placed:

Notes

Physicians:

Plastic/Hand/Reconstructive Surgeons

Allied Health Professionals:

Infectious Diseases Society of America, The, and The HIV Medicine Association

Continents Served
Africa ☑ Asia ☐ Europe ☐ The Americas ☐

Countries Served
Uganda

Address: **66 Canal Center Plaza, Suite 600, Alexandria, VA 22314 U.S.A.**

Phone: **(703) 299-0200** FAX: **(703) 299-0204**

E-Mail: **info@idsociety.org or hivma@idsociety.org** Web: **www.idsociety.org**

Mission: To improve the health of individuals, communities, and society by promoting excellence in patient care, education, research, public health and prevention relating to infectious diseases. Core values include enhancing care of children and adults based on sound scientific evidence; advancing the discipline of infectious diseases as a foundation of medicine and public health; promoting and sharing knowledge to reduce human and societal toll from infectious diseases; advocating for sound and humane public policy; promoting collaboration and cooperation among, and services for, members and other professional colleagues.

Placement opportunities for . . .		Organization/Service Specifics:	
People of only certain faiths?	No	Size of the Organization's Staff:	0-5
Couples: both are health providers?	Yes	Number of providers sent or received/year:	11-20
Couples: only one is a health provider? *1*	Yes	Minimum term of assignment:	4 weeks
Families with children? *2*	Yes	Maximum term of assignment:	9 weeks
Medical students?	No	Is funding available for travel?	Yes
Pre-medical or college students?	No	Are room and board provided?	Yes
Other health professional students?	No	Is any other funding available?	Yes
Doctors in training? *3*	Yes	Is training provided or available?	Yes
Health personnel who are US citizens?	Yes	Is a language other than English required?	No

Health personnel who are non-US citizens?	Yes
Health personnel with no prior experience in developing countries? *4*	Yes
Health personnel who are not current members of your organization?	No

(continued)

Health Professionals Placed:

Physicians:

Infectious Disease Spec.

Allied Health Professionals:

Notes

1. Variable; *2.* Variable; *3.* Only Infectious Disease fellows; *4.* Preference given to those with prior experience.

Intercultural Nursing, Inc.

Address: **39 Pine Ridge Road, Waban, MA 02468-1616 U.S.A.**

Phone: **(617) 965-4856** FAX:

E-Mail: **lbabington@comcast.net** Web:

Continents Served

Africa ☐ Asia ☐ Europe ☐ The Americas ☑

Countries Served

Dominican Republic Haiti

Mission: Intercultural Nursing, Inc. (INI) is a non-profit, charitable organization founded in 1985. INI organizes short-term intercultural immersion opportunities for nurses and other health care professionals to provide care to the ill, underserved, and malnourished in the developing Caribbean nations of Haiti and the Dominican Republic. The trips occur three times each year and are two weeks in length. There are no specific religious requirements, but the missions INI works with are Catholic and Episcopal. Volunteers are responsible for raising the participation fees.

Placement opportunities for . . .	
People of only certain faiths? *1*	No
Couples: both are health providers?	Yes
Couples: only one is a health provider?	Yes
Families with children?	No
Medical students?	Yes
Pre-medical or college students?	Yes
Other health professional students?	Yes
Doctors in training?	Yes
Health personnel who are US citizens?	Yes
Health personnel who are non-US citizens?	Yes
Health personnel with no prior experience in developing countries?	Yes
Health personnel who are not current members of your organization?	Yes

Organization/Service Specifics:	
Size of the Organization's Staff:	0-5
Number of providers sent or received/year:	21-50
Minimum term of assignment:	2 weeks
Maximum term of assignment:	2 months
Is funding available for travel?	No
Are room and board provided? *2*	Yes
Is any other funding available? *3*	No
Is training provided or available?	Yes
Is a language other than English required?	No

Health Professionals Placed:

Physicians:

Physicians; Dermatologists; Emergency Medicine Physicians; Family Practitioners; Infectious Disease Spec.; Internal Medicine GPS & PCP; OB/GYN; Pediatricians

Allied Health Professionals:

Dentists; Nurse Midwives; Nurse Practitioners; Nurses; Nutritionists & Dieticians; Physical & Occupational Therapists

Notes

1. The missions we work with are Catholic and Episcopal; *2.* Room and board are provided by the participation fee; *3.* Volunteers must solicit support from family, friends, churches, etc.

Interface UCSD

Address: **4907 Morena Blvd., Suite 1412, San Diego, CA 92117 U.S.A.**

Phone: **(858) 581-3080** FAX: **(858) 581-3181**

E-Mail: **kmayo@ucsd.edu** Web:

Continents Served

Africa ☐ Asia ☐ Europe ☐ The Americas ☑

Countries Served

Mexico

Mission: Interface coordinates volunteer reconstructive surgery trips to 4 locations in Mexico. Interface makes 8-10 trips per year with 3-4 physicians and 1 resident plastic surgeon, anesthesiologist, and operating room nurse.

(continued)

Placement opportunities for . . .		Organization/Service Specifics:	
People of only certain faiths?	No	Size of the Organization's Staff:	0-5
Couples: both are health providers?	No	Number of providers sent or received/year:	21-50
Couples: only one is a health provider?	No	Minimum term of assignment:	1 day
Families with children?	No	Maximum term of assignment:	5 days
Medical students?	No	Is funding available for travel?	No
Pre-medical or college students?	No	Are room and board provided?	No
Other health professional students?	No	Is any other funding available?	No
Doctors in training?	Yes	Is training provided or available?	No
Health personnel who are US citizens? *1*	Yes	Is a language other than English required? *2*	No
Health personnel who are non-US citizens?	No		
Health personnel with no prior experience in developing countries?	Yes		
Health personnel who are not current members of your organization?	Yes		

Health Professionals Placed:

Physicians:

Anesthesiologists; Plastic/Hand/Reconstructive Surgeons

Allied Health Professionals:

Nurses

Notes

1. Mostly from San Diego area;
2. Spanish helpful.

International Aid, Inc.

Address: **17011 W. Hickory, Spring Lake, MI 49456-9712 U.S.A.**

Phone: **(616) 846-7490**
(800) 968-7490
FAX: **(616) 846-3842**

E-Mail: **volunteer@internationalaid.org**
Web: **www.internationalaid.org**

Continents Served
Africa ✔ Asia ✔ Europe ✔ The Americas ✔

Countries Served
El Salvador; Ghana; Honduras; Philippines; Yugoslavia, former

Mission: International Aid mobilizes caring people, churches, organizations, and businesses to extend Christ's love and mercy to those who suffer. For more than 20 years, we have been providing assistance and medical support to missionaries worldwide, and partnering with churches throughout the United States to reach some of the most desperate countries devastated by war, famine and drought. Founded as an agency committed to supporting missionaries, International Aid serves a global network of institutional and program partners, hospitals, clinics, orphanages, and churches across the globe. Through our missionary assistance, medical support, church-based compassion ministries, and relief and development services, International Aid reaches out to those in need regardless of nationality, ethnicity or creed. Volunteers can serve for 1 week or more. Room and board are provided, but volunteers are reponsible for other funding.

Placement opportunities for . . .		Organization/Service Specifics:	
People of only certain faiths?	No	Size of the Organization's Staff:	51-100
Couples: both are health providers?	Yes	Number of providers sent or received/year:	>200
Couples: only one is a health provider?	Yes	Minimum term of assignment:	1 week
Families with children?	Yes	Maximum term of assignment:	more
Medical students?	No	Is funding available for travel?	No
Pre-medical or college students?	No	Are room and board provided?	Yes
Other health professional students?	Yes	Is any other funding available?	No
Doctors in training?	Yes	Is training provided or available?	No
Health personnel who are US citizens?	Yes	Is a language other than English required?	No
Health personnel who are non-US citizens?	Yes		
Health personnel with no prior experience in developing countries?	Yes		
Health personnel who are not current members of your organization?	Yes		

Health Professionals Placed:

Physicians:

Physicians; Family Practitioners; Internal Medicine GPS & PCP; Ophthalmologists; Optometrists; Pediatricians

Allied Health Professionals:

Dentists; Medical Technicians (lab, X-ray, etc)

Notes

International Children's Heart Foundation

Address: **1750 Madison Ave., Suite 100, Memphis, TN 38104 U.S.A.**

Phone: **(877) 869-4243** FAX: **(901) 432-4243**

E-Mail: **martinapavanic@babyheart.org** Web: **www.babyheart.org**

Mission: The International Children's Heart Foundation is dedicated to helping children with congenital or acquired heart disease in developing countries throughout the world. We serve all children without respect to their race, religion or sex. Our primary goal is to make our services obsolete in the countries that we serve and we strive to educate the health care professionals in the countries where we travel. We have a need to fill out medical teams for 2 week missions and are always in need of highly qualified physicians, nurses, respiratory therapists, and biomedical engineers with specialization in pediatric cardiac surgery and intensive care.

Continents Served

Africa ✔ Asia ✔ Europe ✔ The Americas ✔

Countries Served

Belarus, China, Colombia, Croatia, Jamaica, Nicaragua, Palestine, Peru, Sudan, Ukraine, Uzbekistan, Yugoslavia, former

Placement opportunities for . . .

People of only certain faiths?	No
Couples: both are health providers?	Yes
Couples: only one is a health provider?	No
Families with children?	No
Medical students?	Yes
Pre-medical or college students?	No
Other health professional students?	Yes
Doctors in training?	No
Health personnel who are US citizens?	Yes
Health personnel who are non-US citizens?	Yes
Health personnel with no prior experience in developing countries?	Yes
Health personnel who are not current members of your organization?	Yes

Organization/Service Specifics:

Size of the Organization's Staff:	21-50
Number of providers sent or received/year:	51-100
Minimum term of assignment:	2 weeks
Maximum term of assignment:	2 weeks
Is funding available for travel?	Yes
Are room and board provided?	
Is any other funding available?	No
Is training provided or available?	No
Is a language other than English required?	No

Health Professionals Placed: *1*

Physicians:

Physicians; Cardiologists; General Surgeons

Allied Health Professionals:

Nurse Practitioners; Nurses

Notes

1. We also need respiratory therapists and biomedical engineers with specialization in pediatric cardiac surgery and intensive care.

International Committee of the Red Cross

Address: **19 Avenue de la Paix Geneva, CH1202 Switzerland**

Phone: **41227346001** FAX: **41227332057**

E-Mail: **op_assist_sante.gva@icrc.org** Web: **www.icrc.org/**

Mission: The International Committee of the Red Cross acts to help all victims of war and internal violence, attempting to ensure implementation of humanitarian rules restricting armed violence. ICRC assistance for victims of armed conflict and internal violence seeks to preserve or restore living conditions with a view to reducing dependence on outside aid and enabling victims to maintain an adequate standard of living. It may include food and/or medicine, but usually builds on the capacity to deliver essential services, such as the construction or repair of water supply systems or medical facilities, the training of primary health care staff, surgeons, or orthopaedic technicians, etc. The staff are paid by salary and terms can last between 3 months and 2 years. There are no language requirements, but knowledge of French, Spanish, or other languages can be an asset.

Continents Served

Africa ✔ Asia ✔ Europe ✔ The Americas ✔

Countries Served

Afghanistan, Albania, Angola, Armenia, Burundi, Cambodia, Colombia, Congo, Ethiopia, Haiti, Iraq, Israel, Kenya, Lebanon, Liberia, Mali, Peru, Rwanda, Sierra Leone, Somalia, Sri Lanka, Uganda, USSR, former, Yugoslavia, former, Zaire (DemRepCongo)

(continued)

Placement opportunities for . . .		Organization/Service Specifics:	
People of only certain faiths?	No	Size of the Organization's Staff:	>200
Couples: both are health providers?	No	Number of providers sent or received/year:	>200
Couples: only one is a health provider?	No	Minimum term of assignment:	3 months
Families with children?	No	Maximum term of assignment:	2 years
Medical students?	No	Is funding available for travel?	Yes
Pre-medical or college students?	No	Are room and board provided?	Yes
Other health professional students?	No	Is any other funding available? *2*	Yes
Doctors in training?	No	Is training provided or available?	Yes
Health personnel who are US citizens?	Yes	Is a language other than English required? *3*	No
Health personnel who are non-US citizens?	Yes		
Health personnel with no prior experience in developing countries? *1*	Yes		
Health personnel who are not current members of your organization?	Yes		

Health Professionals Placed:

Physicians:

Physicians; Anesthesiologists; General Surgeons; Internal Medicine GPS & PCP; Orthopedic Surgeons

Allied Health Professionals:

Administrative Health Positions; Medical Technicians (lab, X-ray, etc); Nurses; Nutritionists & Dieticians; Pharmacists; Physical & Occupational Therapists; Prosthetists; Public Health Specialists, Epidemiologists and Health Educators; Water/Sanitation Specialists

Notes

1. Experience is preferred;
2. Personnel are paid by salary;
3. Knowledge of the local language is an asset.

International Cooperation for Development (formerly CIIR Overseas Programme)

Address: **Unit 3, Canonbury Yard, 109a New North Road, London, N1- 7BJ U.K.**

Phone: **00 44 171 354 0883** FAX: **00 44 171 359 0017**

E-Mail: **ciir@ciir.org** Web: **www.ciir.org**

Continents Served

Africa ☑ Asia ☐ Europe ☐ The Americas ☑

Countries Served

Dominican Republic, Ecuador, El Salvador, Haiti, Honduras, Namibia, Nicaragua, Yemen, Zimbabwe

Mission: ICD workers are people who want to share their skills with communities that need them. Each worker is professionally qualified with a minimum of two year's work experience, and often with a background in training. Jobs with ICD are professionally and personally challenging and they can carry great responsibility. But they are also rewarding. Many workers at the end of their contracts say it was an enriching experience that has made a lasting impact on them, and extend their contracts or look for a second posting with us. Today, ICD workers join with local people in Latin America, the Caribbean, Africa, and the Middle East in programs that empower communities and improve their quality of life.

Placement opportunities for . . .		Organization/Service Specifics:	
People of only certain faiths?	No	Size of the Organization's Staff:	51-100
Couples: both are health providers?	No	Number of providers sent or received/year:	21-50
Couples: only one is a health provider?	No	Minimum term of assignment:	2 years
Families with children?	No	Maximum term of assignment:	5 years
Medical students?	No	Is funding available for travel? *1*	Yes
Pre-medical or college students?	No	Are room and board provided?	Yes
Other health professional students?	Yes	Is any other funding available?	Yes
Doctors in training?	No	Is training provided or available?	Yes
Health personnel who are US citizens?	Yes	Is a language other than English required? *2*	No
Health personnel who are non-US citizens?	Yes		
Health personnel with no prior experience in developing countries?	Yes		
Health personnel who are not current members of your organization?	Yes		

(continued)

Health Professionals Placed:

Physicians:

Physicians; Anesthesiologists; Emergency Medicine Physicians; Family Practitioners; General Surgeons; Infectious Disease Spec.; Optometrists; Orthopedic Surgeons; Pediatricians; Plastic/Hand/Reconstructive Surgeons

Allied Health Professionals:

Administrative Health Positions; Dentists; Medical Technicians (lab, X-ray, etc); Nurse Midwives; Nurse Practitioners; Nurses; Nutritionists & Dieticians; Pharmacists; Physical & Occupational Therapists; Physician Assistants; Public Health Specialists, Epidemiologists and Health Educators; Social Workers; Water/Sanitation Specialists

Notes

1. Health care workers sign on for 2-year terms as paid employees with salary and benefits; *2.* Spanish often helpful.

International Eye Foundation, Inc.

Address: **10801 Connecticut Avenue, Kensington, MD 20895 U.S.A.**

Phone: **(240) 290-0263** FAX: **(240) 290-0269**

E-Mail: **ief@iefusa.org** Web: **www.iefusa.org**

Continents Served

Africa ☑ Asia ☐ Europe ☑ The Americas ☑

Countries Served

Albania	Bulgaria	Cameroon
Ethiopia	Guatemala	Guinea-Bissau
Honduras	Malawi	Nigeria

Mission: The International Eye Foundation has been helping people see since 1961. In more than 60 countries around the world, IEF's staff and volunteers have restored the gift of sight for hundreds of thousands of people in the developing world. Through SightReach, IEF's three program areas include (1) SightReach Prevention (targeting cataract, trachoma, "river blindness," and childhood blindness, including vitamin A deficiency/child survival), (2) SightReach Surgical (bringing down the cost of ophthalmic supplies), and (3) SightReach® Management (creating financial self-sufficiency of eye care providers).

Placement opportunities for . . .

People of only certain faiths?	No
Couples: both are health providers?	No
Couples: only one is a health provider?	No
Families with children?	No
Medical students?	No
Pre-medical or college students?	No
Other health professional students?	No
Doctors in training?	No
Health personnel who are US citizens?	Yes
Health personnel who are non-US citizens?	No
Health personnel with no prior experience in developing countries?	No
Health personnel who are not current members of your organization?	Yes

Organization/Service Specifics:

Size of the Organization's Staff:	101-150
Number of providers sent or received/year:	1-5
Minimum term of assignment:	1 week
Maximum term of assignment:	3 weeks
Is funding available for travel? *1*	Yes
Are room and board provided?	Yes
Is any other funding available?	No
Is training provided or available?	No
Is a language other than English required? *2*	No

Health Professionals Placed:

Physicians:

Ophthalmologists

Allied Health Professionals:

Public Health Specialists, Epidemiologists and Health Educators

Notes

1. Funding for travel and room and board are available as part of a grant; *2.* No language is required, but the language of the country of service is preferable.

International Federation of Red Cross and Red Crescent Societies

Address: **PO Box 372, 17 chemin des Crets CH-1211, Geneva 19, Switzerland**

Phone: **41 22 730 4222** FAX: **41 22 733 0395**

E-Mail: **secretariat@ifrc.org** Web: **www.ifrc.org**

Mission: The International Federation is a federation of Red Cross and Red Crescent Societies from more than 176 countries, working together to improve the lives of the world's most vulnerable people. Too many people die as a result of no access to even the most basic health services and elementary health education. Health and community care have become a cornerstone of humanitarian assistance, and accounts for a large part of Red Cross Red Crescent spending. Through these programmes, the Federation aims to enable communities to reduce their vulnerability to disease, and prepare for and respond to public health crises. Service volunteers are usually recruited to well-structured volunteer services which are developed and managed by volunteer and/or programme managers. However, front line service volunteering can also be done by self-managed groups of members or by vulnerable people organized into self-help groups. The form that is best depends on the situation and several forms can coexist in a national society.

Continents Served

Africa ✔ Asia ✔ Europe ✔ The Americas ✔

Countries Served

Afghanistan	Albania	Angola
Australia	Bangladesh	Benin
Burkina Faso	Burundi	Cambodia
China	Comoros	Congo
Costa Rica	Ethiopia	Haiti
Hungary	Iraq	Israel
Ivory Coast	Jordan	Kenya
Korea, North	Madagascar	Malawi
Mongolia	Mozambique	Nepal
Nigeria	Papua-New Guinea	
Romania	Rwanda	Somalia
Sudan	Tanzania	Uganda
USSR, former	Zaire (DemRepCongo)	
Zambia	Zimbabwe	

Placement opportunities for . . .

People of only certain faiths?	No
Couples: both are health providers?	No
Couples: only one is a health provider?	Yes
Families with children?	Yes
Medical students?	No
Pre-medical or college students?	No
Other health professional students?	Yes
Doctors in training?	No
Health personnel who are US citizens?	Yes
Health personnel who are non-US citizens?	Yes
Health personnel with no prior experience in developing countries?	No
Health personnel who are not current members of your organization?	Yes

Organization/Service Specifics:

Size of the Organization's Staff:	>200
Number of providers sent or received/year:	>200
Minimum term of assignment:	3 weeks
Maximum term of assignment:	3 years
Is funding available for travel?	No
Are room and board provided?	Yes
Is any other funding available? *1*	Yes
Is training provided or available?	Yes
Is a language other than English required? *2*	Yes

Health Professionals Placed:

Physicians:

Physicians; Anesthesiologists; Emergency Medicine Physicians; Family Practitioners; General Surgeons; Infectious Disease Spec.; Internal Medicine GPS & PCP; Pediatricians

Allied Health Professionals:

Nutritionists & Dieticians; Public Health Specialists, Epidemiologists and Health Educators; Water/Sanitation Specialists

Notes

1. There is possible support by the Red Cross National Society;
2. For certain projects, Spanish or French is required.

International Federation of Social Workers

Address: **33 rue de l'Athenee, Geneva, 1206 Switzerland**

Phone: **41 22 347 1236** FAX: **41 22 346 8657**

E-Mail: **secr.gen@ifsw.org** Web: **www.ifsw.org**

Mission: The International Federation of Social Workers (IFSW) is a global organization striving for social justice, human rights and social development through the development of social work, best practices and international cooperation between social workers and their professional organizations. IFSW does not generally recruit personnel, but the federation is involved in some projects that send social workers abroad.

Continents Served

Africa ✔ Asia ✔ Europe ✔ The Americas ✔

Countries Served

Albania	Argentina	Australia
Austria	Bahrain	Belgium
Benin	Bolivia	
Bosnia Herzegovina		Brazil
Bulgaria	Canada	Chile
China	Colombia	Croatia
Czech Republic	Denmark	Egypt
Finland	France	Germany
Ghana	Greece	Hong Kong
Hungary	Iceland	Ireland
Israel	Italy	Japan
Kenya	Korea, South	Kuwait
Luxembourg	Macedonia	Malawi
Malaysia	Mauritius	Netherlands
New Zealand	Nicaragua	Niger
Nigeria	Norway	Philippines
Poland	Portugal	Romania
Serbia and Montenegro		Singapore
Slovakia	South Africa	Spain
Sri Lanka	Sweden	Switzerland
Tanzania	Thailand	Turkey
Uganda	United Kingdom	
United States	USSR, former	Vietnam
Zimbabwe		

Placement opportunities for . . .

People of only certain faiths?	No
Couples: both are health providers?	No
Couples: only one is a health provider?	No
Families with children?	No
Medical students?	No
Pre-medical or college students?	No
Other health professional students? *1*	Yes
Doctors in training?	No
Health personnel who are US citizens?	No
Health personnel who are non-US citizens?	No
Health personnel with no prior experience in developing countries?	No
Health personnel who are not current members of your organization?	No

Organization/Service Specifics:

Size of the Organization's Staff:	0-5
Number of providers sent or received/year:	6-10
Minimum term of assignment:	0
Maximum term of assignment:	0
Is funding available for travel? *2*	
Are room and board provided?	
Is any other funding available?	
Is training provided or available?	
Is a language other than English required?	No

Health Professionals Placed:

Physicians:

Allied Health Professionals:

Social Workers

Notes

1. International Federation of Social Workers sometimes sends social workers abroad; *2.* Funding information not available. Social workers should contact the federation directly.

International Health Exchange

Address: **1 Great George Street, London, SW1P 3AA U.K.**
Phone: **44 02 07 233 1100** FAX: **44 02 07 233 3590**
E-Mail: **info@ihe.org.uk** Web: **www.ihe.org.uk/**

Mission: International Health Exchange (IHE) supports health development and humanitarian relief programs in developing countries by providing appropriately experienced people to organizations requiring their skills. IHE is not an operational agency but supports a wide number of UK and European agencies by providing personnel for their operations. IHE works to support initiatives to bring about sustained improvements to people's health in developing countries by providing appropriately experienced people to organizations requiring their skills. Funding and room and board are provided, and while there are no specific language requirements, knowledge of French, Spanish, or Portuguese is desirable.

Continents Served

Africa ✔ Asia ✔ Europe ✔ The Americas ✔

Countries Served

Afghanistan	Albania	Angola
Argentina	Bangladesh	Bolivia
Bosnia and Herzegovina		Botswana
Brazil	Bulgaria	Burkina Faso
Burundi	Cambodia	Chile
China	Colombia	Costa Rica
Croatia	Cuba	Czech Republic
Dominican Republic		Ecuador
Egypt	El Salvador	Ethiopia
Gambia	Ghana	Guatemala
Guinea	Guyana	Haiti
Honduras	India	Iran
Iraq	Jamaica	Kenya
Laos	Lebanon	Lesotho
Liberia	Malawi	Malaysia
Mali	Mexico	Mozambique
Myanmar (Burma)		Nepal
Nicaragua	Nigeria	Pakistan
Papua-New Guinea		Paraguay
Peru	Philippines	Poland
Romania	Rwanda	
Serbia and Montenegro		Sierra Leone
Solomon Islands		Somalia
South Africa	Sri Lanka	Sudan
Swaziland	Tanzania	Thailand
Trinidad and Tobago		Turkey
Uganda	USSR, former	Vanuatu
Vietnam	Yugoslavia, former	
Zaire (DemRepCongo)		Zambia
Zimbabwe		

Placement opportunities for . . .

People of only certain faiths?	No
Couples: both are health providers?	Yes
Couples: only one is a health provider?	Yes
Families with children?	Yes
Medical students?	No
Pre-medical or college students?	No
Other health professional students?	No
Doctors in training?	No
Health personnel who are US citizens?	Yes
Health personnel who are non-US citizens?	Yes
Health personnel with no prior experience in developing countries?	Yes
Health personnel who are not current members of your organization?	Yes

Organization/Service Specifics:

Size of the Organization's Staff:	6-10
Number of providers sent or received/year:	151-200
Minimum term of assignment:	3 months
Maximum term of assignment:	3 years
Is funding available for travel?	Yes
Are room and board provided?	Yes
Is any other funding available? *1*	Yes
Is training provided or available?	Yes
Is a language other than English required? *2*	No

Health Professionals Placed:

Physicians:

Physicians; Anesthesiologists; Emergency Medicine Physicians; General Surgeons; Hematologists; Oncologists; Infectious Disease Spec.; Internal Medicine GPS & PCP; OB/GYN; Ophthalmologists; Oral Surgeons; Pediatricians; Psychiatrists; Pulmonary Specialists; Radiologists

Allied Health Professionals:

Administrative Health Positions; Dentists; Medical Technicians (lab, X-ray, etc); Nurse Midwives; Nurse Practitioners; Nurses; Nutritionists & Dieticians; Paramedics; Pharmacists; Physical & Occupational Therapists; Prosthetists; Psychologists; Public Health Specialists, Epidemiologists and Health Educators; Social Workers; Water/Sanitation Specialists

Notes

1. Funding depends on the post and agency; *2.* Languages are not required, but preferrable, esp. French, Spanish, or Portuguese.

International Health Service

Continents Served			
Africa ☐	Asia ☐	Europe ☐	The Americas ☑

Countries Served
Honduras

Address: **PO Box 44339, St Louis Park Eden Prarie, MN 55344 U.S.A.**

Phone: **(952) 920-0433** FAX: **(952) 920-0433**

E-Mail: **cschraeder@earthlink.net** Web: **www.ihsofmn.org**

Mission: International Health Service is a non-profit international relief organization which provides medical and dental assistance to the people of Honduras and does not charge for services provided. Volunteers can participate in 1 or 2 week trips during the month of February. Volunteers must provide their own funding and Spanish is highly recommended, although not required.

Placement opportunities for . . .	
People of only certain faiths?	No
Couples: both are health providers?	Yes
Couples: only one is a health provider?	Yes
Families with children?	No
Medical students?	Yes
Pre-medical or college students?	Yes
Other health professional students?	Yes
Doctors in training?	Yes
Health personnel who are US citizens?	Yes
Health personnel who are non-US citizens?	Yes
Health personnel with no prior experience in developing countries?	Yes
Health personnel who are not current members of your organization?	Yes

Organization/Service Specifics:	
Size of the Organization's Staff:	0-5
Number of providers sent or received/year:	21-50
Minimum term of assignment:	1 week
Maximum term of assignment:	2 weeks
Is funding available for travel?	No
Are room and board provided?	No
Is any other funding available? *1*	No
Is training provided or available?	Yes
Is a language other than English required? *2*	No

Health Professionals Placed:

Physicians:

Physicians; Anesthesiologists; Emergency Medicine Physicians; Family Practitioners; General Surgeons; Internal Medicine GPS & PCP; Ophthalmologists; Orthopedic Surgeons; Plastic/Hand/Reconstructive Surgeons

Allied Health Professionals:

Dental Hygienists; Dentists; Medical Technicians (lab, X-ray, etc); Nurse Practitioners; Nurses; Paramedics; Pharmacists

Notes

1. Volunteers must pay their own way; *2.* Spanish is highly recommended, but not required.

International Medical Corps

Continents Served			
Africa ☑	Asia ☑	Europe ☑	The Americas ☐

Address: **1919 Santa Monica Blvd, Suite 300, Santa Monica, CA 90404 U.S.A.**

Phone: **(310) 826-7800** FAX: **(310) 442-6622**

E-Mail: **imc@imcworldwide.org** Web: **www.imcworldwide.org**

Countries Served

Afghanistan	Albania	Angola
Armenia	Azerbaijan	Burundi
Cambodia	Chad	Croatia
Eritrea	Ethiopia	Georgia
Honduras	Indonesia	Ingushetia
Kenya	Liberia	Macedonia
Moldova	Mozambique	Namibia
Pakistan	Rwanda	
Serbia and Montenegro		Sierra Leone
Somalia	Sri Lanka	Sudan
Tanzania	Thailand	Uganda
Zaire (DemRepCongo)		Zambia

Mission: International Medical Corps is a global humanitarian nonprofit organization dedicated to saving lives and relieving suffering through health care training and relief programs. Established in 1984 by volunteer US doctors and nurses, IMC is a private, voluntary, nonpolitical, nonsectarian organization. Its mission is to improve the quality of life through health interventions and related activities that build local capacity in areas worldwide where few organizations dare to serve. By offering training and health care to local populations and medical assistance to people at highest risk, and with the flexibility to respond rapidly to emergency situations, IMC rehabilitates devastated health care systems and helps bring them back to self-reliance.

(continued)

Placement opportunities for . . .	
People of only certain faiths?	No
Couples: both are health providers?	Yes
Couples: only one is a health provider?	Yes
Families with children?	No
Medical students?	No
Pre-medical or college students?	No
Other health professional students?	Yes
Doctors in training?	No
Health personnel who are US citizens?	Yes
Health personnel who are non-US citizens?	Yes
Health personnel with no prior experience in developing countries?	Yes
Health personnel who are not current members of your organization?	Yes

Organization/Service Specifics:	
Size of the Organization's Staff:	>200
Number of providers sent or received/year:	101-150
Minimum term of assignment:	6 months
Maximum term of assignment:	
Is funding available for travel?	Yes
Are room and board provided? *1*	Yes
Is any other funding available?	Yes
Is training provided or available?	No
Is a language other than English required? *2*	Yes

Health Professionals Placed:

Physicians:

Physicians; Anesthesiologists; Emergency Medicine Physicians; Family Practitioners; General Surgeons; Infectious Disease Spec.; Internal Medicine GPS & PCP; Nephrologists; OB/GYN; Orthopedic Surgeons; Pediatricians

Allied Health Professionals:

Administrative Health Positions; Nurse Midwives; Nurse Practitioners; Nurses; Nutritionists & Dieticians; Paramedics; Pharmacists; Physician Assistants; Prosthetists; Psychologists; Public Health Specialists, Epidemiologists and Health Educators; Water/Sanitation Specialists

Notes

1. A food allowance is given; *2.* French or Portuguese may be required depending on the country.

International Ministries, American Baptist Churches, USA

Address: **P.O. Box 851, Valley Forge, PA 19482-0851 U.S.A.**

Phone: **(800) 222-3872** FAX: **(610) 768-2115**

E-Mail: **bimvolunteers@abc-usa.org** Web: **www.internationalministries.org**

Continents Served

Africa ☑ Asia ☑ Europe ☐ The Americas ☑

Countries Served

Cambodia, Dominican Republic, Haiti, India, Mexico, Nepal, Nicaragua, Rwanda, South Africa, Thailand, Zaire (DemRepCongo)

Mission: The mission of American Baptist International Ministries is to glorify God in all the earth by crossing cultural boudaries to make disciples of Jesus Christ.
International Ministries sends between 11 and 20 physicans to various countries in Africa, Asia, and the Americas for longer term assignments. Volunteers must serve for a minimum of 5 years. Expenses are paid for and each person is given a living allowance while overseas. Personnel must be part of the American Baptist Church.

Placement opportunities for . . .	
People of only certain faiths? *1*	Yes
Couples: both are health providers?	Yes
Couples: only one is a health provider?	Yes
Families with children?	Yes
Medical students?	No
Pre-medical or college students?	No
Other health professional students?	No
Doctors in training?	No
Health personnel who are US citizens?	Yes
Health personnel who are non-US citizens?	No
Health personnel with no prior experience in developing countries?	Yes
Health personnel who are not current members of your organization?	Yes

Organization/Service Specifics:	
Size of the Organization's Staff:	101-150
Number of providers sent or received/year:	11-20
Minimum term of assignment:	5 years
Maximum term of assignment:	25 years
Is funding available for travel?	Yes
Are room and board provided?	Yes
Is any other funding available? *2*	Yes
Is training provided or available?	Yes
Is a language other than English required? *3*	Yes

Health Professionals Placed:

Physicians:

Physicians; Family Practitioners; General Surgeons; Internal Medicine GPS & PCP; Ophthalmologists

Allied Health Professionals:

Nurses

Notes

1. Volunteers must be from the American Baptist Churches, USA; *2.* A living allowance is provided; *3.* The local langauge of the place of service is needed.

International Nepal Fellowship

Continents Served

Africa ☐ Asia ☑ Europe ☐ The Americas ☐

Countries Served

India Nepal

Address: **P.O. Box 5, Simpani, Pokhara, Nepal**

Phone: **977 [0]61-520 111** FAX: **977 [0]61-520 430**

E-Mail: **recruit@inf.org.np or hq@inf.org.np** Web: **www.inf.org.np**

Mission: INF is a Christian mission which seeks to have a wholistic approach in all its activities, and to be culturally sensitive. INF's work is set out in Five-Year Agreements with the Government of Nepal. Our activities include training; supporting the official health services (with medics, managers, and technicians); community development; facilitating social and economic change, especially in disadvantaged groups; disease control and rehabilitation (leprosy and tuberculosis); drug abuse and AIDS prevention; administration and management. Funding is provided by friends and family of the volunteer, but INF will help find a house and pay basic allowance. Training in Nepali is provided. Volunteers may travel for a minimum of 2 months but can stay for life.

Placement opportunities for . . .

People of only certain faiths? *1*	Yes
Couples: both are health providers?	Yes
Couples: only one is a health provider?	Yes
Families with children?	Yes
Medical students?	Yes
Pre-medical or college students?	Yes
Other health professional students?	Yes
Doctors in training?	Yes
Health personnel who are US citizens?	Yes
Health personnel who are non-US citizens?	Yes
Health personnel with no prior experience in developing countries?	Yes
Health personnel who are not current members of your organization?	Yes

Organization/Service Specifics:

Size of the Organization's Staff:	>200
Number of providers sent or received/year:	21-50
Minimum term of assignment:	2 months
Maximum term of assignment:	life
Is funding available for travel?	No
Are room and board provided?	No
Is any other funding available? *2*	No
Is training provided or available?	Yes
Is a language other than English required? *3*	Yes

Health Professionals Placed:

Physicians:

Physicians; Anesthesiologists; Emergency Medicine Physicians; Family Practitioners; General Surgeons; Infectious Disease Spec.; OB/GYN; Oral Surgeons; Optometrists; Otolaryngologists; Plastic/Hand/Reconstructive Surgeons

Allied Health Professionals:

Administrative Health Positions; Dentists; Medical Technicians (lab, X-ray, etc); Nurse Midwives; Nurse Practitioners; Nurses; Paramedics; Pharmacists; Prosthetists; Psychologists; Public Health Specialists, Epidemiologists and Health Educators; Water/Sanitation Specialists

Notes

1. Volunteers must be Protestant; *2.* Volunteers must raise their own support. INF will help find housing and will pay a basic allowance; *3.* Lessons in Nepali are provided.

International Partnership for Human Development

Continents Served

Africa ☑ Asia ☑ Europe ☑ The Americas ☑

Countries Served

Central African Rep. Congo
Equatorial Guinea Guinea
Moldova Romania

Address: **210 North 21st Street, Unit J, Purcellville, VA 20132 U.S.A.**

Phone: **(540) 751-1630** FAX: **(540) 751-1637**

E-Mail: **iphdhq@iphd.org** Web: **www.iphd.org**

Mission: The purpose for founding the IPHD was to respond to the unmet needs of the poor and those people who aspire to remove the causes of poverty through grassroots or popular efforts of development that go beyond the donor-recipient relationship and instead emphasize partnership and solidarity. The end result will not only be people working together to build a better world, but the attainment of better understanding between peoples, which is seen as a step towards full human development and world peace. The phenomena of poverty are viewed in their global dimensions, with each person and each community becoming the architect of their own development in cooperation with people everywhere.

(continued)

Placement opportunities for . . .

People of only certain faiths?	No
Couples: both are health providers?	Yes
Couples: only one is a health provider?	No
Families with children?	No
Medical students?	Yes
Pre-medical or college students?	No
Other health professional students?	Yes
Doctors in training?	Yes
Health personnel who are US citizens?	Yes
Health personnel who are non-US citizens?	Yes
Health personnel with no prior experience in developing countries?	Yes
Health personnel who are not current members of your organization?	Yes

Organization/Service Specifics:

Size of the Organization's Staff:	21-50
Number of providers sent or received/year:	1-5
Minimum term of assignment:	2 weeks
Maximum term of assignment:	1 month
Is funding available for travel? *1*	Yes
Are room and board provided?	Yes
Is any other funding available?	Yes
Is training provided or available?	No
Is a language other than English required? *2*	Yes

Health Professionals Placed:

Physicians:

Family Practitioners; Infectious Disease Spec.; Ophthalmologists

Allied Health Professionals:

Dentists; Nurse Practitioners; Nurses; Nutritionists & Dieticians; Social Workers; Water/Sanitation Specialists

Notes

1. Funding for travel is sometimes provided; *2.* Language requirements are dependent on the country of service.

International Relief Teams

Address: **3547 Camino del Rio South, Suite C, San Diego, CA 92108 U.S.A.**

Phone: **(619) 284-7979** FAX: **(619) 284-7938**

E-Mail: **info@irtcams.org** Web: **www.irteams.org**

Continents Served

Africa ☐ Asia ☐ Europe ☑ The Americas ☑

Countries Served

Brazil	Ecuador	Indonesia
Romania	Sri Lanka	USSR, former

Mission: International Relief Teams is a non-profit, international relief organization dedicated to organizing volunteer teams to provide non-medical and medical assistance to the victims of disaster and profound poverty worldwide. We rely on the skill and compassion of men and women serving as short-term volunteers, and we provide thousands of people each year. Funding for travel and room and board depends on each project. Volunteers can serve for 1-3 week terms. There are no religious or language requirements.

Placement opportunities for . . .

People of only certain faiths?	No
Couples: both are health providers?	Yes
Couples: only one is a health provider?	No
Families with children?	No
Medical students?	No
Pre-medical or college students?	No
Other health professional students?	No
Doctors in training?	Yes
Health personnel who are US citizens?	Yes
Health personnel who are non-US citizens?	No
Health personnel with no prior experience in developing countries?	Yes
Health personnel who are not current members of your organization?	Yes

Organization/Service Specifics:

Size of the Organization's Staff:	0-5
Number of providers sent or received/year:	21-50
Minimum term of assignment:	1 week
Maximum term of assignment:	3 weeks
Is funding available for travel?	Yes
Are room and board provided?	Yes
Is any other funding available? *1*	Yes
Is training provided or available?	No
Is a language other than English required?	No

Health Professionals Placed:

Physicians:

Emergency Medicine Physicians; OB/GYN; Ophthalmologists; Pediatricians; Plastic/Hand/Reconstructive Surgeons

Allied Health Professionals:

Nurse Midwives; Nurse Practitioners; Nurses; Pharmacists; Respiratory Therapists

Notes

1. All funding, including travel and room and board, is dependent on the project.

International Rescue Committee

Address: **122 East 42nd Street, 12th Floor, New York, NY 10168-1289 U.S.A.**

Phone: **(212) 551-3000**
(212) 551-3082 FAX: **(212) 551-3170**

E-Mail: **irc@theirc.org** Web: **www.theirc.org or www.intrescom.org/**

Mission: Founded in 1933, the International Rescue Committee is the leading non-sectarian, voluntary organization providing relief, protection, and resettlement services for refugees and victims of oppression or violent conflict. Funding is provided for travel and room and board. There is also a montly stipend provided. Volunteers can serve from 1 month to 1 year. There are no religious requirements and language requirements depend on the placement.

Continents Served

Africa ✔ Asia ✔ Europe ✔ The Americas ✔

Countries Served

Afghanistan, Bosnia and Herzegovina, Burundi, Chad, Croatia, Ethiopia, Guinea, Indonesia, Iraq, Kenya, Kosovo, Liberia, Macedonia, Myanmar (Burma), Pakistan, Rwanda, Serbia and Montenegro, Sierra Leone, Sudan, Tanzania, Thailand, United States, Yugoslavia, former, Zaire (DemRepCongo)

Placement opportunities for . . .

People of only certain faiths?	No
Couples: both are health providers?	No
Couples: only one is a health provider?	No
Families with children?	No
Medical students?	No
Pre-medical or college students?	No
Other health professional students?	Yes
Doctors in training?	Yes
Health personnel who are US citizens?	Yes
Health personnel who are non-US citizens?	Yes
Health personnel with no prior experience in developing countries?	No
Health personnel who are not current members of your organization?	Yes

Organization/Service Specifics:

Size of the Organization's Staff:	>200
Number of providers sent or received/year:	21-50
Minimum term of assignment:	1 month
Maximum term of assignment:	1 year
Is funding available for travel?	Yes
Are room and board provided?	Yes
Is any other funding available? *1*	Yes
Is training provided or available?	No
Is a language other than English required? *2*	Yes

Health Professionals Placed:

Physicians:

Physicians; Emergency Medicine Physicians; Infectious Disease Spec.; Internal Medicine GPS & PCP; OB/GYN; Pediatricians

Allied Health Professionals:

Nurse Midwives; Nurse Practitioners; Nutritionists & Dieticians; Pharmacists; Public Health Specialists, Epidemiologists and Health Educators; Social Workers; Water/Sanitation Specialists

Notes

1. A monthly stipend is provided; *2.* Depends on the place of service.

Interplast

Address: **300-B Pioneer Way, Mountain View, CA 94041 U.S.A.**

Phone: **(650) 962-0123**
(888) 467-5278 FAX: **(650) 962-1619**

E-Mail: **Ipnews@interplast.org** Web: **www.interplast.org**

Mission: Interplast's mission is to provide free reconsructive surgery for people in developing nations, and to help improve health care world wide. The organization's goals are to establish, develop, and maintain host-country, domestic-patient, and educational programs with the following objectives: provide direct patient care; provide educational training and medical independence; assist host country medical colleagues toward medical independence; enable recipients of care to become providers of care to new sites.

Continents Served

Africa ☐ Asia ✔ Europe ✔ The Americas ✔

Countries Served

Bangladesh, Bolivia, Brazil, Chile, Cuba, Dominican Republic, Ecuador, El Salvador, Honduras, Jamaica, Mongolia, Myanmar (Burma), Nepal, Nicaragua, Peru, Philippines, Sri Lanka, Thailand, USSR, former, Vietnam

(continued)

Placement opportunities for . . .

People of only certain faiths?	No
Couples: both are health providers?	Yes
Couples: only one is a health provider?	No
Families with children?	No
Medical students?	No
Pre-medical or college students?	No
Other health professional students?	Yes
Doctors in training? *1*	Yes
Health personnel who are US citizens?	Yes
Health personnel who are non-US citizens?	Yes
Health personnel with no prior experience in developing countries?	Yes
Health personnel who are not current members of your organization?	Yes

Organization/Service Specifics:

Size of the Organization's Staff:	11-20
Number of providers sent or received/year:	>200
Minimum term of assignment:	1 week
Maximum term of assignment:	2 weeks
Is funding available for travel?	Yes
Are room and board provided? *2*	Yes
Is any other funding available?	No
Is training provided or available?	No
Is a language other than English required? *3*	No

Health Professionals Placed:

Physicians:

Anesthesiologists; Pediatricians; Plastic/Hand/Reconstructive Surgeons

Allied Health Professionals:

Nurses

Notes

1. If they are accompanied by their attending physician; *2.* Room and board depends on availability and restrictions; *3.* Bilinguals preferred.

InterServe

Address: **P.O. Box 418, Upper Darby, PA 19082-0418 U.S.A.**

Phone: **(610) 352-0581** FAX: **(215) 352-4394**
(800) 809-4440

E-Mail: **info@interserve.org or ot@ludlow.net** Web: **www.interserve.org**

Mission: As an international fellowship committed to serving the Christian Church, InterServe's mission is to contribute directly or indirectly to the making of disciples of Jesus Christ, particularly in countries of south and central Asia, the Gulf, Middle East, and North Africa, and in other countries where there are significant groups of migrants from these countries. InterServe places medical personnel of Christian faiths into countries for both short-term (1 month) and long-term (3 year) appointments. Long term volunteers are required to learn the language of the country they are serving, while there are no language requirements for short term volunteers.

Continents Served

Africa ☑ Asia ☑ Europe ☐ The Americas ☑

Countries Served

Afghanistan, Bahrain, Bangladesh, Bhutan, China, Egypt, Hong Kong, India, Indonesia, Iraq, Jordan, Kuwait, Lebanon, Mongolia, Morocco, Myanmar (Burma), Nepal, Oman, Pakistan, Qatar, Saudi Arabia, Syria, Tunisia, Turkey, United Arab Emirates, Yemen

Placement opportunities for . . .

People of only certain faiths? *1*	Yes
Couples: both are health providers?	Yes
Couples: only one is a health provider?	Yes
Families with children?	Yes
Medical students?	Yes
Pre-medical or college students?	No
Other health professional students?	Yes
Doctors in training?	Yes
Health personnel who are US citizens?	Yes
Health personnel who are non-US citizens?	No
Health personnel with no prior experience in developing countries?	Yes
Health personnel who are not current members of your organization?	Yes

Organization/Service Specifics:

Size of the Organization's Staff:	51-100
Number of providers sent or received/year:	11-20
Minimum term of assignment:	1 month
Maximum term of assignment:	3 years
Is funding available for travel?	No
Are room and board provided?	Yes
Is any other funding available?	No
Is training provided or available?	Yes
Is a language other than English required? *2*	Yes

Health Professionals Placed:

Physicians:

Physicians; Anesthesiologists; Cardiologists; Family Practitioners; General Surgeons; Infectious Disease Spec.; Internal Medicine GPS & PCP; OB/GYN; Ophthalmologists; Optometrists; Pediatricians; Radiologists

Allied Health Professionals:

Administrative Health Positions; Dentists; Medical Technicians (lab, X-ray, etc); Nurse Practitioners; Nurses; Pharmacists; Physical & Occupational Therapists; Physician Assistants; Prosthetists; Public Health Specialists, Epidemiologists and Health Educators; Social Workers; Water/Sanitation Specialists

Notes

1. Volunteers must be Catholic or Protestant; *2.* For long-term assignments, knowledge of the language of the place of service is required. For short-term assignments, there are no language requirements.

INTERTEAM

Continents Served			
Africa ✔	Asia ✔	Europe ☐	The Americas ✔

Countries Served

Bolivia, Colombia, Mozambique, Namibia, Nicaragua, Papua-New Guinea, Peru, Tanzania

Address: **Unter-Geissenstein 10/12 6005, Luzern, CH6000 Switzerland**

Phone: **(041) 360-6722** FAX: **(041) 361-0580**

E-Mail: **info@interteam.ch** Web: **www.interteam.ch**

Mission: INTERTEAM works mainly with the indigenous church and with some State based insititutions in Africa, Asia, and Latin America. They are looking for men and women with good professional skills to encourage community awareness and activities at the grassroots level, as well as providing professional training or further education. Funding and room and board are all provided. Personnel can serve for 3-12 years. German and local languages are required of personnel, as well as Spanish and Portuguese in some cases.

Placement opportunities for . . .

People of only certain faiths?	No
Couples: both are health providers?	Yes
Couples: only one is a health provider?	Yes
Families with children?	Yes
Medical students?	No
Pre-medical or college students?	No
Other health professional students?	No
Doctors in training?	No
Health personnel who are US citizens?	No
Health personnel who are non-US citizens? *1*	Yes
Health personnel with no prior experience in developing countries?	Yes
Health personnel who are not current members of your organization?	Yes

Organization/Service Specifics:

Size of the Organization's Staff:	6-10
Number of providers sent or received/year:	21-50
Minimum term of assignment:	3 years
Maximum term of assignment:	12 years
Is funding available for travel?	Yes
Are room and board provided?	Yes
Is any other funding available? *2*	Yes
Is training provided or available?	Yes
Is a language other than English required? *3*	Yes

Health Professionals Placed:

Physicians:

Allied Health Professionals:

Medical Technicians (lab, X-ray, etc); Nurse Midwives; Nurses; Nutritionists & Dieticians; Paramedics; Public Health Specialists, Epidemiologists and Health Educators; Social Workers; Water/Sanitation Specialists

Notes

1. Only Swiss citizens; *2.* Social security, health insurance, training, and monthly savings for reintegration are all provided; *3.* Language requirements depend on the place of service.

Jesuit Refugee Service

Continents Served			
Africa ✔	Asia ✔	Europe ✔	The Americas ☐

Countries Served

Angola, Burundi, Ethiopia, Guinea, Ivory Coast, Liberia, Mexico, Rwanda, Sudan, Thailand, Yugoslavia, former, Zambia

Address: **1616 P Street NW, Suite 300, Washington, DC 20036-1405 U.S.A.**

Phone: **(202) 462-0400** FAX: **(202) 328-9212**

E-Mail: **international@jrs.net** Web: **usa@jrs.net**

Mission: The Jesuit Refugee Service is an international Catholic organization, at work in over 40 countries, with a mission to accompany, serve, and defend the rights of refugees and forcibly displaced people. The mission given to JRS embraces all who are driven from their homes by conflict, humanitarian disaster, or violation of human rights, following Catholic social teaching which applies the expression "de facto refugee" to many related categories of people. JRS undertakes services at national and regional levels with the support of an international office in Rome. With a priority to working wherever the needs of displaced people are urgent and unattended by others, JRS offers a human and pastoral service to refugees and the communities that host them through a wide range of rehabilitation and relief activities. Services including programs of pastoral care, education for children and adults, social services and counselling, and health care are tailored to meet local needs according to available resources. Funding and room and board are available for 2-year terms of service. The local language of the country of service is required for volunteers.

(continued)

Placement opportunities for . . .

People of only certain faiths? *1*	No
Couples: both are health providers?	No
Couples: only one is a health provider?	
Families with children?	No
Medical students?	No
Pre-medical or college students?	No
Other health professional students?	Yes
Doctors in training?	No
Health personnel who are US citizens?	Yes
Health personnel who are non-US citizens?	Yes
Health personnel with no prior experience in developing countries?	No
Health personnel who are not current members of your organization?	Yes

Organization/Service Specifics:

Size of the Organization's Staff:	>200
Number of providers sent or received/year:	51-100
Minimum term of assignment:	2 years
Maximum term of assignment:	2 years
Is funding available for travel?	Yes
Are room and board provided?	Yes
Is any other funding available? *2*	Yes
Is training provided or available?	Yes
Is a language other than English required? *3*	Yes

Health Professionals Placed:

Physicians:

General Surgeons

Allied Health Professionals:

Nurse Midwives; Nurses; Public Health Specialists, Epidemiologists and Health Educators; Social Workers

Notes

1. No specific religious requirements, "but we are a Catholic organization"; *2.* There is a modest stipend; *3.* Language requirements depend on the local lingua franca.

Johns Hopkins Univ. School of Public Health, Dept. of International Health

Continents Served

Africa ☑ Asia ☑ Europe ☐ The Americas ☑

Countries Served

Bangladesh	Cambodia	Cameroon
Dominican Republic		Egypt
Ethiopia	Haiti	India
Indonesia	Korea, South	Malawi
Nepal	Rwanda	Taiwan
Tanzania	Thailand	Uganda
Vietnam	Zambia	Zimbabwe

Address: **615 North Wolfe St., Baltimore, MD 21205-2179 U.S.A.**

Phone: **(410) 955-3934** FAX: **(410) 955-7159**

E-Mail: **rblack@jhsph.edu** Web: **www.jhsph.edu/dept/ih**

Mission: The Department of International Health at Johns Hopkins seeks to understand health issues and institute realistic means of disease prevention and health protection in underserved populations around the world. To this end, this nondenominational program places nurses, midwives, nutritionists, administrative personnel, public health specialists, and health educators for short terms stays (2-5 weeks) in various regions of Africa, Asia, and the Americas. There are no religious or language requirements.

Placement opportunities for . . .

People of only certain faiths?	No
Couples: both are health providers?	Yes
Couples: only one is a health provider?	Yes
Families with children?	Yes
Medical students?	No
Pre-medical or college students?	No
Other health professional students?	No
Doctors in training?	Yes
Health personnel who are US citizens?	Yes
Health personnel who are non-US citizens?	Yes
Health personnel with no prior experience in developing countries?	No
Health personnel who are not current members of your organization?	No

Organization/Service Specifics:

Size of the Organization's Staff:	>200
Number of providers sent or received/year:	11-20
Minimum term of assignment:	2 weeks
Maximum term of assignment:	5 years
Is funding available for travel?	No
Are room and board provided?	No
Is any other funding available?	No
Is training provided or available?	Yes
Is a language other than English required?	No

Health Professionals Placed:

Physicians:

Allied Health Professionals:

Administrative Health Positions; Nurse Midwives; Nurse Practitioners; Nurses; Nutritionists & Dieticians; Public Health Specialists, Epidemiologists and Health Educators

Notes

Jubilee Volunteer Africa Program of AFRIDEC

Continents Served
Africa ☑ Asia ☐ Europe ☐ The Americas ☐

Countries Served
Kenya South Africa

Address: **P.O. Box 2242-00100 GPO Nairobi, Kenya**
Phone: **254-20-4450517** FAX: **254-721-646624**
E-Mail: **helpdesk@jubileeventures.org** Web: **http://jubileeventures.org/volunteer.html**

Mission: Africa Development Consortium (AFRIDEC) is an international non-profit organization with the mission to work in partnership with local communities to promote community development and nature conservation. AFRIDEC has long-term, short-term and group placement volunteer programs suitable for anyone interested in international volunteer and overseas internships. Work is available in many areas including teaching, medical, etc. Current medical programs are only available in Kenya. Topkins Medical Clinic is one facility where we place volunteers. The clinic provides service to patients from Kimende and neighboring areas within a radius of ten miles from the township.

Placement opportunities for . . .		Organization/Service Specifics:	
People of only certain faiths?	No	Size of the Organization's Staff:	
Couples: both are health providers?	No	Number of providers sent or received/year:	
Couples: only one is a health provider?	No	Minimum term of assignment:	2 weeks
Families with children?	No	Maximum term of assignment:	2 months
Medical students?	Yes	Is funding available for travel?	No
Pre-medical or college students?	Yes	Are room and board provided? *1*	Yes
Other health professional students?	Yes	Is any other funding available?	No
Doctors in training?	Yes	Is training provided or available?	Yes
Health personnel who are US citizens?	Yes	Is a language other than English required?	No
Health personnel who are non-US citizens?	Yes		
Health personnel with no prior experience in developing countries?	Yes		
Health personnel who are not current members of your organization?	Yes		

Health Professionals Placed:

Physicians:

Physicians

Allied Health Professionals:

Nurses; Physician Assistants

Notes

1. Included in cost of program.

Lalmba Association

Continents Served
Africa ☑ Asia ☐ Europe ☐ The Americas ☑

Countries Served
Ethiopia Kenya

Address: **7685 Quartz St., Arvada, CO 80007 U.S.A.**
Phone: **(303) 420-1810** FAX: **(303) 467-1232**
E-Mail: **lalmba@lalmba.org** Web: **www.lalmba.org/**

Mission: Lalmba is committed to the people of Africa on a long term basis. Lalmba provides the medical treatment these people need today, while training and educating them to care for themselves tomorrow. It is a mission of relief and development that makes these people responsible for their own future. Assignments last between 1 and 2 years. Funding, as well as health and life insurance, are provided.

Placement opportunities for . . .		Organization/Service Specifics:	
People of only certain faiths?	No	Size of the Organization's Staff:	0-5
Couples: both are health providers?	Yes	Number of providers sent or received/year:	6-10
Couples: only one is a health provider?	Yes	Minimum term of assignment:	1 year
Families with children?	No	Maximum term of assignment:	2 years
Medical students?	No	Is funding available for travel?	Yes
Pre-medical or college students?	No	Are room and board provided?	Yes
Other health professional students?	No	Is any other funding available? *1*	Yes
Doctors in training?	No	Is training provided or available?	Yes
Health personnel who are US citizens?	Yes	Is a language other than English required?	No
Health personnel who are non-US citizens?	Yes		
Health personnel with no prior experience in developing countries?	Yes		
Health personnel who are not current members of your organization?	Yes		

(continued)

Health Professionals Placed:

Physicians:

Physicians; Family Practitioners; Internal Medicine GPS & PCP; Pediatricians

Allied Health Professionals:

Nurse Midwives; Nurse Practitioners; Nurses; Physician Assistants; Public Health Specialists, Epidemiologists and Health Educators

Notes

1. Health and life insurance are provided.

Lay Mission-Helpers Association

Continents Served

Africa ☑ Asia ☑ Europe ☐ The Americas ☑

Countries Served

American Samoa, Cameroon, Caroline Islands, Ecuador, Ghana, Guatemala, Kenya, Marshall Islands, Thailand, Uganda

Address: **3435 Wilshire Blvd., Suite 1035, Los Angeles, CA 90010 U.S.A.**

Phone: **(213) 368-1870** FAX: **(213) 368-1871**

E-Mail: **info@laymissionhelpers.org** Web: **laymissionhelpers.org**

Mission: We are a Catholic community of lay people called through our baptism to mission. We seek to share in the ministry of Jesus to spread the Good News and work for the Reign of God. We seek to walk with the poor of other countries, sharing our talents, learning from one another, and working together for a just and more compassionate world. We are teachers, nurses, social workers, administrators, secretaries, craftsmen, computer technicians, mechanics, and others who strive to live a simple lifestyle close to the poor. We want to be bridges between the US Catholic communities that send us and the overseas communities that receive us. We work for greater respect, understanding, and solidarity among all peoples. We provide funding and room and board for volunteers who serve for 3 year, renewable terms.

Placement opportunities for . . .		Organization/Service Specifics:	
People of only certain faiths? *1*	Yes	Size of the Organization's Staff:	0-5
Couples: both are health providers?	Yes	Number of providers sent or received/year:	>200
Couples: only one is a health provider?	Yes	Minimum term of assignment:	3 years
Families with children?	Yes	Maximum term of assignment:	renewable
Medical students?	No	Is funding available for travel?	Yes
Pre-medical or college students?	No	Are room and board provided?	Yes
Other health professional students?	No	Is any other funding available? *2*	Yes
Doctors in training?	No	Is training provided or available?	Yes
Health personnel who are US citizens?	Yes	Is a language other than English required?	No
Health personnel who are non-US citizens?	No		
Health personnel with no prior experience in developing countries?	Yes		
Health personnel who are not current members of your organization?	Yes		

Health Professionals Placed:

Physicians:

Allied Health Professionals:

Administrative Health Positions; Nurses; Physician Assistants; Social Workers

Notes

1. Volunteers must be Catholic;
2. Medical insurance is provided.

Liga International, Inc.

Continents Served

Africa ☐ Asia ☐ Europe ☐ The Americas ☑

Countries Served

Mexico, Nicaragua, Peru, Philippines

Address: **1464 N. Fitzgerald Hanger 2, Riolto, CA 92376 U.S.A.**

Phone: **(909) 875-6300** FAX: **(909) 875-6900**

E-Mail: **info@ligainternational.org** Web: **www.ligainternational.org**

Mission: Our organization is structured to provide ongoing medical, dental, and eye care to the poor in rural Mexico. We fly to designated locations once a month from October through June each year. We leave on the first Friday of the month and return on Sunday, making a three-day weekend. This is done 9 times per year. Volunteers can participate as often or as little as they desire; each individual stay would only be three days. Volunteers must fund their own trips; however, most fly in small private aircrafts from California. Total cost per trip in 2004 was approximately $250. Spanish is helpful but not required. *(continued)*

Placement opportunities for . . .		Organization/Service Specifics:	
People of only certain faiths?	No	Size of the Organization's Staff:	0-5
Couples: both are health providers?	Yes	Number of providers sent or received/year:	151-200
Couples: only one is a health provider?	Yes	Minimum term of assignment:	3 days
Families with children?	No	Maximum term of assignment:	
Medical students?	Yes	Is funding available for travel?	No
Pre-medical or college students?	Yes	Are room and board provided?	No
Other health professional students?	Yes	Is any other funding available?	No
Doctors in training?	Yes	Is training provided or available?	Yes
Health personnel who are US citizens?	Yes	Is a language other than English required? *1*	No
Health personnel who are non-US citizens?	Yes		
Health personnel with no prior experience in developing countries?	Yes		
Health personnel who are not current members of your organization?	Yes		

Health Professionals Placed:

Physicians:

Physicians; Anesthesiologists; Cardiologists; Dermatologists; Emergency Medicine Physicians; Endocrinologists; Family Practitioners; General Surgeons; Internal Medicine GPS & PCP; OB/GYN; Ophthalmologists; Optometrists; Orthopedic Surgeons; Pediatricians; Plastic/Hand/Reconstructive Surgeons

Allied Health Professionals:

Dentists; Medical Technicians (lab, X-ray, etc); Nurse Midwives; Nurse Practitioners; Nurses; Paramedics; Pharmacists; Physical & Occupational Therapists; Physician Assistants; Podiatrists; Prosthetists; Social Workers

Notes

1. Spanish is helpful, but not required.

Lighthouse for Christ Mission and Eye Centre

Address: **P.O. Box 8318 Tyler, TX 75711-8318 U.S.A.**

Phone: **(903) 593-2157** FAX: **(903) 849-3504**

E-Mail: **info@lighthouseforchrist.org/ or lfcec@aol.com** Web: **http://lighthouseforchrist.org/**

Continents Served

Africa ☑ Asia ☐ Europe ☐ The Americas ☐

Countries Served

Kenya

Mission: Lighthouse for Christ maintains an eye clinic in Mobasa, Kenya, that sees more than 25,000 patients annually, including 2000 surgeries. Through Lighthouse's efforts, local Kenyans can receive much needed health care while being introduced to and/or educated about the bible. Lighthouse has helped develop churches, a laboratory and modern quest quarters in addition to its eye clinic. Christian volunteer ophthalmologists, optometrists and health personnel are needed for the clinical surgery center.

Placement opportunities for . . .		Organization/Service Specifics:	
People of only certain faiths?	No	Size of the Organization's Staff:	11-20
Couples: both are health providers?	Yes	Number of providers sent or received/year:	11-20
Couples: only one is a health provider?	Yes	Minimum term of assignment:	2 weeks
Families with children?	Yes	Maximum term of assignment:	1 year
Medical students?	Yes	Is funding available for travel?	No
Pre-medical or college students?	No	Are room and board provided?	Yes
Other health professional students? *1*	Yes	Is any other funding available?	No
Doctors in training?	Yes	Is training provided or available? *2*	Yes
Health personnel who are US citizens?	Yes	Is a language other than English required?	No
Health personnel who are non-US citizens?	Yes		
Health personnel with no prior experience in developing countries?			
Health personnel who are not current members of your organization?	Yes		

Health Professionals Placed: *3*

Physicians:

Ophthalmologists; Optometrists

Allied Health Professionals:

Nurses

Notes

1. Nursing students; *2.* Training will be limited to an orientation of the facility and equipment; *3.* Certified assistants.

Loma Linda University International Programs

Continents Served			
Africa ☑	Asia ☑	Europe ☐	The Americas ☑

Countries Served

Address: **11060 Anderson St., Magan Hall Suite 105, Loma Linda, CA 92350 U.S.A.**

Phone: **(909) 558-4420** FAX: **(909) 558-0116**

E-Mail: **globaloutreach@univ univ.llu.edu** Web: **www.llu.edu/inter national/index.html**

Mission: Loma Linda University International Programs operates under the general Conference of Seventh-day Adventist Churches and as a consequence has access to a worldwide network of mission hospitals. It offers physicians short-term and long-term volunteer service opportunities around the world. The Seventh-day Adventist Church has established work in 207 countries. Volunteers must provide their own funding for travel, but room and board are provided.

Placement opportunities for . . .		Organization/Service Specifics:	
People of only certain faiths? *1*	No	Size of the Organization's Staff:	0-5
Couples: both are health providers?	Yes	Number of providers sent or received/year:	1-5
Couples: only one is a health provider?	Yes	Minimum term of assignment:	none
Families with children?	Yes	Maximum term of assignment:	none
Medical students?	Yes	Is funding available for travel?	No
Pre-medical or college students?	No	Are room and board provided?	Yes
Other health professional students?	No	Is any other funding available?	No
Doctors in training?	No	Is training provided or available?	Yes
Health personnel who are US citizens?	Yes	Is a language other than English required?	No
Health personnel who are non-US citizens?	Yes		
Health personnel with no prior experience in developing countries?	Yes		
Health personnel who are not current members of your organization?	Yes		

Health Professionals Placed:

Physicians:

General Surgeons; Orthopedic Surgeons

Allied Health Professionals:

Nurses

Notes

1. Most of our volunteers are Adventist.

Ludhiana Christian Medical College Board USA

Continents Served			
Africa ☐	Asia ☑	Europe ☐	The Americas ☐

Countries Served

India

Address: **1105 Garden of the Gods Road, Colorado Springs, CO 80907 U.S.A.**

Phone: **(719) 272-0200** FAX: **(719) 272-0201**

E-Mail: **ludhianamc@aol.com** Web:

Mission: Our mission is to advance Christian medical education in India as an expression of Christ's healing love, and to promote the work of the Christian Medical College and Hospital in Ludhiana, India. Volunteers travel for a minimum of 3 weeks. Volunteers are responsible for their own funding, although room and board are provided. There are no language or religious requirements.

Placement opportunities for . . .		Organization/Service Specifics:	
People of only certain faiths?	No	Size of the Organization's Staff:	0-5
Couples: both are health providers?	Yes	Number of providers sent or received/year:	11-20
Couples: only one is a health provider?	Yes	Minimum term of assignment:	3 weeks
Families with children?	Yes	Maximum term of assignment:	
Medical students?	No	Is funding available for travel? *2*	No
Pre-medical or college students?	No	Are room and board provided?	Yes
Other health professional students?	No	Is any other funding available?	No
Doctors in training?	Yes	Is training provided or available?	Yes
Health personnel who are US citizens?	Yes	Is a language other than English required?	No
Health personnel who are non-US citizens?	No		
Health personnel with no prior experience in developing countries? *1*	Yes		
Health personnel who are not current members of your organization?	Yes		

(continued)

Health Professionals Placed:

Physicians:

Physicians; Anesthesiologists; Cardiologists; Dermatologists; Emergency Medicine Physicians; Endocrinologists; General Surgeons; Hematologists; Oncologists; Infectious Disease Spec.; Neurologists; Neurosurgeons; OB/GYN; Ophthalmologists; Orthopedic Surgeons; Radiologists

Allied Health Professionals:

Administrative Health Positions; Dentists; Nurses; Public Health Specialists, Epidemiologists and Health Educators

Notes

1. We may possibly consider personnel with no prior experience in developing countries; *2.* Funding for travel is rarely available.

Lumiere Medical Ministries, Inc.

Address: **3816 2 New Hope Rd., Suite 20, Gastonia, NC 28056 U.S.A.**

Phone: **(704) 823-0271** FAX: **(704) 823-0272**

E-Mail: **lmmhaiti@carolina.rr.com** Web: **lovetheycanfeel.org**

Continents Served

Africa ☐ Asia ☐ Europe ☐ The Americas ☐

Countries Served

Haiti

Mission: Lumiere Medical Ministries is a Christian organization that aims to enlighten health care for bodies and provide the light of the Gospel for hearts. Hospital of Light in Haiti has an international staff composed of Haitians, Europeans, and North Americans and provides hospital and out-patient services in surgery and medicine, maternity and child care, pharmacy services, as well as community services such as health education, immunizations, and pre-natal care. Christian volunteers can go for as little as one week or as long as life. There are no language requirements, although French or Creole are very useful. Room and board are provided, but volunteers are responsible for other funding. Medical students may attend with a supervising professor.

Placement opportunities for . . .	
People of only certain faiths? *1*	Yes
Couples: both are health providers?	No
Couples: only one is a health provider?	Yes
Families with children?	Yes
Medical students?	Yes
Pre-medical or college students?	Yes
Other health professional students?	Yes
Doctors in training?	Yes
Health personnel who are US citizens?	Yes
Health personnel who are non-US citizens?	Yes
Health personnel with no prior experience in developing countries?	Yes
Health personnel who are not current members of your organization?	Yes

Organization/Service Specifics:	
Size of the Organization's Staff:	6-10
Number of providers sent or received/year:	51-100
Minimum term of assignment:	1 week
Maximum term of assignment:	life
Is funding available for travel?	No
Are room and board provided? *2*	Yes
Is any other funding available?	No
Is training provided or available?	Yes
Is a language other than English required? *3*	No

Health Professionals Placed:

Physicians:

Physicians; Anesthesiologists; Cardiologists; Dermatologists; Emergency Medicine Physicians; Endocrinologists; Family Practitioners; Gastroenterologists; General Surgeons; Hematologists; Oncologists; Infectious Disease Spec.; Internal Medicine GPS & PCP; Nephrologists; Neurologists; Neurosurgeons; OB/GYN; Ophthalmologists; Oral Surgeons; Optometrists; Orthopedic Surgeons; Otolaryngologists; Pathologists; Pediatricians; Plastic/Hand/Reconstructive Surgeons; Psychiatrists; Pulmonary Specialists; Radiologists; Urologists

Allied Health Professionals:

Administrative Health Positions; Dental Hygienists; Dentists; Medical Technicians (lab, X-ray, etc); Nurse Midwives; Nurse Practitioners; Nurses; Nutritionists & Dieticians; Paramedics; Pharmacists; Physical & Occupational Therapists; Physician Assistants; Podiatrists; Prosthetists; Psychologists; Public Health Specialists, Epidemiologists and Health Educators; Respiratory Therapists; Social Workers; Water/Sanitation Specialists

Notes

1. We are a non-denominational Christian organization; *2.* There is a charge for housing, but it is available on our property; *3.* French Creole.

M.E.D.I.C.O.

Continents Served
Africa ☐ Asia ☐ Europe ☐ The Americas ☑

Countries Served
Honduras Mexico Nicaragua Panama

Address: **2955 Dawn Dr., Suite D, Georgetown, TX 78628 U.S.A.**

Phone: **(512) 930-1893** FAX: **(512) 869-7500**

E-Mail: **info@medico.org** Web: **www.medico.org**

Mission: Our mission is to provide free medical, dental and optometric care and educational services to people in developing countries who have little or no access to basic medical care. Volunteers serve for 1 week and must generally provide their own funding. There are limited scholarships for students. Spanish is helpful, but not required.

Placement opportunities for . . .	
People of only certain faiths?	No
Couples: both are health providers?	Yes
Couples: only one is a health provider?	Yes
Families with children?	No
Medical students?	Yes
Pre-medical or college students?	Yes
Other health professional students?	Yes
Doctors in training?	Yes
Health personnel who are US citizens?	Yes
Health personnel who are non-US citizens?	Yes
Health personnel with no prior experience in developing countries?	Yes
Health personnel who are not current members of your organization?	Yes

Organization/Service Specifics:	
Size of the Organization's Staff:	0-5
Number of providers sent or received/year:	101-150
Minimum term of assignment:	1 week
Maximum term of assignment:	1 week
Is funding available for travel?	No
Are room and board provided?	No
Is any other funding available? *1*	Yes
Is training provided or available?	No
Is a language other than English required? *2*	No

Health Professionals Placed:

Physicians:

Physicians; Anesthesiologists; Dermatologists; Emergency Medicine Physicians; Family Practitioners; General Surgeons; Internal Medicine GPS & PCP; Neurologists; OB/GYN; Optometrists; Orthopedic Surgeons; Pediatricians; Radiologists; Urologists

Allied Health Professionals:

Administrative Health Positions; Dental Hygienists; Dentists; Nurse Practitioners; Nurses; Paramedics; Pharmacists; Physical & Occupational Therapists; Physician Assistants; Podiatrists; Respiratory Therapists; Social Workers

Notes

1. There are limited scholarships available for students; *2.* Spanish is helpful, but not required.

Magee-Womens Hospital

Continents Served
Africa ☐ Asia ☐ Europe ☑ The Americas ☐

Countries Served
Russia Ukraine

Address: **300 Halket Street, Pittsburgh, PA 15213-3180 U.S.A.**

Phone: **(412) 641-1189** FAX: **(412) 641-1202**

E-Mail: **jcooper@mail.magee.edu** Web: **www.magee.edu/**

Mission: To globalize the primary mission of Magee-Womens Hospital: to care for women through programs which advocate dignity, access, education, and quality of service in women's health care. We send volunteers on an individual/internship basis.

Placement opportunities for . . .	
People of only certain faiths?	No
Couples: both are health providers? *1*	No
Couples: only one is a health provider?	No
Families with children?	No
Medical students?	Yes
Pre-medical or college students?	No
Other health professional students?	Yes
Doctors in training?	Yes
Health personnel who are US citizens?	Yes
Health personnel who are non-US citizens?	Yes
Health personnel with no prior experience in developing countries?	Yes
Health personnel who are not current members of your organization?	No

Organization/Service Specifics:	
Size of the Organization's Staff:	11-20
Number of providers sent or received/year:	51-100
Minimum term of assignment:	1 week
Maximum term of assignment:	1 week
Is funding available for travel?	Yes
Are room and board provided?	Yes
Is any other funding available? *2*	Yes
Is training provided or available?	Yes
Is a language other than English required?	No

(continued)

Health Professionals Placed:

Physicians:

Physicians; Anesthesiologists; Cardiologists; Emergency Medicine Physicians; Endocrinologists; Family Practitioners; Gastroenterologists; General Surgeons; Hematologists; Oncologists; Infectious Disease Spec.; Internal Medicine GPS & PCP; OB/GYN; Pathologists; Pediatricians; Plastic/Hand/Reconstructive Surgeons; Psychiatrists; Radiologists

Allied Health Professionals:

Administrative Health Positions; Medical Technicians (lab, X-ray, etc); Nurse Midwives; Nurse Practitioners; Nurses; Nutritionists & Dieticians; Pharmacists; Public Health Specialists, Epidemiologists and Health Educators

Notes

1. Magee-Womens Hospital provides funding for independent projects done on an internship/volunteer basis; *2.* For some programs, "We have funding, but we do not offer subgrants."

Maluti Adventist Hospital (Lesotho)

Address: **P. Bag X019, Ficksburg 9370, South Africa**

Phone: **(082) 820-1303** FAX: **(082) 822-0161**

E-Mail: **hurlow@yebo.co.za or maluti@yebo.co.za** Web:

Continents Served

Africa ☑ Asia ☐ Europe ☐ The Americas ☐

Countries Served

Lesotho

Mission: To relieve the sick and afflicted by scientific medical ministry. To awaken a spirit of inquiry by demonstrating Christian compassion and deep dedication that prompts inquiry as to the motivation. To disseminate light by making known the laws of God pertaining to health of body and soul. To advance reform by precept and example, thus encouraging healthy habits of life. To prepare others to serve by conducting educational and training programs. Volunteers can serve from 2 weeks to 1 year. There are no language or religious requirements. Volunteers are responsible for their own funding, but Maluti Adventist Hospital will provide room and board.

Placement opportunities for . . .	
People of only certain faiths?	No
Couples: both are health providers?	Yes
Couples: only one is a health provider?	Yes
Families with children?	Yes
Medical students?	Yes
Pre-medical or college students?	No
Other health professional students?	Yes
Doctors in training?	Yes
Health personnel who are US citizens?	Yes
Health personnel who are non-US citizens?	Yes
Health personnel with no prior experience in developing countries?	Yes
Health personnel who are not current members of your organization?	Yes

Organization/Service Specifics:	
Size of the Organization's Staff: *1*	51-100
Number of providers sent or received/year:	1-5
Minimum term of assignment:	2 weeks
Maximum term of assignment:	1 year
Is funding available for travel?	No
Are room and board provided?	Yes
Is any other funding available?	No
Is training provided or available?	Yes
Is a language other than English required?	No

Health Professionals Placed:

Physicians:

Physicians; General Surgeons; Internal Medicine GPS & PCP; Ophthalmologists; Optometrists

Allied Health Professionals:

Dentists; Medical Technicians (lab, X-ray, etc); Nurse Midwives; Nurse Practitioners; Nurses; Nutritionists & Dieticians; Pharmacists; Physical & Occupational Therapists

Notes

1. Last contacted in 11/02. Did not respond to inquiry in 2/05.

Management Sciences for Health

Address: **784 Memorial Drive, Cambridge, MA 02139 U.S.A.**

Phone: **(617) 250-9500** FAX: **(617) 250-9090**

E-Mail: **development@msh.org** Web: **www.msh.org**

Mission: MSH works collaboratively with health care policy-makers, managers, providers, and consumers to help close the gap between knowledge and action in the field of public health. We seek to increase the effectiveness, efficiency, and sustainability of health and family planning services by improving their management, to promote access to these services, and to influence public policy. MSH activities focus on educating health care managers, providers, and consumers through training, pulications, electronic media, and conferences; applying practical management skills to public health problems in both the public and private sectors; strengthening the technical and management capabilities of individuals and institutions through collaborative work and training programs; and discovering, applying, and replicating innovations in health management. MSH also provides technical assistance in six areas of expertise: drug management, family planning and reproductive health, management information systems, management training, health financing, and primary health care.

Continents Served

Africa ✔ Asia ✔ Europe ✔ The Americas ✔

Countries Served

Afghanistan	Algeria	Angola
Bangladesh	Benin	Bhutan
Bolivia	Brazil	Burkina Faso
Cambodia	Cameroon	Chad
Dominican Republic		Egypt
El Salvador	Ethiopia	Gambia
Ghana	Guatemala	Guinea
Guinea-Bissau	Haiti	Honduras
India	Indonesia	Japan
Kenya	Liberia	Madagascar
Malawi	Mali	Mauritania
Mexico	Morocco	Mozambique
Nepal	Nicaragua	Niger
Nigeria	Papua-New Guinea	
Peru	Philippines	Romania
Senegal	Sierra Leone	South Africa
Tanzania	Uganda	United States
USSR, former	Zaire (DemRepCongo)	
Zambia	Zimbabwe	

Placement opportunities for . . .

People of only certain faiths?	No
Couples: both are health providers?	Yes
Couples: only one is a health provider?	Yes
Families with children?	Yes
Medical students?	No
Pre-medical or college students?	No
Other health professional students? *1*	Yes
Doctors in training?	No
Health personnel who are US citizens?	Yes
Health personnel who are non-US citizens?	Yes
Health personnel with no prior experience in developing countries?	No
Health personnel who are not current members of your organization?	Yes

Organization/Service Specifics:

Size of the Organization's Staff:	>200
Number of providers sent or received/year:	>200
Minimum term of assignment:	9 months
Maximum term of assignment:	5 years
Is funding available for travel?	No
Are room and board provided?	No
Is any other funding available?	No
Is training provided or available?	No
Is a language other than English required? *2*	Yes

Health Professionals Placed:

Physicians:

Allied Health Professionals:

Public Health Specialists, Epidemiologists and Health Educators

Notes

1. Primarily public health students; *2.* French or Spanish may be required for some assignments.

Maryknoll Mission Association of the Faithful

Address: **P.O. Box 307, Maryknoll, NY 10545 U.S.A.**

Phone: **(914) 762-6364** FAX: **(914) 762-7031**
(800) 818-5276

E-Mail: **kwright@mkl-mmaf.org or or admissions@mklm.org** Web: **www.maryknoll .org/**

Mission: We are doctors, nurses, teachers, social workers, pastoral agents, community organizers and others who join our lives to those of the poor, marginalized, and oppressed people of the earth. With them we strive for justice, peace and fullness of life. We are a branch of the Maryknoll movement and share in its commitment to global mission. We are open to receiving all health care professionals.

Continents Served

Africa ✔ Asia ✔ Europe ☐ The Americas ✔

Countries Served

Bolivia	Brazil	Cambodia
Chile	East Timor	El Salvador
Japan	Kenya	Mexico
Nepal	Panama	Peru
Tanzania	Thailand	Venezuela
Vietnam	Zimbabwe	

(continued)

Placement opportunities for . . .

People of only certain faiths? *1*	Yes
Couples: both are health providers?	Yes
Couples: only one is a health provider?	Yes
Families with children?	Yes
Medical students?	No
Pre-medical or college students?	No
Other health professional students?	No
Doctors in training?	Yes
Health personnel who are US citizens?	Yes
Health personnel who are non-US citizens? *2*	No
Health personnel with no prior experience in developing countries?	Yes
Health personnel who are not current members of your organization?	Yes

Organization/Service Specifics:

Size of the Organization's Staff:	21-50
Number of providers sent or received/year:	>200
Minimum term of assignment:	3.5 years
Maximum term of assignment:	no max
Is funding available for travel?	Yes
Are room and board provided?	Yes
Is any other funding available? *3*	Yes
Is training provided or available?	Yes
Is a language other than English required? *4*	Yes

Health Professionals Placed:

Physicians:

Not specified

Allied Health Professionals:

Not specified

Notes

1. Maryknoll is a Catholic missionary organization; *2.* If they are permanent residents; *3.* Health care, personal allowance, food allowence, other living expenses are provided; *4.* Language requirements dependent on the country of service.

Maua Methodist Hospital

Address: **P.O. Box 63 Maua - Meru North, Kenya, E. Africa**

Phone: **011 25 41 672 1003** FAX: **011 25 41 672 1121**

E-Mail: **mckhosp@net2000ke.com, mckhosp@africaonline.co.ke** Web:

Continents Served

Africa ☑ Asia ☐ Europe ☐ The Americas ☐

Countries Served

Kenya

Mission: Maua Methodist Hospital is a 150-bed hospital serving the Igembe, Ntonyiri and Mutuati divisions of the Nyambene District, and is run by the Methodist Church in Kenya. There are two general medical/surgical wards for men and women, two pediatric wards, an isolation ward and maternity ward, which has about 3,500–4,000 deliveries annually. There is an outpatient department with dental and ophthalmic clinics, and an active community health department, with several mobile clinics providing child development screening, immunization, antenatal and family planning services. There is also a nurse training school, training registered nurses, with an intake of 16 students per year. Maua Methodist Hospital offers "hands on" experience to students, who will be expected to be first in the assessment and evaluation of patients, and who will do night and weekend call in rotation with our clinical officers (physician's assistants), with a doctor always available as a supervisor. There are usually 4-5 doctors at Maua, although this varies from time to time.

Placement opportunities for . . .

People of only certain faiths?	No
Couples: both are health providers?	Yes
Couples: only one is a health provider?	Yes
Families with children? *1*	Yes
Medical students?	Yes
Pre-medical or college students?	No
Other health professional students?	Yes
Doctors in training?	Yes
Health personnel who are US citizens?	Yes
Health personnel who are non-US citizens?	Yes
Health personnel with no prior experience in developing countries?	Yes
Health personnel who are not current members of your organization?	Yes

Organization/Service Specifics:

Size of the Organization's Staff: *1*	>200
Number of providers sent or received/year:	11-20
Minimum term of assignment:	6 weeks
Maximum term of assignment:	none
Is funding available for travel?	No
Are room and board provided? *2*	Yes
Is any other funding available?	No
Is training provided or available?	Yes
Is a language other than English required?	No

(continued)

Health Professionals Placed:

Physicians:

Physicians; Family Practitioners; General Surgeons; Infectious Disease Spec.; Internal Medicine GPS & PCP; OB/GYN; Ophthalmologists; Oral Surgeons; Orthopedic Surgeons; Otolaryngologists; Pathologists; Pediatricians; Plastic/Hand/Reconstructive Surgeons; Psychiatrists; Pulmonary Specialists; Radiologists

Allied Health Professionals:

Dental Hygienists; Dentists; Medical Technicians (lab, X-ray, etc); Nurse Midwives; Nurse Practitioners; Nurses; Paramedics; Pharmacists; Physical & Occupational Therapists; Physician Assistants; Prosthetists; Water/Sanitation Specialists

Notes

1. Last contacted on 12/02. No response to inquiry in 2/05.
2. Furnished dormitory rooms with kitchens and bathrooms are available.

Medecins Sans Frontieres / Doctors Without Borders USA

Continents Served

Africa ✔ Asia ✔ Europe ✔ The Americas ✔

Countries Served

Address: **333 7th Avenue, 2nd Floor, New York, NY 10001-5004 U.S.A.**

Phone: **(212) 679-6800** FAX: **(212) 679-7016**

E-Mail: **doctors@newyork.msf.org** Web: **www.msf.org or www.doctorswithoutborders.org**

Mission: Médecins Sans Frontières (Doctors Without Borders) provides aid and medical assistance to people victimized by war, epidemic diseases, natural and manmade disasters, and those without health care. MSF believes all people have the right to health care regardless of race, religion, social or political affiliations. MSF provides primary health care, mental health care, surgeries, rehabilitation of hospitals and clinics, nutrition and sanitation programs, training local medical personnel, and the treatment of chronic diseases such as TB, malaria, sleeping sickness, and AIDS.

Placement opportunities for . . .	
People of only certain faiths?	No
Couples: both are health providers?	No
Couples: only one is a health provider?	No
Families with children?	No
Medical students?	No
Pre-medical or college students?	No
Other health professional students?	Yes
Doctors in training?	No
Health personnel who are US citizens?	Yes
Health personnel who are non-US citizens?	Yes
Health personnel with no prior experience in developing countries?	Yes
Health personnel who are not current members of your organization?	Yes

Organization/Service Specifics:		
Size of the Organization's Staff:		>200
Number of providers sent or received/year:		>200
Minimum term of assignment:	*1*	6 months
Maximum term of assignment:		
Is funding available for travel?		Yes
Are room and board provided?		Yes
Is any other funding available?	*2*	Yes
Is training provided or available?		Yes
Is a language other than English required?	*3*	No

Health Professionals Placed:

Physicians:

Physicians; Anesthesiologists; Emergency Medicine Physicians; Family Practitioners; General Surgeons; Neurologists; Pediatricians; Psychiatrists

Allied Health Professionals:

Nurses; Water/Sanitation Specialists

Notes

1. Six weeks for surgeons and anesthesiologists; *2.* Monthly stipend provided; *3.* Second language helpful.

Medical Aid for Palestinians

Continents Served

Africa ☐ Asia ✔ Europe ☐ The Americas ☐

Countries Served

Israel Lebanon

Address: **33a Islington Park Street, London, N11QB U.K.**

Phone: **44 (0) 20 7226 4114** FAX: **44 (0) 20 7226 0880**

E-Mail: **admin@map-uk.org** Web: **www.map-uk.org/**

Mission: Medical Aid for Palestinians (MAP) is an independent, non-political British charity established in 1984 to alleviate the medical and humanitarian needs of the Palestinian people. MAP aims to deliver basic healthcare to those Palestinian refugees displaced from their homes and those whose living conditions have deteriorated markedly as a result of the Israeli-Palestinian conflict.

(continued)

Placement opportunities for . . .

People of only certain faiths?	No
Couples: both are health providers?	Yes
Couples: only one is a health provider?	No
Families with children?	No
Medical students?	No
Pre-medical or college students?	No
Other health professional students?	No
Doctors in training?	No
Health personnel who are US citizens?	Yes
Health personnel who are non-US citizens?	Yes
Health personnel with no prior experience in developing countries?	Yes
Health personnel who are not current members of your organization?	Yes

Organization/Service Specifics:

Size of the Organization's Staff:	21-50
Number of providers sent or received/year:	21-50
Minimum term of assignment:	6 months
Maximum term of assignment:	2 years
Is funding available for travel?	Yes
Are room and board provided?	Yes
Is any other funding available? *1*	Yes
Is training provided or available?	No
Is a language other than English required?	No

Health Professionals Placed:

Physicians:

Physicians; Family Practitioners; Internal Medicine GPS & PCP; Nephrologists; OB/GYN; Pediatricians

Allied Health Professionals:

Administrative Health Positions; Medical Technicians (lab, X-ray, etc); Nurse Midwives; Nurse Practitioners; Nurses; Paramedics; Physical & Occupational Therapists; Public Health Specialists, Epidemiologists and Health Educators

Notes

1. Salary, medical insurance, and resettlement allowance are part of the funding.

Medical Ambassadors International

Address: **P.O. Box 576645, Modesto, CA 95357-6645 U.S.A.**

Phone: **(209) 524-0600** FAX: **(209) 571-3538**
(888) 403-0600

E-Mail: **info@med-amb.org** Web: **www.med-amb.org**

Continents Served

Africa ☑ Asia ☑ Europe ☑ The Americas ☑

Countries Served

Guatemala, India, Kenya, USSR, former, Venezuela

Mission: Under the Lordship of Jesus Christ, Medical Ambassadors recruits, trains, and supports national leaders among developing peoples to take responsibility to reach their own people physically and spiritually. Committed to an integrated ministry, Medical Ambassadors equips nationals in basic preventive and curative medical care, as well as training them to evangelize and disciple their neighbors. The results are healthier families, self-reliant communities, and stronger churches—new and exisiting—with a clearly defined ministry and mission. Volunteers can serve for short term (2 weeks) to longer term (4 years) assignments. There are no language requirements. Volunteers are responsible for raising their own funding.

Placement opportunities for . . .

People of only certain faiths? *1*	Yes
Couples: both are health providers?	Yes
Couples: only one is a health provider?	Yes
Families with children?	Yes
Medical students?	No
Pre-medical or college students?	No
Other health professional students?	Yes
Doctors in training?	No
Health personnel who are US citizens?	Yes
Health personnel who are non-US citizens?	Yes
Health personnel with no prior experience in developing countries?	Yes
Health personnel who are not current members of your organization?	Yes

Organization/Service Specifics:

Size of the Organization's Staff:	
Number of providers sent or received/year:	
Minimum term of assignment:	2 weeks
Maximum term of assignment:	4 years
Is funding available for travel?	No
Are room and board provided?	No
Is any other funding available?	No
Is training provided or available?	Yes
Is a language other than English required?	No

Health Professionals Placed:

Physicians:

Physicians; Family Practitioners; Internal Medicine GPS & PCP

Allied Health Professionals:

Dentists; Nurses; Nutritionists & Dieticians; Physician Assistants

Notes

1. Volunteers must be Protestant.

Medical Care Development International Division

Continents Served

Africa ✔ Asia ✔ Europe ☐ The Americas ✔

Countries Served

Angola, Benin, Central African Rep., Guinea, Ivory Coast, Madagascar, Mali, Mozambique, Saudi Arabia, Sierra Leone, South Africa, Swaziland, Tunisia, Vietnam

Address: **8401 Colesville Road, Silver Springs, MD 20910 U.S.A.**

Phone: **(301) 562-1920** FAX: **(301) 562-1921**

E-Mail: **mcdi@mcd.org** Web: **http://mcdi.mcd.org/index.html or mcd.org**

Mission: MCD's mission is to improve the health and well-being of people. We will do this in partnership with communities, organizations and governments. We pledge to develop and operate creative, compassionate, and practical programs that result in the delivery of services that will improve health status. There is a minimum time commitment for 2 weeks and personnel can serve for up to 2 years. For some placements, French, Spanish, or Portuguese may be required. Funding is provided.

Placement opportunities for . . .

People of only certain faiths?	No
Couples: both are health providers?	Yes
Couples: only one is a health provider?	Yes
Families with children?	Yes
Medical students?	Yes
Pre-medical or college students?	No
Other health professional students?	Yes
Doctors in training?	No
Health personnel who are US citizens?	Yes
Health personnel who are non-US citizens?	Yes
Health personnel with no prior experience in developing countries?	No
Health personnel who are not current members of your organization?	Yes

Organization/Service Specifics:

Size of the Organization's Staff:	51-100
Number of providers sent or received/year:	51-100
Minimum term of assignment:	2 weeks
Maximum term of assignment:	2 years
Is funding available for travel?	Yes
Are room and board provided?	Yes
Is any other funding available?	Yes
Is training provided or available? *1*	Yes
Is a language other than English required? *2*	Yes

Health Professionals Placed:

Physicians:

Physicians; Emergency Medicine Physicians; Family Practitioners; General Surgeons; Infectious Disease Spec.; Internal Medicine GPS & PCP; OB/GYN; Pediatricians

Allied Health Professionals:

Administrative Health Positions; Nurse Midwives; Nurse Practitioners; Nurses; Paramedics; Public Health Specialists, Epidemiologists and Health Educators; Social Workers; Water/Sanitation Specialists

Notes

1. Research and work materials are provided; *2.* French, Spanish, or Portuguese may be required for some placements.

Medical Ministry International

Continents Served

Africa ✔ Asia ✔ Europe ✔ The Americas ✔

Countries Served

Afghanistan, Armenia, Belize, Benin, Brazil, Bulgaria, Burundi, Cambodia, China, Costa Rica, Dominican Republic, Ecuador, El Salvador, Eritrea, Ghana, Guatemala, Haiti, Honduras, Hungary, India, Ivory Coast, Jamaica, Liberia, Mexico, Mongolia, Morocco, Mozambique, Nepal, Nicaragua, Nigeria, Pakistan, Papua-New Guinea, Paraguay, Peru, Philippines, Poland, Romania, Rwanda, Swaziland, Thailand, Uganda, USSR, former, Vietnam, Zaire (DemRepCongo), Zimbabwe

Address: **P.O. Box 1339, Allen, TX 75013 U.S.A.**

Phone: **(972) 727-5864** FAX: **(972) 727-7810**

E-Mail: **mmitx@mmint.org** Web: **www.mmint.org**

Mission: MMI is the world's largest, short term, volunteer Christian medical mission with 1500 annual participants from North America. We are an interdenominational non-profit organization welcoming all health care professionals to volunteer in short-term projects to provide health care to the poor in developing countries. Volunteers pay a participation fee (US $875 for 2 weeks, $660 for 1 week) plus airfare, gather and carry medical supplies. This healing ministry strengthens village churches and enhances missions outreach in our participants' home churches.

(continued)

Placement opportunities for . . .

People of only certain faiths? *1*	Yes
Couples: both are health providers?	Yes
Couples: only one is a health provider?	Yes
Families with children? *2*	Yes
Medical students?	Yes
Pre-medical or college students?	Yes
Other health professional students?	Yes
Doctors in training?	Yes
Health personnel who are US citizens?	Yes
Health personnel who are non-US citizens?	Yes
Health personnel with no prior experience in developing countries?	Yes
Health personnel who are not current members of your organization?	Yes

Organization/Service Specifics:

Size of the Organization's Staff:	21-50
Number of providers sent or received/year:	>200
Minimum term of assignment:	1 week
Maximum term of assignment:	2 weeks
Is funding available for travel?	No
Are room and board provided?	No
Is any other funding available? *2*	No
Is training provided or available?	
Is a language other than English required? *3*	No

Health Professionals Placed:

Physicians:

Physicians; Anesthesiologists; Cardiologists; Dermatologists; Emergency Medicine Physicians; Family Practitioners; Gastroenterologists; General Surgeons; Infectious Disease Spec.; Internal Medicine GPS & PCP; Nephrologists; Neurologists; Neurosurgeons; OB/GYN; Ophthalmologists; Oral Surgeons; Optometrists; Orthopedic Surgeons; Otolaryngologists; Pathologists; Pediatricians; Plastic/Hand/Reconstructive Surgeons; Psychiatrists; Pulmonary Specialists; Radiologists; Urologists

Allied Health Professionals:

Administrative Health Positions; Dental Hygienists; Dentists; Medical Technicians (lab, X-ray, etc); Nurse Midwives; Nurse Practitioners; Nurses; Nutritionists & Dieticians; Paramedics; Pharmacists; Physical & Occupational Therapists; Physician Assistants; Prosthetists; Public Health Specialists, Epidemiologists and Health Educators; Respiratory Therapists; Water/Sanitation Specialists

Notes

1. MMI is a Christian organization, but others are welcome to participate; *2.* Children must be older than 13; *3.* Volunteers must raise their own funds; *4.* Other languages are not required but helpful.

Medical Missionaries of Mary

Address: **563 Minneford Avenue City Island, Bronx, NY 10464 U.S.A.**

Phone: **(718) 885-0945** FAX: **(718) 885-0010**

E-Mail: **mmmci@aol.com** Web: **www.medical-missionaries.com**

Continents Served

Africa ☑ Asia ☐ Europe ☐ The Americas ☑

Countries Served

Angola	Benin	Brazil
Ethiopia	Honduras	Kenya
Malawi	Mexico	Nigeria
Rwanda	Tanzania	Uganda

Mission: Medical Missionaries of Mary take a holistic approach to health care. In line with the policies of the World Health Organization—especially since the Alma Ata Declaration of 1978—we have placed great emphasis on Community-based Health Care. This takes our mobile teams to many remote villages in Africa and in Central and South America, and to sprawling urban slums, where local health workers join us in helping people to take care of their health in a sustainable way at low cost.

Placement opportunities for . . .

People of only certain faiths? *1*	No
Couples: both are health providers?	Yes
Couples: only one is a health provider?	Yes
Families with children?	Yes
Medical students?	Yes
Pre-medical or college students?	Yes
Other health professional students?	Yes
Doctors in training?	Yes
Health personnel who are US citizens?	Yes
Health personnel who are non-US citizens?	Yes
Health personnel with no prior experience in developing countries?	Yes
Health personnel who are not current members of your organization?	Yes

Organization/Service Specifics:

Size of the Organization's Staff:	>200
Number of providers sent or received/year:	6-10
Minimum term of assignment:	2 years
Maximum term of assignment:	3 years
Is funding available for travel?	
Are room and board provided?	Yes
Is any other funding available?	
Is training provided or available?	
Is a language other than English required? *2*	Yes

Health Professionals Placed: *3*

Physicians:

Physicians; Internal Medicine GPS & PCP; OB/GYN

Allied Health Professionals:

Nurse Midwives; Nurse Practitioners

Notes

1. No religious requirements, but volunteers are usually Catholic; *2.* Language requirements are dependant on the country; *3.* Placements are treated on an individual basis.

Medicine for Humanity

Address: **15821 Ventura Blvd., Suite 645, Encino, CA 91436 U.S.A.**

Phone: **(818) 455-4071** FAX: **(818) 784-9437**

E-Mail: **debby@medicineforhumnaity.org** Web: **www.medicineforhumanity.org/**

Continents Served

Africa ✔ Asia ✔ Europe ✔ The Americas ✔

Countries Served

Bangladesh	Costa Rica	Croatia
Kenya	Malawi	Mexico
Mongolia	Nepal	Panama
Philippines	Poland	South Africa
Taiwan	Tanzania	United States
Uzbekistan		

Mission: With over 38 countries in desperate need of modern medical care, Medicine for Humanity is striving to bring to developing countries not only screening and prevention of cervical cancer, but also comprehensive curative treatment. The main mission of Medicine for Humanity spans the following points: Committed to the belief that quality healthcare is a basic human right; Committed to providing a continuously expanding opportunity for caring, involved humanitarians and foundations to participate in programs that will change humanity and expand the possibilities for future generations to live better and more satisfying lives; In the face of the ever-changing environment of modern healthcare, providing an opportunity for volunteer physicians and nurses to share in a collaborative freedom that transcends academic institutions and national borders; Offer the world's healthcare infrastructure the opportunity to provide products and services in under-served areas of the globe; Offer collaborative partners and volunteers the unprecedented opportunity to directly impact the future of humanity.

To date, Medicine for Humanity has served and made a difference in the lives of women in five developing countries and their mission is still young. With proper financial backing, adequate numbers of volunteers and an unfortunate number of women who are in need of treatment, Medicine for Humanity will continue to fulfill its vision of bringing quality health care to women throughout the world.

Placement opportunities for . . .

People of only certain faiths?	No
Couples: both are health providers?	No
Couples: only one is a health provider?	No
Families with children?	No
Medical students?	No
Pre-medical or college students?	No
Other health professional students?	No
Doctors in training?	Yes
Health personnel who are US citizens?	Yes
Health personnel who are non-US citizens?	Yes
Health personnel with no prior experience in developing countries?	Yes
Health personnel who are not current members of your organization?	Yes

Organization/Service Specifics:

Size of the Organization's Staff:	6-10
Number of providers sent or received/year:	21-50
Minimum term of assignment:	2 weeks
Maximum term of assignment:	2 weeks
Is funding available for travel?	Yes
Are room and board provided?	Yes
Is any other funding available?	No
Is training provided or available?	No
Is a language other than English required?	No

Health Professionals Placed:

Physicians:

Physicians; Anesthesiologists; OB/GYN; Pathologists

Allied Health Professionals:

Notes

Medicine for Peace

Address: **2732 Unicorn Lane NW, Washington, DC 20015 U.S.A.**

Phone: **(202) 362-9121** FAX: **(202) 362-6797**

E-Mail: **medforpeace@aol.com** Web: **www.medpeace.org/**

Continents Served

Africa ☐ Asia ✔ Europe ✔ The Americas ✔

Countries Served

Bosnia and Herzegovina	El Salvador
Haiti	Iraq

Mission: Medicine for Peace strives to provide medical care and humanitarian assistance to children who are victims of war. Medicine for Peace has helped children in El Salvador, Bosnia, Iraq, Haiti and the United States. We are a voluntary organization in which doctors, nurses, engineers, and dedicated individuals selflessly donate time, energy and resources to achieve our common goals of providing medical aid to children in need.

(continued)

Placement opportunities for . . .		Organization/Service Specifics:	
People of only certain faiths?	No	Size of the Organization's Staff:	0-5
Couples: both are health providers?	No	Number of providers sent or received/year:	11-20
Couples: only one is a health provider?	No	Minimum term of assignment:	2 weeks
Families with children?	No	Maximum term of assignment:	1 month
Medical students? *1*	Yes	Is funding available for travel?	Yes
Pre-medical or college students?	No	Are room and board provided?	Yes
Other health professional students?	No	Is any other funding available?	No
Doctors in training?	No	Is training provided or available?	Yes
Health personnel who are US citizens?	Yes	Is a language other than English required?	No
Health personnel who are non-US citizens?			No
Health personnel with no prior experience in developing countries? *2*			Yes
Health personnel who are not current members of your organization?			Yes

Health Professionals Placed:

Physicians:

Physicians; Emergency Medicine Physicians; Family Practitioners; General Surgeons; Hematologists; Oncologists; Infectious Disease Spec.; Internal Medicine GPS & PCP; OB/GYN; Pediatricians; Plastic/Hand/Reconstructive Surgeons; Psychiatrists

Allied Health Professionals:

Nurse Midwives; Nurse Practitioners; Nurses; Nutritionists & Dieticians; Physical & Occupational Therapists; Public Health Specialists, Epidemiologists and Health Educators; Social Workers; Water/Sanitation Specialists

Notes

1. Select projects are available; *2.* Some overseas experience preferable but not necessary.

Memisa Medicus Mundi

Address: **P.O. Box 61, Rotterdam, AB3000 Netherlands**

Phone: **(010) 206-4646** FAX: **(010) 206-4647**

E-Mail: **recruit@memisa.nl or info@memisa.nl** Web: **www.drik.net/memisa/**

Mission: Founded in the Netherlands 73 years ago, Memisa is one of Europes' largest Third World medical aid charities. Memisa Medicus Mundi is a private Dutch organization active in the area of providing professional (basic) health care in developing countries. Memisa works together with local partner organizations in 21 countries in Africa, Asia, and Latin America and provides staffing assistance by sending out about 150 experts each year specialized in the field of health care.

Continents Served

Africa ☑ Asia ☑ Europe ☐ The Americas ☑

Countries Served

Afghanistan, Angola, Benin, Cambodia, Cameroon, Ethiopia, Ghana, Haiti, Kenya, Malawi, Mozambique, Papua-New Guinea, Rwanda, Somalia, Tanzania, Uganda, Zaire (DemRepCongo), Zambia, Zimbabwe

Placement opportunities for . . .		Organization/Service Specifics:	
People of only certain faiths?	No	Size of the Organization's Staff:	>200
Couples: both are health providers?	Yes	Number of providers sent or received/year:	101-150
Couples: only one is a health provider?	Yes	Minimum term of assignment:	3 years
Families with children?	Yes	Maximum term of assignment:	3 years
Medical students?	No	Is funding available for travel?	Yes
Pre-medical or college students?	No	Are room and board provided?	Yes
Other health professional students?	No	Is any other funding available?	Yes
Doctors in training?	No	Is training provided or available?	No
Health personnel who are US citizens?	No	Is a language other than English required?	No
Health personnel who are non-US citizens?			Yes
Health personnel with no prior experience in developing countries?			No
Health personnel who are not current members of your organization?			Yes

Health Professionals Placed:

Physicians:

Physicians; Emergency Medicine Physicians; Pediatricians

Allied Health Professionals:

Pharmacists; Public Health Specialists, Epidemiologists and Health Educators

Notes

Mennonite Central Committee

Address: **21 South 12th Street, P.O. Box 500, Akron, PA 17501-0500 U.S.A.**

Phone: **(717) 859-1151** **(888) 563-4676** FAX: **(717) 859-2171**

E-Mail: **mailbox@mcc.org** Web: **www.mcc.org**

Mission: Mennonite Central Committee is an agency of the Mennonite and Brethren in Christ Churches in North America. MCC seeks to demonstrate God's love through committed women and men who work among people suffering from poverty, conflict, oppression and natural disaster. Overseas MCC is involved in development work such as education, health and agriculture, peace and justice issues, relief work and job creation, among other things. It also operates Ten Thousand Villages, which purchases crafts from developing world artisans and craftspersons for sale in North America. MCC seeks Christians who believe strongly in nonviolence for relatively long term (3 years or more) stays in numerous different countries throughout the world. Languages appropriate for the region may be required, but MCC does provide language study courses for participants.

Continents Served

Africa ☑ Asia ☑ Europe ☑ The Americas ☑

Countries Served

Angola, Bangladesh, Bolivia, Bosnia and Herzegovina, Botswana, Brazil, Burkina Faso, Burundi, Cambodia, Canada, Chad, China, Colombia, Congo, Costa Rica, Croatia, Cuba, Egypt, El Salvador, Ethiopia, Germany, Guatemala, Haiti, Honduras, India, Indonesia, Iran, Iraq, Ireland, Israel, Jamaica, Japan, Jordan, Kenya, Laos, Lebanon, Lesotho, Mexico, Mozambique, Nepal, Nicaragua, Nigeria, Paraguay, Peru, Philippines, Rwanda, Serbia and Montenegro, Somalia, South Africa, Sudan, Swaziland, Switzerland, Syria, Tanzania, Thailand, Uganda, United States, USSR, former, Vietnam, Zambia, Zimbabwe

Placement opportunities for . . .

People of only certain faiths? *1*	Yes
Couples: both are health providers?	Yes
Couples: only one is a health provider?	Yes
Families with children?	Yes
Medical students?	No
Pre-medical or college students?	No
Other health professional students?	Yes
Doctors in training?	No
Health personnel who are US citizens?	Yes
Health personnel who are non-US citizens?	Yes
Health personnel with no prior experience in developing countries?	Yes
Health personnel who are not current members of your organization?	Yes

Organization/Service Specifics:

Size of the Organization's Staff:	>200
Number of providers sent or received/year:	11-20
Minimum term of assignment:	3 years
Maximum term of assignment:	unlimited
Is funding available for travel?	Yes
Are room and board provided?	Yes
Is any other funding available? *2*	Yes
Is training provided or available?	Yes
Is a language other than English required? *3*	Yes

Health Professionals Placed:

Physicians:

Family Practitioners; General Surgeons

Allied Health Professionals:

Nurse Practitioners; Nurses; Nutritionists & Dieticians; Public Health Specialists, Epidemiologists and Health Educators; Social Workers; Water/Sanitation Specialists

Notes

1. Volunteers must be Christian; *2.* Health coverage, life insurance, limited educational loan assistance; *3.* Sometimes there are language requirements. Language study is available.

Mercy Ships

Address: **P.O. Box 2020, Garden Valley, TX 75771-2020 U.S.A.**

Phone: **(903) 939-7000** FAX: **(903) 939-7110** **(903) 882-0336**

E-Mail: **info@mercyships.org** Web: **www.mercyships.org**

Mission: Mercy Ships operates ocean-going vessels to bring physical and spiritual healing to the poor and needy around the world. Following Christ's example, Mercy Ships serves nations through medical care, relief, community development, training, and evangelism. Volunteers must be Christians and they can serve between 2 weeks and 1 year. Any volunteers serving for more than 1 year must attend a discipleship training school. There are no language requirements, and while training is provided, volunteers must provided their own expenses for travel and room and board.

Continents Served

Africa ☑ Asia ☐ Europe ☐ The Americas ☑

Countries Served

American Samoa, Benin, Brazil, China, Cook Islands, Cuba, Dominican Republic, El Salvador, Estonia, Faroe Islands, Fiji, Gambia, Ghana, Grenada, Guatemala, Guinea, Guinea-Bissau, Haiti, Honduras, Ivory Coast, Jamaica, Korea, South, La Tria, Latvia, Lithuania, Madagascar, Mexico, New Caledonia, Nicaragua, Papua-New Guinea, Philippines, Pitcairn Island, Poland, Samoa, Senegal, Sierra Leone, Solomon Islands, South Africa, Togo, Tonga, Trinidad and Tobago, USSR, former, Vanuatu

Placement opportunities for . . .

People of only certain faiths? *1*	Yes
Couples: both are health providers?	Yes
Couples: only one is a health provider?	Yes
Families with children? *2*	Yes
Medical students? *3*	No
Pre-medical or college students? *3*	No
Other health professional students? *4*	No
Doctors in training?	No
Health personnel who are US citizens?	Yes
Health personnel who are non-US citizens?	Yes
Health personnel with no prior experience in developing countries? *5*	Yes
Health personnel who are not current members of your organization?	Yes

Organization/Service Specifics:

Size of the Organization's Staff:	>200
Number of providers sent or received/year:	>200
Minimum term of assignment:	2 weeks
Maximum term of assignment:	1 year
Is funding available for travel?	No
Are room and board provided?	No
Is any other funding available?	No
Is training provided or available?	No
Is a language other than English required?	No

Health Professionals Placed:

Physicians:

Physicians; Anesthesiologists; Cardiologists; Dermatologists; Emergency Medicine Physicians; Endocrinologists; Family Practitioners; Gastroenterologists; General Surgeons; Hematologists; Oncologists; Infectious Disease Spec.; Internal Medicine GPS & PCP; OB/GYN; Ophthalmologists; Oral Surgeons; Optometrists; Orthopedic Surgeons; Otolaryngologists; Pathologists; Pediatricians; Plastic/Hand/Reconstructive Surgeons; Psychiatrists; Radiologists; Urologists

Allied Health Professionals:

Administrative Health Positions; Dental Hygienists; Dentists; Medical Technicians (lab, X-ray, etc); Nurse Midwives; Nurse Practitioners; Nurses; Nutritionists & Dieticians; Paramedics; Pharmacists; Physical & Occupational Therapists; Physician Assistants; Podiatrists; Prosthetists; Psychologists; Public Health Specialists, Epidemiologists and Health Educators; Respiratory Therapists; Social Workers; Water/Sanitation Specialists

Notes

1. We are a non-denominational Christian organization; *2.* Family opportunities are with land-based teams; *3.* We are unable to use students; *4.* Health care professionals must be certified and currently licenesed; *5.* Nurses must have previous experience.

Mexican Medical Ministries

Continents Served			
Africa ☐	Asia ☐	Europe ☐	The Americas ☑

Countries Served
Mexico

Address: **251 Landis Avenue, Chula Vista, CA 91910-2628 U.S.A.**

Phone: **(619) 420-9750** FAX: **(619) 420-9570**

E-Mail: **info@mexicanmedical.com** Web: **www.mexicanmedical.com**

Mission: Mexican Medical Ministries is an interdenominational, non-profit organization and a member of the Evangelical Council for Financial Accountability. Health care services are provided through hospitals, clinics and free mobile clinics which travel to remote areas. Evangelism is extended through Vacation Bible School, film and door-to-door ministries, bible studies, and support of local churches. Low cost, or no-cost health care is provided to meet the physical needs of people, and to draw people in to talk about their spiritual life needs and concerns, and to then present the Gospel of Jesus Christ to them. Clinics and hospitals are constructed, developed, established, and expanded as needed in Mexico, in conjunction with our national sister non-profit organizations, and staffed and operated by nationals. Many American and Canadian doctors, nurses, dentists, and specialists donate their services to help these national doctors to meet the various needs of the people.

Placement opportunities for . . .

People of only certain faiths? *1*	Yes
Couples: both are health providers?	Yes
Couples: only one is a health provider?	Yes
Families with children?	Yes
Medical students?	Yes
Pre-medical or college students?	No
Other health professional students?	Yes
Doctors in training?	Yes
Health personnel who are US citizens?	Yes
Health personnel who are non-US citizens?	Yes
Health personnel with no prior experience in developing countries?	Yes
Health personnel who are not current members of your organization?	Yes

Organization/Service Specifics:

Size of the Organization's Staff:	101-150
Number of providers sent or received/year:	21-50
Minimum term of assignment:	1 week
Maximum term of assignment:	2 years
Is funding available for travel?	No
Are room and board provided?	Yes
Is any other funding available?	No
Is training provided or available? *2*	Yes
Is a language other than English required? *3*	Yes

Health Professionals Placed:

Physicians:

Physicians; Anesthesiologists; Emergency Medicine Physicians; Family Practitioners; General Surgeons; Internal Medicine GPS & PCP; OB/GYN; Ophthalmologists; Optometrists; Plastic/Hand/Reconstructive Surgeons; Urologists

Allied Health Professionals:

Dentists; Medical Technicians (lab, X-ray, etc); Nurses; Prosthetists

Notes

1. Volunteers must be evangelical, born-again Christians; *2.* Training is available on site; *3.* Spanish is required.

Michigan State University Institute for International Health

Continents Served			
Africa ☑	Asia ☑	Europe ☑	The Americas ☑

Countries Served

Brazil	Bulgaria	China
Dominican Republic		Greece
Haiti	Indonesia	Jamaica
Japan	Malawi	Mexico
Philippines	Romania	Sweden
Thailand	United Arab Emirates	
Zimbabwe		

Address: **B-320 West Fee Hall, Michigan State University, East Lansing, MI 48824-1315 U.S.A.**

Phone: **(517) 353-8992** FAX: **(517) 355-1894**

E-Mail: **iih@msu.edu** Web: **www.msu.edu/unit/iih**

Mission: The Institute of International Health was established at Michigan State University in January 1987 to marshal university resources to address problems of world health and to serve as a center for information on world health issues. The IIH is a focal point at MSU for facilitating faculty and student research and academic interests in international health and for international health projects overseas. The IIH works with the health-related colleges, as well as with social and agricultural scientists, nutritionists, and a variety of interdisciplinary units, to foster and coordinate research, education, and development at the international level. Collaboration with these units enhances the IIH's ability to provide inputs to the health sector in its broadest sense, from the medical sciences to nutrition and from the sociocultural correlates of health to the effects of the environment on human health. The IIH collaborates with more than 36 MSU-affiliated community hospitals throughout the State of Michigan that are used for the clinical training of our medical students. These hospitals contribute health experts for IIH's overseas projects and hospital-based training for visiting foreign health professionals. *(continued)*

Placement opportunities for . . .		Organization/Service Specifics:	
People of only certain faiths?	No	Size of the Organization's Staff:	0-5
Couples: both are health providers?	No	Number of providers sent or received/year:	11-20
Couples: only one is a health provider?	No	Minimum term of assignment:	1 week
Families with children?	No	Maximum term of assignment:	2 years
Medical students?	No	Is funding available for travel?	No
Pre-medical or college students?	Yes	Are room and board provided?	No
Other health professional students?	No	Is any other funding available? *2*	No
Doctors in training?	No	Is training provided or available?	Yes
Health personnel who are US citizens?	Yes	Is a language other than English required?	No
Health personnel who are non-US citizens?	No		
Health personnel with no prior experience in developing countries?	No		
Health personnel who are not current members of your organization? *1*	No		

Health Professionals Placed:

Physicians:

Physicians; Emergency Medicine Physicians; Endocrinologists; Infectious Disease Spec.

Allied Health Professionals:

Public Health Specialists, Epidemiologists and Health Educators; Water/Sanitation Specialists

Notes

1. We generally send personnel who are affiliated with Michigan State University; *2.* We have funds available, but these are for MSU staff and students who are participating in MSU programs or projects.

Mima Foundation, Inc.

Address: **PO Box 7133, Jupiter, FL 33468-7133 U.S.A.**

Phone: **(561) 747-3334** FAX: **(561) 747-2535**

E-Mail: **mimafoundation@bellsouth.net** Web: **www.mimafoundation.com**

Continents Served

Africa ☐ Asia ☐ Europe ☐ The Americas ☑

Countries Served

Bolivia Peru

Mission: The Mima philosophy is twofold: to provide medical care to indigent populations and underserved individuals who cannot otherwise access health care and to share medical knowledge with health care providers to ensure continuity of care. MIMA sends short term teams of health care professionals to Bolivia and Peru. There are no religious or language requirements. Funding for travel and room and board are provided by the volunteer.

Placement opportunities for . . .		Organization/Service Specifics:	
People of only certain faiths?	No	Size of the Organization's Staff:	21-50
Couples: both are health providers?	Yes	Number of providers sent or received/year:	21-50
Couples: only one is a health provider?	Yes	Minimum term of assignment:	1 week
Families with children?	Yes	Maximum term of assignment:	2 weeks
Medical students?	Yes	Is funding available for travel?	No
Pre-medical or college students?	Yes	Are room and board provided?	No
Other health professional students?	Yes	Is any other funding available?	No
Doctors in training?	Yes	Is training provided or available?	No
Health personnel who are US citizens?	Yes	Is a language other than English required?	No
Health personnel who are non-US citizens?	Yes		
Health personnel with no prior experience in developing countries?	Yes		
Health personnel who are not current members of your organization?	Yes		

Health Professionals Placed:

Notes

Physicians:

Physicians; Anesthesiologists; Family Practitioners; General Surgeons; Infectious Disease Spec.; Internal Medicine GPS & PCP; OB/GYN; Ophthalmologists; Oral Surgeons; Optometrists; Orthopedic Surgeons; Otolaryngologists; Pediatricians; Plastic/Hand/Reconstructive Surgeons; Urologists

Allied Health Professionals:

Administrative Health Positions; Dental Hygienists; Dentists; Nurse Practitioners; Nurses; Physician Assistants; Podiatrists; Public Health Specialists, Epidemiologists and Health Educators

Minnesota International Health Volunteers

Continents Served
Africa ☑ Asia ☑ Europe ☐ The Americas ☑

Countries Served
Haiti, Kenya, Nicaragua, Somalia, Thailand, Uganda

Address: **122 West Franklin Avenue, Suite 522, Minneapolis, MN 55404-2480 U.S.A.**

Phone: **(612) 871-3759** FAX: **(612) 230-3257**

E-Mail: **info@mihv.org** Web: **www.mihv.org**

Mission: The mission of MIHV is to:

I. Improve community health by creating and nurturing primary, self-sustainable health care projects around the world; and

II. Create partnerships for learning among the U.S. and host country volunteers and communtiy members.

MIHV sends out very few U.S. staff and volunteers, but train and utilize several hundred host country volunteers, and about 30 staff. Volunteers can serve for a minimum of 2 months and funding is provided.

Placement opportunities for . . .	
People of only certain faiths?	No
Couples: both are health providers?	Yes
Couples: only one is a health provider?	Yes
Families with children?	Yes
Medical students?	Yes
Pre-medical or college students?	Yes
Other health professional students?	Yes
Doctors in training?	Yes
Health personnel who are US citizens?	Yes
Health personnel who are non-US citizens?	Yes
Health personnel with no prior experience in developing countries?	Yes
Health personnel who are not current members of your organization?	Yes

Organization/Service Specifics:	
Size of the Organization's Staff:	6-10
Number of providers sent or received/year:	1-5
Minimum term of assignment:	2 month
Maximum term of assignment:	4 years
Is funding available for travel?	Yes
Are room and board provided?	Yes
Is any other funding available? *1*	Yes
Is training provided or available?	Yes
Is a language other than English required? *2*	Yes

Health Professionals Placed:

Physicians:

Physicians; Pediatricians

Allied Health Professionals:

Administrative Health Positions; Public Health Specialists, Epidemiologists and Health Educators

Notes

1. Personnel are paid per diem or by salary; *2.* Spanish or African languages may be helpful.

Mission Doctors Association

Continents Served
Africa ☑ Asia ☑ Europe ☐ The Americas ☑

Countries Served
Cameroon, Ecuador, Papua-New Guinea, Thailand, Uganda

Address: **3435 Wilshire Blvd., Suite 1035, Los Angeles, CA 90010 U.S.A.**

Phone: **(213) 368-1875** FAX: **(213) 368-1871**

E-Mail: **missiondrs@earthlink.net** Web: **www.MissionDoctors.org**

Mission: Mission Doctors Association was established in 1959, since that time MDA has assisted physicians serving in Africa, Papua New Guinea and Thailand. We have long term (2-3 years) and short term (1-2 month) programs. Funding for travel and room and board is provided. There are no language requirements, but personnel must be Catholic.

Placement opportunities for . . .	
People of only certain faiths? *1*	Yes
Couples: both are health providers?	Yes
Couples: only one is a health provider?	Yes
Families with children?	Yes
Medical students?	No
Pre-medical or college students?	No
Other health professional students?	Yes
Doctors in training?	No
Health personnel who are US citizens?	Yes
Health personnel who are non-US citizens?	No
Health personnel with no prior experience in developing countries?	Yes
Health personnel who are not current members of your organization?	Yes

Organization/Service Specifics:	
Size of the Organization's Staff:	0-5
Number of providers sent or received/year:	1-5
Minimum term of assignment:	1 month
Maximum term of assignment:	2 years
Is funding available for travel?	Yes
Are room and board provided?	Yes
Is any other funding available? *2*	Yes
Is training provided or available?	Yes
Is a language other than English required?	No

(continued)

Health Professionals Placed:

Physicians:

Physicians; Anesthesiologists; Cardiologists; Dermatologists; Emergency Medicine Physicians; Endocrinologists; Family Practitioners; Gastroenterologists; General Surgeons; Hematologists; Oncologists; Infectious Disease Spec.; Internal Medicine GPS & PCP; Nephrologists; Neurologists; Neurosurgeons; OB/GYN; Ophthalmologists; Oral Surgeons; Otolaryngologists; Pathologists; Pediatricians; Psychiatrists; Pulmonary Specialists; Radiologists; Urologists

Allied Health Professionals:

Administrative Health Positions; Public Health Specialists, Epidemiologists and Health Educators

Notes

1. Volunteers must be Catholic; *2.* There is a small stipend available.

Moi University Faculty of Health Sciences

Continents Served

Africa ☑ Asia ☐ Europe ☐ The Americas ☐

Countries Served

Kenya

Address: **1001 West 10th Street, WD/OPW M200, Indianapolis, IN 46206 USA**

Phone: **(317) 630-6455** FAX: **(317) 630-7066**

E-Mail: **reinterz@iupui.edu** Web: **http://medicine.iupui.edu/kenya/program.html**

Mission: Since 1989, Indiana University School of Medicine has been involved in a collaborative educational project with Moi University Faculty of Health Sciences (MUFHS) in Eldoret, Kenya. As Kenya's second medical school, MUFHS possesses an innovative curriculum focused on problem-based learning and community-based health care. The primary goals of the IUSM-MUFHS program are to enhance medical education at both institutions, to promote collegial relationships between American and Kenyan medical doctors and students, and to develop leaders in health care in Kenya and the United States. This partnership helps satisfy Moi University's need for additional academic instructors, while also creating new professional and personal development opportunities for Indiana University medical faculty, staff, and students.

Placement opportunities for . . .

People of only certain faiths?	No
Couples: both are health providers?	Yes
Couples: only one is a health provider?	Yes
Families with children?	Yes
Medical students?	Yes
Pre-medical or college students?	Yes
Other health professional students?	Yes
Doctors in training?	Yes
Health personnel who are US citizens?	Yes
Health personnel who are non-US citizens?	Yes
Health personnel with no prior experience in developing countries?	Yes
Health personnel who are not current members of your organization?	Yes

Organization/Service Specifics:

Size of the Organization's Staff:	51-100
Number of providers sent or received/year:	6-10
Minimum term of assignment:	12 weeks
Maximum term of assignment:	3 years
Is funding available for travel?	No
Are room and board provided?	No
Is any other funding available?	No
Is training provided or available?	Yes
Is a language other than English required?	No

Health Professionals Placed:

Physicians:

Physicians; Anesthesiologists; Cardiologists; Dermatologists; Emergency Medicine Physicians; Endocrinologists; Family Practitioners; Gastroenterologists; General Surgeons; Hematologists; Oncologists; Infectious Disease Spec.; Internal Medicine GPS & PCP; Nephrologists; Neurologists; Neurosurgeons; OB/GYN; Ophthalmologists; Oral Surgeons; Optometrists; Orthopedic Surgeons; Otolaryngologists; Pathologists; Pediatricians; Plastic/Hand/Reconstructive Surgeons; Psychiatrists; Pulmonary Specialists; Radiologists; Urologists

Allied Health Professionals:

Administrative Health Positions; Dental Hygienists; Dentists; Medical Technicians (lab, X-ray, etc); Nurse Midwives; Nurse Practitioners; Nurses; Nutritionists & Dieticians; Paramedics; Pharmacists; Physical & Occupational Therapists; Physician Assistants; Podiatrists; Prosthetists; Psychologists; Public Health Specialists, Epidemiologists and Health Educators; Respiratory Therapists; Social Workers; Water/Sanitation Specialists

Notes

Mountain Mover's Missions International

Continents Served			
Africa ☐	Asia ☐	Europe ☐	The Americas ☑

Address: **Bario Las Brisis Danli, El Paraiso, Honduras**

Phone: **(011) 505-732-2718 or (505) 732-3049** FAX: **(011) 504-883-2347**

E-Mail: **kathy_rubio2@yahoo.com** Web: **www.geocities/com/clinica_eya/formerindex**

Countries Served
Honduras Nicaragua

Mission: Mountain Mover's Missions International is a program dedicated to the health, welfare and love for the poor people of Central America. It was started as a result of Hurricane Mitch in 1998. At that time Kathy Rubio was one of very few Americans working here. There is a clinic that is being built in Danli, Honduras, and there are medical brigades planned for many different locations within Honduras and Nicaragua. We are in need of volunteering doctors and medical personal, Medical student groups.

Placement opportunities for . . .	
People of only certain faiths?	No
Couples: both are health providers?	Yes
Couples: only one is a health provider?	Yes
Families with children?	No
Medical students?	Yes
Pre-medical or college students?	Yes
Other health professional students?	Yes
Doctors in training?	Yes
Health personnel who are US citizens?	Yes
Health personnel who are non-US citizens?	
Health personnel with no prior experience in developing countries?	Yes
Health personnel who are not current members of your organization?	Yes

Organization/Service Specifics:	
Size of the Organization's Staff:	0-5
Number of providers sent or received/year:	6-10
Minimum term of assignment:	2 weeks
Maximum term of assignment:	1 year
Is funding available for travel?	No
Are room and board provided?	No
Is any other funding available?	No
Is training provided or available?	Yes
Is a language other than English required? *1*	No

Health Professionals Placed:

Physicians:

All physician specialties

Allied Health Professionals:

All allied health professionals

Notes

1. Spanish helpful.

National Eye Care Project for Armenia

Continents Served			
Africa ☐	Asia ☑	Europe ☐	The Americas ☐

Address: **P.O. Box 4275, Laguna Beach, CA 92652 U.S.A.**

Phone: **(949) 493-5411** FAX: **(949) 497-2483**

E-Mail: **eyeproject@aol.com** Web:

Countries Served
Armenia

Mission: To make 21st century eye care available and affordable to every Armenian. Volunteers can serve between 10 days and 1 month. Armenian or Russian would be helpful, but neither is required.

Placement opportunities for . . .	
People of only certain faiths?	No
Couples: both are health providers?	Yes
Couples: only one is a health provider?	No
Families with children?	No
Medical students?	No
Pre-medical or college students?	No
Other health professional students?	No
Doctors in training?	No
Health personnel who are US citizens?	Yes
Health personnel who are non-US citizens?	Yes
Health personnel with no prior experience in developing countries?	Yes
Health personnel who are not current members of your organization?	Yes

Organization/Service Specifics:	
Size of the Organization's Staff:	0-5
Number of providers sent or received/year:	1-5
Minimum term of assignment:	10 days
Maximum term of assignment:	1 month
Is funding available for travel?	No
Are room and board provided?	Yes
Is any other funding available?	No
Is training provided or available?	No
Is a language other than English required? *1*	No

Health Professionals Placed:

Physicians:

Ophthalmologists

Allied Health Professionals:

Notes

1. Armenian or Russian would be helpful.

National Health Service Corps, Recruitment Program

Address: **Bureau of Primary Health Care, DHHS, Parklawn Building, 5600 Fishers Lane, Rockville, MD 20857 U.S.A.**

Phone: **(800) 221-9393** FAX: **(301) 594-4076** **(310) 594-5008**

E-Mail: **nhsc@hrsa.gov** Web: **www.bphc.hrsa.gov/nhsc/**

Continents Served

Africa ☐ Asia ☐ Europe ☐ The Americas ☑

Countries Served

United States

Mission: The National Health Service Corps is a program of the Federal Health Resources and Services Administration's Bureau of Primary Health Care, which is the focal point for providing primary health care to underserved and vulnerable populations. The NHSC assists underserved US communities through the development, recruitment, and retention of community-responsive, culturally competent, primary care clinicians dedicated to practicing in health professional shortage areas.

Placement opportunities for . . .	
People of only certain faiths?	No
Couples: both are health providers?	Yes
Couples: only one is a health provider?	Yes
Families with children?	Yes
Medical students?	Yes
Pre-medical or college students?	No
Other health professional students?	Yes
Doctors in training?	Yes
Health personnel who are US citizens?	Yes
Health personnel who are non-US citizens?	No
Health personnel with no prior experience in developing countries?	No
Health personnel who are not current members of your organization?	Yes

Organization/Service Specifics:	
Size of the Organization's Staff:	>200
Number of providers sent or received/year:	>200
Minimum term of assignment:	2 years
Maximum term of assignment:	4 years
Is funding available for travel?	No
Are room and board provided?	No
Is any other funding available? *1*	Yes
Is training provided or available?	No
Is a language other than English required?	No

Health Professionals Placed:

Physicians:

Physicians; Family Practitioners; Internal Medicine GPS & PCP; OB/GYN; Pediatricians; Psychiatrists

Allied Health Professionals:

Dental Hygienists; Dentists; Nurse Practitioners; Nurses; Physician Assistants; Social Workers

Notes

1. Some individuals may qualify for loan repayment.

New Missions In Haiti

Address: **P.O. Box 2727, Orlando, FL 32802 U.S.A.**

Phone: **(800) 937-4248** FAX: **(407) 240-1962**

E-Mail: **info@newmissions.org** Web: **newmissions.org**

Continents Served

Africa ☐ Asia ☐ Europe ☐ The Americas ☑

Countries Served

Dominican Republic Haiti

Mission: The New Missions in Haiti strive to establish and maintain a place of worship for our Almighty God and the Lord Jesus Christ, and to promote Christian fellowship and edification. They minister the general community by providing churches, schools, clinics, and feeding stations, and by teaching other skills helpful to the people of Haiti and the Dominican Republic. One of the missions' components is their medical clinics, which are staffed with Christian health workers. They administer care from basic first aid to disease prevention for children and their families.

Placement opportunities for . . .	
People of only certain faiths?	No
Couples: both are health providers?	Yes
Couples: only one is a health provider?	Yes
Families with children?	No
Medical students?	Yes
Pre-medical or college students?	Yes
Other health professional students?	Yes
Doctors in training?	Yes
Health personnel who are US citizens?	Yes
Health personnel who are non-US citizens?	Yes
Health personnel with no prior experience in developing countries?	Yes
Health personnel who are not current members of your organization?	Yes

Organization/Service Specifics:	
Size of the Organization's Staff:	0-5
Number of providers sent or received/year:	>200
Minimum term of assignment:	varies
Maximum term of assignment:	varies
Is funding available for travel?	No
Are room and board provided?	No
Is any other funding available?	No
Is training provided or available?	No
Is a language other than English required?	No

(continued)

Health Professionals Placed:

Physicians:

Not specified

Allied Health Professionals:

Not specified

Notes

Nicaraguan Children's Fund

Continents Served

Africa ☐ Asia ☐ Europe ☐ The Americas ☑

Countries Served

Address: **850 Aspen Circle, Oxnard, CA 93030 U.S.A.**

Phone: **(805) 985-6866** FAX: **(805) 985-6866**

E-Mail: **nicachildfund@juno.com** Web:

Mission: The Nicaraguan Children's Fund works in remote areas of Nicaragua to provide health care and other assistance to children in need. We ask volunteers to be flexible, and fit into many roles other than their given profession. We work in remote areas that can be physically taxing.

Placement opportunities for . . .	
People of only certain faiths?	No
Couples: both are health providers?	Yes
Couples: only one is a health provider?	Yes
Families with children?	Yes
Medical students? *1*	Yes
Pre-medical or college students? *1*	Yes
Other health professional students?	Yes
Doctors in training? *1*	Yes
Health personnel who are US citizens?	Yes
Health personnel who are non-US citizens?	Yes
Health personnel with no prior experience in developing countries?	Yes
Health personnel who are not current members of your organization?	Yes

Organization/Service Specifics:	
Size of the Organization's Staff:	6-10
Number of providers sent or received/year:	11-20
Minimum term of assignment:	10 days
Maximum term of assignment:	4
Is funding available for travel?	No
Are room and board provided?	No
Is any other funding available?	No
Is training provided or available?	No
Is a language other than English required? *2*	No

Health Professionals Placed:

Physicians:

All physician specialties

Allied Health Professionals:

All allied health professionals

Notes

1. Only as assistants; *2.* Spanish very helpful.

North American Baptist Conference Missions

Continents Served

Africa ☑ Asia ☐ Europe ☐ The Americas ☐

Countries Served

Cameroon

Address: **1 South 210 Summit Ave., Oakbrook Terrace, IL 60181 U.S.A.**

Phone: **(630) 495-2000** FAX: **(630) 495-3301**

E-Mail: **serve@nabconf.org or NABMissions@nabconf.org** Web: **www.nabconference.org**

Mission: The North American Baptist Conference (NABC) is a family of over 400 churches with more than 73,000 members in the United States and Canada. North American Baptists are a diverse group of believers representing many cultures and languages. NABC offers volunteer mission work to baptist medical personnel in Cameroon, in association with the Cameroon Baptist Convention. The convention has grown significantly in recent years with an extensive medical ministry, flourishing ministry to women, theological education, colleges, high schools, primary schools, a school for the blind and a school of nursing are included in the overall ministry.

(continued)

Placement opportunities for . . .		Organization/Service Specifics:	
People of only certain faiths? *1*	Yes	Size of the Organization's Staff:	>200
Couples: both are health providers?	Yes	Number of providers sent or received/year:	11-20
Couples: only one is a health provider?	Yes	Minimum term of assignment:	2 weeks
Families with children?	Yes	Maximum term of assignment:	2 years
Medical students?	Yes	Is funding available for travel?	No
Pre-medical or college students?	No	Are room and board provided?	Yes
Other health professional students?	No	Is any other funding available?	No
Doctors in training?	Yes	Is training provided or available?	Yes
Health personnel who are US citizens?	Yes	Is a language other than English required?	No
Health personnel who are non-US citizens?	Yes		
Health personnel with no prior experience in developing countries?	Yes		
Health personnel who are not current members of your organization?	Yes		

Health Professionals Placed: *2*

Physicians:

Physicians

Allied Health Professionals:

Dentists; Medical Technicians (lab, X-ray, etc); Nurse Practitioners; Nurses; Physician Assistants

Notes

1. Baptists; *2.* Also need public health care workers.

Northwest Medical Teams International, Inc.

Address: **P.O. Box 10, Portland, OR 97207 U.S.A.**

Phone: **(503) 624-1000** **(800) 959-4325** FAX: **(503) 624-1001**

E-Mail: **volunteermail@nwmti.org or info@nwmti.org** Web: **www.nwmedicalteams.org**

Mission: The mission of Northwest Medical Teams International is to demonstrate the love of Christ to people affected by disaster, conflict and poverty. Volunteers can stay for as little as 1 week and up to 6 months. There are no religious requirements, but Spanish is required for volunteers serving in Peru.

Continents Served

Africa ☑ Asia ☑ Europe ☑ The Americas ☑

Countries Served

Bosnia and Herzegovina; Burkina Faso; Cambodia; Cameroon; China; El Salvador; Eritrea; Ethiopia; Gabon; Guatemala; Honduras; Iraq; Ivory Coast; Kazakhstan; Liberia; Macedonia; Mali; Mexico; Moldova; Nicaragua; Niger; Peru; Romania; Serbia and Montenegro; Ukraine; Uzbekistan; Vietnam; Yugoslavia, former; Zaire (DemRepCongo)

Placement opportunities for . . .		Organization/Service Specifics:	
People of only certain faiths?	No	Size of the Organization's Staff:	51-100
Couples: both are health providers?	Yes	Number of providers sent or received/year:	>200
Couples: only one is a health provider?	Yes	Minimum term of assignment:	1 week
Families with children?	No	Maximum term of assignment:	6 months
Medical students?	No	Is funding available for travel?	No
Pre-medical or college students?	No	Are room and board provided?	No
Other health professional students?	No	Is any other funding available? *1*	Yes
Doctors in training?		Is training provided or available?	Yes
Health personnel who are US citizens?	Yes	Is a language other than English required? *2*	Yes
Health personnel who are non-US citizens?	No		
Health personnel with no prior experience in developing countries?	Yes		
Health personnel who are not current members of your organization?	Yes		

Health Professionals Placed:

Physicians:

Physicians; Anesthesiologists; Emergency Medicine Physicians; Family Practitioners; General Surgeons; Internal Medicine GPS & PCP; Neurosurgeons; OB/GYN; Ophthalmologists; Oral Surgeons; Optometrists; Orthopedic Surgeons; Pediatricians; Plastic/Hand/Reconstructive Surgeons; Psychiatrists

Allied Health Professionals:

Administrative Health Positions; Dental Hygienists; Dentists; Medical Technicians (lab, X-ray, etc); Nurse Midwives; Nurse Practitioners; Nurses; Paramedics; Physical & Occupational Therapists; Physician Assistants; Prosthetists; Psychologists; Public Health Specialists, Epidemiologists and Health Educators

Notes

1. Limited funding available for medical supplies and disaster relief teams; *2.* Spanish required for volunteers traveling to Peru.

Notre Dame India Mission

Continents Served
Africa ☑ Asia ☑ Europe ☐ The Americas ☐

Countries Served
India

Address: **13000 Auburn Rd., Chardon, OH 44024 U.S.A.**
Phone: **(440) 270-1160** FAX: **(440) 279-1167**
E-Mail: **ndim@ndec.org** Web: **ndindiamission.org**

Mission: Notre Dame India Mission is a non-profit organization of the Sisters of Notre Dame of Chardo, Ohio. Rooted in the mission of Jesus and the charism of St. Julie Billiart, the staff works to assist the Notre Dame missionaries ministering in India. Through prayer, service, and financial support, the staff and donors help the Sisters proclaim to the people of India that God is a good, loving, and provident Father. Volunteer terms last between 1 month and 1 year. Room and board are provided, but travel expenses are not.

Placement opportunities for . . .		Organization/Service Specifics:	
People of only certain faiths?	No	Size of the Organization's Staff:	6-10
Couples: both are health providers?	Yes	Number of providers sent or received/year:	
Couples: only one is a health provider?	Yes	Minimum term of assignment:	1 month
Families with children?	No	Maximum term of assignment:	1 year
Medical students?	Yes	Is funding available for travel?	No
Pre-medical or college students?	Yes	Are room and board provided? *1*	Yes
Other health professional students?	Yes	Is any other funding available?	No
Doctors in training?	Yes	Is training provided or available? *2*	Yes
Health personnel who are US citizens?	Yes	Is a language other than English required?	No
Health personnel who are non-US citizens?	Yes		
Health personnel with no prior experience in developing countries?	Yes		
Health personnel who are not current members of your organization?	Yes		

Health Professionals Placed:

Physicians:

Physicians

Allied Health Professionals:

Nurses

Notes

1. Room provided on a case by case basis; *2.* There is training available on site.

Omni Med

Continents Served
Africa ☑ Asia ☑ Europe ☐ The Americas ☑

Countries Served
Belize Guyana Kenya Thailand

Address: **81 Wyman St., #1, Waban, MA 02468 U.S.A.**
Phone: **(617) 332-9614** FAX: **(617) 332-6623**
E-Mail: **ejoneil@omnimed.org** Web: **www.omnimed.org**

Mission: "Fulfilling the essential calling of the medical profession: To improve the health of all people." Omni Med works in Belize, Kenya, Guyana, and Thailand to raise the standard of care through health education and other innovative program ventures. We send doctors to teach indigenous health providers in all sites, coordinate medical supply donations in Kenya, train village health stations' staff in northeast Thailand, and run a cervical cancer screening program and an HIV/AIDS education program in Guyana. We also publish a guide on international health service, maintaining a current database on organizations. A CME course on health volunteerism is planned for 2006. Following Albert Schweitzer's "Reverence for Life," Omni Med believes we can collectively improve the health of the world's poor through a better understanding of the mechanisms of poverty and direct action through health volunteerism.

Placement opportunities for . . .		Organization/Service Specifics:	
People of only certain faiths?	No	Size of the Organization's Staff:	6-10
Couples: both are health providers?	Yes	Number of providers sent or received/year:	11-20
Couples: only one is a health provider?	Yes	Minimum term of assignment:	1 week
Families with children?	No	Maximum term of assignment:	4 weeks
Medical students? *1*	Yes	Is funding available for travel?	No
Pre-medical or college students?	No	Are room and board provided?	Yes
Other health professional students?	No	Is any other funding available?	No
Doctors in training?	Yes	Is training provided or available?	Yes
Health personnel who are US citizens?	Yes	Is a language other than English required?	No
Health personnel who are non-US citizens?	Yes		
Health personnel with no prior experience in developing countries?	Yes		
Health personnel who are not current members of your organization?	Yes		

(continued)

Health Professionals Placed:

Physicians:

Physicians; Anesthesiologists; Cardiologists; Dermatologists; Emergency Medicine Physicians; Endocrinologists; Family Practitioners; Gastroenterologists; General Surgeons; Hematologists; Oncologists; Infectious Disease Spec.; Internal Medicine GPS & PCP; Nephrologists; Neurologists; Neurosurgeons; OB/GYN; Ophthalmologists; Oral Surgeons; Orthopedic Surgeons; Otolaryngologists; Pathologists; Pediatricians; Plastic/Hand/Reconstructive Surgeons; Psychiatrists; Pulmonary Specialists; Radiologists; Urologists

Allied Health Professionals:

Administrative Health Positions; Nurse Practitioners; Nurses; Physician Assistants

Notes

1. Sporadic involvement; should increase in the future.

Operation Blessing, Medical Division

Address: **977 Centerville Turnpike, Virginia Beach, VA 23463 U.S.A.**

Phone: **(757) 226-3902**
(757) 226-3401

FAX: **(757) 226-3657**
(757) 226-3411

E-Mail: **operationblessing@ob.org**

Web: **www.ob.org/programs/medical_services/index.asp**

Mission: Operation Blessing International's (OBI's) medical teams combine compassionate care and medical expertise to change lives. The chief tool for providing same day medical, dental, and surgical services is the Flying Hospital. This L-1011 jet aircraft is a fully equipped outpatient medical facility dedicated to addressing the unmet medical needs of underserved populations around the world. The Flying Hospital enables OBI medical teams to work closely with national healthcare professionals and workers to provide education and training. Medical services offered will vary depending on the composition of the volunteer medical teams and patients' needs.

Continents Served

Africa ☑ Asia ☑ Europe ☑ The Americas ☑

Countries Served

Afghanistan	Argentina	Brazil
Chile	China	Colombia
Costa Rica	Cuba	El Salvador
Finland	Guatemala	Haiti
Honduras	India	Israel
Korea, North	Mexico	Mongolia
Nicaragua	Pakistan	Panama
Peru	Philippines	Romania
Rwanda	Thailand	United States
USSR, former	Venezuela	Vietnam
Zaire (DemRepCongo)		

Placement opportunities for . . .

People of only certain faiths? *1*	No
Couples: both are health providers?	Yes
Couples: only one is a health provider?	Yes
Families with children?	No
Medical students?	Yes
Pre-medical or college students?	Yes
Other health professional students?	Yes
Doctors in training?	Yes
Health personnel who are US citizens?	Yes
Health personnel who are non-US citizens?	Yes
Health personnel with no prior experience in developing countries?	Yes
Health personnel who are not current members of your organization?	Yes

Organization/Service Specifics:

Size of the Organization's Staff:	11-20
Number of providers sent or received/year:	>200
Minimum term of assignment:	1 week
Maximum term of assignment:	1 month
Is funding available for travel?	No
Are room and board provided?	Yes
Is any other funding available? *2*	Yes
Is training provided or available?	Yes
Is a language other than English required?	No

Health Professionals Placed:

Physicians:

Physicians; Anesthesiologists; Cardiologists; Dermatologists; Emergency Medicine Physicians; Endocrinologists; Family Practitioners; Gastroenterologists; General Surgeons; Hematologists; Oncologists; Internal Medicine GPS & PCP; Neurosurgeons; OB/GYN; Ophthalmologists; Oral Surgeons; Optometrists; Orthopedic Surgeons; Otolaryngologists; Pediatricians; Plastic/Hand/Reconstructive Surgeons; Psychiatrists; Radiologists; Urologists

Allied Health Professionals:

Dental Hygienists; Dentists; Medical Technicians (lab, X-ray, etc); Nurse Practitioners; Nurses; Nutritionists & Dieticians; Paramedics; Pharmacists; Physical & Occupational Therapists; Physician Assistants; Psychologists; Public Health Specialists, Epidemiologists and Health Educators

Notes

1. There are no religious restrictions, although OB is an Evangelical Protestant mission; *2.* Volunteers are responsible for raising part of the costs.

Operation Luz del Sol

Continents Served
Africa ☐ Asia ☐ Europe ☐ The Americas ☑

Countries Served
Dominican Republic

Address: **1145 19th Street, N.W., Suite 802, Washington, D.C. 20036 U.S.A.**

Phone: **(202) 467-6700** FAX: **(202) 296-7545**

E-Mail: **jwilliamlittle@erols.com** Web:

Mission: Operation Luz del Sol is one of sixteen agencies that make up RSVP—the Reconstructive Surgeons Volunteer Program. The organization provides medical treatment to poor children and families in the Americas. It is only open to residents at Georgetown University.

Placement opportunities for . . .	
People of only certain faiths?	No
Couples: both are health providers?	No
Couples: only one is a health provider?	No
Families with children?	No
Medical students?	No
Pre-medical or college students?	No
Other health professional students?	No
Doctors in training?	Yes
Health personnel who are US citizens?	Yes
Health personnel who are non-US citizens?	Yes
Health personnel with no prior experience in developing countries?	Yes
Health personnel who are not current members of your organization?	Yes

Organization/Service Specifics:	
Size of the Organization's Staff:	0-5
Number of providers sent or received/year:	11-20
Minimum term of assignment:	10 days
Maximum term of assignment:	10 days
Is funding available for travel?	Yes
Are room and board provided?	Yes
Is any other funding available?	No
Is training provided or available?	Yes
Is a language other than English required?	No

Health Professionals Placed:

Physicians:

Oral Surgeons; Orthopedic Surgeons; Otolaryngologists; Plastic/Hand/Reconstructive Surgeons; Urologists

Allied Health Professionals:

Nurses; Physician Assistants

Notes

Operation Rainbow

Continents Served
Africa ☐ Asia ☑ Europe ☐ The Americas ☑

Countries Served

Armenia	China	Ecuador
El Salvador	Guatemala	Haiti
Honduras	Mexico	Nicaragua
Peru	Philippines	
Trinidad and Tobago		USSR, former
Vietnam		

Address: **3411 Richmond Avenue, Suite 333, Houston, TX 77046 U.S.A.**

Phone: **(713) 960-7800** FAX: **(713) 960-7803**

E-Mail: **info@operationrainbow.org** Web: **www.operationrainbow.org**

Mission: Operation Rainbow organizes, funds, and oversees an international service program in which volunteer health care teams provide free reconstructive surgery to indigent children patients in medically underserved countries. By caring for these children, Operation Rainbow volunteers and donors are proud ambassadors of goodwill—not only to the patients themselves, but also to their families, their communities, and in a broader sense, to their homelands. Travel is provided for nurses and CRNAs only. All other personnel must provide their own funding. Trips last between 1-3 weeks, and while there are no language requirements, Spanish is helpful for some assignments.

Placement opportunities for . . .	
People of only certain faiths?	No
Couples: both are health providers?	Yes
Couples: only one is a health provider?	Yes
Families with children?	No
Medical students?	Yes
Pre-medical or college students?	Yes
Other health professional students?	Yes
Doctors in training?	Yes
Health personnel who are US citizens?	Yes
Health personnel who are non-US citizens?	Yes
Health personnel with no prior experience in developing countries?	Yes
Health personnel who are not current members of your organization?	Yes

Organization/Service Specifics:		
Size of the Organization's Staff:		0-5
Number of providers sent or received/year:		>200
Minimum term of assignment:		1 weeks
Maximum term of assignment:		2 weeks
Is funding available for travel?	*1*	Yes
Are room and board provided?		Yes
Is any other funding available?		No
Is training provided or available?		No
Is a language other than English required?	*2*	No

(continued)

Health Professionals Placed:

Physicians:

Physicians; Anesthesiologists; General Surgeons; Oral Surgeons; Orthopedic Surgeons; Plastic/Hand/Reconstructive Surgeons

Allied Health Professionals:

Dentists; Nurses; Social Workers

Notes

1. Funding for travel is available for nurses and CRNAs only;
2. Spanish is helpful for some assignments.

Operation Smile International

Address: **6435 Tidewater Drive, Norfolk, VA 23509 U.S.A.**

Phone: **(757) 321-7645** FAX: **(757) 321-7660**

E-Mail: **info@operationsmile.org** Web: **www.operationsmile.org**

Mission: Operation Smile is a private, not-for-profit volunteer medical services organization providing reconstructive surgery and related health care to indigent children and young adults in developing countries and the United States. Operation Smile provides education and training around the world to physicians and other health care professionals to achieve long-term self-sufficiency. Trips are relatively short, between 1-3 weeks. Funding for travel and room and board are provided, although there is a team fee. Operation Smile has no language or religious requirements.

Continents Served

Africa ✔ Asia ✔ Europe ✔ The Americas ✔

Countries Served

Belarus	Brazil	China
Colombia	Ecuador	Honduras
Kenya	Morocco	Nicaragua
Panama	Philippines	Russia
Thailand	United States	Venezuela
Vietnam		

Placement opportunities for . . .	
People of only certain faiths?	No
Couples: both are health providers?	Yes
Couples: only one is a health provider?	No
Families with children?	No
Medical students?	Yes
Pre-medical or college students?	No
Other health professional students?	No
Doctors in training?	Yes
Health personnel who are US citizens?	Yes
Health personnel who are non-US citizens?	Yes
Health personnel with no prior experience in developing countries?	Yes
Health personnel who are not current members of your organization?	Yes

Organization/Service Specifics:	
Size of the Organization's Staff:	21-50
Number of providers sent or received/year:	>200
Minimum term of assignment:	2 week
Maximum term of assignment:	3 weeks
Is funding available for travel?	Yes
Are room and board provided?	Yes
Is any other funding available?	No
Is training provided or available?	Yes
Is a language other than English required?	No

Health Professionals Placed:

Physicians:

Physicians; Anesthesiologists; Emergency Medicine Physicians; Otolaryngologists; Plastic/Hand/Reconstructive Surgeons

Allied Health Professionals:

Administrative Health Positions; Dentists; Nurses; Nutritionists & Dieticians; Paramedics; Physical & Occupational Therapists; Psychologists; Respiratory Therapists

Notes

Operation USA

Address: **8320 Melrose Avenue, Suite 200, Los Angeles, CA 90069 U.S.A.**

Phone: **(323) 658-8876** FAX: **(323) 653-7846**

E-Mail: **stan@opusa.org** Web: **www.opusa.org**

Mission: Operation USA is an international relief and development agency founded in 1979 which has delivered over $135 million in donated high-priority relief supplies to 82 countries. Operation USA's mission is to solicit corporate in-kind contributions of goods and services and match them with established needs in both disaster areas and long term development projects. We establish partnerships with indigenous and international non-governmental organizations to obtain assistance with needs assessment, implementation and evaluation. This method is used in responding to all types of disasters as well as for long term development projects.

Continents Served

Africa ☑ Asia ☑ Europe ☑ The Americas ☑

Countries Served

Albania, Angola, Bangladesh, Bolivia, Bosnia and Herzegovina, Brazil, Cambodia, China, Congo, Costa Rica, Croatia, Cuba, Ecuador, El Salvador, Ethiopia, Guatemala, Honduras, Hong Kong, India, Israel, Jamaica, Jordan, Korea, North, Laos, Lebanon, Liberia, Malaysia, Mexico, Mozambique, Myanmar (Burma), Nepal, Nicaragua, Panama, Philippines, Poland, Romania, Rwanda, Somalia, South Africa, Sri Lanka, Sudan, Thailand, United States, Vietnam, Yugoslavia, former, Zaire (DemRepCongo)

Placement opportunities for . . .

People of only certain faiths?	No
Couples: both are health providers?	No
Couples: only one is a health provider?	No
Families with children?	No
Medical students?	No
Pre-medical or college students?	No
Other health professional students?	Yes
Doctors in training?	No
Health personnel who are US citizens?	Yes
Health personnel who are non-US citizens?	Yes
Health personnel with no prior experience in developing countries?	No
Health personnel who are not current members of your organization?	Yes

Organization/Service Specifics:

Size of the Organization's Staff:	6-10
Number of providers sent or received/year:	21-50
Minimum term of assignment:	1 week
Maximum term of assignment:	2 weeks
Is funding available for travel?	No
Are room and board provided?	No
Is any other funding available?	No
Is training provided or available?	No
Is a language other than English required? *1*	Yes

Health Professionals Placed:

Physicians:

Physicians; Hematologists; Oncologists; Ophthalmologists; Orthopedic Surgeons; Pediatricians; Plastic/Hand/Reconstructive Surgeons; Psychiatrists

Allied Health Professionals:

Prosthetists; Psychologists

Notes

1. Spanish or French may be required.

Our Little Brothers and Sisters

Address: **1210 Hillside Terrace, Alexandria, VA 22302 U.S.A.**

Phone: **(703) 836-1233** FAX: **(703) 836-3554**

E-Mail: **olbsus@olbsus.org** Web: **www.nphamigos.org**

Continents Served

Africa ☐ Asia ☐ Europe ☐ The Americas ☑

Countries Served

El Salvador, Guatemala, Haiti, Honduras, Mexico, Nicaragua

Mission: Our Little Brothers and Sisters, also known as Nuestros Pequeños Hermanos (NPH), is a charitable organization serving orphaned and abandoned children in Latin America and the Caribbean. The mission is to provide shelter, food, clothing, health care, and education in a Christian family environment based on unconditional acceptance and love, sharing, working and responsibility. A worldwide community of donors, staff, and volunteers enables NPH to help the children become caring and productive citizens of their countries.

(continued)

Placement opportunities for . . .		Organization/Service Specifics:	
People of only certain faiths?	No	Size of the Organization's Staff:	11-20
Couples: both are health providers?	Yes	Number of providers sent or received/year:	11-20
Couples: only one is a health provider?	Yes	Minimum term of assignment:	1 Year
Families with children?	Yes	Maximum term of assignment:	5 Years
Medical students?	No	Is funding available for travel?	No
Pre-medical or college students?	Yes	Are room and board provided?	Yes
Other health professional students?	Yes	Is any other funding available? *1*	Yes
Doctors in training?	Yes	Is training provided or available?	No
Health personnel who are US citizens?	Yes	Is a language other than English required? *2*	Yes

Health personnel who are non-US citizens?	Yes
Health personnel with no prior experience in developing countries?	Yes
Health personnel who are not current members of your organization?	Yes

Health Professionals Placed:

Physicians:

Physicians; Family Practitioners; Internal Medicine GPS & PCP; Pediatricians

Allied Health Professionals:

Dentists; Nurse Practitioners; Nurses; Pharmacists; Physician Assistants

Notes

1. A stipend is available; *2.* Spanish or French may be required for some assignments.

P.C.E.A. Chogoria Hospital

Address: **P.O. Box 35 Chogoria, Kenya, E. Africa**

Phone: **254 0166 22620** FAX: **254 0166 22122**

E-Mail: **chogoria@africaonline.co.ke** Web:

Continents Served

Africa ☑ Asia ☐ Europe ☐ The Americas ☐

Countries Served

Kenya

Mission: Presbyterian Church of East Africa-Chogoria Hospital is located on the eastern slopes of Mount Kenya. Its catchment area comprises a population of 450,000. The hospital consists of medical, surgical, pediatric, and maternity wards (312 beds), a busy outpatient department with dental and eye units, and a community health department, which maintains 32 rural clinics and an extensive network of community volunteers. On average, the hospital is staffed by eight doctors, three clinical officers, and 100 nurses (enrolled and registered). Medical staff together with support staff number over 500. The hospital has a nursing training school. Chogoria Hospital is owned by the Presbyterian Church of East Africa (PCEA). As a mission hospital it is founded on a strong Christian philosophy. Staff are expected to be sympathetic and respectful to this approach.

Placement opportunities for . . .		Organization/Service Specifics:	
People of only certain faiths? *1*	Yes	Size of the Organization's Staff: *2*	>200
Couples: both are health providers?	Yes	Number of providers sent or received/year:	11-20
Couples: only one is a health provider?	No	Minimum term of assignment:	6 weeks
Families with children?	Yes	Maximum term of assignment:	4 years
Medical students?	Yes	Is funding available for travel?	No
Pre-medical or college students?	No	Are room and board provided?	Yes
Other health professional students?	No	Is any other funding available? *3*	Yes
Doctors in training?	No	Is training provided or available?	Yes
Health personnel who are US citizens?	Yes	Is a language other than English required?	No

Health personnel who are non-US citizens?	Yes
Health personnel with no prior experience in developing countries?	No
Health personnel who are not current members of your organization?	Yes

Health Professionals Placed:

Physicians:

General Surgeons; OB/GYN; Pediatricians

Allied Health Professionals:

Dentists; Pharmacists

Notes

1. Volunteers must be Christians or sympathetic to the Christian faith; *2.* Last contacted on 05/01. No response to inquiry in 2/05; *3.* A small living expense allowance is provided.

P.C.E.A. Kikuyu Hospital

Address: **P.O. Box 45 Kikuyu, Kenya, E. Africa**

Phone: **254 0154 32412** FAX: **254 0154 32413**

E-Mail: **pceagenhosp@maf.org** Web:

Continents Served

Africa ☑ Asia ☐ Europe ☐ The Americas ☐

Countries Served

Kenya

Mission: Kikuyu Hospital is the oldest mission hospital in Kenya, established in 1908 by Scottish Presbyterian Missionaries. At Thogoto, they set up a center to teach boys to read and write, a Bible teaching center and a first aid center which is now the hospital, operated by the Presbyterian Church of East Africa. The hospital serves patients from the semi-rural area 25km from the center of Nairobi, from the city, and from many other parts of Kenya. Patients also come from neighboring countries. For more information, you can also contact the Wilson Rehabilitation Foundation, 1424 Hartford Ave., Maryville, TN 37803. (423)681-7500. cgdurham@juno.com.

Placement opportunities for . . .		Organization/Service Specifics:	
People of only certain faiths? *1*	No	Size of the Organization's Staff: *2*	>200
Couples: both are health providers?	Yes	Number of providers sent or received/year:	51-100
Couples: only one is a health provider?	Yes	Minimum term of assignment: *3*	2 weeks
Families with children?	Yes	Maximum term of assignment:	no limit
Medical students?	Yes	Is funding available for travel?	No
Pre-medical or college students?	No	Are room and board provided?	Yes
Other health professional students?	Yes	Is any other funding available?	No
Doctors in training?	Yes	Is training provided or available?	Yes
Health personnel who are US citizens?	Yes	Is a language other than English required?	No
Health personnel who are non-US citizens?	Yes		
Health personnel with no prior experience in developing countries?	Yes		
Health personnel who are not current members of your organization?	Yes		

Health Professionals Placed:

Physicians:

Physicians; Anesthesiologists; Cardiologists; Dermatologists; Emergency Medicine Physicians; Endocrinologists; Family Practitioners; Gastroenterologists; General Surgeons; Hematologists; Oncologists; Infectious Disease Spec.; Internal Medicine GPS & PCP; Nephrologists; Neurologists; Neurosurgeons; OB/GYN; Oral Surgeons; Orthopedic Surgeons; Otolaryngologists; Pathologists; Pediatricians; Plastic/Hand/ Reconstructive Surgeons; Pulmonary Specialists; Radiologists; Urologists

Allied Health Professionals:

Administrative Health Positions; Medical Technicians (lab, X-ray, etc); Nurse Midwives; Nurse Practitioners; Nurses; Nutritionists & Dieticians; Pharmacists; Physical & Occupational Therapists; Physician Assistants; Prosthetists; Public Health Specialists, Epidemiologists and Health Educators; Respiratory Therapists; Social Workers; Water/Sanitation Specialists

Notes

1. We are a Christian organization but not exclusive; *2.* Last contacted on 05/01. No response to inquiry in 2/05; *3.* Minimum stays depend on the medical specialty of the provider.

P.C.E.A. Tumutumu Hospital

Address: **Private Bag Karatina, Kenya, E. Africa**

Phone: **254 0171 72033** FAX: **254 0171 72656**

E-Mail: **tumutumu@africa online.co.ke** Web:

Continents Served

Africa ☑ Asia ☐ Europe ☐ The Americas ☐

Countries Served

Kenya

Mission: PCEA Tumutumu Hospital is one of the three mission hospitals in Kenya sponsored by the Presbyterian Church of East Africa. Our 203 bed facility in the central highlands of Kenya serves some 200,000 local residents, most of whom are rural peasants. Modest fees are charged for service which account for 80% of our operating expenses. Obviously, without volunteer physicians many now served could not be.

(continued)

Placement opportunities for . . .		**Organization/Service Specifics:**	
People of only certain faiths? *1*	Yes	Size of the Organization's Staff: *2*	>200
Couples: both are health providers?	Yes	Number of providers sent or received/year:	
Couples: only one is a health provider?	Yes	Minimum term of assignment: *3*	8 weeks
Families with children?	Yes	Maximum term of assignment:	
Medical students?	Yes	Is funding available for travel?	No
Pre-medical or college students?	Yes	Are room and board provided?	Yes
Other health professional students?	Yes	Is any other funding available? *4*	Yes
Doctors in training?	Yes	Is training provided or available?	Yes
Health personnel who are US citizens?	Yes	Is a language other than English required?	No
Health personnel who are non-US citizens?	Yes		
Health personnel with no prior experience in developing countries?	Yes		
Health personnel who are not current members of your organization?	Yes		

Health Professionals Placed:

Physicians:

Physicians; Family Practitioners; General Surgeons; Internal Medicine GPS & PCP; OB/GYN; Pediatricians

Allied Health Professionals:

Administrative Health Positions; Dental Hygienists; Medical Technicians (lab, X-ray, etc); Nurse Midwives; Nurse Practitioners; Nurses; Nutritionists & Dieticians; Paramedics; Pharmacists; Physical & Occupational Therapists; Physician Assistants; Public Health Specialists, Epidemiologists and Health Educators; Water/Sanitation Specialists

Notes

1. Volunteers must be Christian;
2. Last contacted on 05/01. No response to inquiry in 2/05;
3. 8 week minimum for students, 12 week minimum for staff;
4. Maintenance allowance is provided for staff.

P.R.A.Y. (Project Rescue of Amazon Youth)

Address: **1006 8th St., Wamego, KS 66547 U.S.A.**

Phone: **(785) 456-1677** FAX:

E-Mail: **saverysally@hotmail.com** Web: **www.praymission.com**

Continents Served

Africa ☐ Asia ☐ Europe ☐ The Americas ☑

Countries Served

Brazil

Mission: P.R.A.Y. provides an emergency children's shelter for abused, neglected, orphaned, abondoned, and homeless children. We now have a brand new medical clinic to serve our children and the many nearby children and mothers who live without basic medical care. There are no language requirements although knowledge of Portuguese is preferred. There is a minimum of 1 month commitment, although there is no maximum term of stay.

Placement opportunities for . . .		**Organization/Service Specifics:**	
People of only certain faiths?	No	Size of the Organization's Staff:	6-10
Couples: both are health providers?	Yes	Number of providers sent or received/year:	6-10
Couples: only one is a health provider?	Yes	Minimum term of assignment:	1 month
Families with children?	Yes	Maximum term of assignment:	
Medical students?	Yes	Is funding available for travel?	No
Pre-medical or college students?	No	Are room and board provided? *1*	Yes
Other health professional students?	Yes	Is any other funding available?	No
Doctors in training?	Yes	Is training provided or available?	No
Health personnel who are US citizens?	Yes	Is a language other than English required? *2*	No
Health personnel who are non-US citizens?	Yes		
Health personnel with no prior experience in developing countries?	Yes		
Health personnel who are not current members of your organization?	Yes		

(continued)

Health Professionals Placed:

Physicians:

Physicians; Anesthesiologists; Cardiologists; Dermatologists; Emergency Medicine Physicians; Endocrinologists; Family Practitioners; Gastroenterologists; General Surgeons; Hematologists; Oncologists; Infectious Disease Spec.; Internal Medicine GPS & PCP; Nephrologists; Neurologists; Neurosurgeons; OB/GYN; Ophthalmologists; Oral Surgeons; Optometrists; Orthopedic Surgeons; Otolaryngologists; Pediatricians; Plastic/Hand/Reconstructive Surgeons; Psychiatrists; Pulmonary Specialists; Radiologists; Urologists

Allied Health Professionals:

Dental Hygienists; Dentists; Medical Technicians (lab, X-ray, etc); Nurse Midwives; Nurse Practitioners; Nurses; Nutritionists & Dieticians; Paramedics; Pharmacists; Physical & Occupational Therapists; Physician Assistants; Podiatrists; Prosthetists; Psychologists; Public Health Specialists, Epidemiologists and Health Educators; Respiratory Therapists; Social Workers

Notes

1. There is a small charge of $15 per week for room and board;
2. No requirements, but we request that volunteers know a little bit of Portuguese.

Palestine Children's Relief Fund

Address: **PO Box 1926, Kent, OH 44240 U.S.A.**

Phone: **(330) 678-2645** FAX: **(330) 678-2661**

E-Mail: **pcrf@pcrf.net** Web: **www.pcrf.net**

Continents Served

Africa ☐ Asia ☑ Europe ☐ The Americas ☐

Countries Served

Lebanon Palestine

Mission: Established in 1992, the Palestine Children's Relief Fund (PCRF) is a US-based, nonprofit, tax-exempt charity, dedicated to helping Arab children in need of life-saving medical care not available in their homelands. Although the PCRF was initially established to help provide advanced medical care in the United States to Palestinian children injured during the intifada, our work has expanded. We now provide medical care for Arab children from other parts of the Middle East including Iraq, Lebanon, Syria, Egypt, and Jordan. Over the past several years, the PCRF intensified its efforts and expanded its activities.

Placement opportunities for . . .	
People of only certain faiths?	No
Couples: both are health providers?	Yes
Couples: only one is a health provider?	No
Families with children?	No
Medical students?	No
Pre-medical or college students?	No
Other health professional students?	No
Doctors in training?	Yes
Health personnel who are US citizens?	Yes
Health personnel who are non-US citizens?	Yes
Health personnel with no prior experience in developing countries?	Yes
Health personnel who are not current members of your organization?	

Organization/Service Specifics:	
Size of the Organization's Staff:	6-10
Number of providers sent or received/year:	>200
Minimum term of assignment:	1 week
Maximum term of assignment:	6 months
Is funding available for travel?	Yes
Are room and board provided?	Yes
Is any other funding available?	No
Is training provided or available?	No
Is a language other than English required?	No

Health Professionals Placed:

Physicians:

Physicians; Anesthesiologists; Cardiologists; Emergency Medicine Physicians; Endocrinologists; Hematologists; Oncologists; Neurosurgeons; OB/GYN; Ophthalmologists; Oral Surgeons; Orthopedic Surgeons; Otolaryngologists; Pediatricians; Plastic/Hand/Reconstructive Surgeons; Radiologists; Urologists

Allied Health Professionals:

Nurses; Physical & Occupational Therapists; Prosthetists

Notes

Palms Australia

Address: **P.O. Box 54, Croydon Park, NSW 2133 Australia**

Phone: **9642 0558** FAX: **9742 5607**

E-Mail: **palms@palms.org.au** Web: **http://homepages.ihug.com.au/~paulian/**

Mission: PALMS aims to foster greater cultural understanding and links between Australians and other global communities, provide the skills of Australians to communities and groups where those skills make a sustainable improvement to the quality of life for people oppressed and dispossessed by cultures that divide, assist Australians to come to a better understanding of the economic, social, and cultural aspirations of people living simply, and to enter into partnership with the people, to work for a just and sustainable international economic order, and assist volunteers to achieve greater self-reliance, independence, spiritual insight and personal development that will develop their appreciation of the value of living in community. Travel expenses and room and board are provided for people who make a 2-3 year commitment. There are no language or religious requirements.

Continents Served

Africa ☑ Asia ☑ Europe ☐ The Americas ☐

Countries Served

Angola	Australia	Benin
Burkina Faso	Burundi	Cambodia
Cameroon	Central African Rep.	
Chad	Comoros	Congo
Gambia	Ghana	Guinea
Guinea-Bissau	Indonesia	Ivory Coast
Kenya	Laos	Liberia
Madagascar	Malawi	Malaysia
Mali	Mauritania	Mauritius
Mozambique	Myanmar (Burma)	
New Zealand	Niger	Nigeria
Papua-New Guinea		Philippines
Rwanda	Senegal	Seychelles
Sierra Leone	Singapore	
Solomon Islands		Somalia
Tanzania	Thailand	Togo
Uganda	Vietnam	
Zaire (DemRepCongo)		Zambia
Zimbabwe		

Placement opportunities for . . .

People of only certain faiths? *1*	No
Couples: both are health providers?	Yes
Couples: only one is a health provider?	Yes
Families with children?	Yes
Medical students?	No
Pre-medical or college students?	No
Other health professional students?	No
Doctors in training?	Yes
Health personnel who are US citizens?	No
Health personnel who are non-US citizens?	Yes
Health personnel with no prior experience in developing countries?	Yes
Health personnel who are not current members of your organization?	Yes

Organization/Service Specifics:

Size of the Organization's Staff:	0-5
Number of providers sent or received/year:	1-5
Minimum term of assignment: *2*	2 years
Maximum term of assignment:	3 years
Is funding available for travel?	Yes
Are room and board provided?	Yes
Is any other funding available? *3*	Yes
Is training provided or available?	Yes
Is a language other than English required?	No

Health Professionals Placed:

Physicians:

Internal Medicine GPS & PCP

Allied Health Professionals:

Nurse Practitioners

Notes

1. All are welcome, but the organization has Catholic ethics; *2.* Shorter assignments are available for special situations; *3.* Insurance, travel expenses, and health care are provided.

Pan American Health Organization

Address: **525 23rd St., N.W., Washington, DC 20037 U.S.A.**

Phone: **(202) 974-3000** FAX: **(202) 974-3663**

E-Mail: **pahef@paho.org** Web: **www.paho.org**

Mission: PAHO is an international public health agency with more than 90 years of experience in working to improve health and living standards of the countries of the Americas. PAHO serves as the specialized organization for health of the Inter-American System. It also serves as the regional office for the Americas of the World Health Organization and enjoys international recognition as part of the United Nations System. PAHO promotes primary health care strategies, which reach people in their communities, to extend health services to all and to increase efficiency in the use of scarce resources. It assists countries in fighting old diseases that have re-emerged, such as cholera, dengue and tuberculosis, and new diseases such as the spreading AIDS epidemic, providing technical cooperation including education and social communications support, promoting work with non-governmental organizations, and support for programs to prevent transmission of communicable diseases. The organization is also involved in prevention of chronic diseases such as diabetes and cancer, which are increasingly affecting the populations of developing countries in the Americas.

Continents Served

Africa ☐ Asia ☐ Europe ☐ The Americas ☑

Countries Served

Antigua and Barbuda, Argentina, Aruba, Bahamas, Barbados, Belize, Bermuda, Bolivia, Brazil, Canada, Cayman Islands, Chile, Colombia, Costa Rica, Cuba, Dominica, Dominican Republic, Ecuador, El Salvador, Grenada, Guadeloupe, Guatemala, Guyana, Haiti, Honduras, Jamaica, Martinique, Mexico, Montserrat, Netherlands, Nicaragua, Panama, Paraguay, Peru, Puerto Rico, St. Kitts, St. Lucia, St. Vincent, Suriname, Trinidad and Tobago, Turks and Caicos Islands, United States, Uruguay, Venezuela, Virgin Islands

Placement opportunities for . . .

People of only certain faiths?	No
Couples: both are health providers?	No
Couples: only one is a health provider?	Yes
Families with children?	Yes
Medical students?	No
Pre-medical or college students?	No
Other health professional students?	Yes
Doctors in training?	Yes
Health personnel who are US citizens?	Yes
Health personnel who are non-US citizens?	Yes
Health personnel with no prior experience in developing countries?	No
Health personnel who are not current members of your organization?	Yes

Organization/Service Specifics:

Size of the Organization's Staff:		>200
Number of providers sent or received/year:		>200
Minimum term of assignment:		1 week
Maximum term of assignment:		life
Is funding available for travel?		Yes
Are room and board provided?		No
Is any other funding available?	*1*	Yes
Is training provided or available?		Yes
Is a language other than English required?	*2*	Yes

Health Professionals Placed:

Physicians:

Physicians; Emergency Medicine Physicians; Infectious Disease Spec.; Ophthalmologists; Oral Surgeons; Pediatricians; Psychiatrists

Allied Health Professionals:

Administrative Health Positions; Dentists; Nurse Midwives; Nurse Practitioners; Nurses; Psychologists; Water/Sanitation Specialists

Notes

1. Salary and other expenses are provided; *2.* French, Spanish, or Portuguese required depending on the country.

Partners of the Americas

Address: **1424 K Street, NW, Suite 700, Washington, DC 20005 U.S.A.**

Phone: **(202) 628-3300** FAX: **(202) 628-3306**

E-Mail: **info@partners.net** Web: **www.partners.net/**

Mission: Partners of the Americas (Partners) is a network of citizens from Latin America, the Caribbean and the United States, who volunteer to work together to improve the lives of people across the region, through nonpolitical, community-based activities. Besides providing technical assistance and training to communities in Latin America, the Caribbean and the U.S., Partners' network of volunteers promote collaboration in the region's social and economic development through working relationships among professionals and institutions across the hemisphere. The two sides of a partnership work together to carry out a wide range of activities to improve food supplies, deliver health services, provide job training to young people, protect the region's natural resources and safeguard the rights of women and children. There is a minimum two week commitment. Portuguese may be required for some assignments.

Continents Served

Africa ☐ Asia ☐ Europe ☐ The Americas ☑

Countries Served

Argentina	Barbados	Belize
Bolivia	Brazil	Chile
Colombia	Costa Rica	
Dominican Republic		Ecuador
El Salvador	Guatemala	Guyana
Haiti	Honduras	Jamaica
Mexico	Nicaragua	Panama
Paraguay	Peru	
Trinidad and Tobago		United States
Uruguay	Venezuela	

Placement opportunities for . . .

People of only certain faiths?	No
Couples: both are health providers?	Yes
Couples: only one is a health provider?	Yes
Families with children?	No
Medical students?	Yes
Pre-medical or college students?	Yes
Other health professional students?	Yes
Doctors in training?	Yes
Health personnel who are US citizens?	Yes
Health personnel who are non-US citizens?	Yes
Health personnel with no prior experience in developing countries?	Yes
Health personnel who are not current members of your organization?	Yes

Organization/Service Specifics:

Size of the Organization's Staff:		21-50
Number of providers sent or received/year:		>200
Minimum term of assignment:		2 weeks
Maximum term of assignment:		
Is funding available for travel?		Yes
Are room and board provided?		Yes
Is any other funding available?		No
Is training provided or available?		Yes
Is a language other than English required?	*1*	Yes

Health Professionals Placed:

Physicians:

Not specified

Allied Health Professionals:

Not specified

Notes

1. Portuguese may be required for some assignments.

PAZAPA

Address: **c/o Siloe Foundation, 82 Rodeo Avenue, Sausalito, CA U.S.A.**

Phone: **(415) 331-1639** FAX: **(415) 331-7767**

E-Mail: **peterc@siloe.org** Web: **www.siloe.org/index.html**

Continents Served

Africa ☐ Asia ☐ Europe ☐ The Americas ☑

Countries Served

Haiti

Mission: PAZAPA provides surgery, orthopedic devices, physical therapy, and rehabilitation for physically handicapped children at no cost to the children's families. Operations are provided for children with club feet, knee and hip problems, cleft palate, hand deformities, etc, by French, Canadian, and American volunteer surgeons, as well as by resident Haitian surgeons at l'Hopital Ste. Croix in Léogane, the St. Vincent Center for the Handicapped in Port-au-Prince, and the St. Michel Hospital in Jacmel.

(continued)

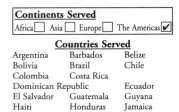

Placement opportunities for . . .		Organization/Service Specifics:	
People of only certain faiths?	No	Size of the Organization's Staff:	21-50
Couples: both are health providers?	Yes	Number of providers sent or received/year:	11-20
Couples: only one is a health provider?	Yes	Minimum term of assignment:	none
Families with children?	No	Maximum term of assignment:	none
Medical students? *1*	Yes	Is funding available for travel?	No
Pre-medical or college students? *1*	Yes	Are room and board provided? *2*	Yes
Other health professional students?	Yes	Is any other funding available?	No
Doctors in training? *1*	Yes	Is training provided or available?	No
Health personnel who are US citizens?	Yes	Is a language other than English required? *3*	No
Health personnel who are non-US citizens?	Yes		
Health personnel with no prior experience in developing countries?	Yes		
Health personnel who are not current members of your organization?	Yes		

Health Professionals Placed: *4*

Physicians:

Physicians; Anesthesiologists; Cardiologists; Dermatologists; Emergency Medicine Physicians; Family Practitioners; General Surgeons; Infectious Disease Spec.; Internal Medicine GPS & PCP; Ophthalmologists; Oral Surgeons; Orthopedic Surgeons; Pediatricians; Plastic/Hand/Reconstructive Surgeons

Allied Health Professionals:

Dentists; Medical Technicians (lab, X-ray, etc); Nurse Practitioners; Nurses; Pharmacists; Physical & Occupational Therapists; Physician Assistants

Notes

1. To assist only; *2.* Paid for by volunteers; *3.* Spanish helpful; *4.* Other specialists should inquire as well.

Peacework: Volunteer Medical Projects

Address: **209 Otey St., Blacksburg, VA 24060-7426 U.S.A.**

Phone: **(800) 272-5519** FAX: **(540) 953-3904**

E-Mail: **mail@peacework.org** Web: **www.peacework.org**

Continents Served

Africa ✔ Asia ✔ Europe ✔ The Americas ✔

Countries Served

Belize Guyana Honduras

Mission: Peacework offers work projects throughout the year to locations such as Mexico, Russia, Cuba, El Salvador, the Dominican Republic, Ghana, Costa Rica, Vietnam, Nicaragua, and Honduras. Volunteer programs are typically focused on development of community infrastructure (homes, schools, clinics, etc). Peacework Medical Projects are 2-week primary care clinics in areas of great need. Urgent, emergent, and chronic needs are addressed, as well as basic health education and some cancer and HIV screening. Typical costs for a volunteers are around $1600, inclusive of airfare and all in-country needs.

Placement opportunities for . . .		Organization/Service Specifics:	
People of only certain faiths?	No	Size of the Organization's Staff:	0-5
Couples: both are health providers?	Yes	Number of providers sent or received/year:	11-20
Couples: only one is a health provider?	Yes	Minimum term of assignment:	2 weeks
Families with children?	No	Maximum term of assignment:	2 weeks
Medical students?	Yes	Is funding available for travel?	No
Pre-medical or college students?	Yes	Are room and board provided?	Yes
Other health professional students?	Yes	Is any other funding available?	No
Doctors in training?	Yes	Is training provided or available?	No
Health personnel who are US citizens?	Yes	Is a language other than English required?	No
Health personnel who are non-US citizens?	No		
Health personnel with no prior experience in developing countries?	Yes		
Health personnel who are not current members of your organization?	Yes		

Health Professionals Placed:

Physicians:

Not specified

Allied Health Professionals:

Not specified

Notes

Physicians for Human Rights

Address: **Two Arrow Street, Suite 301, Cambridge, MA 02138 U.S.A.**

Phone: **(617) 695-0041** FAX: **(617) 301-4250**

E-Mail: **phrusa@phrusa.org** Web: **www.phrusa.org**

Continents Served

Africa ☐ Asia ☐ Europe ☐ The Americas ☑

Countries Served

Bosnia, Herzegovina; Cyprus; El Salvador; Georgia; Iraq; Israel; Mexico; Mozambique; Palestine; Rwanda; Thailand; Uganda; United States

Mission: Physicians for Human Rights (PHR), a Nobel prize winning NGO, has promoted health by protecting human rights since 1986. We believe that human rights are essential preconditions for the health and well-being of all people. Using medical and scientific methods, we investigate and expose violations of human rights worldwide and we work to stop them. We support institutions that hold perpetrators of human rights abuses, including health professionals, accountable for their actions. We educate health professionals and medical, public health and nursing students and organize them to become active in supporting a movement for human rights and creating a culture of human rights in the medical and scientific professions. Volunteers can work on an as-needed basis. There are no language requirements, although language skills can be helpful. We operate the Asylum Network which depends on the volunteer support of physicians, psychologists and social workers who conduct medical and psychological examinations of foreigners seeking asylum in the U.S.

Placement opportunities for . . .

People of only certain faiths?	No
Couples: both are health providers?	Yes
Couples: only one is a health provider?	Yes
Families with children?	Yes
Medical students?	Yes
Pre-medical or college students?	Yes
Other health professional students?	
Doctors in training?	
Health personnel who are US citizens?	Yes
Health personnel who are non-US citizens?	No
Health personnel with no prior experience in developing countries?	Yes
Health personnel who are not current members of your organization?	Yes

Organization/Service Specifics:

Size of the Organization's Staff:	21-50
Number of providers sent or received/year:	101-150
Minimum term of assignment: *1*	
Maximum term of assignment:	
Is funding available for travel?	No
Are room and board provided?	No
Is any other funding available?	No
Is training provided or available? *2*	Yes
Is a language other than English required? *3*	No

Health Professionals Placed:

Physicians:

Physicians; Emergency Medicine Physicians; Internal Medicine GPS & PCP; OB/GYN; Psychiatrists

Allied Health Professionals:

Dentists; Psychologists; Social Workers

Notes

1. Volunteers work as needed; *2.* Training is available for asylum evaluations; *3.* There are no requirements, but language skills are helpful.

Physicians for Peace

Address: **229 West Bute St., Suite 200, Norfolk, VA 23510 U.S.A.**

Phone: **(757) 625-7569** FAX: **(757) 625-7680**

E-Mail: **admin@physiciansforpeace.org, or info@** Web: **www.physiciansforpeace.org**

Continents Served

Africa ☑ Asia ☑ Europe ☐ The Americas ☑

Countries Served *2*

Bolivia; Costa Rica; Dominican Republic; Egypt; El Salvador; Guatemala; Haiti; Israel; Jordan; Nicaragua; Nigeria; Palestine; Philippines; Syria; Turkey; Yemen

Mission: Physicians for Peace was founded to promote international friendships and peace through medicine and is dedicated to improving health care through continuing medical education utilizing the donated services of volunteer professionals. It has conducted more than 200 educational missions, usually ranging from 10 days to two weeks, in the Middle East, Central America, Africa, eastern Europe, the Caribbean, and Asia. Its volunteer physicians teach instructors at local medical schools. Volunteers can travel for 1-2 week assignments. Travel and room and board expenses are provided. There are no language or religious requirements for volunteers.

(continued)

Placement opportunities for . . .

People of only certain faiths?	No
Couples: both are health providers?	Yes
Couples: only one is a health provider?	Yes
Families with children?	
Medical students?	Yes
Pre-medical or college students?	Yes
Other health professional students?	Yes
Doctors in training?	Yes
Health personnel who are US citizens?	Yes
Health personnel who are non-US citizens?	Yes
Health personnel with no prior experience in developing countries?	Yes
Health personnel who are not current members of your organization?	Yes

Organization/Service Specifics:

Size of the Organization's Staff:	0-5
Number of providers sent or received/year:	21-50
Minimum term of assignment:	1 week
Maximum term of assignment: *1*	2 weeks
Is funding available for travel? *3*	Yes
Are room and board provided?	Yes
Is any other funding available?	No
Is training provided or available?	No
Is a language other than English required?	No

Health Professionals Placed:

Physicians:

Cardiologists; Infectious Disease Spec.; Nephrologists; OB/GYN; Ophthalmologists; Orthopedic Surgeons; Otolaryngologists; Pediatricians; Plastic/Hand/Reconstructive Surgeons; Pulmonary Specialists; Urologists

Allied Health Professionals:

Dentists; Medical Technicians (lab, X-ray, etc); Nurses; Physical & Occupational Therapists; Physician Assistants

Notes

1. The average mission is 10 days long; *2.* The countries where programs take place vary according to need; *3.* Funding is available for physicians, but most choose to pay their own way.

Presbyterian Church USA, Mission Service Recruitment

Address: **100 Witherspoon Street, Louisville, KY 40202-1396 U.S.A.**

Phone: **(888) 728-7228 x2530** FAX: **(502) 569-8963**

E-Mail: **msr@ctr.pcusa.org or DBLee@ctr.pcusa.org** Web: **www.pcusa.org/msr**

Mission: The International Health Ministries Office of the Presbyterian Church (USA) coordinates the ministries of the denomination in international health and development. The church's concern focuses particularly upon serving the poorest of the poor and helping them to attain health and wholeness. Through more than 150 years in health ministries the PC(USA) has learned that health is more important than absence of physical illness and disease; health cannot be pursued apart from the culture and conditions under which one lives; lasting changes in the health status of communities can best be realized through ministries in partnership with indigenous churches and through development of national leadership; a comprehensive health care system requires an integrated system of referral hospitals, health centers and clinics, and well-trained community health workers working together to achieve health for all. Volunteers must be Christian and can serve for 2-3 year terms. Travel and room and board are provided and there are some salaried positions available.

Continents Served

Africa ✔ Asia ✔ Europe ✔ The Americas ✔

Countries Served

Afghanistan, Albania, Angola, Argentina, Australia, Austria, Bangladesh, Barbados, Belgium, Benin, Bolivia, Botswana, Brazil, Bulgaria, Burundi, Cambodia, Cameroon, Central African Rep., Chad, Chile, China, Colombia, Congo, Costa Rica, Cuba, Czech Republic, Denmark, Dominican Republic, Ecuador, Egypt, El Salvador, Ethiopia, Finland, France, Gambia, Germany, Ghana, Greece, Guatemala, Guinea, Guinea-Bissau, Haiti, Honduras, Hong Kong, Hungary, India, Indonesia, Iraq, Ireland, Israel, Italy, Jamaica, Japan, Jordan, Kenya, Korea, South, Laos, Lebanon, Lesotho, Liberia, Madagascar, Malawi, Malaysia, Mali, Mauritania, Mauritius, Mexico, Mozambique, Myanmar (Burma), Nepal, Netherlands, New Zealand, Nicaragua, Niger, Nigeria, Norway, Pakistan, Papua-New Guinea, Paraguay, Peru, Philippines, Portugal, Romania, Rwanda, Senegal, Sierra Leone, Singapore, Somalia, South Africa, Spain, Sri Lanka, Sudan, Swaziland, Sweden, Switzerland, Syria, Taiwan, Tanzania, Thailand, Togo, Trinidad and Tobago, Turkey, Uganda, United Kingdom, United States, Uruguay, USSR, former, Vanuatu, Venezuela, Vietnam, Yugoslavia, former, Zaire (DemRepCongo), Zambia, Zimbabwe

(continued)

Placement opportunities for . . .

People of only certain faiths? *1*	Yes
Couples: both are health providers?	Yes
Couples: only one is a health provider?	Yes
Families with children?	Yes
Medical students?	Yes
Pre-medical or college students?	Yes
Other health professional students?	No
Doctors in training?	Yes
Health personnel who are US citizens?	Yes
Health personnel who are non-US citizens?	No
Health personnel with no prior experience in developing countries?	Yes
Health personnel who are not current members of your organization?	Yes

Organization/Service Specifics:

Size of the Organization's Staff:	>200
Number of providers sent or received/year:	
Minimum term of assignment:	2 years
Maximum term of assignment:	3 years
Is funding available for travel?	Yes
Are room and board provided?	Yes
Is any other funding available? *2*	Yes
Is training provided or available?	Yes
Is a language other than English required?	No

Health Professionals Placed:

Physicians:

Physicians; Family Practitioners; General Surgeons; Infectious Disease Spec.; Pediatricians; Psychiatrists

Allied Health Professionals:

Psychologists; Public Health Specialists, Epidemiologists and Health Educators; Social Workers

Notes

1. Volunteers must be Christian; *2.* There are some salaried positions.

Project AmaZon

Address: **PO Box 913 Morton, IL 61550 U.S.A.**

Phone: **(309) 263-2299** FAX: **(309) 263-2299**

E-Mail: **dove@dpc.net** Web: **www.projectamazon.org/index.html**

Continents Served

Africa ☐ Asia ☐ Europe ☐ The Americas ☑

Countries Served

Brazil

Mission: Project Amazon (PAZ) is a non-profit Christian organization with the vision to develop a nationally led church planting movement in the Amazon Basin. PAZ provides health care to the people of Brazil on its river boats and in the jungles and communities. PAZ also provides training to local health care personnel to help ensure that basic health care perpetuates in the region. All volunteers must agree not to smoke or drink alcohol while working on mission.

Placement opportunities for . . .

People of only certain faiths? *1*	Yes
Couples: both are health providers?	Yes
Couples: only one is a health provider?	Yes
Families with children?	No
Medical students?	Yes
Pre-medical or college students?	Yes
Other health professional students?	Yes
Doctors in training?	Yes
Health personnel who are US citizens?	Yes
Health personnel who are non-US citizens?	No
Health personnel with no prior experience in developing countries?	Yes
Health personnel who are not current members of your organization?	Yes

Organization/Service Specifics:

Size of the Organization's Staff:	0-5
Number of providers sent or received/year:	6-10
Minimum term of assignment:	1 week
Maximum term of assignment:	3 weeks
Is funding available for travel?	No
Are room and board provided?	No
Is any other funding available?	No
Is training provided or available?	No
Is a language other than English required?	No

Health Professionals Placed:

Physicians:

All physician specialties

Allied Health Professionals:

All allied health professionals

Notes

1. Christian.

Project Concern International: OPTIONS

Continents Served			
Africa ✔	Asia ✔	Europe ✔	The Americas ✔

Countries Served

Bolivia	El Salvador	Ghana
Guatemala	Honduras	India
Indonesia	Mexico	Nicaragua
Romania	United States	Zambia

Address: **5151 Murphy Canyon Rd, Suite 320, San Diego, CA 92123 U.S.A.**

Phone: **(858) 279-9690** FAX: **(858) 694-0294**

E-Mail: **postmaster@projectconcern.org** Web: **www.projectconcern.org/**

Mission: Project Concern International provides parents and our worldwide partners with medical training, support and health care crucial to protecting the well being of children and families. Project Concern programs save lives by ensuring basic medical care, halting the spread of infectious disease, feeding the hungry, helping keep families small, safeguarding the health of communities along the US-Mexico border, and ensuring clean water. OPTIONS links health and development specialists with programs, hospitals, and clinics worldwide. Project Concern's efficient programs provide health care to more than 3,000,000 people each year. Volunteers can serve for short terms (2 weeks) to longer terms (2 years). There are no religious requirements and language requirements vary. There is no funding available for travel, but room and board are provided. OPTIONS also publishes a bi-monthly newsletter listing service opportunities for a number of health professionals.

Placement opportunities for . . .	
People of only certain faiths?	No
Couples: both are health providers?	Yes
Couples: only one is a health provider?	Yes
Families with children?	Yes
Medical students?	Yes
Pre-medical or college students?	No
Other health professional students?	Yes
Doctors in training?	Yes
Health personnel who are US citizens?	Yes
Health personnel who are non-US citizens?	Yes
Health personnel with no prior experience in developing countries?	Yes
Health personnel who are not current members of your organization?	Yes

Organization/Service Specifics:	
Size of the Organization's Staff:	0-5
Number of providers sent or received/year:	151-200
Minimum term of assignment:	2 weeks
Maximum term of assignment:	2 years
Is funding available for travel?	No
Are room and board provided?	Yes
Is any other funding available?	Yes
Is training provided or available?	Yes
Is a language other than English required? *1*	Yes

Health Professionals Placed:

Physicians:

Anesthesiologists; Cardiologists; Dermatologists; Infectious Disease Spec.; Internal Medicine GPS & PCP; Ophthalmologists; Optometrists; Orthopedic Surgeons

Allied Health Professionals:

Administrative Health Positions; Dental Hygienists; Dentists; Nurse Midwives; Nurse Practitioners; Nurses; Nutritionists & Dieticians; Paramedics; Pharmacists; Physician Assistants

Notes

1. Language requirements depend on the country of service.

Project Hope / People to People Health Foundation

Continents Served			
Africa ✔	Asia ✔	Europe ✔	The Americas ✔

Countries Served

Address: **255 Carter Hall Lane, Millwood, VA 22646 U.S.A.**

Phone: **(540) 837-2100 or (800) 544-HOPE** FAX: **(540) 837-9052 (540) 837-1813**

E-Mail: **recruitment@projecthope.org** Web: **www.projhope.org**

Mission: "It is Project HOPE's mission to achieve sustainable advances in health care around the world by implementing health education programs, conducting health policy research, and providing humanitarian assistance in areas of need; thereby contributing to human dignity, promoting international understanding, and enhancing social and economic development. The essence of Project HOPE is teaching; the basis is partnership. Identifiable to many by the S.S. HOPE, the world's first peacetime hospital ship, Project HOPE now conducts land-based medical training and health care education programs on five continents, including North America."

(continued)

Placement opportunities for . . .		**Organization/Service Specifics:**	
People of only certain faiths?	No	Size of the Organization's Staff:	>200
Couples: both are health providers?	Yes	Number of providers sent or received/year:	51-100
Couples: only one is a health provider?	Yes	Minimum term of assignment:	3 days
Families with children?	Yes	Maximum term of assignment:	None
Medical students?	No	Is funding available for travel?	Yes
Pre-medical or college students?	No	Are room and board provided?	Yes
Other health professional students?	No	Is any other funding available?	No
Doctors in training?	Yes	Is training provided or available?	Yes
Health personnel who are US citizens?	Yes	Is a language other than English required?	No
Health personnel who are non-US citizens?	Yes		
Health personnel with no prior experience in developing countries? *1*	Yes		
Health personnel who are not current members of your organization?	Yes		

Health Professionals Placed:

Physicians:

Physicians; Anesthesiologists; Cardiologists; Dermatologists; Emergency Medicine Physicians; Endocrinologists; Family Practitioners; Gastroenterologists; General Surgeons; Hematologists; Oncologists; Infectious Disease Spec.; Internal Medicine GPS & PCP; Nephrologists; OB/GYN; Oral Surgeons; Pediatricians; Pulmonary Specialists

Allied Health Professionals:

Dentists; Medical Technicians (lab, X-ray, etc); Nurse Midwives; Nurse Practitioners; Nurses; Nutritionists & Dieticians; Pharmacists; Physical & Occupational Therapists; Physician Assistants; Respiratory Therapists; Social Workers

Notes

1. Experience is sometimes required.

Project Open Hearts

Address: **14262 Jubilee Trl, Pine, CO 80470 U.S.A.**

Phone: **(303) 816-2736** FAX:

E-Mail: **info@poh.org** Web: **www.poh.org/index.html**

Continents Served

Africa ☑ Asia ☑ Europe ☑ The Americas ☐

Countries Served

Kazakhstan	Kenya	Mongolia
Palestine	Poland	Tanzania

Mission: Since 1994, Project Open Hearts has provided specialized cardiac services to many foreign countries. Volunteers work with foreign medical staff to provide first-hand surgical training, assistance with diagnostic procedures, and an on-going exchange of knowledge to continue the education process. The ultimate goal is to promote self sufficiency for the foreign medical staffs. We have an ongoing need for anesthesiologists, perfusionists, cardiologists, and OB-GYN doctors and nurses.

Placement opportunities for . . .		**Organization/Service Specifics:**	
People of only certain faiths?	No	Size of the Organization's Staff:	6-10
Couples: both are health providers?	Yes	Number of providers sent or received/year:	21-50
Couples: only one is a health provider?	No	Minimum term of assignment:	1 week
Families with children?	No	Maximum term of assignment:	
Medical students?	No	Is funding available for travel?	No
Pre-medical or college students?	No	Are room and board provided?	Yes
Other health professional students?	No	Is any other funding available?	No
Doctors in training?	No	Is training provided or available?	No
Health personnel who are US citizens?	Yes	Is a language other than English required? *1*	No
Health personnel who are non-US citizens?	Yes		
Health personnel with no prior experience in developing countries?	Yes		
Health personnel who are not current members of your organization?	Yes		

Health Professionals Placed: *2*

Physicians:

Anesthesiologists; Cardiologists; General Surgeons; OB/GYN

Allied Health Professionals:

Nurse Practitioners; Nurses

Notes

1. Foreign languages can be useful depending on project location;
2. Clinical engineers needed.

Project ORBIS International, Inc.

Address: **520 8th Avenue, 11th Floor, New York, NY 10018**

Phone: **(646) 674-5500** FAX: **(646) 674-5599**

E-Mail: **info@ny.orbis.org** Web: **www.orbis.org/**

Continents Served

Africa ☑ Asia ☑ Europe ☑ The Americas ☑

Countries Served

Bangladesh	Canada	China
Cuba	El Salvador	Ethiopia
Guinea	Guyana	Hong Kong
India	Mongolia	
Myanmar (Burma)		Nepal
Paraguay	Peru	Singapore
Syria	Taiwan	
Trinidad and Tobago		United States
USSR, former		Vietnam
Yugoslavia, former		

Mission: ORBIS is a non-profit humanitarian organization dedicated to fighting blindness worldwide through health education and hands-on training for opthalmologists, nurses, biomedical technicians, and health care workers. Since 1982, ORBIS has carried out more than 300 programs in over 70 countries. Programs take place in the ORBIS aircraft, a DC-10 jet converted into a fully equipped eye surgery hospital and teaching facility, and in local hospitals. Each week visiting volunteer doctors join ORBIS's 25 member international medical team to demonstrate surgery and share their skills hands-on with host country medical personnel. Volunteer assisgnments range from short term (3 weeks) to longer term (2 years). Travel and room and board are paid for and personnel receive a per diem stipend.

Placement opportunities for . . .

People of only certain faiths?	No
Couples: both are health providers?	Yes
Couples: only one is a health provider?	
Families with children?	No
Medical students?	No
Pre-medical or college students?	No
Other health professional students?	No
Doctors in training?	No
Health personnel who are US citizens?	Yes
Health personnel who are non-US citizens?	Yes
Health personnel with no prior experience in developing countries?	Yes
Health personnel who are not current members of your organization?	Yes

Organization/Service Specifics:

Size of the Organization's Staff:	51-100
Number of providers sent or received/year:	
Minimum term of assignment:	3 weeks
Maximum term of assignment:	2 years
Is funding available for travel?	Yes
Are room and board provided?	Yes
Is any other funding available? *1*	Yes
Is training provided or available?	Yes
Is a language other than English required?	No

Health Professionals Placed:

Physicians:

Anesthesiologists; Ophthalmologists

Allied Health Professionals:

Administrative Health Positions; Nurses

Notes

1. A per diem stipend is provided.

Project Skye

Address: **2941 Greenwood Dr., Joplin, MO 64804 U.S.A.**

Phone: **(417) 781-0951** FAX: **(417) 623-3387**

E-Mail: Web:

Continents Served

Africa ☐ Asia ☐ Europe ☐ The Americas ☑

Countries Served

Ecuador	El Salvador	Guatemala
Honduras	Peru	

Mission: Project Skye's purpose is to enhance a child's chance of survival in his or her world. This organization is dependent on supplies donated by St. John's Regional Medical Center. Volunteers can travel for 1 week assignments. There are no religious or language requirements. Volunteers are responsible for their own travel and room and board expenses.

Placement opportunities for . . .

People of only certain faiths?	No
Couples: both are health providers?	Yes
Couples: only one is a health provider?	No
Families with children?	No
Medical students?	No
Pre-medical or college students?	No
Other health professional students?	No
Doctors in training?	No
Health personnel who are US citizens?	Yes
Health personnel who are non-US citizens?	No
Health personnel with no prior experience in developing countries?	Yes
Health personnel who are not current members of your organization?	Yes

Organization/Service Specifics:

Size of the Organization's Staff:	0-5
Number of providers sent or received/year:	11-20
Minimum term of assignment:	1 week
Maximum term of assignment:	1 week
Is funding available for travel?	No
Are room and board provided?	No
Is any other funding available?	No
Is training provided or available?	No
Is a language other than English required?	No

(continued)

Health Professionals Placed:

Physicians:

Physicians

Allied Health Professionals:

Notes

PROMESA

Continents Served			
Africa ☐	Asia ☐	Europe ☐	The Americas ☑

Countries Served

Honduras

Address: **20 Kent St, Lower Level, Brookline, MA 02445 U.S.A.**

Phone: **(617) 730-4470** FAX: **(617) 730-4474**

E-Mail: **ljstern@partners.org** Web: **none**

Mission: The mission of PROMESA is to improve the health status, knowledge and self-reliance of the people of the Yeguare Region of Honduras by developing partner projects with families, communities and community based organizations and by training providers to understand the challenges and opportunities in providing health care in a developing country. The principles of the project reflect the basic premise that we can all learn from one another as we work towards these mutual goals, that we think creatively, encourage participation and learn by doing. Trips range from 1-6 months and there are no religious requirements for volunteers. Knowledge of Spanish is a requirement and volunteers must provide their own expenses.

Placement opportunities for . . .	
People of only certain faiths?	No
Couples: both are health providers?	Yes
Couples: only one is a health provider?	No
Families with children?	No
Medical students?	Yes
Pre-medical or college students?	No
Other health professional students?	Yes
Doctors in training?	Yes
Health personnel who are US citizens?	Yes
Health personnel who are non-US citizens?	Yes
Health personnel with no prior experience in developing countries?	No
Health personnel who are not current members of your organization?	Yes

Organization/Service Specifics:		
Size of the Organization's Staff:		0-5
Number of providers sent or received/year:		11-20
Minimum term of assignment:		1 month
Maximum term of assignment:		6 months
Is funding available for travel?		No
Are room and board provided?		No
Is any other funding available?		No
Is training provided or available?		Yes
Is a language other than English required?	*1*	Yes

Health Professionals Placed:

Physicians:

Emergency Medicine Physicians; Internal Medicine GPS & PCP; Pediatricians

Allied Health Professionals:

Dentists; Nurse Midwives; Nurses; Water/Sanitation Specialists

Notes

1. Spanish is required.

Remote Area Medical

Continents Served			
Africa ☐	Asia ☑	Europe ☐	The Americas ☑

Countries Served

Brazil, Dominican Republic, Guatemala, Guyana, Haiti, India, Mexico, United States, Venezuela

Address: **1834 Beech Street, Knoxville, TN 37920 U.S.A.**

Phone: **(865) 579-1530** FAX: **(865) 609-1876**

E-Mail: **ram@ramusa.org** Web: **www.ramusa.org**

Mission: Remote Area Medical (RAM) is a nonprofit, all volunteer medical relief corps serving remote and impoverished areas of the United States and abroad. RAM teams have completed over 260 expeditions and have provided $10 million of free medical, dental, eye, and veterinary care. Care is delivered to remote places, such as Amerindian Villages in South America, tiny mountain towns tucked away in Appalachia, and Native American reservations. Medical, premedical, and veterinary students are welcome provided that they are accompanied by an MD or DVM. Volunteer assignments range from 1 week to 6 months. Room and board are provided, although volunteers are responsible for their own travel expenses.

(continued)

Placement opportunities for . . .

People of only certain faiths?	No
Couples: both are health providers?	Yes
Couples: only one is a health provider?	Yes
Families with children?	No
Medical students? *1*	Yes
Pre-medical or college students? *1*	Yes
Other health professional students? *1*	Yes
Doctors in training?	Yes
Health personnel who are US citizens?	Yes
Health personnel who are non-US citizens?	Yes
Health personnel with no prior experience in developing countries?	Yes
Health personnel who are not current members of your organization?	Yes

Organization/Service Specifics:

Size of the Organization's Staff:	6-10
Number of providers sent or received/year:	>200
Minimum term of assignment:	1 week
Maximum term of assignment:	6 months
Is funding available for travel?	No
Are room and board provided? *2*	Yes
Is any other funding available?	No
Is training provided or available? *3*	Yes
Is a language other than English required? *4*	No

Health Professionals Placed:

Physicians:

Physicians; Anesthesiologists; Cardiologists; Dermatologists; Emergency Medicine Physicians; Endocrinologists; Family Practitioners; Gastroenterologists; General Surgeons; Hematologists; Oncologists; Infectious Disease Spec.; Internal Medicine GPS & PCP; OB/GYN; Ophthalmologists; Oral Surgeons; Optometrists; Orthopedic Surgeons; Otolaryngologists; Pediatricians; Plastic/Hand/Reconstructive Surgeons; Radiologists

Allied Health Professionals:

Administrative Health Positions; Dental Hygienists; Dentists; Medical Technicians (lab, X-ray, etc); Nurse Practitioners; Nurses; Nutritionists & Dieticians; Paramedics; Pharmacists; Physician Assistants; Public Health Specialists, Epidemiologists and Health Educators; Respiratory Therapists; Social Workers; Water/Sanitation Specialists

Notes

1. Med students, pre-med students, and other health professional students must be accompanied by an MD; *2.* Room and board are usually provided; *3.* There is limited training on the job; *4.* No language requirements, but interpreters are essential.

Saint Joseph's Medical Center, Family Practice Residency Program, Int'l Health Track

Address: **837 E. Cedar St., Suite 125, South Bend, IN 46617 U.S.A.**

Phone: **(574) 237-7637** FAX: **(574) 472-6088**

E-Mail: **ericsonk@sjrmc.com or residencyweb@sjrmc.com** Web: **www.saintjosephresidency.com/inthealth/**

Continents Served

Africa ☑ Asia ☑ Europe ☑ The Americas ☑

Countries Served

Argentina, Belize, Chile, Ecuador, Grenada, Guatemala, Guyana, Haiti, Honduras, Jamaica, Kenya, Malawi, Nepal, Nicaragua, Nigeria, Papua-New Guinea, Paraguay, Peru, Philippines, Tanzania, Trinidad and Tobago

Mission: The International Health Track (IHT) is a unique feature of the Saint Joseph's Family Practice Residency Program. It is an optional opportunity for residents interested in international health and healthcare for the medically underserved. The residency program offers financial assistance for a one- to two-week rotation the first year and two- to eight-week rotation in the second and third year in a medically underserved area in North America or overseas. Funding for travel and room and board is provided. There are no language or religious requirements.

Placement opportunities for . . .

People of only certain faiths?	No
Couples: both are health providers?	Yes
Couples: only one is a health provider?	Yes
Families with children?	Yes
Medical students?	No
Pre-medical or college students?	No
Other health professional students?	No
Doctors in training?	Yes
Health personnel who are US citizens?	Yes
Health personnel who are non-US citizens?	No
Health personnel with no prior experience in developing countries?	Yes
Health personnel who are not current members of your organization?	No

Organization/Service Specifics:

Size of the Organization's Staff:	0-5
Number of providers sent or received/year:	1-5
Minimum term of assignment:	2 weeks
Maximum term of assignment:	2 months
Is funding available for travel?	Yes
Are room and board provided?	Yes
Is any other funding available?	Yes
Is training provided or available?	Yes
Is a language other than English required?	No

(continued)

Health Professionals Placed:

Physicians:

Family Practitioners

Allied Health Professionals:

Notes

Salesian Missions

Continents Served

Africa ✔ Asia ☐ Europe ☐ The Americas ✔

Countries Served

Address: **2 Lefevre Lane, PO Box 30, New Rochelle, NY 10802-0030 U.S.A.**

Phone: **(914) 633-8344** FAX: **(914) 633-7404**

E-Mail: **slm@salesianmissions.org** Web: **http://salesianmissions.org**

Mission: Salesian Missions is a Catholic organization that seeks people of all Christian traditions. Funding is available for travel with a one-year minimum commitment. Shorter term commitments can also be accomodated by special-term arrangement. Salesian Missions serves 122 countries in various ways.

Placement opportunities for . . .

People of only certain faiths?	No
Couples: both are health providers?	Yes
Couples: only one is a health provider?	No
Families with children?	No
Medical students?	No
Pre-medical or college students?	No
Other health professional students?	Yes
Doctors in training?	No
Health personnel who are US citizens?	Yes
Health personnel who are non-US citizens?	No
Health personnel with no prior experience in developing countries?	Yes
Health personnel who are not current members of your organization?	Yes

Organization/Service Specifics:

Size of the Organization's Staff:	0-5
Number of providers sent or received/year:	1-5
Minimum term of assignment:	1 year
Maximum term of assignment:	3 year
Is funding available for travel?	Yes
Are room and board provided?	Yes
Is any other funding available?	No
Is training provided or available?	Yes
Is a language other than English required? *1*	Yes

Health Professionals Placed:

Physicians:

Family Practitioners; Internal Medicine GPS & PCP; Pediatricians

Allied Health Professionals:

Nurses; Social Workers

Notes

1. Conversational knowledge of language of country of service is required.

Sanyati Baptist Hospital, Baptist Convention of Zimbabwe

Continents Served

Africa ✔ Asia ☐ Europe ☐ The Americas ☐

Countries Served

Zimbabwe

Address: **P.O. BOX 250 Sanyati, Zimbabwe, Africa**

Phone: **Zim-68-72412** FAX:

E-Mail: **pboone@healthnet.zw** Web:

Mission: Sanyati Baptist Hospital strives to provide Christ-centered and excellent medical care to the people of our area of Zimbabwe. Volunteers are most often Baptists, although they will accept anyone who holds to Judeo-Christian precepts. Housing is provided for US $100/person/month or $150/couple/month. Volunteers need to pay for transport from/to Harare, a three-hour journey by car (longer by local bus). Renting a vehicle is very expensive. There is a minimum of 2 weeks and a maximum of 2 years in service.

(continued)

Placement opportunities for . . .	
People of only certain faiths? *1*	No
Couples: both are health providers?	Yes
Couples: only one is a health provider?	Yes
Families with children?	Yes
Medical students?	Yes
Pre-medical or college students?	No
Other health professional students?	No
Doctors in training?	Yes
Health personnel who are US citizens?	Yes
Health personnel who are non-US citizens?	Yes
Health personnel with no prior experience in developing countries?	Yes
Health personnel who are not current members of your organization?	Yes

Organization/Service Specifics:	
Size of the Organization's Staff:	51-100
Number of providers sent or received/year:	11-20
Minimum term of assignment:	2 weeks
Maximum term of assignment:	2 years
Is funding available for travel?	No
Are room and board provided? *2*	No
Is any other funding available?	No
Is training provided or available?	No
Is a language other than English required?	No

Health Professionals Placed:

Physicians:

Physicians; Emergency Medicine Physicians; Family Practitioners; General Surgeons; Infectious Disease Spec.; Internal Medicine GPS & PCP; OB/GYN; Ophthalmologists; Oral Surgeons; Orthopedic Surgeons; Otolaryngologists; Pediatricians; Urologists

Allied Health Professionals:

Dentists

Notes

1. Prefer Baptists but accept anyone who will respect traditional Judaeo-Christian precepts; *2.* Room is provided for a maintenance fee.

School Sisters of St. Francis

Address: **1501 South Layton Blvd., Milwaukee, WI 53215 U.S.A.**

Phone: **(414) 384-4105** FAX: **(414) 384-1950**

E-Mail: **generalate@sssf.org** Web: **www.sssf.org**

Mission: The School Sisters of St. Francis Mission is "to witness to the good news of Jesus and the presence of the reign of God as we enter into the lives and needs of people, especially the poor… Our focus is giving, healing and defending life."—Response in Faith

At the present time, we have requests for professional men and woman, age 23 and older, with at least one year's work experience, to work in North and Central America and Africa.

Continents Served

Africa ☑ Asia ☐ Europe ☑ The Americas ☑

Countries Served

Costa Rica, Germany, Guatemala, Honduras, India, Nicaragua, Switzerland, United States

Placement opportunities for . . .	
People of only certain faiths? *1*	Yes
Couples: both are health providers?	Yes
Couples: only one is a health provider?	Yes
Families with children?	Yes
Medical students?	Yes
Pre-medical or college students?	
Other health professional students?	Yes
Doctors in training?	No
Health personnel who are US citizens?	Yes
Health personnel who are non-US citizens?	No
Health personnel with no prior experience in developing countries?	Yes
Health personnel who are not current members of your organization?	Yes

Organization/Service Specifics:	
Size of the Organization's Staff:	>200
Number of providers sent or received/year:	21-50
Minimum term of assignment:	varies
Maximum term of assignment:	varies
Is funding available for travel? *2*	No
Are room and board provided?	Yes
Is any other funding available?	Yes
Is training provided or available?	Yes
Is a language other than English required? *3*	Yes

Health Professionals Placed:

Physicians:

Physicians; Emergency Medicine Physicians; Family Practitioners; General Surgeons; Hematologists; Oncologists; Infectious Disease Spec.; Internal Medicine GPS & PCP; OB/GYN; Ophthalmologists; Optometrists; Pediatricians; Radiologists

Allied Health Professionals:

Administrative Health Positions; Dental Hygienists; Dentists; Medical Technicians (lab, X-ray, etc); Nurse Midwives; Nurse Practitioners; Nurses; Pharmacists; Physical & Occupational Therapists; Physician Assistants; Podiatrists; Social Workers; Water/Sanitation Specialists

Notes

1. Christians of all denominations are welcome; *2.* Small stipend possible; *3.* Spanish.

Selian Lutheran Hospital

Continents Served

Africa ☑ Asia ☐ Europe ☐ The Americas ☐

Countries Served

Tanzania

Address: **P.O. Box 3164 Arusha, Tanzania, E. Africa**

Phone: **255 27 2503726** FAX:

E-Mail: **selianlh@habari.co.tz** Web: **http://selianlh.habari.co.tz/**

Mission: The mission of Selian Lutheran Hospital is to serve, treat, and minister to the whole person, in body, mind, and spirit. Selian Lutheran Hospital strives to attain this mission by providing competent and compassionate medical care, by promoting health development through community health projects, and by proclaiming the gospel of Jesus Christ. Volunteers must be Catholic or Protestant and Swahili is a required language.

Placement opportunities for . . .

People of only certain faiths? *1*	Yes
Couples: both are health providers?	Yes
Couples: only one is a health provider?	Yes
Families with children?	Yes
Medical students?	Yes
Pre-medical or college students?	Yes
Other health professional students?	No
Doctors in training?	Yes
Health personnel who are US citizens?	Yes
Health personnel who are non-US citizens?	No
Health personnel with no prior experience in developing countries?	Yes
Health personnel who are not current members of your organization?	Yes

Organization/Service Specifics:

Size of the Organization's Staff:	101-150
Number of providers sent or received/year:	1-5
Minimum term of assignment:	8 weeks
Maximum term of assignment:	
Is funding available for travel?	No
Are room and board provided?	Yes
Is any other funding available?	No
Is training provided or available?	Yes
Is a language other than English required? *2*	Yes

Health Professionals Placed:

Physicians:

Physicians

Allied Health Professionals:

Nurse Midwives; Nurse Practitioners

Notes

1. Volunteers must be Catholic or Protestant; *2.* Swahili is required.

Seva Foundation

Continents Served

Africa ☑ Asia ☑ Europe ☐ The Americas ☐

Countries Served

Cambodia, India, Macau, Nepal, Tanzania, Tibet

Address: **1876 5th St., Berkeley, CA 94710 U.S.A.**

Phone: **(510) 845-7382** FAX: **(510) 845-7410**

E-Mail: **admin@seva.org** Web: **www.seva.org**

Mission: Seva works to prevent blindness by supporting locally run programs in underserved communities. Seva emphasizes research, service and evaluation of community-based methods to provide high quality, high volume, and low cost cataract surgery. This effort has focused on two main partnerships: one with the Aravind Eye Hospital in India, the world's largest eye care program and the other with the Nepal Blindness Program. Volunteers can travel for 2-week to 1-year assignments. There are no religious or language requirements. While room and board are provided, volunteers must pay for their own travel expenses.

Placement opportunities for . . .

People of only certain faiths?	No
Couples: both are health providers?	Yes
Couples: only one is a health provider?	Yes
Families with children?	No
Medical students?	No
Pre-medical or college students?	No
Other health professional students?	Yes
Doctors in training? *1*	Yes
Health personnel who are US citizens?	Yes
Health personnel who are non-US citizens?	Yes
Health personnel with no prior experience in developing countries?	No
Health personnel who are not current members of your organization?	Yes

Organization/Service Specifics:

Size of the Organization's Staff:	11-20
Number of providers sent or received/year:	151-200
Minimum term of assignment:	2 weeks
Maximum term of assignment:	1 year
Is funding available for travel?	No
Are room and board provided?	Yes
Is any other funding available?	No
Is training provided or available?	No
Is a language other than English required?	No

(continued)

Health Professionals Placed:

Physicians:

Infectious Disease Spec.; Ophthalmologists; Pediatricians

Allied Health Professionals:

Nutritionists & Dieticians; Paramedics; Public Health Specialists, Epidemiologists and Health Educators; Social Workers

Notes

1. Fellows only.

SIM USA

Address: **P.O. Box 7900, Charlotte, NC 28241 U.S.A.**

Phone: **(704) 588-4300**
(800) 521-6449
FAX: **(704) 587-1518**

E-Mail: **postmaster@simusa.sim.org** Web: **www.sim.org**

Mission: The purpose of SIM is to glorify God by planting, strengthening, and partnering with churches around the world as we evangelize the unreached, minister to human need, disciple believers into churches, and equip churches to fulfill Christ's Commission. Volunteers can serve for shorter terms (4 weeks) to longer terms (9 months). There are no language requirements, but volunteers must be Protestants, committed to spreading the Gospel. Travel expenses must be provided by the volunteer, but room and board are provided by SIM.

Continents Served

Africa ☑ Asia ☑ Europe ☐ The Americas ☑

Countries Served

Angola	Benin	Burkina Faso
Chile	Ecuador	Ethiopia
Ghana	India	Liberia
Mongolia	Namibia	Nepal
Niger	Nigeria	Paraguay
Peru	South Africa	Zambia

Placement opportunities for . . .	
People of only certain faiths? *1*	Yes
Couples: both are health providers?	Yes
Couples: only one is a health provider?	Yes
Families with children?	No
Medical students?	Yes
Pre-medical or college students?	Yes
Other health professional students?	Yes
Doctors in training?	Yes
Health personnel who are US citizens?	Yes
Health personnel who are non-US citizens?	No
Health personnel with no prior experience in developing countries?	Yes
Health personnel who are not current members of your organization?	Yes

Organization/Service Specifics:	
Size of the Organization's Staff:	>200
Number of providers sent or received/year:	51-100
Minimum term of assignment:	4 weeks
Maximum term of assignment:	9 months
Is funding available for travel?	No
Are room and board provided?	Yes
Is any other funding available?	No
Is training provided or available?	Yes
Is a language other than English required?	No

Health Professionals Placed:

Physicians:

Physicians; General Surgeons; OB/GYN; Ophthalmologists; Plastic/Hand/Reconstructive Surgeons

Allied Health Professionals:

Nurses; Pharmacists; Physical & Occupational Therapists

Notes

1. Volunteers must be Protestant.

Siméus Foundation, The

Address: **812 South 5th Avenue Mansfield, TX U.S.A.**

Phone: **(817) 473-5246** FAX: **(817) 473-7886**

E-Mail: **vdickey@simeus foundation.org** Web: **www.simeus foundation.org**

Continents Served

Africa ☐ Asia ☐ Europe ☐ The Americas ☑

Countries Served

Haiti

Mission: The Siméus Foundation strives to improve the standard of living for the poor of Haiti by providing essential medical care, clean water, education, nutritional services, and clothing. The Siméus Foundation engages the community in all of our initiatives so that the projects are self-sustaining and provide the community with jobs and a sense of pride. The Siméus Foundation opened a full-time medical clinic in Pont-Sondé, Haiti which employees Haitian doctors on a permanent basis but still depends and benefits from the efforts of volunteer healtcare workers worldwide.

(continued)

Placement opportunities for . . .	
People of only certain faiths?	No
Couples: both are health providers?	Yes
Couples: only one is a health provider?	Yes
Families with children?	No
Medical students?	Yes
Pre-medical or college students?	Yes
Other health professional students?	Yes
Doctors in training?	Yes
Health personnel who are US citizens?	Yes
Health personnel who are non-US citizens?	Yes
Health personnel with no prior experience in developing countries?	Yes
Health personnel who are not current members of your organization?	Yes

Organization/Service Specifics:	
Size of the Organization's Staff:	0-5
Number of providers sent or received/year:	11-20
Minimum term of assignment: *1*	2 days
Maximum term of assignment:	none
Is funding available for travel?	No
Are room and board provided?	Yes
Is any other funding available?	No
Is training provided or available?	Yes
Is a language other than English required? *2*	

Health Professionals Placed:

Physicians:

All physician specialties

Allied Health Professionals:

All allied health professionals

Notes

1. Usually 5 days-1 week;
2. Creole or French helpful and some level of literacy recommended.

Sister Community Alliances: Ouelessebougou-Utah Alliance

Continents Served
Africa ☑ Asia ☐ Europe ☐ The Americas ☐

Countries Served
Mali

Address: **10 West 100 South, Suite 605, Salt Lake City, UT 84101 U.S.A.**

Phone: **(801) 983-6254** FAX: **(801) 978-9565**

E-Mail: **info@sistercommunity.org** Web: **www.sistercommunity.org**

Mission: The Ouelessebougou-Utah Alliance is committed to assist the people of the Ouelessebougou Region in Mali, West Africa, through a long-term development relationship. The Alliance works in partnership with village citizens to achieve their economic, health care, and community development objectives, and provides the opportunity for both cultures to learn from the other's family and social relationships. French skills are helpful for short term assignments (1 week) and are required for long term assignments (6 months). Room and board are provided, but volunteers must pay for their own travel expenses.

Placement opportunities for . . .	
People of only certain faiths?	No
Couples: both are health providers?	Yes
Couples: only one is a health provider?	Yes
Families with children?	No
Medical students?	Yes
Pre-medical or college students?	No
Other health professional students?	Yes
Doctors in training?	Yes
Health personnel who are US citizens?	Yes
Health personnel who are non-US citizens?	Yes
Health personnel with no prior experience in developing countries?	Yes
Health personnel who are not current members of your organization?	Yes

Organization/Service Specifics:	
Size of the Organization's Staff:	6-10
Number of providers sent or received/year:	6-10
Minimum term of assignment:	1 weeks
Maximum term of assignment:	6 months
Is funding available for travel?	No
Are room and board provided?	Yes
Is any other funding available?	No
Is training provided or available?	Yes
Is a language other than English required? *1*	Yes

Health Professionals Placed:

Physicians:

Physicians; Anesthesiologists; Emergency Medicine Physicians; General Surgeons; Infectious Disease Spec.; OB/GYN; Ophthalmologists; Oral Surgeons; Optometrists; Plastic/Hand/Reconstructive Surgeons

Allied Health Professionals:

Dental Hygienists; Medical Technicians (lab, X-ray, etc); Nurse Practitioners; Nurses; Pharmacists; Physician Assistants; Public Health Specialists, Epidemiologists and Health Educators; Water/Sanitation Specialists

Notes

1. French language skills are helpful for short-term assignments and required for long-term assignments.

SkillShare International

Continents Served
Africa ☑ Asia ☑ Europe ☐ The Americas ☐

Countries Served
Botswana, India, Lesotho, Mozambique, Namibia, South Africa, Swaziland, Tanzania, Uganda

Address: **126 New Walk Leicester, LEI 7JA U.K.**
Phone: **+44 (0) 116 254-1862** FAX: **+44 (0) 116 254-2614**
E-Mail: **info@skillshare.org** Web: **www.skillshare.org**

Mission: SkillShare International works for sustainable development in partnership with people and communities in nine countries: Botswana, Lesotho, India, Mozambique, Namibia, Swaziland, South Africa, Tanzania, and Uganda. Communities come to SkillShare International with specific needs, and SkillShare seeks to provide a route for those needs to be fulfilled. The bulk of SkillShare's work is in education and vocational training, agriculture, health, HIV and AIDS, engineering and planning, the environment and income generation initiatives. These incorporate rural development, empowering disadvantaged groups and improving opportunities for young people. SkillShare prefers to place UK or European health care providers for relatively long (1 year and more) stays. There are no religious requirements, and language requirements depend upon posting.

Placement opportunities for . . .	
People of only certain faiths?	No
Couples: both are health providers?	Yes
Couples: only one is a health provider?	Yes
Families with children?	No
Medical students?	No
Pre-medical or college students?	No
Other health professional students?	Yes
Doctors in training?	No
Health personnel who are US citizens?	No
Health personnel who are non-US citizens? *1*	Yes
Health personnel with no prior experience in developing countries?	Yes
Health personnel who are not current members of your organization?	Yes

Organization/Service Specifics:	
Size of the Organization's Staff:	21-50
Number of providers sent or received/year:	6-10
Minimum term of assignment:	1 year
Maximum term of assignment: *2*	2 years
Is funding available for travel?	Yes
Are room and board provided?	Yes
Is any other funding available? *3*	Yes
Is training provided or available?	Yes
Is a language other than English required? *4*	Yes

Health Professionals Placed:

Physicians:

Physicians; Family Practitioners; Internal Medicine GPS & PCP

Allied Health Professionals:

Nurse Midwives; Nurses; Physical & Occupational Therapists; Public Health Specialists, Epidemiologists and Health Educators

Notes

1. Perference to UK or European citizens as the interview process is lengthy; *2.* Two-year terms can be extended, depending on the program; *3.* Annual stipend of approximately £1500 is provided; *4.* Language requirements depend on the placement.

Sons of Mary Missionary Society

Continents Served
Africa ☐ Asia ☑ Europe ☐ The Americas ☑

Countries Served
Honduras, Peru, Philippines, Venezuela

Address: **567 Salem End Road, Framingham, MA 01702-5599 U.S.A.**
Phone: **(508) 879-2541** FAX: **(508) 879-7667**
E-Mail: **kevin@sonsofmary.com** Web: **www.sonsofmary.com**

Mission: The Sons of Mary Missionaries, founded by Father Edward F. Garesche in 1952, strives to bring and discover the healing love of Jesus Christ through medical, catechetical and social apostolates. Working in smaller villages in the Americas, these missionaries spread the love of God by healing the sick and the poor.

(continued)

Placement opportunities for . . .

People of only certain faiths? *1*	Yes
Couples: both are health providers?	Yes
Couples: only one is a health provider?	No
Families with children?	No
Medical students?	No
Pre-medical or college students?	No
Other health professional students?	No
Doctors in training?	Yes
Health personnel who are US citizens?	No
Health personnel who are non-US citizens?	No
Health personnel with no prior experience in developing countries?	Yes
Health personnel who are not current members of your organization?	No

Organization/Service Specifics:

Size of the Organization's Staff:	21-50
Number of providers sent or received/year:	1-5
Minimum term of assignment:	1 year
Maximum term of assignment:	3 years
Is funding available for travel?	No
Are room and board provided?	Yes
Is any other funding available?	No
Is training provided or available?	No
Is a language other than English required? *2*	Yes

Health Professionals Placed:

Physicians:

Physicians

Allied Health Professionals:

Nurses; Public Health Specialists, Epidemiologists and Health Educators; Social Workers

Notes

1. Catholic; *2.* Tagalog (Preferred).

Special Olympics, Inc.

Address: **1133 19th Street, N.W., Washington, DC 20036-3604 U.S.A.**

Phone: **(202) 628-3630** FAX: **(202) 824-0200**

E-Mail: **mwagner@specialolympics.org** Web: **www.specialolympics.org**

Continents Served

Africa ☑ Asia ☑ Europe ☑ The Americas ☑

Countries Served

1

Mission: Special Olympics empowers people with intellectual disabilities to realize their full potential and develop their skills through year-round sports training and competition. The Special Olympics Healthy Athletes initiative was developed because Special Olympics athletes cannot participate successfully in their sport unless they maintain good fitness and are in good health. During a Health Athletes event, Special Olympics athletes receive a variety of free health screenings and services provided by volunteer health care professionals in a series of clinics conducted in a welcoming, fun environment. Volunteer health care professionals and students are trained to provide the screenings in an effort to educate the professional community about the health needs and abilities of persons with intellectual and developmental disabilities.

Placement opportunities for . . .

People of only certain faiths?	No
Couples: both are health providers?	Yes
Couples: only one is a health provider?	Yes
Families with children?	Yes
Medical students?	Yes
Pre-medical or college students?	
Other health professional students?	Yes
Doctors in training?	Yes
Health personnel who are US citizens?	Yes
Health personnel who are non-US citizens?	Yes
Health personnel with no prior experience in developing countries?	Yes
Health personnel who are not current members of your organization?	Yes

Organization/Service Specifics:

Size of the Organization's Staff:	>200
Number of providers sent or received/year:	>200
Minimum term of assignment:	1 week
Maximum term of assignment:	
Is funding available for travel?	No
Are room and board provided?	No
Is any other funding available?	No
Is training provided or available?	Yes
Is a language other than English required?	No

Health Professionals Placed:

Physicians:

Physicians; Emergency Medicine Physicians; Endocrinologists; Family Practitioners; Gastroenterologists; General Surgeons; Infectious Disease Spec.; Internal Medicine GPS & PCP; Nephrologists; Neurologists; Ophthalmologists; Oral Surgeons; Optometrists; Orthopedic Surgeons; Otolaryngologists; Pediatricians

Allied Health Professionals:

Dental Hygienists; Dentists; Medical Technicians (lab, X-ray, etc); Nurse Practitioners; Nurses; Nutritionists & Dieticians; Paramedics; Physical & Occupational Therapists; Physician Assistants; Podiatrists; Public Health Specialists, Epidemiologists and Health Educators; Respiratory Therapists; Social Workers

Notes

1. Countries not specified.

St. Francis Hospital

Address: **Private Bag 11 Katete, Zambia, Africa**

Phone: **(260) 625-2210** FAX: **(260) 625-2278**

E-Mail: **stfrhosp@zmnet.zm** Web:

Continents Served

Africa ☑ Asia ☐ Europe ☐ The Americas ☐

Countries Served

Zambia

Mission: St. Francis Hospital, Katete, Zambia is a very busy 350 bed general hospital, jointly administered by the Anglican and Roman Catholic churches. It is in the hilly Eastern province of Zambia where most people live by subsistence agriculture. It has two nursing schools—one for general nursing and one for midwifery—and is the centre of a network of fourteen rural clinics which serve a population of 157,000. It also acts as referral center for surgery for the whole of the province of one million people. Students can volunteer for a minimum of 6 weeks while more qualified personnel must stay for a minimum of 3 months. Room and board are provided, but volunteers must provide their own travel expenses. There are no religious or language requirements.

Placement opportunities for . . .		Organization/Service Specifics:	
People of only certain faiths?	No	Size of the Organization's Staff: *1*	>200
Couples: both are health providers?	Yes	Number of providers sent or received/year:	6-10
Couples: only one is a health provider?	Yes	Minimum term of assignment: *2*	6 weeks
Families with children?	Yes	Maximum term of assignment:	
Medical students?	Yes	Is funding available for travel?	No
Pre-medical or college students?	Yes	Are room and board provided?	Yes
Other health professional students?	Yes	Is any other funding available?	No
Doctors in training?	Yes	Is training provided or available?	Yes
Health personnel who are US citizens?	Yes	Is a language other than English required?	No
Health personnel who are non-US citizens?	Yes		
Health personnel with no prior experience in developing countries?	Yes		
Health personnel who are not current members of your organization?	Yes		

Health Professionals Placed:

Physicians:

Physicians; Family Practitioners; General Surgeons; Internal Medicine GPS & PCP; OB/GYN; Ophthalmologists; Pediatricians

Allied Health Professionals:

Dentists; Medical Technicians (lab, X-ray, etc); Nurse Midwives; Nurse Practitioners; Nurses; Pharmacists; Physical & Occupational Therapists; Physician Assistants

Notes

1. Did not reply to email inquiry 2/05; *2.* There is a 6-week minimum for students, 3-month minimum for qualified personnel.

St. John's Medical College

Address: **Sarjapur Road Bangalore 560 034, Karnataka India**

Phone: **(080) 553-0724** FAX: **91 80 25 53 1786**

E-Mail: Web:

Continents Served

Africa ☐ Asia ☑ Europe ☐ The Americas ☐

Countries Served

India

Mission: St. John's Medical College was founded by the Catholic Bishops of India. Part of St. John's National Academy of Health Sciences, it has a nursing college, a 1200 bed hospital and an Institute for Para-Medical Training programs. Our thrust is on service to the underpriviledged of our country and students are trained with this mission in mind. We also have a well structured syllabus in Medical Ethics for both medical and nursing students.

Placement opportunities for . . .		Organization/Service Specifics:	
People of only certain faiths?	No	Size of the Organization's Staff: *1*	>200
Couples: both are health providers?	No	Number of providers sent or received/year:	>200
Couples: only one is a health provider?	No	Minimum term of assignment:	4 weeks
Families with children?	No	Maximum term of assignment:	8 weeks
Medical students?	Yes	Is funding available for travel?	No
Pre-medical or college students?	No	Are room and board provided?	No
Other health professional students?	Yes	Is any other funding available?	No
Doctors in training?	Yes	Is training provided or available?	Yes
Health personnel who are US citizens?	Yes	Is a language other than English required?	No
Health personnel who are non-US citizens?	Yes		
Health personnel with no prior experience in developing countries?	Yes		
Health personnel who are not current members of your organization?	Yes		

(continued)

Health Professionals Placed:

Physicians:

Physicians; Anesthesiologists; Cardiologists; Dermatologists; Endocrinologists; Family Practitioners; Gastroenterologists; General Surgeons; Hematologists; Oncologists; Infectious Disease Spec.; Internal Medicine GPS & PCP; Nephrologists; Neurologists; Neurosurgeons; OB/GYN; Ophthalmologists; Oral Surgeons; Orthopedic Surgeons; Otolaryngologists; Pathologists; Pediatricians; Plastic/Hand/Reconstructive Surgeons; Psychiatrists; Pulmonary Specialists; Radiologists; Urologists

Allied Health Professionals:

Administrative Health Positions; Dentists; Medical Technicians (lab, X-ray, etc); Nurse Midwives; Nurses; Nutritionists & Dieticians; Paramedics; Pharmacists; Physical & Occupational Therapists; Psychologists; Public Health Specialists, Epidemiologists and Health Educators; Social Workers; Water/Sanitation Specialists

Notes

1. Last contacted 08/02.

St. Jude Hospital

Address: **Box 331, Vieux Fort, St. Lucia, West Indies**

Phone: **(809) 454-6041** FAX:

E-Mail: Web: **www.stjudeswebsite.org**

Continents Served

Africa ☐ Asia ☐ Europe ☐ The Americas ☑

Countries Served

St. Lucia

Mission: St. Jude Hospital, operating under the principles of the Catholic Church, is a health care facility that will render inpatient and outpatient care consisting of primary and specialty services with a medical education component including medical students, residents and other professional entities. St. Jude will function as a good employer recognizing the dignity and value of all staff irrespective of position at the hospital. Additionally, as business entity within the Vieux Fort Area and St. Lucia, St. Jude will operate within the parameters of good business principles and ethics.

Placement opportunities for . . .

People of only certain faiths?	No
Couples: both are health providers?	Yes
Couples: only one is a health provider?	Yes
Families with children?	Yes
Medical students?	Yes
Pre-medical or college students?	No
Other health professional students?	No
Doctors in training?	Yes
Health personnel who are US citizens?	Yes
Health personnel who are non-US citizens?	Yes
Health personnel with no prior experience in developing countries?	Yes
Health personnel who are not current members of your organization?	Yes

Organization/Service Specifics:

Size of the Organization's Staff: *1*	>200
Number of providers sent or received/year:	51-100
Minimum term of assignment:	1 month
Maximum term of assignment:	1 year
Is funding available for travel?	No
Are room and board provided?	Yes
Is any other funding available?	No
Is training provided or available?	Yes
Is a language other than English required?	No

Health Professionals Placed:

Physicians:

Physicians; Anesthesiologists; Cardiologists; Dermatologists; Emergency Medicine Physicians; Endocrinologists; Family Practitioners; General Surgeons; Internal Medicine GPS & PCP; OB/GYN; Ophthalmologists; Oral Surgeons; Optometrists; Orthopedic Surgeons; Pathologists; Pediatricians; Psychiatrists; Radiologists; Urologists

Allied Health Professionals:

Administrative Health Positions; Dental Hygienists; Dentists; Medical Technicians (lab, X-ray, etc); Nurse Midwives; Nurse Practitioners; Nurses; Paramedics; Pharmacists; Physical & Occupational Therapists; Physician Assistants; Prosthetists; Psychologists

Notes

1. Last contacted 4/04.

St. Mary's Hospital, Vunapope

Continents Served
Africa ☐ Asia ☑ Europe ☐ The Americas ☐

Countries Served
Papua-New Guinea

Address: **P.O. Box 58, Kokopo, Papua New Guinea**

Phone: **0116759828301** FAX: **0116759828301**

E-Mail: **stmarys@online.net.pg** Web:

Mission: St. Mary's Hospital is a two hundred bed private hospital providing general medical care to supplement nearby government hospitals. Doctors are essentially expats, with yearly turnover. Because of increasing problems in the government health program, there is increasing urgency for this hopital to continue in the region for some years to come. Travel expenses are paid for in certain cases, and room, but not board, is provided. There are no religious or language requirements, although Pidgin English is widely spoken.

Placement opportunities for . . .

People of only certain faiths?	No
Couples: both are health providers? *2*	Yes
Couples: only one is a health provider?	Yes
Families with children? *3*	Yes
Medical students?	Yes
Pre-medical or college students?	No
Other health professional students?	No
Doctors in training?	No
Health personnel who are US citizens?	Yes
Health personnel who are non-US citizens?	Yes
Health personnel with no prior experience in developing countries?	Yes
Health personnel who are not current members of your organization?	Yes

Organization/Service Specifics:

Size of the Organization's Staff: *1*	0-5
Number of providers sent or received/year:	1-5
Minimum term of assignment: *4*	6 months
Maximum term of assignment:	life
Is funding available for travel? *5*	Yes
Are room and board provided? *6*	Yes
Is any other funding available? *7*	Yes
Is training provided or available?	No
Is a language other than English required?	No

Health Professionals Placed:

Physicians:

Physicians; Family Practitioners; General Surgeons; OB/GYN

Allied Health Professionals:

Dental Hygienists; Dentists; Medical Technicians (lab, X-ray, etc)

Notes

1. Last contacted 8/02. No reply 2/05; *2.* Depends on the specialty; *3.* Depends on the age of the children; *4.* Short-term assignments only. Must pay their own way; *5.* In selected cases; *6.* Room only is provided; *7.* Doctors receive a stipend from the state.

Surfer's Medical Association

Continents Served
Africa ☐ Asia ☑ Europe ☐ The Americas ☐

Countries Served
Fiji

Address: **Box 1210, Aptos, CA 95001 U.S.A.**

Phone: **(831) 684-0916** FAX:

E-Mail: **SMACentral@aol.com** Web: **www.damoon.net/sma/index.html**

Mission: The Surfer's Medical Association is an international organization of surfers committed to helping all surfers be healthier. The organization consists of surfing physicians and other health professionals, and scientists (surfers interested in the health and medical aspects of surfing). During annual conferences on the Fijian island of Tavarua, SMA conducts clinics and gives medical updates on the health problems of surfers to local health care workers.

Placement opportunities for . . .

People of only certain faiths?	No
Couples: both are health providers?	Yes
Couples: only one is a health provider?	Yes
Families with children?	No
Medical students?	No
Pre-medical or college students?	No
Other health professional students?	No
Doctors in training?	No
Health personnel who are US citizens?	Yes
Health personnel who are non-US citizens?	Yes
Health personnel with no prior experience in developing countries?	Yes
Health personnel who are not current members of your organization?	Yes

Organization/Service Specifics:

Size of the Organization's Staff:	0-5
Number of providers sent or received/year:	6-10
Minimum term of assignment: *1*	1 week
Maximum term of assignment: *1*	2 weeks
Is funding available for travel?	No
Are room and board provided?	No
Is any other funding available?	No
Is training provided or available?	No
Is a language other than English required?	No

(continued)

Health Professionals Placed:

Physicians:

Not specified

Allied Health Professionals:

Not specified

Notes

1. Depends on conference length.

Surgical Eye Expeditions International (S.E.E.), Inc.

Address: **27 E. De La Guerra St., Suite C-2, Santa Barbara, CA 93101 U.S.A.**

Phone: **(800) 208-6733** **(805) 963-3303** FAX: **(805) 965-3564**

E-Mail: **info@seeintl.org or seeintl@seeintl.org** Web: **www.seeintl.org**

Mission: Founded in 1974, Surgical Eye Expeditions (S.E.E.) International Inc., a non-profit organization, provides free opthalmic medical, surgical, and educational services by volunteer professionals to benefit disadvantaged, sight-impaired individuals in the United States and throughout the world. Volunteers can travel for 1-week assignments. Room and board are sometimes provided, although volunteers are responsible for their own travel expenses. There are no language or religious requirements.

Continents Served

Africa ✔ Asia ✔ Europe ✔ The Americas ✔

Countries Served

Brazil	Bulgaria	China
El Salvador	Ethiopia	Fiji
Ghana	Guatemala	Haiti
Honduras	India	Jamaica
Kenya	Mexico	
Myanmar (Burma)		Nepal
Nigeria	Panama	
Papua-New Guinea		Peru
Philippines	Romania	Rwanda
Sierra Leone	Solomon Islands	
Tanzania	Thailand	Tonga
Vanuatu	Vietnam	Zambia
Zimbabwe		

Placement opportunities for . . .

People of only certain faiths?		No
Couples: both are health providers?		Yes
Couples: only one is a health provider?	*1*	Yes
Families with children?		Yes
Medical students?		No
Pre-medical or college students?		No
Other health professional students?		No
Doctors in training?		No
Health personnel who are US citizens?		Yes
Health personnel who are non-US citizens?		Yes
Health personnel with no prior experience in developing countries?		Yes
Health personnel who are not current members of your organization?		Yes

Organization/Service Specifics:

Size of the Organization's Staff:		6-10
Number of providers sent or received/year:		>200
Minimum term of assignment:	*2*	1 week
Maximum term of assignment:	*2*	1 week
Is funding available for travel?		No
Are room and board provided?	*3*	Yes
Is any other funding available?	*4*	No
Is training provided or available?		No
Is a language other than English required?	*5*	No

Health Professionals Placed: *6*

Physicians:

Physicians; Anesthesiologists; Emergency Medicine Physicians; Family Practitioners; General Surgeons; Internal Medicine GPS & PCP; Neurologists; Pediatricians

Allied Health Professionals:

Nurse Practitioners; Nurses

Notes

1. Each medical volunteer is placed strictly according to need. Although a situation could arise where a medically trained couple could serve together, it is rare; *2.* Assignments are 1-2 weeks; *3.* Room and board are sometimes provided; *4.* Monthly stipend provided; *5.* Second languages are helpful; *6.* Surgeons and anesthesiologists only asked to serve a minimum of six weeks.

Surgical Medical Assistance Relief Teams

Address: **P.O. 444, Springhill, KS 66083 U.S.A.**

Phone: **(913) 338-1234**
(913) 814-3700
FAX: **(913) 338-2890**

E-Mail: **teresa.searcy@smart teams.org**
Web: **www.smartteams.org/**

Continents Served
Africa ☐ Asia ☐ Europe ☐ The Americas ☑

Countries Served
El Salvador Guatemala Honduras

Mission: Surgical Medical Assistance Relief Teams (S.M.A.R.T.) provides surgical, medical and dental services to over 25,000 needy children in Honduras, Guatemala, El Salvador, and Ecuador. Health care volunteers are always needed. Past volunteers maintain that their time spent on a S.M.A.R.T. trip ranks as one of the most rewarding experiences of their medical career.

Placement opportunities for . . .	
People of only certain faiths?	No
Couples: both are health providers?	Yes
Couples: only one is a health provider?	Yes
Families with children? *1*	Yes
Medical students?	Yes
Pre-medical or college students?	Yes
Other health professional students?	Yes
Doctors in training?	Yes
Health personnel who are US citizens?	Yes
Health personnel who are non-US citizens?	Yes
Health personnel with no prior experience in developing countries?	Yes
Health personnel who are not current members of your organization?	Yes

Organization/Service Specifics:	
Size of the Organization's Staff:	0-5
Number of providers sent or received/year:	101-150
Minimum term of assignment:	5 days
Maximum term of assignment:	5 days
Is funding available for travel?	No
Are room and board provided?	Yes
Is any other funding available?	No
Is training provided or available?	No
Is a language other than English required? *2*	No

Health Professionals Placed: *3*

Physicians:

Physicians; Anesthesiologists; Cardiologists; Family Practitioners; General Surgeons; Neurologists; OB/GYN; Ophthalmologists; Oral Surgeons; Orthopedic Surgeons; Pediatricians; Urologists

Allied Health Professionals:

Dentists; Nurses

Notes

1. 13 yrs or older; *2.* Spanish is very helpful; *3.* Other speciality health care workers encouraged to apply. Chiropractors also needed.

Surgicorps International

Address: **1471 Glen Ave, Glenshaw, PA 15116 U.S.A.**

Phone: **(724) 443-5115**
FAX: **(724) 443-5129**

E-Mail: **info@surgicorps.org**
Web: **www.surgicorps.org/index2.html**

Continents Served
Africa ☑ Asia ☑ Europe ☐ The Americas ☑

Countries Served
Brazil Guatemala India
Paraguay South Africa Tanzania
Vietnam

Mission: Surgicorps International is a non-profit organization based out of Pittsburgh which travels to offer surgical services to indigent patients in need worldwide. The teams aim to provide training to local healthcare professionals in addition to providing medical services. Surgicorps organizes 2-3 trips each year with 20 volunteers (medical and some non-medical) needed for each trip.

Placement opportunities for . . .	
People of only certain faiths?	No
Couples: both are health providers?	Yes
Couples: only one is a health provider?	Yes
Families with children?	No
Medical students?	Yes
Pre-medical or college students?	Yes
Other health professional students?	Yes
Doctors in training?	Yes
Health personnel who are US citizens?	Yes
Health personnel who are non-US citizens?	No
Health personnel with no prior experience in developing countries?	Yes
Health personnel who are not current members of your organization?	Yes

Organization/Service Specifics:	
Size of the Organization's Staff:	0-5
Number of providers sent or received/year:	21-50
Minimum term of assignment:	1 week
Maximum term of assignment:	15 days
Is funding available for travel?	No
Are room and board provided?	No
Is any other funding available?	No
Is training provided or available?	Yes
Is a language other than English required?	No

(continued)

Health Professionals Placed:

Physicians:

Physicians; Anesthesiologists; General Surgeons; Oral Surgeons; Plastic/Hand/Reconstructive Surgeons

Allied Health Professionals:

Nurses; Physical & Occupational Therapists; Physician Assistants

Notes

Trinity Health International

Address: **34605 Twelve Mile Road, Farmington Hills, MI 48331-3293 U.S.A.**

Phone: **(248) 489-6100** FAX: **(248) 489-6102**

E-Mail: **International@trinity-health.org** Web: **www.mercyinternational.com/**

Mission: Trinity Health, fomerly Holy Cross Health System and Mercy Health Services, is one of the largest non-profit Catholic healthcare systems in the United States. It conducts over 150 projects in 39 undeveloped and developed countries in Africa, Asia, the Americas, and Europe. Services include but are not limited to technical assistance, hospital management, consulting services, and training programs. There are no religious or language restrictions. Trinity Health seeks health providers who can be staffed on projects for short (1 week) to longer term (3 year) stays.

Continents Served

Africa ✔ Asia ✔ Europe ✔ The Americas ✔

Countries Served

Argentina	Australia	Bahamas
Bahrain	Brazil	
Caroline Islands		Croatia
Cuba	Egypt	Fiji
Guam	Guyana	India
Ireland	Jordan	Kenya
Korea, South	Kuwait	Lithuania
Malaysia	Marshall Islands	
Mexico	Nauru	New Zealand
Nicaragua	Northern Mariana Isl.	
Palau	Palestine	Russia
Samoa	Saudi Arabia	Sri Lanka
Tanzania	Trinidad and Tobago	
Ukraine	United Kingdom	
United States	Zimbabwe	

Placement opportunities for . . .

People of only certain faiths?	No
Couples: both are health providers?	Yes
Couples: only one is a health provider?	Yes
Families with children?	Yes
Medical students?	No
Pre-medical or college students?	No
Other health professional students?	Yes
Doctors in training?	No
Health personnel who are US citizens?	Yes
Health personnel who are non-US citizens?	Yes
Health personnel with no prior experience in developing countries?	Yes
Health personnel who are not current members of your organization?	Yes

Organization/Service Specifics:

Size of the Organization's Staff:	11-20
Number of providers sent or received/year:	>200
Minimum term of assignment:	1 week
Maximum term of assignment:	3 years
Is funding available for travel? *1*	Yes
Are room and board provided?	Yes
Is any other funding available?	Yes
Is training provided or available?	Yes
Is a language other than English required? *2*	No

Health Professionals Placed:

Physicians:

Physicians; Family Practitioners

Allied Health Professionals:

Administrative Health Positions; Public Health Specialists, Epidemiologists and Health Educators

Notes

1. Funding for travel is mostly provided; *2.* There are no language requirements, but language skills are helpful.

Tulane University School of Public Health and Tropical Medicine

Address: **1440 Canal St., Suite 2200, New Orleans, LA 70112 U.S.A.**

Phone: **(504) 988-3655** FAX: **(504) 988-3653**

E-Mail: **pjessop@tulane.edu** Web: **www.tulane.edu/~inhl/inhl.htm**

Continents Served

Africa ☑ Asia ☑ Europe ☐ The Americas ☑

Countries Served

Costa Rica	Cuba	Guatemala
Kenya	Rwanda	South Africa
Sri Lanka	Thailand	Zimbabwe

Mission: The Department of International Health and Development is dedicated to improving the health status of populations throughout the world. The teaching and research programs emphasize interdisciplinary, creative problem-solving in the health and social sectors. The teaching program addresses the needs of young and mid-career professionals who intend to work outside the United States, with international organizations, or in multicultural contexts. The curriculum and applied learning opportunities draw upon Tulane's extensive overseas research, technical assistance work, and more than twenty years of experience in providing leadership training in international health to students from around the world.

Placement opportunities for . . .

People of only certain faiths?	No
Couples: both are health providers?	Yes
Couples: only one is a health provider?	Yes
Families with children?	Yes
Medical students?	Yes
Pre-medical or college students?	No
Other health professional students?	Yes
Doctors in training?	Yes
Health personnel who are US citizens?	Yes
Health personnel who are non-US citizens?	Yes
Health personnel with no prior experience in developing countries?	Yes
Health personnel who are not current members of your organization? *1*	No

Organization/Service Specifics:

Size of the Organization's Staff:	21-50
Number of providers sent or received/year:	151-200
Minimum term of assignment:	300 hours
Maximum term of assignment:	
Is funding available for travel?	No
Are room and board provided?	No
Is any other funding available?	No
Is training provided or available?	Yes
Is a language other than English required?	No

Health Professionals Placed:

Physicians:

Physicians; Emergency Medicine Physicians; Infectious Disease Spec.; Internal Medicine GPS & PCP; OB/GYN; Pediatricians; Psychiatrists

Allied Health Professionals:

Administrative Health Positions; Nurse Midwives; Nurse Practitioners; Nurses; Nutritionists & Dieticians; Psychologists; Public Health Specialists, Epidemiologists and Health Educators; Respiratory Therapists; Social Workers

Notes

1. All personnel must be from Tulane.

UCSD, Division of International Health

Address: **UCSD School of Medicine, 0622,9500 Gilman Drive, La Jolla, CA 92093-0622 U.S.A.**

Phone: **(858) 822-6468** FAX: **(858) 534-4642**

E-Mail: **jevera@ucsd.edu** Web: **medicine.ucsd.edu/fpm/ihccm/**

Mission: University of California at San Diego, Division of International Health provides overseas placement opportunities for students interested in International Health. Students travel for three-month rotations. Expenses are not paid for, but training is available. The language of the host country is a requirement.

Continents Served

Africa ✔ Asia ✔ Europe ✔ The Americas ✔

Countries Served

Argentina, Australia, Austria, Barbados, Belgium, Belize, Bolivia, Bosnia and Herzegovina, Botswana, Brazil, Canada, Chile, China, Colombia, Costa Rica, Cuba, Denmark, Ecuador, Egypt, El Salvador, Finland, France, Germany, Greece, Guatemala, Honduras, Hong Kong, Hungary, India, Indonesia, Ireland, Israel, Italy, Jamaica, Japan, Jordan, Kenya, Korea, South, Kuwait, Lesotho, Madagascar, Mexico, Nepal, Netherlands, New Zealand, Nicaragua, Norway, Panama, Papua-New Guinea, Peru, Philippines, Poland, Seychelles, Singapore, South Africa, Spain, Sweden, Switzerland, Taiwan, Tanzania, Thailand, Tunisia, Turkey, Uganda, United Kingdom, United States, USSR, former, Venezuela, Vietnam

Placement opportunities for . . .

People of only certain faiths?	No
Couples: both are health providers?	No
Couples: only one is a health provider?	No
Families with children?	No
Medical students?	Yes
Pre-medical or college students?	No
Other health professional students?	No
Doctors in training?	Yes
Health personnel who are US citizens?	No
Health personnel who are non-US citizens?	No
Health personnel with no prior experience in developing countries?	Yes
Health personnel who are not current members of your organization?	Yes

Organization/Service Specifics:

Size of the Organization's Staff:	>200
Number of providers sent or received/year:	11-20
Minimum term of assignment:	3 months
Maximum term of assignment:	3 months
Is funding available for travel?	No
Are room and board provided?	No
Is any other funding available?	No
Is training provided or available?	Yes
Is a language other than English required? *1*	Yes

Health Professionals Placed:

Physicians:

Physicians; Family Practitioners

Allied Health Professionals:

Nurse Midwives; Nurse Practitioners; Nurses; Paramedics; Public Health Specialists, Epidemiologists and Health Educators

Notes

1. The host country language is required.

Unite for Sight

Continents Served	
Africa ✔	Asia ✔
Europe ✔	The Americas ✔

Countries Served

Armenia	Benin	Cameroon
Ghana	India	Malawi
Nicaragua	Panama	Peru
Sierra Leone	Tanzania	Thailand

Address: **31 Brookwood Dr., Newtown, CT 06470 U.S.A.**

Phone: **(203) 417-6968** FAX:

E-Mail: **JStaple@uniteforsight.org** Web: **www.uniteforsight.org**

Mission: Unite for Sight includes more than 4,000 volunteers in 90 chapters throughout the world. Volunteers prescribe eyeglasses, screen for disease and coordinate and fund diagnosis, treatment, and surgery by doctors. Volunteers also implement educational programs for children and adults about good eye health and preventing blindness. Opthamologists are always in need and optometrists are welcome to participate for one week or more. In addition to doctors, programs are open to premedical and medical students, public health professionals, nurses, graduate students, and non-medical volunteers. Must be 18 years or older for program participation.

Placement opportunities for . . .

People of only certain faiths?	No
Couples: both are health providers?	Yes
Couples: only one is a health provider?	Yes
Families with children?	No
Medical students?	Yes
Pre-medical or college students?	Yes
Other health professional students?	Yes
Doctors in training?	Yes
Health personnel who are US citizens?	Yes
Health personnel who are non-US citizens?	Yes
Health personnel with no prior experience in developing countries?	Yes
Health personnel who are not current members of your organization?	Yes

Organization/Service Specifics:

Size of the Organization's Staff:	>200
Number of providers sent or received/year:	151-200
Minimum term of assignment:	1 week
Maximum term of assignment:	2 months
Is funding available for travel?	No
Are room and board provided?	No
Is any other funding available?	No
Is training provided or available?	Yes
Is a language other than English required? *1*	No

Health Professionals Placed:

Physicians:

Ophthalmologists; Optometrists

Allied Health Professionals:

Notes

1. A need for a foreign language may arise depending on location served.

Univ. of Wisconsin Med., Office of International Health Affairs, US Committee for Scientific Cooperation With Vietnam

Continents Served	
Africa ☐	Asia ✔
Europe ✔	The Americas ✔

Countries Served

Address: **1760 Medical Sciences Center, 1300 University Ave. Madison, WI 53706 U.S.A.**

Phone: **(608) 263-4150** FAX: **(608) 262-2327**

E-Mail: **jlladins@facstaff.wisc.edu** Web:

Mission: The University of Wisconsin's International Health Exchange (IHE) is a student founded, student operated program to allow medical students and health care professionals the opportunity to apply their interests in international health toward the development and organization of projects and events. A major tenant of IHE is the exchange of ideas, as well as the exchange of material supplies, with an emphasis on the continuing relationship with Madison's Sister Cities of Vilnius, Lithuania, and Arcatao, El Salvador; yet not limited to these areas. Length of service terms range from 8-12 weeks. There are no language or religious requirements, and while travel expenses are not paid for by the school, room and board are provided.

(continued)

Placement opportunities for . . .		Organization/Service Specifics:	
People of only certain faiths?	No	Size of the Organization's Staff:	>200
Couples: both are health providers?	Yes	Number of providers sent or received/year:	11-20
Couples: only one is a health provider?	Yes	Minimum term of assignment:	8 weeks
Families with children?	Yes	Maximum term of assignment:	3 months
Medical students?	Yes	Is funding available for travel?	No
Pre-medical or college students?	No	Are room and board provided?	Yes
Other health professional students?	No	Is any other funding available?	No
Doctors in training?	Yes	Is training provided or available?	Yes
Health personnel who are US citizens?	Yes	Is a language other than English required?	No
Health personnel who are non-US citizens?	Yes		
Health personnel with no prior experience in developing countries?	Yes		
Health personnel who are not current members of your organization?	Yes		

Health Professionals Placed:

Notes

Physicians:

Physicians; Anesthesiologists; Emergency Medicine Physicians; Endocrinologists; General Surgeons; Hematologists; Oncologists; Infectious Disease Spec.; Internal Medicine GPS & PCP; Neurologists; Ophthalmologists; Orthopedic Surgeons; Pathologists; Plastic/Hand/Reconstructive Surgeons

Allied Health Professionals:

Administrative Health Positions; Nurse Midwives; Nurse Practitioners; Public Health Specialists, Epidemiologists and Health Educators

---

Universidad de Chile, Facultad de Medicina

Continents Served

Africa ☐ Asia ☐ Europe ☐ The Americas ☑

Address: **PO Box 13898 Correo 21 Santiago, Chile**

Phone: **(562) 678-6401** FAX: **(562) 777-4890**

E-Mail: Web: **www.med.uchile.cl**

Countries Served

Chile

Mission: This is a faculty of Medicine. Its mission includes (1) teaching undergraduate and graduate students in the following health care professions: medicine, nursery, midwifery, occupational therapy, nutritionists, physical therapy, and medical technicians. (They also give masters and graduate degrees in medical science.); (2) biomedical research; and (3) community action.

Placement opportunities for . . .		Organization/Service Specifics:	
People of only certain faiths?	No	Size of the Organization's Staff: *1*	>200
Couples: both are health providers?	No	Number of providers sent or received/year:	>200
Couples: only one is a health provider?	No	Minimum term of assignment:	
Families with children?		Maximum term of assignment:	
Medical students?	Yes	Is funding available for travel?	No
Pre-medical or college students? *1*		Are room and board provided?	No
Other health professional students?	Yes	Is any other funding available?	No
Doctors in training?	Yes	Is training provided or available?	Yes
Health personnel who are US citizens?	No	Is a language other than English required? *2*	Yes
Health personnel who are non-US citizens?	No		
Health personnel with no prior experience in developing countries?	No		
Health personnel who are not current members of your organization?	No		

Health Professionals Placed:

Physicians:

Physicians; Anesthesiologists; Cardiologists; Dermatologists; Emergency Medicine Physicians; Endocrinologists; Family Practitioners; Gastroenterologists; General Surgeons; Hematologists; Oncologists; Infectious Disease Spec.; Internal Medicine GPS & PCP; Nephrologists; Neurologists; Neurosurgeons; OB/GYN; Ophthalmologists; Oral Surgeons; Orthopedic Surgeons; Otolaryngologists; Pathologists; Pediatricians; Plastic/Hand/Reconstructive Surgeons; Psychiatrists; Pulmonary Specialists; Radiologists; Urologists

Allied Health Professionals:

Administrative Health Positions; Medical Technicians (lab, X-ray, etc); Nurse Midwives; Nurse Practitioners; Nurses; Nutritionists & Dieticians; Pharmacists; Physical & Occupational Therapists; Prosthetists; Psychologists; Public Health Specialists, Epidemiologists and Health Educators; Respiratory Therapists; Social Workers

Notes

1. No contact since 11/02;
2. Spanish.

University of Cincinnati, College of Medicine, Dept. of Family Medicine

Continents Served
Africa ☐ Asia ☐ Europe ☐ The Americas ☑

Address: **3235 Eden Ave., Cincinnati, OH 45267 U.S.A.**

Phone: **(513) 558-4021** FAX: **(513) 558-4111**

E-Mail: **susmanjl@fammed.uc.edu** Web: **www.familymedicine.uc.edu**

Countries Served
Brazil Honduras

Mission: Rotations are available through the University of Cincinnati College of Medicine at Hombro a Hombro Clinic in Santa Lucia, Honduras. Residents and medical students afford great assistance to two Honduran physicians at the clinic. Exposure to tropical diseases, orthopedics, obstetrics, trauma, and primary care is afforded at this site. People of all faiths are welcome, and while there are no language requirements, knowledge of Spanish is desirable. Travel expenses are not provided, and room, but not board, is covered.

Placement opportunities for . . .

People of only certain faiths?	No
Couples: both are health providers?	Yes
Couples: only one is a health provider?	Yes
Families with children?	Yes
Medical students?	Yes
Pre-medical or college students?	No
Other health professional students?	Yes
Doctors in training?	Yes
Health personnel who are US citizens?	Yes
Health personnel who are non-US citizens?	Yes
Health personnel with no prior experience in developing countries?	Yes
Health personnel who are not current members of your organization?	Yes

Organization/Service Specifics:

Size of the Organization's Staff:		6-10
Number of providers sent or received/year:		51-100
Minimum term of assignment:		2 weeks
Maximum term of assignment:		1 year
Is funding available for travel?		No
Are room and board provided?	*1*	Yes
Is any other funding available?		No
Is training provided or available?		Yes
Is a language other than English required?	*2*	No

Health Professionals Placed:

Physicians:

Physicians; Anesthesiologists; Internal Medicine GPS & PCP; Oral Surgeons; Pediatricians

Allied Health Professionals:

Administrative Health Positions; Dentists; Medical Technicians (lab, X-ray, etc); Nurse Practitioners; Nurses; Pharmacists; Physician Assistants; Public Health Specialists, Epidemiologists and Health Educators; Water/Sanitation Specialists

Notes

1. Only room is available;
2. Spanish is not required, but desirable.

University of Illinois at Chicago College of Nursing, Global Health Leadership Office

Continents Served
Africa ☑ Asia ☑ Europe ☑ The Americas ☑

Address: **845 S. Damen Ave., Room 1160, Chicago, IL 60612-7350 U.S.A.**

Phone: **(312) 996-0621** **(312) 996-7800** FAX: **(312) 996-8945**

E-Mail: **ghlo@uic.edu** Web: **www.uic.edu/nursing/ghlo/**

Countries Served

Bahrain	Botswana	Brazil
Burkina Faso	Canada	Chile
Colombia	Denmark	Egypt
Hong Kong	Indonesia	Israel
Japan	Jordan	Korea, South
Lithuania	Malawi	Nigeria
Pakistan	Poland	South Africa
Swaziland	Switzerland	Taiwan
Thailand	United Kingdom	
United States		

Mission: The Global Health Leadership Office (GHLO) staff seeks to provide opportunities for nurses of all countries to improve the quality of nursing and health care. We expect nurses to assume positions of leadership in education, practice, research, and policy in order to ensure the participation of community members in accessible, affordable, and essential health care. We are a WHO collaborating center for the international development of primary health care—so we primarily match students and faculty to requests for exchanges, research projects, consolation, short term study, or graduate degree programs.

(continued)

Placement opportunities for . . .		Organization/Service Specifics:	
People of only certain faiths?	No	Size of the Organization's Staff:	151-200
Couples: both are health providers?	No	Number of providers sent or received/year:	11-20
Couples: only one is a health provider?	No	Minimum term of assignment: *2*	vary
Families with children?	No	Maximum term of assignment:	vary
Medical students?	No	Is funding available for travel?	Yes
Pre-medical or college students?	No	Are room and board provided?	Yes
Other health professional students? *1*	Yes	Is any other funding available? *3*	Yes
Doctors in training?	No	Is training provided or available?	Yes
Health personnel who are US citizens?	Yes	Is a language other than English required? *4*	Yes
Health personnel who are non-US citizens?	Yes		
Health personnel with no prior experience in developing countries?	Yes		
Health personnel who are not current members of your organization?	Yes		

Health Professionals Placed:

Physicians:

Allied Health Professionals:

Nurse Midwives; Nurse Practitioners; Nurses

Notes

1. Nursing students; *2.* Depends on funding and requirements of project; *3.* Grants may be available; *4.* Language requirements depend on the host site.

University of Illinois College of Medicine at Rockford

Address: **1601 Parkview Ave., Rockford, IL 61107 U.S.A.**

Phone: **(815) 395-0600** FAX: **(815) 395-5887**

E-Mail: **BuzS@uic.edu** Web: **www.uirockford.com/info/affiliations_who.asp**

Continents Served

Africa ☐ Asia ☑ Europe ☑ The Americas ☑

Countries Served

India	Iran	Israel
Italy	Jamaica	Malaysia
Nepal	Sri Lanka	Thailand
USSR, former		

Mission: The University of Illinois College of Medicine trains medical students and family practice residents to serve in Jamaica, the countries of the former USSR, as well as countries in Southern and Southeast Asia. It is a collaborating research center of the WHO with a strong focus in primary care and public health. Length of stay for medical students and family practice residents is short-term (1-2 weeks). Involvement is restricted to people affiliated with the University.

Placement opportunities for . . .		Organization/Service Specifics:	
People of only certain faiths?	No	Size of the Organization's Staff:	>200
Couples: both are health providers?	No	Number of providers sent or received/year:	1-5
Couples: only one is a health provider?	Yes	Minimum term of assignment:	1 week
Families with children?	No	Maximum term of assignment:	6 weeks
Medical students?	Yes	Is funding available for travel? sometimes	Yes
Pre-medical or college students?	No	Are room and board provided?	No
Other health professional students?	No	Is any other funding available? *1*	No
Doctors in training?	Yes	Is training provided or available?	Yes
Health personnel who are US citizens?	Yes	Is a language other than English required?	No
Health personnel who are non-US citizens?	No		
Health personnel with no prior experience in developing countries?	Yes		
Health personnel who are not current members of your organization?	No		

Health Professionals Placed:

Physicians:

Physicians; Anesthesiologists; Cardiologists; Dermatologists; Emergency Medicine Physicians; Endocrinologists; Family Practitioners; Gastroenterologists; General Surgeons; Hematologists; Oncologists; Infectious Disease Spec.; Internal Medicine GPS & PCP; Nephrologists; Neurologists; Neurosurgeons; OB/GYN; Ophthalmologists; Oral Surgeons; Orthopedic Surgeons; Otolaryngologists; Pathologists; Pediatricians; Plastic/Hand/Reconstructive Surgeons; Psychiatrists; Pulmonary Specialists; Radiologists; Urologists

Allied Health Professionals:

Nurse Practitioners; Psychologists; Public Health Specialists, Epidemiologists and Health Educators; Social Workers

Notes

1. Sometimes funding and room/board are provided.

University of Nebraska Medical Center, Office of International Programs and Studies

Continents Served			
Africa ☐	Asia ☐	Europe ☐	The Americas ☑

Countries Served

Ecuador	Guatemala	Jamaica
Mexico	Nicaragua	Venezuela

Address: **Nebraska Medical Center, 42nd and Dewey, Omaha, NE 68198-5735 U.S.A.**

Phone: **(402) 559-6414** FAX: **(402) 559-2923**

E-Mail: **international@unmc.edu or globalmc@unmc.edu** Web: **www.unmc.edu/isp**

Mission: The Office of International Programs and Studies at the University of Nebraska Medical Center sponsors short term (4 weeks to 3 months) stays in Guatemala, Nicaragua, and Jamaica for physicians, medical students, and nurse practitioners. The programs provide opportunities for students and health care professionals to experience onsite exposure to health care in an underdeveloped country, as well as cultural and linguistic immersion. Participants are required to have at least some level of prior Spanish knowledge for Guatemala and Nicaragua, and to provide their own funding for all expenses. There are no religious restrictions.

Placement opportunities for . . .

People of only certain faiths?	No
Couples: both are health providers?	Yes
Couples: only one is a health provider?	Yes
Families with children?	No
Medical students?	Yes
Pre-medical or college students?	No
Other health professional students?	Yes
Doctors in training?	Yes
Health personnel who are US citizens?	Yes
Health personnel who are non-US citizens?	Yes
Health personnel with no prior experience in developing countries?	Yes
Health personnel who are not current members of your organization?	Yes

Organization/Service Specifics:

Size of the Organization's Staff:	>200
Number of providers sent or received/year:	51-100
Minimum term of assignment:	4 weeks
Maximum term of assignment:	3 months
Is funding available for travel?	No
Are room and board provided?	No
Is any other funding available?	No
Is training provided or available?	No
Is a language other than English required? *1*	Yes

Health Professionals Placed:

Physicians:

Physicians; Emergency Medicine Physicians; Family Practitioners; Infectious Disease Spec.; Internal Medicine GPS & PCP

Allied Health Professionals:

Nurse Practitioners

Notes

1. Some knowledge of Spanish is required for Guatemala and Nicaragua.

University of Virginia, Center for Global Health

Continents Served			
Africa ☑	Asia ☑	Europe ☐	The Americas ☑

Countries Served

Bangladesh	Brazil	China
Ghana	Mexico	Philippines
South Africa		

Address: **P.O. Box 801379, Room 3146, Bldg MR-4, Lane Road, UVA Health System, Charlottesville, VA 22908 U.S.A.**

Phone: **(434) 924-5242** FAX: **(434) 977-5323**

E-Mail: **guerrant@Virginia.edu or lorntz@virginia.edu** Web: **www.healthsystem.virginia.edu/internet/cgh**

Mission: Health, a universal value, transcends geo-political boundaries and provides an unassailable basis for improving human and international relationships. The mission of the Office of International Health, therefore, is to foster mutually beneficial education, research, and services in the health professions, especially in the health problems of the disadvantaged around the world.

(continued)

Placement opportunities for . . .		Organization/Service Specifics:	
People of only certain faiths?	No	Size of the Organization's Staff:	>200
Couples: both are health providers?	No	Number of providers sent or received/year:	51-100
Couples: only one is a health provider?	No	Minimum term of assignment:	8 weeks
Families with children?	No	Maximum term of assignment:	12 weeks
Medical students?	Yes	Is funding available for travel?	Yes
Pre-medical or college students?	Yes	Are room and board provided?	No
Other health professional students?	Yes	Is any other funding available?	No
Doctors in training?	Yes	Is training provided or available?	Yes
Health personnel who are US citizens?	Yes	Is a language other than English required? *1*	Yes
Health personnel who are non-US citizens?	Yes		
Health personnel with no prior experience in developing countries?	No		
Health personnel who are not current members of your organization?	No		

Health Professionals Placed:

Physicians:

Anesthesiologists; Cardiologists; General Surgeons; Infectious Disease Spec.; Orthopedic Surgeons; Plastic/Hand/Reconstructive Surgeons

Allied Health Professionals:

Nurses

Notes

1. Language requirements depend on the country of service.

University of Zimbabwe

Address: **P. O. Box MP167, Mt. Pleasant Harare, Zimbabwe, Africa**

Phone: **(263) 430-3211** FAX:

E-Mail: Web: **www.uz.ac.zw**

Continents Served

Africa ☑ Asia ☐ Europe ☐ The Americas ☐

Countries Served

Zimbabwe

Mission: The hospital at the University of Zimbabwe welcomes volunteer health care providers at its site in Avondale Harare, Zimbabwe.

Placement opportunities for . . .		Organization/Service Specifics:	
People of only certain faiths?	No	Size of the Organization's Staff:	101-150
Couples: both are health providers?	Yes	Number of providers sent or received/year:	?
Couples: only one is a health provider?	Yes	Minimum term of assignment:	0
Families with children?	Yes	Maximum term of assignment:	0
Medical students?	Yes	Is funding available for travel?	No
Pre-medical or college students?	Yes	Are room and board provided?	No
Other health professional students?	Yes	Is any other funding available? *1*	Yes
Doctors in training?	Yes	Is training provided or available?	Yes
Health personnel who are US citizens?	Yes	Is a language other than English required? *2*	No
Health personnel who are non-US citizens?	Yes		
Health personnel with no prior experience in developing countries?	Yes		
Health personnel who are not current members of your organization?	Yes		

Health Professionals Placed:

Physicians:

Physicians; Anesthesiologists; Cardiologists; Dermatologists; Emergency Medicine Physicians; Endocrinologists; Family Practitioners; Gastroenterologists; General Surgeons; Hematologists; Oncologists; Infectious Disease Spec.; Internal Medicine GPS & PCP; Nephrologists; Neurologists; Neurosurgeons; OB/GYN; Ophthalmologists; Oral Surgeons; Optometrists; Orthopedic Surgeons; Otolaryngologists; Pathologists; Pediatricians; Plastic/Hand/Reconstructive Surgeons; Psychiatrists; Pulmonary Specialists; Radiologists; Urologists

Allied Health Professionals:

Administrative Health Positions; Dental Hygienists; Dentists; Medical Technicians (lab, X-ray, etc); Nurse Midwives; Nurse Practitioners; Nurses; Nutritionists & Dieticians; Paramedics; Pharmacists; Physical & Occupational Therapists; Physician Assistants; Podiatrists; Prosthetists; Psychologists; Public Health Specialists, Epidemiologists and Health Educators; Respiratory Therapists

Notes

1. Passage travel for prospective employees of the University of Zimbabwe; *2.* No specific lengths are prescribed.

Uplift Internationale

Continents Served			
Africa ☐	Asia ☑	Europe ☐	The Americas ☐

Countries Served
Philippines

Address: **P.O. Box 582, Wheat Ridge, CO 80034 U.S.A.**

Phone: **(303) 707-1361** FAX: **(303) 703-4840**

E-Mail: **info@upliftinternationale.org** Web: **upliftinternationale.org**

Mission: Uplift Internationale aims to give a life-changing gift to children with facial deformities by mending faces one child at a time. Uplift Internationale is a non-profit organization whose objectives include the recruitment of self-funded healthcare practitioners to participate in patient care in rural Philippines, as well as share know-how with local colleagues at a host public-funded hospital. Uplift Internationale operates in the Philippines where 1 in 5 Filipinos live without receiving basic medical care. There are no religious requirements and volunteers can travel on 1 or 2 week trips of an organized annual mission.

Placement opportunities for . . .

People of only certain faiths?	No
Couples: both are health providers?	Yes
Couples: only one is a health provider?	Yes
Families with children?	Yes
Medical students?	Yes
Pre-medical or college students?	Yes
Other health professional students?	Yes
Doctors in training?	Yes
Health personnel who are US citizens?	Yes
Health personnel who are non-US citizens?	Yes
Health personnel with no prior experience in developing countries?	Yes
Health personnel who are not current members of your organization?	Yes

Organization/Service Specifics:

Size of the Organization's Staff:	0-5
Number of providers sent or received/year:	11-20
Minimum term of assignment:	1 week
Maximum term of assignment:	2 weeks
Is funding available for travel?	No
Are room and board provided?	No
Is any other funding available?	No
Is training provided or available?	No
Is a language other than English required?	No

Health Professionals Placed:

Physicians:

Anesthesiologists; Family Practitioners; Internal Medicine GPS & PCP; Oral Surgeons; Otolaryngologists; Pediatricians; Plastic/Hand/Reconstructive Surgeons

Allied Health Professionals:

Dental Hygienists; Dentists; Nurses; Physician Assistants

Notes

Mission teams are customarily organized by early summer of the year before the mission trip, which takes place in late February.

UTMB-WHO Collaborating Center for Training in International Health

Continents Served			
Africa ☐	Asia ☐	Europe ☐	The Americas ☑

Countries Served

Address: **301 University Boulevard, Primary Care Pavilion, Suite 2.258, Galveston, TX 77555-1123 U.S.A.**

Phone: **(409) 772-0637** FAX: **(409) 772-9865**

E-Mail: **jksmith@utmb.edu or jmessex@utmb.edu** Web: **ctih.utmb.edu**

Mission: The Center caters to the needs of students and faculty who seek collaborative opportunities with colleagues in the American, African, Eastern Mediterranean, European, South East Asian, and Western Pacific Regions of the WHO. Priority, however, will be given to forging linkages and building partnerships in countries of the Western hemisphere; and "twinning arrangements" are possible as a modality of technical cooperation between selected small island communities in the Caribbean, for example, and some matched underserved areas of Texas.

(continued)

Placement opportunities for . . .

People of only certain faiths?	No
Couples: both are health providers?	Yes
Couples: only one is a health provider?	
Families with children?	No
Medical students?	Yes
Pre-medical or college students?	
Other health professional students?	Yes
Doctors in training?	Yes
Health personnel who are US citizens?	Yes
Health personnel who are non-US citizens?	Yes
Health personnel with no prior experience in developing countries?	Yes
Health personnel who are not current members of your organization?	Yes

Organization/Service Specifics:

Size of the Organization's Staff:	0-5
Number of providers sent or received/year:	1-5
Minimum term of assignment:	8 weeks
Maximum term of assignment:	2 years
Is funding available for travel?	No
Are room and board provided? *1*	Yes
Is any other funding available?	No
Is training provided or available?	No
Is a language other than English required? *2*	Yes

Health Professionals Placed:

Physicians:

Dermatologists; OB/GYN

Allied Health Professionals:

Medical Technicians (lab, X-ray, etc); Nurse Midwives; Public Health Specialists, Epidemiologists and Health Educators

Notes

1. Room and board are provided on some programs; *2.* Spanish is sometimes required.

Vietnam ENT Mission

Address: **UTMB, Dept. of Otolaryngology, Galveston, TX 77555 U.S.A.**

Phone: **(409) 772-2704** FAX: **(409) 772-1715**

E-Mail: **bbailey@utmb.edu** Web:

Continents Served

Africa ☐ Asia ☑ Europe ☐ The Americas ☑

Countries Served

Cuba Vietnam

Mission: Volunteer ENT specialists will teach and provide modern educational resources and medical technology needed to modernize ENT training and patient care in Vietnam and Cuba. Trips are 2 weeks long. Training but not funding is provided. There are no language or religious requirements.

Placement opportunities for . . .

People of only certain faiths?	No
Couples: both are health providers?	Yes
Couples: only one is a health provider?	Yes
Families with children?	Yes
Medical students?	No
Pre-medical or college students?	No
Other health professional students?	Yes
Doctors in training?	Yes
Health personnel who are US citizens?	Yes
Health personnel who are non-US citizens?	No
Health personnel with no prior experience in developing countries?	Yes
Health personnel who are not current members of your organization?	Yes

Organization/Service Specifics:

Size of the Organization's Staff:	0-5
Number of providers sent or received/year:	11-20
Minimum term of assignment:	2 weeks
Maximum term of assignment:	2 weeks
Is funding available for travel?	No
Are room and board provided?	No
Is any other funding available?	No
Is training provided or available?	Yes
Is a language other than English required?	No

Health Professionals Placed:

Physicians:

Physicians; Otolaryngologists

Allied Health Professionals:

Notes

Virginia Children's Connection, Dept. of Plastic & Reconstructive Surgery

Continents Served
Africa ☐ Asia ☑ Europe ☐ The Americas ☐

Countries Served
India

Address: **PO Box 800376, Charlottesville, VA 22908 U.S.A.**
Phone: **(434) 924-5068** FAX: **(434) 924-1333**
E-Mail: **tjg6f@virginia.edu or tjg6f@hscmail.mcc.virginia.edu** Web:

Mission: For ten years, a team of plastic surgeons and anesthesiologists from the University of Virginia Health Sciences Center have gone to Giridih in the Chotanagpur Hills of South Bihar to perform what many of their patients, primarily children, consider to be reconstructive miracles. This is the Virginia Children's Connection. Over the course of these five visits, the team of physicians and nurses have performed literally hundreds of surgical procedures. The primary pool of patients have been children with cleft lips and cleft palates, and burn patients, among the more physically disfiguring and at the same time treatable medical conditions found in India. In recent years, Indian medicine has developed surgical capabilities to deal with these conditions, but in a common and painful irony the world over, it is a capability primarily available in urban centers, and incredibly less so for the rural poor of an economically depressed place like Giridih.

Placement opportunities for . . .

People of only certain faiths?	No
Couples: both are health providers?	Yes
Couples: only one is a health provider?	No
Families with children?	No
Medical students?	Yes
Pre-medical or college students?	Yes
Other health professional students?	Yes
Doctors in training?	Yes
Health personnel who are US citizens?	Yes
Health personnel who are non-US citizens?	Yes
Health personnel with no prior experience in developing countries?	Yes
Health personnel who are not current members of your organization?	Yes

Organization/Service Specifics:

Size of the Organization's Staff:	0-5
Number of providers sent or received/year:	
Minimum term of assignment:	2 weeks
Maximum term of assignment:	3 weeks
Is funding available for travel?	Yes
Are room and board provided?	Yes
Is any other funding available?	No
Is training provided or available?	No
Is a language other than English required?	No

Health Professionals Placed:

Physicians:

Physicians; Anesthesiologists; Ophthalmologists; Pediatricians; Plastic/Hand/Reconstructive Surgeons

Allied Health Professionals:

Dentists; Nurse Practitioners; Nurses

Notes

Visions in Action

Continents Served
Africa ☑ Asia ☐ Europe ☐ The Americas ☑

Countries Served

Burkina Faso	Mexico	South Africa
Tanzania	Uganda	Zimbabwe

Address: **2710 Ontario Rd. NW, Washington, DC 20009 U.S.A.**
Phone: **(202) 625-7402** FAX: **(202) 588-9344**
E-Mail: **visions@visionsinaction.org** Web: **www.visionsinaction.org**

Mission: Visions in Action is an international nonprofit organization offering 6- and 12-month volunteer positions in Mexico and five African countries. A 9-week summer program focusing on appropriate technology is also offered in Tanzania. Positions are available with nonprofit development organizations, research institutes, health clinics, community groups, and news organizations. Visions in Action operates primarily on volunteer energy, though it has 15 permanent staff based in the United States, Africa, and Latin America, and another dozen orientation leaders and language instructors who are hired on a short-term basis to facilitate a specific country's orientation. It seeks individuals for relatively short term (6 month–1 year) stays in countries in Africa and the Americas.

(continued)

Placement opportunities for . . .

People of only certain faiths?	No
Couples: both are health providers?	Yes
Couples: only one is a health provider?	Yes
Families with children?	Yes
Medical students?	Yes
Pre-medical or college students?	Yes
Other health professional students?	Yes
Doctors in training?	Yes
Health personnel who are US citizens?	Yes
Health personnel who are non-US citizens?	Yes
Health personnel with no prior experience in developing countries?	Yes
Health personnel who are not current members of your organization?	Yes

Organization/Service Specifics:

Size of the Organization's Staff:	11-20
Number of providers sent or received/year:	>200
Minimum term of assignment:	6 months
Maximum term of assignment:	1 year
Is funding available for travel? *1*	No
Are room and board provided? *1*	No
Is any other funding available? *1*	No
Is training provided or available? *2*	Yes
Is a language other than English required? *3*	No

Health Professionals Placed:

Physicians:

Infectious Disease Spec.; Internal Medicine GPS & PCP; Pediatricians

Allied Health Professionals:

Nurse Midwives; Nurse Practitioners; Nurses; Nutritionists & Dieticians; Physical & Occupational Therapists; Psychologists; Public Health Specialists, Epidemiologists and Health Educators; Social Workers

Notes

1. Lodging is organized for a tax deductible program fee and $50 stipend; *2.* Cultural/Orientation training (not medical/technical training) is provided; *3.* 4 of the programs require only English. One requires French, and one Spanish.

Voluntary Service Overseas Canada

Address: **806-151 Slater Street, Ottawa, ON K1P 5H3, Canada**

Phone: **(888) 876-2911**
(613) 234-1364 FAX: **(613) 234-1444**

E-Mail: **inquiry@vsocan.org** Web: **www.vsocan.org**

Continents Served

Africa ☑ Asia ☑ Europe ☑ The Americas ☐

Countries Served

Mission: VSO Canada is part of the Voluntary Service Overseas international development agency. VSO recruits volunteers with a wide range of skills, in response to requests from our overseas partners. VSO aims to support disadvantaged people in fulfilling their rights to physical, mental and social health, and improving their access to good quality essential services. VSO recruits health care workers from a range of professions and our need for health-care professionals is ongoing.

Placement opportunities for . . .

People of only certain faiths?	No
Couples: both are health providers?	Yes
Couples: only one is a health provider?	Yes
Families with children?	Yes
Medical students?	No
Pre-medical or college students?	No
Other health professional students?	No
Doctors in training?	Yes
Health personnel who are US citizens?	Yes
Health personnel who are non-US citizens?	Yes
Health personnel with no prior experience in developing countries?	Yes
Health personnel who are not current members of your organization?	Yes

Organization/Service Specifics:

Size of the Organization's Staff:	21-50
Number of providers sent or received/year:	21-50
Minimum term of assignment:	1 year
Maximum term of assignment:	2 years
Is funding available for travel?	Yes
Are room and board provided?	Yes
Is any other funding available?	No
Is training provided or available?	Yes
Is a language other than English required?	No

Health Professionals Placed:

Physicians:

Anesthesiologists; General Surgeons; Infectious Disease Spec.; Internal Medicine GPS & PCP; OB/GYN; Pediatricians; Psychiatrists; Radiologists

Allied Health Professionals:

Administrative Health Positions; Dentists; Medical Technicians (lab, X-ray, etc); Nurse Midwives; Nurse Practitioners; Nurses; Pharmacists; Physical & Occupational Therapists; Physician Assistants; Psychologists; Public Health Specialists, Epidemiologists and Health Educators; Social Workers; Water/Sanitation Specialists

Notes

Volunteer Missionary Movement

Continents Served
Africa ☑ Asia ☐ Europe ☐ The Americas ☑

Address: **5980 West Loomis Rd., Greendale, WI 53129 U.S.A.**
Phone: **(414) 423-8660** FAX: **(414) 423-8964**
E-Mail: **info@vmmusa.org** Web: **www.vmmusa.org**

Countries Served

Canada	El Salvador	Guatemala
Kenya	Uganda	United States

Mission: The Volunteer Missionary Movement sends volunteer Christian lay missioners, who are from the United States or Canada and 23 years or older with at least a year of work experience, to service-oriented ministries in Central America, the United States, and Africa for periods of at least two years. VMM is an international community of Christians with its origins in the Catholic tradition.

Placement opportunities for . . .

People of only certain faiths? *1*	Yes
Couples: both are health providers?	Yes
Couples: only one is a health provider?	Yes
Families with children?	Yes
Medical students?	Yes
Pre-medical or college students?	Yes
Other health professional students?	Yes
Doctors in training?	Yes
Health personnel who are US citizens?	Yes
Health personnel who are non-US citizens?	Yes
Health personnel with no prior experience in developing countries?	Yes
Health personnel who are not current members of your organization?	

Organization/Service Specifics:

Size of the Organization's Staff:	0-5
Number of providers sent or received/year:	>200
Minimum term of assignment:	2 years
Maximum term of assignment:	
Is funding available for travel?	Yes
Are room and board provided?	Yes
Is any other funding available?	Yes
Is training provided or available?	Yes
Is a language other than English required? *2*	Yes

Health Professionals Placed: *3*

Physicians:

All physician specialists

Allied Health Professionals:

All allied health professionals

Notes

1. Catholic, Protestant; *2.* Spanish; *3.* The type of health care provider sought by the Volunteer Missionary Movement varies from location to location and year to year.

Volunteer Optometric Service to Humanity (VOSH) International

Continents Served
Africa ☑ Asia ☑ Europe ☑ The Americas ☑

Address: **111 Linda Lane, Lake Mary, FL 32746-4208 U.S.A.**
Phone: **(407) 328-5825** FAX: **(407) 302-6046**
E-Mail: **ccovington@cfl.rr.com** Web: **www.vosh.org**

Mission: The primary mission of VOSH is to facilitate the provision of vision care worldwide where it is not affordable or attainable. VOSH International helps accomplish this goal by serving as a coordinating body to affiliated Chapters and other humanitarian organizations. Volunteers can serve for up to 2 week terms and must pay for their own expenses, although room and board is sometimes provided. VOSH has no religious or language requirements.

Countries Served

Albania	Barbados	Belize
Bulgaria	China	Colombia
Costa Rica	Cuba	
Dominican Republic		Ecuador
El Salvador	Ghana	Guatemala
Guyana	Haiti	Honduras
India	Jamaica	Kenya
Mexico	Mongolia	Morocco
Nepal	Nicaragua	Nigeria
Panama	Paraguay	Peru
Poland	Romania	South Africa
Tanzania	Thailand	
Trinidad and Tobago		Turkey
United States	USSR, former	Venezuela
Vietnam	Yugoslavia, former	

(continued)

Placement opportunities for . . .		**Organization/Service Specifics:**	
People of only certain faiths?	No	Size of the Organization's Staff:	0-5
Couples: both are health providers?	Yes	Number of providers sent or received/year:	>200
Couples: only one is a health provider?	Yes	Minimum term of assignment:	1 week
Families with children? *1*	Yes	Maximum term of assignment:	2 weeks
Medical students?	Yes	Is funding available for travel?	No
Pre-medical or college students?	Yes	Are room and board provided? *2*	Yes
Other health professional students?	Yes	Is any other funding available?	No
Doctors in training?	Yes	Is training provided or available?	Yes
Health personnel who are US citizens?	Yes	Is a language other than English required?	No

Health personnel who are non-US citizens?	Yes
Health personnel with no prior experience in developing countries?	Yes
Health personnel who are not current members of your organization?	Yes

Health Professionals Placed:

Physicians:

Physicians; Family Practitioners; Ophthalmologists; Optometrists

Allied Health Professionals:

Dentists; Nurse Practitioners

Notes

1. Teens; *2.* Room and board is sometimes provided.

Volunteers in Medical Missions

Address: **Box 756, 265 South Cove Rd., Seneca, SC 29679 U.S.A.**

Phone: **(864) 885-9023** **(800) 615-8695** FAX: **(864) 885-9411**

E-Mail: **missions@vimm.org** Web: **www.vimm.org**

Mission: Volunteers in Medical Missions will minister to the physical and spiritual needs of children and adults in developing countries throughout the world and will provide opportunities for Christian medical professionals and other volunteers to experience mission first-hand. Volunteers can take 1-2 week trips to various countries around the world. Partial funding is provided through a scholarship fund, and room and board are both provided for volunteers through the program fee.

Continents Served

Africa ✔ Asia ✔ Europe ✔ The Americas ✔

Countries Served

China, Dominican Republic, Ecuador, El Salvador, Guatemala, Haiti, Honduras, Hungary, India, Mexico, Mongolia, Nicaragua, Panama, Peru, Philippines, Romania, Suriname, Tanzania, Trinidad and Tobago, Uganda, Vietnam, Zambia, Zimbabwe

Placement opportunities for . . .		**Organization/Service Specifics:**	
People of only certain faiths? *1*	Yes	Size of the Organization's Staff:	0-5
Couples: both are health providers?	Yes	Number of providers sent or received/year:	>200
Couples: only one is a health provider?	Yes	Minimum term of assignment:	1 week
Families with children?	Yes	Maximum term of assignment:	2 weeks
Medical students?	Yes	Is funding available for travel?	No
Pre-medical or college students?	Yes	Are room and board provided?	Yes
Other health professional students?	Yes	Is any other funding available? *2*	Yes
Doctors in training?	Yes	Is training provided or available?	No
Health personnel who are US citizens?	Yes	Is a language other than English required?	No

Health personnel who are non-US citizens?	Yes
Health personnel with no prior experience in developing countries?	Yes
Health personnel who are not current members of your organization?	Yes

Health Professionals Placed:

Physicians:

Physicians

Allied Health Professionals:

Notes

1. Christians; *2.* There is a scholarship fund.

VSO

Address: **317 Putney Bridge Road, London, SW15 2PN U.K.**

Phone: **44 20 87807200** FAX: **44 2087807300**

E-Mail: **enquiry@vso.org.uk** Web: **www.vso.org.uk/**

Mission: VSO is an international development charity that works through volunteers. We enable people aged 17-70 to share their skills and experiences with local communities in the developing world. We passionately believe we can make a difference in tackling poverty by helping people to realize their potential. Ours is a very individual 'people to people' approach to development. Our overriding goal is to help individuals learn from each other—and consequently benefit the communities and countries in which they live. But above all, we are realistic in our expectations. We purposefully harness our resources to long-term objectives and focus on sustainable development rather than the short-term relief of certain problems. Therefore, there is a minimum of 6 months commitment for volunteers. Travel expenses and room and board are provided. There are no language or religious requirements.

Continents Served

Africa ✔ Asia ✔ Europe ✔ The Americas ☐

Countries Served

Bhutan	Cambodia	China
Gambia	Ghana	Guinea-Bissau
India	Indonesia	Kenya
Laos	Malawi	Mongolia
Nepal	Nigeria	Pakistan
Papua-New Guinea		Philippines
Romania	Sierra Leone	
Solomon Islands		South Africa
Sri Lanka	Tanzania	Thailand
Uganda	USSR, former	Vietnam
Zambia	Zimbabwe	

Placement opportunities for . . .

People of only certain faiths?	No
Couples: both are health providers?	Yes
Couples: only one is a health provider?	Yes
Families with children?	No
Medical students?	No
Pre-medical or college students?	No
Other health professional students?	No
Doctors in training?	No
Health personnel who are US citizens?	Yes
Health personnel who are non-US citizens?	Yes
Health personnel with no prior experience in developing countries?	Yes
Health personnel who are not current members of your organization?	Yes

Organization/Service Specifics:

Size of the Organization's Staff:	>200
Number of providers sent or received/year:	51-100
Minimum term of assignment:	6 months
Maximum term of assignment:	2 years
Is funding available for travel?	Yes
Are room and board provided?	Yes
Is any other funding available? *1*	Yes
Is training provided or available?	Yes
Is a language other than English required?	No

Health Professionals Placed:

Physicians:

Family Practitioners; Radiologists

Allied Health Professionals:

Administrative Health Positions; Dentists; Medical Technicians (lab, X-ray, etc); Nurse Midwives; Nurses; Nutritionists & Dieticians; Physical & Occupational Therapists; Public Health Specialists, Epidemiologists and Health Educators; Social Workers

Notes

1. Allowances are provided.

Women's Commission for Refugee Women and Children

Address: **122 East 42nd St., 12th Floor, New York, NY 10168-1289 U.S.A.**

Phone: **(212) 551-3088**
(212) 551-3000 FAX: **(212) 551-3180**

E-Mail: **info@womens commission.org** Web: **www.womenscommission.org**

Continents Served

Africa ✔ Asia ✔ Europe ☐ The Americas ☐

Countries Served

Afghanistan	Chad	Colombia
Rwanda	Sudan	Thailand
Uganda		

Mission: The Women's Commission is an expert resource and advocacy organization that monitors the care of refugee women and children. It speaks out on issues of concern to refugee and displaced women, children and adolescents, who have a critical perspective in bringing about change, but often do not have access to governments and policy makers. It also provides opportunities for refugee women and youth to speak for themselves through briefings, testimony, participation in field assignments and international conferences.

(continued)

Placement opportunities for . . .		Organization/Service Specifics:	
People of only certain faiths?	No	Size of the Organization's Staff:	11-20
Couples: both are health providers?	No	Number of providers sent or received/year:	1-5
Couples: only one is a health provider?	No	Minimum term of assignment:	2 weeks
Families with children?	No	Maximum term of assignment:	3 months
Medical students?	No	Is funding available for travel?	No
Pre-medical or college students?	No	Are room and board provided?	No
Other health professional students?	No	Is any other funding available?	No
Doctors in training?	No	Is training provided or available?	Yes
Health personnel who are US citizens?	No	Is a language other than English required? *1*	No
Health personnel who are non-US citizens?	No		
Health personnel with no prior experience in developing countries?	No		
Health personnel who are not current members of your organization?	No		

Health Professionals Placed:

Physicians:

Allied Health Professionals:

Public Health Specialists, Epidemiologists and Health Educators

Notes

1. Language requirements depend on the placement.

World Association for Children and Parents

Address: **315 South Second Street, Renton, WA 98055 U.S.A.**

Phone: **(206) 575-4550** **(800) 732-1887** FAX: **(206) 575-4148**

E-Mail: **wacap@wacap.org** Web: **www.wacap.org/**

Continents Served

Africa ☐ Asia ☑ Europe ☑ The Americas ☐

Countries Served

China, India, Korea, South, Romania, Russia, Thailand

Mission: World Association for Children and Parents (WACAP), founded in 1976, is one of the most respected and experienced international nonprofit adoption agencies in the United States. We've placed more than 8,000 children with loving adoptive parents. We've also provided food, medical care and education to over 160,000 children in nine countries. World Association for Children and Parents (WACAP) has an ongoing project in China, the Peony Project, aimed at improving educational and medical services for children with disabilities living in orphanages and in the surrounding communities. WACAP is seeking volunteer occupational therapists, physical therapists and special education teachers to support the ongoing integration of Western rehabilitation and educational philosophies and techniques with the existing programs for children with disabilities.

Placement opportunities for . . .		Organization/Service Specifics:	
People of only certain faiths?	No	Size of the Organization's Staff:	21-50
Couples: both are health providers? *1*		Number of providers sent or received/year:	11-20
Couples: only one is a health provider?		Minimum term of assignment:	3 months
Families with children?		Maximum term of assignment:	none
Medical students?	No	Is funding available for travel?	Yes
Pre-medical or college students?	No	Are room and board provided?	Yes
Other health professional students?	No	Is any other funding available? *2*	Yes
Doctors in training?	No	Is training provided or available?	Yes
Health personnel who are US citizens?	Yes	Is a language other than English required?	No
Health personnel who are non-US citizens?	Yes		
Health personnel with no prior experience in developing countries?	Yes		
Health personnel who are not current members of your organization?	Yes		

Health Professionals Placed:

Physicians:

Allied Health Professionals:

Physical & Occupational Therapists; Social Workers

Notes

1. Depends on needs and time served; *2.* The Peony Project will arrange and provide travel, lodging and a daily living stipend in China for volunteers.

World Concern

Address: **19303 Fremont Avenue North, Seattle, WA 98133 U.S.A.**

Phone: **(800) 755-5022** FAX: **(206) 546-7269**

E-Mail: **info@worldconcern.org** Web: **www.worldconcern.org**

Continents Served

Africa ✔ Asia ✔ Europe ✔ The Americas ✔

Countries Served

Bolivia	Cambodia	Haiti
Kenya	Laos	
Myanmar (Burma)	Peru	Sudan
Thailand	Uganda	
Uzbekistan	Vietnam	

Mission: World Concern is an international Christian relief and development organization serving more than four million people in 27 countries each year. Founded in 1955, World Concern is strengthening families and helping people become self-reliant through food and work programs. Our mission is to overcome human suffering through emergency relief, rehabilitation, and long-term development programs so that familites and individuals can be in the right relationship with God, with one another and with creation. World Concern supports projects and personnel in 22 countries in the areas of food security, primary health care, income generation and education. The projects serve more than four million poor and oppressed people annually.

Placement opportunities for . . .

People of only certain faiths? *1*	Yes
Couples: both are health providers?	Yes
Couples: only one is a health provider?	Yes
Families with children?	Yes
Medical students?	Yes
Pre-medical or college students?	No
Other health professional students?	Yes
Doctors in training?	Yes
Health personnel who are US citizens?	Yes
Health personnel who are non-US citizens?	Yes
Health personnel with no prior experience in developing countries?	Yes
Health personnel who are not current members of your organization?	Yes

Organization/Service Specifics:

Size of the Organization's Staff:	21-50
Number of providers sent or received/year:	>200
Minimum term of assignment:	6 months
Maximum term of assignment:	
Is funding available for travel?	No
Are room and board provided?	No
Is any other funding available?	No
Is training provided or available?	No
Is a language other than English required? *2*	No

Health Professionals Placed:

Physicians:

Physicians

Allied Health Professionals:

Dentists; Nurses; Public Health Specialists, Epidemiologists and Health Educators; Water/Sanitation Specialists

Notes

1. Volunteers must be Christian;
2. Language requirements depend on the project.

World Emergency Relief

Address: **2270 Camino Vida Rable, Suite D, Carlsbad, CA 92009 U.S.A.**

Phone: **(760) 930-8001** **(888) 484-4543** FAX: **(760) 930-9085**

E-Mail: **info@wer-us.org** Web: **www.worldemergency.org**

Continents Served

Africa ✔ Asia ✔ Europe ✔ The Americas ✔

Countries Served

Argentina	Bosnia and Herzegovina	
Brazil	Burundi	China
Colombia	Congo	
Dominican Republic		Guatemala
Honduras	Hong Kong	India
Jamaica	Kenya	Liberia
Mauritania	Mexico	Nicaragua
Peru	Philippines	Romania
Thailand	Uganda	USSR, former
Yugoslavia, former	Zaire (DemRepCongo)	

Mission: World Emergency Relief is an interdenominational fellowship of Christians worldwide, working together to help people in need, especially children and their families. Personnel must share Christian (conservative) views. Lengths of stay in various regions range from 2 weeks to 3 years. Different health provider types are used by the organization; prosthetists are in particularly high demand. Language requirements depend upon location.

(continued)

Placement opportunities for . . .

People of only certain faiths? *1*	No
Couples: both are health providers?	Yes
Couples: only one is a health provider?	Yes
Families with children?	No
Medical students?	Yes
Pre-medical or college students?	Yes
Other health professional students?	Yes
Doctors in training?	Yes
Health personnel who are US citizens?	Yes
Health personnel who are non-US citizens?	Yes
Health personnel with no prior experience in developing countries?	Yes
Health personnel who are not current members of your organization?	Yes

Organization/Service Specifics:

Size of the Organization's Staff:	11-20
Number of providers sent or received/year:	51-100
Minimum term of assignment:	2 weeks
Maximum term of assignment:	3 years
Is funding available for travel?	Yes
Are room and board provided?	Yes
Is any other funding available?	No
Is training provided or available?	Yes
Is a language other than English required? *2*	Yes

Health Professionals Placed:

Physicians:

Physicians; Emergency Medicine Physicians; Internal Medicine GPS & PCP; OB/GYN; Pediatricians; Plastic/Hand/Reconstructive Surgeons

Allied Health Professionals:

Nurse Midwives; Nurse Practitioners; Nurses; Prosthetists; Public Health Specialists, Epidemiologists and Health Educators

Notes

1. No specific religious requirements, but volunteers must share Christian values; *2.* Language requirements depend on the country of service.

World Gospel Mission

Address: **3783 State Road 18 East, P.O. Box 948, Marion, IN 46952-0948 U.S.A.**

Phone: **(765) 664-7331** FAX: **(765) 671-7230**

E-Mail: **wgm@wgm.org** Web: **www.wgm.org**

Mission: With 325 missionaries and support staff serving on five continents, World Gospel Mission is committed to making Christ known to people all over the world. Ministries include church planting, evangelism, discipleship, education, medical care, community health/development, agriculture, rescue missions, aviation, and literature. Health care personnel seeking to serve abroad through WGM must be of the Protestant faith. Minimum assignments are short-term, and maximum are lifelong. There are no language requirements.

Continents Served

Africa ✔ Asia ✔ Europe ✔ The Americas ✔

Countries Served

Argentina	Bolivia	Burundi
Honduras	Hungary	India
Japan	Kenya	Mexico
Papua-New Guinea		Paraguay
St. Croix	Taiwan	Tanzania
Uganda	Ukraine	United States

Placement opportunities for . . .

People of only certain faiths? *1*	Yes
Couples: both are health providers?	Yes
Couples: only one is a health provider?	Yes
Families with children?	Yes
Medical students? *2*	Yes
Pre-medical or college students?	No
Other health professional students?	Yes
Doctors in training?	No
Health personnel who are US citizens?	Yes
Health personnel who are non-US citizens?	Yes
Health personnel with no prior experience in developing countries?	Yes
Health personnel who are not current members of your organization?	Yes

Organization/Service Specifics:

Size of the Organization's Staff:	>200
Number of providers sent or received/year:	11-20
Minimum term of assignment:	2 months
Maximum term of assignment:	career
Is funding available for travel?	No
Are room and board provided?	No
Is any other funding available? *3*	No
Is training provided or available?	Yes
Is a language other than English required?	No

Health Professionals Placed:

Physicians:

Physicians; Emergency Medicine Physicians; Family Practitioners; General Surgeons; Internal Medicine GPS & PCP; Pediatricians

Allied Health Professionals:

Administrative Health Positions; Medical Technicians (lab, X-ray, etc); Nurse Midwives; Nurses; Physician Assistants; Public Health Specialists, Epidemiologists and Health Educators

Notes

1. Protestant; *2.* Sometimes. *3.* Missionaries raise all their support for travel and ministry.

World Hearing Network

Address: **Denver Ear Associates PC, 799 E Hampden Ave, #510, Englewood, CO 80110 U.S.A.**

Phone: **(303) 788-7880** FAX: **(303) 788-7883**

E-Mail: **NPyle@TheCNI.org** Web: **www.thecni.org/hearing/world.htm**

Continents Served

Africa ☐ Asia ☐ Europe ☐ The Americas ☑

Countries Served

Costa Rica, Ecuador, Honduras, Jamaica, Mexico, Peru, Vietnam

Mission: The World Hearing Network, as part of the Colorado Neurological Institute, seeks to help alleviate hearing loss and disease of the ear worldwide by empowering local doctors and audiologists and transferring state-of-the-art medical knowledge, tools, and training. Volunteers of any faith are sent on 20 missions to Third World countries including Peru, Ecuador, Costa Rica, Vietnam, Honduras, Mexico, and Jamaica. Currently, the World Hearing Network is not accepting new applications. However, interested applicants may be placed on a waiting list for future placements.

Placement opportunities for . . .

People of only certain faiths?	No
Couples: both are health providers?	Yes
Couples: only one is a health provider?	Yes
Families with children?	No
Medical students?	Yes
Pre-medical or college students?	Yes
Other health professional students?	No
Doctors in training?	Yes
Health personnel who are US citizens?	Yes
Health personnel who are non-US citizens?	Yes
Health personnel with no prior experience in developing countries?	Yes
Health personnel who are not current members of your organization?	Yes

Organization/Service Specifics:

Size of the Organization's Staff:	0-5
Number of providers sent or received/year:	11-20
Minimum term of assignment:	2 weeks
Maximum term of assignment:	4 weeks
Is funding available for travel?	Yes
Are room and board provided?	Yes
Is any other funding available? *1*	No
Is training provided or available?	Yes
Is a language other than English required?	No

Health Professionals Placed:

Physicians:

Physicians; Anesthesiologists; Cardiologists; Dermatologists; Emergency Medicine Physicians; Endocrinologists; Family Practitioners; Gastroenterologists; General Surgeons; Hematologists; Oncologists; Infectious Disease Spec.; Internal Medicine GPS & PCP; Nephrologists; Neurologists; Neurosurgeons; OB/GYN; Ophthalmologists; Oral Surgeons; Orthopedic Surgeons; Otolaryngologists; Pathologists; Pediatricians; Plastic/Hand/Reconstructive Surgeons; Pulmonary Specialists; Radiologists; Urologists

Allied Health Professionals:

Nurses

Notes

1. Funding availability varies with the program and budget. We have funded expenses for the Belize program but will likely not continue this practice in the future.

World Medical Mission

Address: **P.O. Box 3000, Boone, NC 28607 U.S.A.**

Phone: **(828) 262-1980** FAX: **(828) 266-1053**

E-Mail: **wmminfo@samaritan.org or projectinfo@samaritan.org** Web: **www.samaritanspurse.org**

Continents Served

Africa ☑ Asia ☑ Europe ☑ The Americas ☑

Countries Served

Albania, Bangladesh, Botswana, Brazil, China, Dominican Republic, Ecuador, Egypt, Ethiopia, Guatemala, Haiti, Honduras, India, Kenya, Mongolia, Mozambique, Papua-New Guinea, Russia, Rwanda, Sudan, Tanzania, Uganda, Ukraine, United States, Vietnam, Zambia

Mission: World Medical Mission, the medical ministry of Samaritan's Purse, provides evangelical mission hospitals and clinics with the resources they need—equipment, supplies, and Christian physicians and biomedical technicians—to treat their patients while standing as a shining witness of God's love through Jesus Christ. Wherever we serve, the Gospel is faithfully presented through hospital chaplains, Christian literature, films, audio tapes, and other means. In 2002, we sent doctors, dentists, and other medical professionals on 315 assignments to 42 locations in 27 countries. We also traveled to 9 countries installing or repairing critically needed equipment, and we shipped more than $2 million worth of medical supplies and equipment to facilities in 54 countries. The motivation behind all our efforts is to go and "heal the sick who are there and tell them, 'The kingdom of God is near you'" (Luke 10:9, NIV). In remote areas around the world, missionary medicine is one of the most effective means of evangelism available. Each year the hospitals we serve are used by God to lead thousands of people to faith in Jesus Christ. WMM will coordinate the mission trip and match interests, abilities, and time frame with a hospital. *(continued)*

Placement opportunities for . . .	
People of only certain faiths? *1*	Yes
Couples: both are health providers?	Yes
Couples: only one is a health provider?	Yes
Families with children?	Yes
Medical students?	No
Pre-medical or college students?	No
Other health professional students?	No
Doctors in training?	Yes
Health personnel who are US citizens?	Yes
Health personnel who are non-US citizens?	Yes
Health personnel with no prior experience in developing countries?	Yes
Health personnel who are not current members of your organization?	Yes

Organization/Service Specifics:	
Size of the Organization's Staff: *2*	
Number of providers sent or received/year:	>200
Minimum term of assignment:	2 months
Maximum term of assignment:	
Is funding available for travel?	No
Are room and board provided?	Yes
Is any other funding available?	No
Is training provided or available?	Yes
Is a language other than English required?	No

Health Professionals Placed:

Physicians:

Physicians

Allied Health Professionals:

Dentists

Notes

1. Christian; *2.* Organization did not respond to inquiries; information from Web site.

World Mission Prayer League

Address: **232 Clifton Ave., Minneapolis, MN 55403 U.S.A.**

Phone: **(612) 871-6843** FAX: **(612) 871-6844**

E-Mail: **wmpl@wmpl.org** Web: **www.wmpl.org**

Mission: The World Mission Prayer League is a Lutheran community committed to knowing Christ, praying for the advancement of His Kingdom, sharing the Gospel and ourselves with those who do not know Him, and encouraging Christians everywhere in the global task. Volunteers can travel for a minimum of 6 week terms. Long-term personnel must be Lutheran, whereas short-term personnel must be Christian. Funding for travel is not included, but room and board are provided.

Continents Served

Africa ☑ Asia ☑ Europe ☑ The Americas ☑

Countries Served

Afghanistan	Bangladesh	Bolivia
Ecuador	Eritrea	Kenya
Mexico	Mongolia	Nepal
Pakistan	Peru	Philippines
Romania		

Placement opportunities for . . .	
People of only certain faiths? *1*	Yes
Couples: both are health providers?	Yes
Couples: only one is a health provider?	Yes
Families with children?	Yes
Medical students?	Yes
Pre-medical or college students?	Yes
Other health professional students?	Yes
Doctors in training?	Yes
Health personnel who are US citizens?	Yes
Health personnel who are non-US citizens?	Yes
Health personnel with no prior experience in developing countries?	Yes
Health personnel who are not current members of your organization?	Yes

Organization/Service Specifics:	
Size of the Organization's Staff:	11-20
Number of providers sent or received/year:	>200
Minimum term of assignment:	6 weeks
Maximum term of assignment:	
Is funding available for travel?	No
Are room and board provided? *2*	Yes
Is any other funding available?	No
Is training provided or available? *3*	Yes
Is a language other than English required? *4*	Yes

Health Professionals Placed:

Physicians:

Physicians; Family Practitioners; General Surgeons; Internal Medicine GPS & PCP; OB/GYN; Pediatricians

Allied Health Professionals:

Nurse Midwives; Nurse Practitioners; Nurses; Public Health Specialists, Epidemiologists and Health Educators

Notes

1. Long-term personnel must be specifically Lutheran Christian. Short-term must be Christian; *2.* Room, but not necessarily board, is provided; *3.* Some on site training is provided; *4.* No language requirements for volunteers serving less than a year.

World Rehabilitation Fund, Inc.

Address: **57 W. 57th Street, Suite 1101, New York, NY 10019 U.S.A.**

Phone: **(212) 207-8374** FAX:

E-Mail: **wrfnewyork@msn.com** Web: **www.worldrehabfund.org**

Continents Served

Africa ✔ Asia ✔ Europe ✔ The Americas ✔

Countries Served

Cambodia, Dominican Republic, Kazakhstan, Lebanon, Mozambique, Sierra Leone, Uzbekistan

Mission: The World Rehabilitation Fund is a world-wide, non-profit organization of physicians, therapists, technicians and specialists who are dedicated to relieving the misery caused by war, natural disaster, and disease. Volunteers can serve for a minimum 1 week term. Both travel expenses and room and board are provided. There are no language or religious requirements.

Placement opportunities for . . .	
People of only certain faiths?	No
Couples: both are health providers?	Yes
Couples: only one is a health provider?	No
Families with children?	No
Medical students?	No
Pre-medical or college students?	No
Other health professional students?	Yes
Doctors in training?	No
Health personnel who are US citizens?	Yes
Health personnel who are non-US citizens?	Yes
Health personnel with no prior experience in developing countries?	No
Health personnel who are not current members of your organization?	Yes

Organization/Service Specifics:		
Size of the Organization's Staff:		6-10
Number of providers sent or received/year:		>200
Minimum term of assignment:		1 week
Maximum term of assignment:		
Is funding available for travel?		No
Are room and board provided?		
Is any other funding available?	*1*	No
Is training provided or available?		No
Is a language other than English required?	*2*	No

Health Professionals Placed:

Physicians:

Physicians

Allied Health Professionals:

Physical & Occupational Therapists; Prosthetists; Psychologists; Public Health Specialists, Epidemiologists and Health Educators; Social Workers

Notes

1. No additional funding unless the volunteer receives a grant;
2. Language of the country of service is desirable but not required.

World Vision International

Address: **800 West Chestnut Avenue, Monrovia, CA 91061-3198 U.S.A.**

Phone: **(626) 303-8811** FAX: **(626) 301-7786**

E-Mail: **lcasazza@worldvision.org, or newsvision@wvi.org** Web: **www.wvi.org**

Mission: World Vision is a Christian organization that serves indigent children in 89 countries by providing community-based relief and development programs. It places physicians of any religion on a long-term basis in countries in Africa, Europe, the Americas, and Asia. World Vision is involved in disaster relief to many parts of the world. Assignments range from 1-2 years, and personnel receive a salary plus benefits. French or Portuguese may be required.

Continents Served

Africa ✔ Asia ✔ Europe ✔ The Americas ✔

Countries Served

Albania	Angola	Armenia
Australia	Austria	Bangladesh
Bosnia and Herzegovina		Brazil
Burundi	Cambodia	Canada
Chad	Chile	China
Colombia	Costa Rica	
Dominican Republic		Ecuador
El Salvador	Eritrea	Ethiopia
Finland	Germany	Ghana
Guatemala	Haiti	Honduras
Hong Kong	India	Indonesia
Ireland	Japan	Jordan
Kenya	Korea, North	Korea, South
Laos	Lebanon	Lesotho
Liberia	Macedonia	Malawi
Malaysia	Mali	Mauritania
Mexico	Mongolia	Mozambique
Nepal	Netherlands	New Zealand
Niger	Peru	Philippines
Romania	Rwanda	Senegal
Sierra Leone	Singapore	Somalia
South Africa	Sri Lanka	Sudan
Swaziland	Switzerland	Syria
Taiwan	Tanzania	Thailand
Uganda	United Kingdom	
United States	USSR, former	Vanuatu
Venezuela	Vietnam	
Yugoslavia, former		Zimbabwe

Placement opportunities for . . .

People of only certain faiths?	No
Couples: both are health providers?	No
Couples: only one is a health provider?	No
Families with children?	No
Medical students?	No
Pre-medical or college students?	No
Other health professional students?	Yes
Doctors in training?	No
Health personnel who are US citizens?	No
Health personnel who are non-US citizens?	No
Health personnel with no prior experience in developing countries?	No
Health personnel who are not current members of your organization?	No

Organization/Service Specifics:

Size of the Organization's Staff:	>200
Number of providers sent or received/year:	6-10
Minimum term of assignment:	1 year
Maximum term of assignment:	2 years
Is funding available for travel?	Yes
Are room and board provided?	Yes
Is any other funding available? *1*	Yes
Is training provided or available?	No
Is a language other than English required? *2*	Yes

Health Professionals Placed:

Physicians:

Physicians; Internal Medicine GPS & PCP

Allied Health Professionals:

Nurse Midwives; Nurses; Nutritionists & Dieticians; Public Health Specialists, Epidemiologists and Health Educators; Water/Sanitation Specialists

Notes

1. Salary plus benefits; *2.* French or Portuguese.

World Vision, Inc.

Address: **PO Box 9716, Federal Way, WA 98063 U.S.A.**

Phone: **(253) 815-1000** FAX: **(253) 815-3343**
(888) 511-6548

E-Mail: **info@worldvision.org** Web: **www.worldvision.org**

Mission: World Vision is an international partnership of Christians, whose mission is to follow our Lord and Savior Jesus Christ in working with the poor and oppressed to promote human transformation, seek justice, and bear witness to the good news of the Kingdom of God. World Vision, Inc. seeks Christian personnel to serve for 1-2 year terms. Employees of World Vision, Inc. are paid by salary plus benefits.

Continents Served

Africa ✔ Asia ✔ Europe ✔ The Americas ✔

Countries Served

Afghanistan	Angola	Brazil
Burundi	Cambodia	Colombia
Congo	El Salvador	Ethiopia
India	Indonesia	Iraq
Israel	Korea, North	Laos
Liberia	Mali	Mongolia
Mozambique	Myanmar (Burma)	
Niger	Rwanda	Sierra Leone
Somalia	Sudan	Taiwan
Uganda	United States	USSR, former
Venezuela	Vietnam	
Zaire (DemRepCongo)		

Placement opportunities for . . .

People of only certain faiths? *1*	Yes
Couples: both are health providers?	No
Couples: only one is a health provider?	Yes
Families with children?	Yes
Medical students?	No
Pre-medical or college students?	No
Other health professional students?	No
Doctors in training?	No
Health personnel who are US citizens?	Yes
Health personnel who are non-US citizens?	Yes
Health personnel with no prior experience in developing countries?	No
Health personnel who are not current members of your organization?	Yes

Organization/Service Specifics:

Size of the Organization's Staff:	>200
Number of providers sent or received/year:	6-10
Minimum term of assignment:	1 year
Maximum term of assignment:	2 years
Is funding available for travel?	Yes
Are room and board provided?	Yes
Is any other funding available? *2*	Yes
Is training provided or available?	No
Is a language other than English required? *3*	Yes

Health Professionals Placed:

Physicians:

Physicians; Internal Medicine GPS & PCP

Allied Health Professionals:

Nurse Midwives; Nurses; Nutritionists & Dieticians; Public Health Specialists, Epidemiologists and Health Educators; Water/Sanitation Specialists

Notes

1. Personnel must be Christian; *2.* Personnel receive salary plus benefits; *3.* Language requirements are dependent on the assignment.

World Witness—The Associate Reformed Presbyterian Church

Address: **1 Cleveland St., Suite 220, Greenville, SC 29601 U.S.A.**

Phone: **(864) 233-5226** FAX: **(864) 233-5326**

E-Mail: **worldwitness@worldwitness.org** Web: **www.worldwitness.org**

Continents Served

Africa ☐ Asia ✔ Europe ✔ The Americas ✔

Countries Served

Germany Mexico Pakistan Russia

Mission: World Witness is the Board of Foreign Missions of the Associate Reformed Presbyterian Church. World Witness is dedicated to serving other nations as disciples of Christ. Trips can be short term (1 week), or personnel can become career missionaries through World Witness. There are no language requirements, and while most volunteers are Protestant, World Witness is open to accepting other people who are comfortable working in a Christian environment. World Witness is a fund-raising organization.

(continued)

Placement opportunities for . . .

People of only certain faiths? *1*	Yes
Couples: both are health providers?	Yes
Couples: only one is a health provider?	Yes
Families with children?	Yes
Medical students?	No
Pre-medical or college students?	No
Other health professional students?	Yes
Doctors in training?	Yes
Health personnel who are US citizens?	Yes
Health personnel who are non-US citizens?	No
Health personnel with no prior experience in developing countries?	Yes
Health personnel who are not current members of your organization?	Yes

Organization/Service Specifics:

Size of the Organization's Staff:	11-20
Number of providers sent or received/year:	21-50
Minimum term of assignment:	1 week
Maximum term of assignment:	
Is funding available for travel?	No
Are room and board provided?	No
Is any other funding available?	No
Is training provided or available?	Yes
Is a language other than English required?	No

Health Professionals Placed:

Physicians:

Physicians; Orthopedic Surgeons; Plastic/Hand/Reconstructive Surgeons

Allied Health Professionals:

Nurses

Notes

1. Volunteers are Protestant, although others able to work in a Christian environment would be considered.

Worldwide Evangelization for Christ (WEC) International

Address: **P.O. Box 1707, 709 Pennsylvania Ave, Fort Washington, PA 19034-8707 U.S.A.**

Phone: **(215) 646-2322** FAX: **(215) 646-6202**
(888) 646-6202

E-Mail: **info@wec-usa.org or trekusa@wectrek.org** Web: **www.wec-int.org**

Mission: Worldwide Evangelization for Christ (WEC) International is a Christian evangelical organization that provides outreach to 130 ethnic groups without a church of their own. WEC is recruiting teams today for each ethnic group. Teams will learn the language, immerse themselves in the culture, make friends, pray for openings to introduce their friends to Jesus, and form groups of disciples. Members of teams may become involved in translating the scriptures, cooperating with someone who is, or teaching. WEC currently seeks individuals for short- (1 week) to long-term stays.

Continents Served

Africa ✔ Asia ✔ Europe ✔ The Americas ✔

Countries Served

Afghanistan, Burkina Faso, Cambodia, Chad, China, Equatorial Guinea, Gambia, Ghana, Guatemala, Guinea-Bissau, Ivory Coast, Jordan, Liberia, Mexico, Mongolia, Nepal, Senegal, South Africa, Spain, Turkey, United Arab Emirates, USSR, former, Yemen, Zaire (DemRepCongo)

Placement opportunities for . . .

People of only certain faiths? *1*	Yes
Couples: both are health providers?	Yes
Couples: only one is a health provider?	Yes
Families with children?	Yes
Medical students?	Yes
Pre-medical or college students?	Yes
Other health professional students?	Yes
Doctors in training?	Yes
Health personnel who are US citizens?	Yes
Health personnel who are non-US citizens?	Yes
Health personnel with no prior experience in developing countries?	Yes
Health personnel who are not current members of your organization?	Yes

Organization/Service Specifics:

Size of the Organization's Staff:	21-50
Number of providers sent or received/year:	>200
Minimum term of assignment:	1 week
Maximum term of assignment:	No Maximum
Is funding available for travel?	No
Are room and board provided?	No
Is any other funding available?	No
Is training provided or available? *2*	No
Is a language other than English required? *3*	Yes

(continued)

Health Professionals Placed:

Physicians:

Physicians; Anesthesiologists; Cardiologists; Dermatologists; Emergency Medicine Physicians; Endocrinologists; Family Practitioners; Gastroenterologists; General Surgeons; Hematologists; Oncologists; Infectious Disease Spec.; Internal Medicine GPS & PCP; Nephrologists; Neurologists; Neurosurgeons; OB/GYN; Ophthalmologists; Oral Surgeons; Optometrists; Orthopedic Surgeons; Otolaryngologists; Pathologists; Pediatricians; Plastic/Hand/Reconstructive Surgeons; Psychiatrists; Pulmonary Specialists; Radiologists; Urologists

Allied Health Professionals:

Administrative Health Positions; Dental Hygienists; Dentists; Medical Technicians (lab, X-ray, etc); Nurse Midwives; Nurse Practitioners; Nurses; Nutritionists & Dieticians; Paramedics; Pharmacists; Physical & Occupational Therapists; Physician Assistants; Podiatrists; Prosthetists; Psychologists; Public Health Specialists, Epidemiologists and Health Educators; Respiratory Therapists; Social Workers; Water/Sanitation Specialists

Notes

1. Volunteers must be Evangelical Protestant; *2.* There is mission training provided, but not medical training; *3.* Language requirements depend on the country and length of service.

Zuma Memorial Hospital

Address: **Irrua Edd State, Nigeria, Africa**

Phone: **055 97300** FAX:

E-Mail: Web:

Continents Served

Africa ☑ Asia ☐ Europe ☐ The Americas ☐

Countries Served

Nigeria

Mission: Zuma Memorial Hospital in Irrua, with a population of about 65,000, was founded in 1950 in rural Nigeria. Today it has 120 beds, a maternity ward, and a school of midwifery. Volunteers can serve for a minimum of 6 weeks. There are no language or religious requirements and volunteers must provide their own expenses.

Placement opportunities for . . .	
People of only certain faiths?	No
Couples: both are health providers?	Yes
Couples: only one is a health provider?	No
Families with children?	No
Medical students?	Yes
Pre-medical or college students?	No
Other health professional students?	No
Doctors in training?	Yes
Health personnel who are US citizens?	Yes
Health personnel who are non-US citizens?	Yes
Health personnel with no prior experience in developing countries?	Yes
Health personnel who are not current members of your organization?	Yes

Organization/Service Specifics:	
Size of the Organization's Staff: *1*	21-50
Number of providers sent or received/year:	1-5
Minimum term of assignment:	6 weeks
Maximum term of assignment:	Optional
Is funding available for travel?	No
Are room and board provided?	No
Is any other funding available?	No
Is training provided or available?	Yes
Is a language other than English required?	No

Health Professionals Placed:

Physicians:

Physicians; General Surgeons; OB/GYN; Ophthalmologists

Allied Health Professionals:

Notes

1. Last contacted on 12/02. No response to inquiry in 2/05.

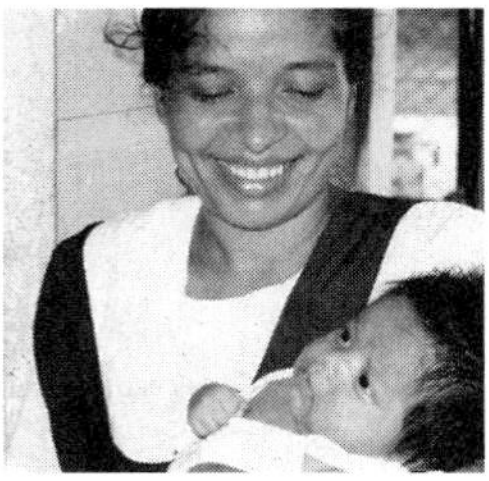

Chapter 4

Cross-Referencing Guide to the Database

Judging by what I have learned about men and women, I am convinced that far more idealistic aspiration exists than is ever evident. Just as the rivers we see are much less numerous than the underground streams, so the idealism that is visible is minor compared to what men and women carry in their hearts, unreleased or scarcely released. Mankind is waiting and longing for those who can accomplish the task of untying what is knotted and bringing the underground waters to the surface.

—Albert Schweitzer

History will be our judge, but what's written is up to us. Who we are, who we've been, what we want to be remembered for. We can't say our generation didn't know how to do it. And we can't say our generation didn't have reason to do it. It's up to us.

—Bono

In the introduction to Chapter 3, I introduced our database of international health service opportunities. In this chapter, we provide the organizations' responses to the specific questions we asked. This cross-referencing information should help you to narrow your search to the organizations that will comprise the best fit for you. Please refer back to the introduction to Chapter 3 if you are unclear as to how to make the most out of the information that follows.

By searching through the lists in this section, you will quickly be able to find organizations that seek those in your particular area in health care, those that send health providers for the time that you have available, those that work in the world regions you prefer to travel to, and so on. Most of the data we collected are reproduced here, in a format that should help you answer the questions most important in serving internationally. Not all the data could fit, however. Those requiring further information can check on the status of the database at www.omnimed.org. The organizations listed in this chapter are organized into the following categories:

- Does your organization have opportunities for the following allied health professionals:

- Do you send health personnel to the following continents:

(Specific country listings are available at www.omnimed.org.)

Once you have found the organizations that best fit your needs and interests, please refer to Chapter 3 or Chapter 5 for concise organizational profiles. Then contact each organization, talk with at least three volunteers that have served through them, and consider posing some of the questions raised in the introduction to Chapter 3.

Organizations seeking couples in which both members are health practitioners

ACCESS
Action Against Hunger
Adventist Development and Relief Agency International
Africa Inland Mission, International
African Inter-Mennonite Mission
Africare
Aid for International Medicine
Ak' Tenamit
Aloha Medical Missions (AMM)
Amazon-Africa Aid and Fundacao Esperanca
Amazon-Africa Aid Organization (3AO)
American Jewish World Service
American Leprosy Missions Inc.
American Physicians Fellowship for Medicine in Israel
American Refugee Committee
Ann Foundation Inc
APUSAN-USA
Archdiocesan Health Care Network for Catholic Charities
Armenian Eye Care Project
ASAPROSAR: The Salvadoran Association for Rural Health
Associate Reformed Presbyterian Church, World Witness
Associazione Italiana 'Amici Raoul Follereau'

Bairo Pite Clinic
Baptist General Conference
Baptist Medical and Dental Mission International
Baptist Medical Missions International
Baptist Mid Missions
Beeve Foundation for World Eye and Health, The
Ben Gurion University of the Negev
Board of World Mission of the Moravian Church
Boston International Foundation for Medical Education
Boston University School of Medicine, Section of Preventive Medicine and Epidemiology
Bread for the World (Brot fur die Welt)
Bridges to Community, Inc.

Cameroon Baptist Convention Health Board
Campus Crusade for Christ International
Canvasback Missions, Inc.
Cape Cares
Cape Verde Care Agency, Inc.
CardioStart International, Inc.
Casa Clinica de la Mujer
Catholic Medical Mission Board, Inc.
Catholic Network of Volunteer Service
CB International
CERT International (Christian Emergency Relief Team)
Children's Cross Connection, International
Children's Medical Mission
Christian Dental Missions
Christian Dental Society
Christian Medical and Dental Associations-Global Health Outreach
Christian Mission of Pignon Inc.
Church of the Nazarene World Mission Division
Clinica Evangelica Morava Elective
Clínica Maxena
College of Medicine, Malawi
Comitato Collaborazione Medica (Doctors for Developing Countries)
Commonwealth Health Center
Community of Caring
Complete Basic Health 2000
CONCERN
CONCERN America
Cross-Cultural Solutions
CrossWorld
Crudem Foundation
Curamericas

Dental Health International
DePauw University Winter Term in Service
DoCare International, Inc.
Doctors for Global Health
Doctors of the World

Edmundite Missions Corps
Emergency International, Inc.
Esperanca, Inc.
Evangelical Alliance Mission (TEAM World)
Evangelical Free Church of America Mission
Evangelical Lutheran Church in America

Father Carr's Place 2B
Feed the Children
Fellowship of Associates of Medical Evangelism
Filipino-American Medical Inc.
Flying Samaritans
FOCUS Inc.
Foundation for International Medical Relief of Children
Foundation of Compassionate American Samaritans
Friends Lugulu Hospital
Friends Without a Border
Fulbright Scholar Award, Council for the International Exchange of Students

General Baptist International
General Board of Global Ministries / The United Methodist Church
General Dept. of World Missions, The Wesleyan Church
Global Operations & Development
Global Outreach International
Global Service Corps/Earth Island Institute

Organizations seeking couples in which both members are health practitioners *(continued)*

Global Volunteers

Grace Ministries International

Grokha Association of Social Health

Guinea Development Foundation, Inc.

Haitian Health Clinic, Inc.

Hands Together, Inc.

Harlem Hospital, Plastic Surgery Program

HBS Foundation, Inc. / Hopital Bon Samaritain

Healing the Children Northeast, Inc.

Health Alliance International

Health and Child Survival Fellows Program

Health Teams International

Health Volunteers Overseas

Helen Keller International

Helping Hands Health Education

Helps International

Hillside Healthcare Center

Himalayan Health Exchange

Himalayan HealthCare Inc.

Honduras Outreach, Inc

Hope Alliance

Hope Worldwide

Hospital Albert Schweitzer

Infectious Diseases Society of America, The, and The HIV Medicine Association

Intercultural Nursing, Inc.

International Aid, Inc.

International Children's Heart Foundation

International Health Exchange

International Health Service

International Medical Corps

International Ministries, American Baptist Churches, USA

International Nepal Fellowship

International Partnership for Human Development

International Relief Teams

Interplast

InterServe

INTERTEAM

Johns Hopkins Univ. School of Public Health, Dept. of International Health

Lalmba Association

Lay Mission-Helpers Association

Liga International, Inc.

Lighthouse for Christ Mission and Eye Centre

Loma Linda University International Programs

Ludhiana Christian Medical College Board USA

M.E.D.I.C.O.

Maluti Adventist Hospital (Lesotho)

Management Sciences for Health

Maryknoll Mission Association of the Faithful

Maua Methodist Hospital

Medical Aid for Palestinians

Medical Ambassadors International

Medical Care Development International Division

Medical Ministry International

Medical Missionaries of Mary

Medical Teams International, Inc.

Memisa Medicus Mundi

Mennonite Central Committee

Mercy Ships

Mexican Medical Ministries

Mima Foundation, Inc.

Minnesota International Health Volunteers

Mission Doctors Association

Moi University Faculty of Health Sciences

Mountain Movers Missions Intl

National Eye Care Project for Armenia

National Health Service Corps, Recruitment Program

New Missions In Haiti

Nicaraguan Children's Fund

North American Baptist Conference Missions

Northwest Medical Teams International, Inc.

Notre Dame India Mission

Omni Med

Operation Blessing, Medical Division

Operation Rainbow

Operation Smile International

Our Little Brothers and Sisters

P.C.E.A. Chogoria Hospital

P.C.E.A. Kikuyu Hospital

P.C.E.A. Tumutumu Hospital

P.R.A.Y. (Project Rescue of Amazon Youth)

Palestine Children's Relief Fund

Palms Australia

Pan American Medical Mission Foundation

Partners of the Americas

PAZAPA

Peacework: Volunteer Medical Projects

Physicians for Human Rights

Physicians for Peace

Presbyterian Church USA, Mission Service Recruitment

Project AmaZon

Project Concern International: OPTIONS

Project Hope / People to People Health Foundation

Project Open Hearts

Project ORBIS International, Inc.

Project Skye

PROMESA

Remote Area Medical

Saint Joseph's Medical Center, Family Practice Residency Program, Int'l Health Track

Organizations seeking couples in which both members are health practitioners *(continued)*

Salesian Missions

Sanyati Baptist Hospital, Baptist Convention of Zimbabwe

School Sisters of Saint Francis

Selian Lutheran Hospital

Seva Foundation

Simeus Foundation, The

SIM USA

Sister Community Alliances: Ouelessebougou-Utah Alliance

SkillShare International

Sons of Mary Missionary Society

Special Olympics, Inc.

St. Francis' Hospital

St. Jude Hospital

St. Mary's Hospital, Vunapope

Surfer's Medical Association

Surgical Eye Expeditions International (S.E.E.), Inc.

Surgical Medical Assistance Relief Teams

Surgicorps International

Trinity Health International

Tulane University School of Public Health and Tropical Medicine

Unite For Sight

Univ. of Wisconsin Med., Office of International Health Affairs

University of Cincinnati College of Medicine, Dept. of Family Medicine

University of Nebraska Medical Center, Office of International Programs and Studies

University of Zimbabwe

Uplift Internationale

US Committee for Scientific Cooperation with Vietnam

UTMB-WHO Collaborating Center for Training in International Health

Vietnam ENT Mission

Virginia Children's Connection, Dept. of Plastic. & Recon. Surgery

Visions in Action

Voluntary Missionary Movement

Voluntary Service Overseas Canada

Volunteer Missionary Movement

Volunteer Optometric Service to Humanity (VOSH) International

Volunteers in Medical Missions

VSO

WEC International

World Concern

World Emergency Relief

World Gospel Mission

World Hearing Network

World Medical Mission

World Mission Prayer League

World Rehabilitation Fund, Inc.

World Witness - the Associate Reformed Presbyterian Church

Zuma Memorial Hospital

Organizations seeking couples in which neither is a health practitioner

Advocates for Youth

Albert Schweitzer Fellowship

American Baptist Board of International Ministries

American College of Nurse-Midwives

American-Nicaraguan Foundation, Inc.

Amigos de las Americas

Anderson University School of Nursing

Armenian Social Transition Program

Canadian Society for International Health

Capiz Emmanuel Hospital

Chanet Community Organization

Child Family Health International

Children's Heartlink

Children-Surgical Aid International

Christian Medical College (Vellore, India) Board

Christoffel-Blindenmission EV

Duke University Medical Center, Division of Infectious Diseases and Int'l Health

FIENS Foundation of International Education in Neurological Surgery

Florida Association for Volunteer Action in the Caribbean and the Americas (FAVACA)

Foundation Human Nature (MeHiPro)

Friends of Liberia, Inc.

Global Health Action, Inc. (formerly INSA, The International Service Association for Health, Inc.)

Harvard University School of Public Health, Dept. of Population and Int'l Health

Indochina Surgical Educational Exchange

Instituto de Medicina Tropical Alexander Von Humboldt

Interface UCSD

International Committee of the Red Cross

International Cooperation for Development (formerly CIIR Overseas Programme)

International Eye Foundation, Inc.

International Federation of Red Cross and Red Crescent Societies

International Federation of Social Workers

International Rescue Committee

Organizations seeking couples in which neither is a health practitioner *(continued)*

Jesuit Refugee Service

Jubilee Volunteer Africa Program of AFRIDEC

Lumiere Medical Ministries, Inc.

Magee-Womens Hospital

MAP International

Medecins Sans Frontieres / Doctors Without Borders USA

Medicine for Humanity

Medicine for Peace

Michigan State University Institute for International Health

Operation Luz del Sol

Operation USA

Outreach International

OXFAM America

Oxfam Great Britain

Pan American Health Organization

Project Pacer International, LTD.

S.E.E. International

Save the Children Federation

St. John's Medical College

State Univ. of New York, Health Science Center at Brooklyn

UCSD, Division of International Health

Universidad de Chile, Facultad de Medicina

University of Illinois at Chicago College of Nursing, Global Health Leadership Office

University of Illinois College of Medicine at Rockford

University of Virginia, Center for Global Health

West Virginia University, Byrd Health Sciences Center International Health Program

Women's Commission for Refugee Women and Children

World Vision International

World Vision, Inc.

Organizations seeking couples in which one member is and one is not a health practitioner

Action Against Hunger

Adventist Development and Relief Agency International

Africa Inland Mission, International

Africare

Aid for International Medicine

Ak' Tenamit

Alice Springs Rural District, Dept. of Health & Community Services

Aloha Medical Missions (AMM)

Amazon-Africa Aid and Fundacao Esperanca

Amazon-Africa Aid Organization (3AO)

American Dental Association

American Dentists for Foreign Service

American Jewish World Service

American Leprosy Missions Inc.

American Refugee Committee

Ann Foundation Inc

APUSAN-USA

Armenian Eye Care Project

ASAPROSAR: The Salvadoran Association for Rural Health

Associate Reformed Presbyterian Church, World Witness

Associazione Italiana 'Amici Raoul Follereau'

Baptist General Conference

Baptist Medical and Dental Mission International

Baptist Medical Missions International

Baptist Mid Missions

Beeve Foundation for World Eye and Health, The

Blessings International

Board of World Mission of the Moravian Church

Boston International Foundation for Medical Education

Boston University School of Medicine, Section of Preventive Medicine and Epidemiology

Bread for the World (Brot fur die Welt)

Bridges to Community, Inc.

Cameroon Baptist Convention Health Board

Campus Crusade for Christ International

Canvasback Missions, Inc.

Cape Cares

Cape Verde Care Agency, Inc.

CardioStart International, Inc.

Casa Clinica de la Mujer

Catholic Medical Mission Board, Inc.

Catholic Network of Volunteer Service

CB International

Centre Medical Evangelique de Nyankunde

CERT International (Christian Emergency Relief Team)

Childreach PLAN International

Children's Medical Mission

Choice

Christian Dental Missions

Christian Dental Society

Christian Foundation for Children and Aging

Christian Medical and Dental Associations-Global Health Outreach

Christian Mission of Pignon Inc.

Christoffel-Blindenmission EV

Organizations seeking couples in which one member is and one is not a health practitioner *(continued)*

Church of the Nazarene World Mission Division

College of Medicine, Malawi

Comitato Collaborazione Medica (Doctors for Developing Countries)

Committee for Health Rights In the Americas

Commonwealth Health Center

Community of Caring

Complete Basic Health 2000

CONCERN

CONCERN America

Cooperative for American Relief Everywhere, Inc.

Covenant House

Cross-Cultural Solutions

CrossWorld

Crudem Foundation

Curamericas

DePauw University Winter Term in Service

DoCare International, Inc.

Doctors for Global Health

Doctors of the World

Edmundite Missions Corps

Estonian American Fund for Economic Education, Inc.

Evangelical Alliance Mission (TEAM World)

Evangelical Free Church of America Mission

Evangelical Lutheran Church in America

Father Carr's Place 2B

Fellowship of Associates of Medical Evangelism

Filipino-American Medical Inc.

Flying Physicians Association

FOCUS Inc.

Foundation for International Medical Relief of Children

Foundation for International Scientific Cooperation

Foundation of Compassionate American Samaritans

Fresh Start Surgical Gifts, Inc.

Friends Lugulu Hospital

Friends United Meeting - Friends Lugulu Hospital

Friends United Meeting, World Missions

Fulbright Scholar Award, Council for the International Exchange of Students

General Baptist International

General Board of Global Ministries / The United Methodist Church

General Dept. of World Missions, The Wesleyan Church

Global Operations & Development

Global Outreach International

Global Service Corps/Earth Island Institute

Global Volunteers

Grace Ministries International

Guinea Development Foundation, Inc.

Haitian Health Clinic, Inc.

Hands Together, Inc.

HBS Foundation, Inc. / Hopital Bon Samaritain

Health Alliance International

Health and Child Survival Fellows Program

Health Teams International

Health Volunteers Overseas

Helen Keller International

Helping Hands Health Education

Helps International

Himalayan Health Exchange

Honduras Outreach, Inc

Hope Alliance

Hope Worldwide

Hospital Albert Schweitzer

Humanity International, Inc.

Infectious Diseases Society of America, The, and The HIV Medicine Association

INTER-AID Inc. International Christian Aid

Intercultural Nursing, Inc.

International Aid, Inc.

International Federation of Red Cross and Red Crescent Societies

International Health Exchange

International Health Service

International Medical Corps

International Ministries, American Baptist Churches, USA

International Nepal Fellowship

International Volunteer Registry - Foundation of the American Academy of Ophthalmology

InterServe

INTERTEAM

Johns Hopkins Univ. School of Public Health, Dept. of International Health

Lalmba Association

Lay Mission-Helpers Association

Liga International, Inc.

Lighthouse for Christ Mission and Eye Centre

Loma Linda University International Programs

Ludhiana Christian Medical College Board USA

Lumiere Medical Ministries, Inc.

M.E.D.I.C.O.

Maluti Adventist Hospital (Lesotho)

Management Sciences for Health

Maryknoll Mission Association of the Faithful

Maua Methodist Hospital

Organizations seeking couples in which one member is and one is not a health practitioner *(continued)*

Medical Ambassadors International

Medical Care Development International Division

Medical Ministry International

Medical Missionaries of Mary

Medical Teams International, Inc.

Memisa Medicus Mundi

Mennonite Central Committee

Mercy Ships

Mexican Medical Ministries

Mima Foundation, Inc.

Minnesota International Health Volunteers

Mission Doctors Association

Moi University Faculty of Health Sciences

Mountain Movers Missions Intl

National Health Service Corps, Recruitment Program

New Missions In Haiti

Nicaraguan Children's Fund

North American Baptist Conference Missions

Northwest Medical Teams International, Inc.

Notre Dame India Mission

Omni Med

Operation Blessing, Medical Division

Operation Rainbow

Our Little Brothers and Sisters

P.C.E.A. Kikuyu Hospital

P.C.E.A. Tumutumu Hospital

P.R.A.Y. (Project Rescue of Amazon Youth)

Palms Australia

Pan American Health Organization

Pan American Medical Mission Foundation

Partners of the Americas

PAZAPA

Peacework: Volunteer Medical Projects

Physicians for Human Rights

Physicians for Peace

Pontificia Univ. Catolica de Chile, Facultad de Medicina

Presbyterian Church USA, Mission Service Recruitment

Project AmaZon

Project Concern International: OPTIONS

Project Hope / People to People Health Foundation

Remote Area Medical

Saint Joseph's Medical Center, Family Practice Residency Program, Int'l Health Track

Sanyati Baptist Hospital, Baptist Convention of Zimbabwe

School Sisters of Saint Francis

Selian Lutheran Hospital

Seva Foundation

Simeus Foundation, The

SIM USA

Sister Community Alliances: Ouelessebougou-Utah Alliance

SkillShare International

Special Olympics, Inc.

St. Francis' Hospital

St. Jude Hospital

St. Mary's Hospital, Vunapope

Surfer's Medical Association

Surgical Eye Expeditions International (S.E.E.), Inc.

Surgical Medical Assistance Relief Teams

Surgicorps International

Trans-World Overseas Employment Service

Trinity Health International

Tulane University School of Public Health and Tropical Medicine

UN Volunteers for Peace and Development

Unite For Sight

Univ. of Wisconsin Med., Office of International Health Affairs

University of Cincinnati College of Medicine, Dept. of Family Medicine

University of Illinois College of Medicine at Rockford

University of Nebraska Medical Center, Office of International Programs and Studies

University of Zimbabwe

Uplift Internationale

US Committee for Scientific Cooperation with Vietnam

Vietnam ENT Mission

Visions in Action

Voluntary Missionary Movement

Voluntary Service Overseas Canada

Volunteer Missionary Movement

Volunteer Optometric Service to Humanity (VOSH) International

Volunteers in Medical Missions

VSO

Wake Forest University Medical Center, Bowman Gray School of Medicine

WEC International

West Virginia Department of Health

World Concern

World Emergency Relief

World Gospel Mission

World Hearing Network

World Medical Mission

World Mission Prayer League

World Vision, Inc.

World Witness - the Associate Reformed Presbyterian Church

Organizations seeking families with children

Adventist Development and Relief Agency International

Africa Inland Mission, International

African Inter-Mennonite Mission

Africare

Alice Springs Rural District, Dept. of Health & Community Services

American Academy of Pediatrics, Office of International Health

American Dental Association

American Leprosy Missions Inc.

Associate Reformed Presbyterian Church, World Witness

Associazione Italiana 'Amici Raoul Follereau'

Baptist General Conference

Baptist Medical and Dental Mission International

Baptist Mid Missions

Blessings International

Boston University School of Medicine, Section of Preventive Medicine and Epidemiology

Bread for the World (Brot fur die Welt)

Cameroon Baptist Convention Health Board

CardioStart International, Inc.

Casa Clinica de la Mujer

Catholic Medical Mission Board, Inc.

Catholic Network of Volunteer Service

CB International

Centre Medical Evangelique de Nyankunde

CERT International (Christian Emergency Relief Team)

Childreach PLAN International

Children's Medical Mission

Choice

Christian Dental Missions

Christian Dental Society

Christian Foundation for Children and Aging

Christian Medical and Dental Associations-Global Health Outreach

Christoffel-Blindenmission EV

Church of the Nazarene World Mission Division

College of Medicine, Malawi

Comitato Collaborazione Medica (Doctors for Developing Countries)

Commonwealth Health Center

Community of Caring

Complete Basic Health 2000

CONCERN

CONCERN America

Cooperative for American Relief Everywhere, Inc.

Cross-Cultural Solutions

CrossWorld

DoCare International, Inc.

Doctors of the World

Edmundite Missions Corps

Evangelical Alliance Mission (TEAM World)

Evangelical Free Church of America Mission

Father Carr's Place 2B

Fellowship of Associates of Medical Evangelism

Foundation for International Medical Relief of Children

Foundation for International Scientific Cooperation

Fresh Start Surgical Gifts, Inc.

Friends Lugulu Hospital

Friends United Meeting - Friends Lugulu Hospital

Friends United Meeting, World Missions

Fulbright Scholar Award, Council for the International Exchange of Students

General Baptist International

General Board of Global Ministries / The United Methodist Church

General Dept. of World Missions, The Wesleyan Church

Global Operations & Development

Global Outreach International

Global Service Corps/Earth Island Institute

Grace Ministries International

HBS Foundation, Inc. / Hopital Bon Samaritain

Health Alliance International

Health and Child Survival Fellows Program

Health Teams International

Health Volunteers Overseas

Helen Keller International

Hope Worldwide

Hospital Albert Schweitzer

Infectious Diseases Society of America, The, and The HIV Medicine Association

Instituto de Medicina Tropical Alexander Von Humboldt

Instituto de Medicina Tropical Alexander Von Humboldt

INTER-AID Inc. International Christian Aid

International Aid, Inc.

International Federation of Red Cross and Red Crescent Societies

International Health Exchange

International Ministries, American Baptist Churches, USA

International Nepal Fellowship

International Volunteer Registry - Foundation of the American Academy of Ophthalmology

InterServe

INTERTEAM

Johns Hopkins Univ. School of Public Health, Dept. of International Health

Lay Mission-Helpers Association

Lighthouse for Christ Mission and Eye Centre

Organizations seeking families with children *(continued)*

Loma Linda University International Programs

Loyd Christian Health Ministries Inc.

Ludhiana Christian Medical College Board USA

Lumiere Medical Ministries, Inc.

Maluti Adventist Hospital (Lesotho)

Management Sciences for Health

Maryknoll Mission Association of the Faithful

Maua Methodist Hospital

Medical Ambassadors International

Medical Care Development International Division

Medical Ministry International

Medical Missionaries of Mary

Memisa Medicus Mundi

Mennonite Central Committee

Mercy Ships

Mexican Medical Ministries

Mima Foundation, Inc.

Minnesota International Health Volunteers

Mission Doctors Association

Moi University Faculty of Health Sciences

National Health Service Corps, Recruitment Program

Nicaraguan Children's Fund

North American Baptist Conference Missions

Our Little Brothers and Sisters

P.C.E.A. Chogoria Hospital

P.C.E.A. Kikuyu Hospital

P.C.E.A. Tumutumu Hospital

P.R.A.Y. (Project Rescue of Amazon Youth)

Palms Australia

Pan American Health Organization

Physicians for Human Rights

Pontificia Univ. Catolica de Chile, Facultad de Medicina

Presbyterian Church USA, Mission Service Recruitment

Project Concern International: OPTIONS

Project Hope / People to People Health Foundation

Saint Joseph's Medical Center, Family Practice Residency Program, Int'l Health Track

Sanyati Baptist Hospital, Baptist Convention of Zimbabwe

School Sisters of Saint Francis

Selian Lutheran Hospital

Special Olympics, Inc.

St. Francis' Hospital

St. Jude Hospital

St. Mary's Hospital, Vunapope

Surgical Eye Expeditions International (S.E.E.), Inc.

Surgical Medical Assistance Relief Teams

Trans-World Overseas Employment Service

Trinity Health International

Tulane University School of Public Health and Tropical Medicine

UN Volunteers for Peace and Development

Univ. of Wisconsin Med., Office of International Health Affairs

University of Cincinnati College of Medicine, Dept. of Family Medicine

University of Zimbabwe

Uplift Internationale

US Committee for Scientific Cooperation with Vietnam

Vietnam ENT Mission

Visions in Action

Voluntary Missionary Movement

Voluntary Service Overseas Canada

Volunteer Missionary Movement

Volunteer Optometric Service to Humanity (VOSH) International

Volunteers in Medical Missions

Wake Forest University Medical Center, Bowman Gray School of Medicine

WEC International

West Virginia Department of Health

World Concern

World Gospel Mission

World Medical Mission

World Mission Prayer League

World Vision, Inc.

World Witness - the Associate Reformed Presbyterian Church

Organizations seeking medical students

ACCESS

Adventist Development and Relief Agency International

Africa Inland Mission, International

Africare

Ak' Tenamit

Albert Schweitzer Fellowship

Aloha Medical Missions (AMM)

American Dentists for Foreign Service

American Jewish World Service

American Leprosy Missions Inc.

American Physicians Fellowship for Medicine in Israel

Ann Foundation Inc

APUSAN-USA

Armenian Eye Care Project

Organizations seeking medical students *(continued)*

Associate Reformed Presbyterian Church, World Witness

Bairo Pite Clinic

Baptist General Conference

Baptist Medical and Dental Mission International

Baptist Mid Missions

Beeve Foundation for World Eye and Health, The

Ben Gurion University of the Negev

Board of World Mission of the Moravian Church

Boston International Foundation for Medical Education

Boston University School of Medicine, Section of Preventive Medicine and Epidemiology

Bridges to Community, Inc.

CAM International

Cameroon Baptist Convention Health Board

Canadian Society for International Health

Cape Cares

Cape Verde Care Agency, Inc.

Capiz Emmanuel Hospital

CardioStart International, Inc.

Casa Clinica de la Mujer

Catholic Network of Volunteer Service

CB International

CERT International (Christian Emergency Relief Team)

Chanet Community Organization

Child Family Health International

Children's Cross Connection, International

Christian Dental Society

Christian Medical College (Vellore, India) Board

Christian Mission of Pignon Inc.

Church of the Nazarene World Mission Division

College of Medicine, Malawi

Community of Caring

Complete Basic Health 2000

Cross-Cultural Solutions

CrossWorld

DoCare International, Inc.

Doctors for Global Health

Duke University Medical Center, Division of Infectious Diseases and Int'l Health

Edmundite Missions Corps

Emergency International, Inc.

Evangelical Alliance Mission (TEAM World)

Evangelical Free Church of America Mission

Evangelical Lutheran Church in America

Father Carr's Place 2B

Fellowship of Associates of Medical Evangelism

Foundation for International Medical Relief of Children

Foundation Human Nature (MeHiPro)

Foundation of Compassionate American Samaritans

Friends Lugulu Hospital

Friends Without a Border

General Baptist International

General Board of Global Ministries / The United Methodist Church

Global Operations & Development

Global Outreach International

Global Service Corps/Earth Island Institute

Global Volunteers

Guinea Development Foundation, Inc.

Haitian Health Clinic, Inc.

Hands Together, Inc.

HBS Foundation, Inc. / Hopital Bon Samaritain

Health Alliance International

Health Teams International

Helen Keller International

Helping Hands Health Education

Helps International

Hillside Healthcare Center

Himalayan Health Exchange

Honduras Outreach, Inc

Hope Alliance

Hope Worldwide

Intercultural Nursing, Inc.

International Children's Heart Foundation

International Health Service

International Nepal Fellowship

International Partnership for Human Development

InterServe

Jubilee Volunteer Africa Program of AFRIDEC

Liga International, Inc.

Lighthouse for Christ Mission and Eye Centre

Loma Linda University International Programs

Lumiere Medical Ministries, Inc.

M.E.D.I.C.O.

Magee-Womens Hospital

Maluti Adventist Hospital (Lesotho)

Maua Methodist Hospital

Medical Care Development International Division

Medical Ministry International

Medical Missionaries of Mary

Medicine for Peace

Mexican Medical Ministries

Mima Foundation, Inc.

Minnesota International Health Volunteers

Moi University Faculty of Health Sciences

Mountain Movers Missions Intl

National Health Service Corps, Recruitment Program

Organizations seeking medical students *(continued)*

New Missions In Haiti

Nicaraguan Children's Fund

North American Baptist Conference Missions

Notre Dame India Mission

Omni Med

Operation Blessing, Medical Division

Operation Rainbow

Operation Smile International

P.C.E.A. Chogoria Hospital

P.C.E.A. Kikuyu Hospital

P.C.E.A. Tumutumu Hospital

P.R.A.Y. (Project Rescue of Amazon Youth)

Partners of the Americas

PAZAPA

Peacework: Volunteer Medical Projects

Physicians for Human Rights

Physicians for Peace

Presbyterian Church USA, Mission Service Recruitment

Project AmaZon

Project Concern International: OPTIONS

PROMESA

Remote Area Medical

Sanyati Baptist Hospital, Baptist Convention of Zimbabwe

School Sisters of Saint Francis

Selian Lutheran Hospital

Simeus Foundation, The

SIM USA

Sister Community Alliances: Ouelessebougou-Utah Alliance

Special Olympics, Inc.

St. Francis' Hospital

St. John's Medical College

St. Jude Hospital

St. Mary's Hospital, Vunapope

Surgical Medical Assistance Relief Teams

Surgicorps International

Tulane University School of Public Health and Tropical Medicine

UCSD, Division of International Health

Unite For Sight

Univ. of Wisconsin Med., Office of International Health Affairs

Universidad de Chile, Facultad de Medicina

University of Cincinnati College of Medicine, Dept. of Family Medicine

University of Illinois College of Medicine at Rockford

University of Nebraska Medical Center, Office of International Programs and Studies

University of Virginia, Center for Global Health

University of Zimbabwe

Uplift Internationale

US Committee for Scientific Cooperation with Vietnam

UTMB-WHO Collaborating Center for Training in International Health

Virginia Children's Connection, Dept. of Plastic. & Recon. Surgery

Visions in Action

Volunteer Missionary Movement

Volunteer Optometric Service to Humanity (VOSH) International

Volunteers in Medical Missions

WEC International

World Concern

World Emergency Relief

World Gospel Mission

World Hearing Network

World Mission Prayer League

Zuma Memorial Hospital

Organizations seeking pre-medical or college students

ACCESS

Adventist Development and Relief Agency International

Africa Inland Mission, International

Aloha Medical Missions (AMM)

American Leprosy Missions Inc.

Amigos de las Americas

Ann Foundation Inc

APUSAN-USA

Armenian Eye Care Project

Bairo Pite Clinic

Baptist General Conference

Baptist Medical and Dental Mission International

Ben Gurion University of the Negev

Board of World Mission of the Moravian Church

Bridges to Community, Inc.

CAM International

Canadian Society for International Health

Cape Cares

CardioStart International, Inc.

Catholic Network of Volunteer Service

CB International

Centre Medical Evangelique de Nyankunde

CERT International (Christian Emergency Relief Team)

Child Family Health International

Children's Cross Connection, International

Christian Mission of Pignon Inc.

Community of Caring

Complete Basic Health 2000

Organizations seeking pre-medical or college students *(continued)*

Cross-Cultural Solutions

DoCare International, Inc.
Doctors for Global Health

Edmundite Missions Corps
Evangelical Free Church of America Mission

Father Carr's Place 2B
Fellowship of Associates of Medical Evangelism
Foundation for Integrated Education and Development
Foundation Human Nature (MeHiPro)
Foundation of Compassionate American Samaritans
Friends Without a Border

General Baptist International
General Board of Global Ministries / The United Methodist Church
Global Operations & Development
Global Outreach International
Global Service Corps/Earth Island Institute
Global Volunteers
Guinea Development Foundation, Inc.

Hands Together, Inc.
HBS Foundation, Inc. / Hopital Bon Samaritain
Health Teams International
Helping Hands Health Education
Himalayan Health Exchange
Honduras Outreach, Inc
Hope Alliance

Intercultural Nursing, Inc.
International Health Service
International Nepal Fellowship

Jubilee Volunteer Africa Program of AFRIDEC

Liga International, Inc.
Lumiere Medical Ministries, Inc.

M.E.D.I.C.O.
Medical Ministry International
Medical Missionaries of Mary
Michigan State University Institute for International Health
Mima Foundation, Inc.
Minnesota International Health Volunteers
Moi University Faculty of Health Sciences
Mountain Movers Missions Intl

Nicaraguan Children's Fund
Notre Dame India Mission

Operation Blessing, Medical Division
Operation Rainbow
Our Little Brothers and Sisters

P.C.E.A. Tumutumu Hospital
Partners of the Americas
PAZAPA
Peacework: Volunteer Medical Projects
Physicians for Human Rights
Physicians for Peace
Presbyterian Church USA, Mission Service Recruitment
Project AmaZon

Remote Area Medical

Save the Children Federation
Selian Lutheran Hospital
Simeus Foundation, The
SIM USA
Special Olympics, Inc.
St. Francis' Hospital
Surgical Medical Assistance Relief Teams
Surgicorps International

Unite For Sight
University of Virginia, Center for Global Health
University of Zimbabwe
Uplift Internationale

Virginia Children's Connection, Dept. of Plastic. & Recon. Surgery
Visions in Action
Voluntary Missionary Movement
Volunteer Missionary Movement
Volunteer Optometric Service to Humanity (VOSH) International
Volunteers in Medical Missions

WEC International
World Emergency Relief
World Hearing Network
World Mission Prayer League

Organizations seeking other health professional students

ACCESS
Action Against Hunger
Adventist Development and Relief Agency International
Africa Inland Mission, International
Africare
Aid for International Medicine
Ak' Tenamit
Aloha Medical Missions (AMM)
Amazon-Africa Aid Organization (3AO)
American Baptist Board of International Ministries
American College of Nurse-Midwives
American Jewish World Service
American Refugee Committee
Amigos de las Americas
Anderson University School of Nursing

Organizations seeking other health professional students *(continued)*

Ann Foundation Inc

APUSAN-USA

Associate Reformed Presbyterian Church, World Witness

Bairo Pite Clinic

Baptist General Conference

Baptist Medical and Dental Mission International

Baptist Mid Missions

Ben Gurion University of the Negev

Blessings International

Board of World Mission of the Moravian Church

Boston University School of Medicine, Section of Preventive Medicine and Epidemiology

Bridges to Community, Inc.

CAM International

Cameroon Baptist Convention Health Board

Canadian Society for International Health

Canvasback Missions, Inc.

Cape Cares

Cape Verde Care Agency, Inc.

Casa Clinica de la Mujer

Catholic Network of Volunteer Service

CB International

CERT International (Christian Emergency Relief Team)

Chanet Community Organization

Child Family Health International

Childreach PLAN International

Children's Cross Connection, International

Children's Heartlink

Christian Dental Missions

Christian Dental Society

Christian Foundation for Children and Aging

Christian Medical College (Vellore, India) Board

Christian Mission of Pignon Inc.

Church of the Nazarene World Mission Division

Comitato Collaborazione Medica (Doctors for Developing Countries)

Commonwealth Health Center

Community of Caring

Complete Basic Health 2000

Cross-Cultural Solutions

CrossWorld

Crudem Foundation

DoCare International, Inc.

Doctors for Global Health

Edmundite Missions Corps

Edward A. Ulzen Memorial Foundation (EAUMF)

Emergency International, Inc.

Esperanca, Inc.

Evangelical Alliance Mission (TEAM World)

Evangelical Free Church of America Mission

Father Carr's Place 2B

Feed the Children

Fellowship of Associates of Medical Evangelism

Filipino-American Medical Inc.

Flying Doctors of America

Flying Samaritans

Foundation for International Medical Relief of Children

Foundation Human Nature (MeHiPro)

Foundation of Compassionate American Samaritans

Friends Without a Border

General Baptist International

General Board of Global Ministries / The United Methodist Church

Global Operations & Development

Global Outreach International

Global Service Corps/Earth Island Institute

Global Volunteers

Grace Ministries International

Grokha Association of Social Health

Guinea Development Foundation, Inc.

Haitian Health Clinic, Inc.

Hands Together, Inc.

HBS Foundation, Inc. / Hopital Bon Samaritain

Healing the Children Northeast, Inc.

Health Alliance International

Health and Child Survival Fellows Program

Health Teams International

Health Volunteers Overseas

Helen Keller International

Helping Hands Health Education

Helps International

Hillside Healthcare Center

Himalayan Health Exchange

Honduras Outreach, Inc

Hope Alliance

Hope Worldwide

Hospital Albert Schweitzer

Intercultural Nursing, Inc.

International Aid, Inc.

International Children's Heart Foundation

International Cooperation for Development (formerly CIIR Overseas Programme)

International Federation of Red Cross and Red Crescent Societies

International Federation of Social Workers

International Health Service

International Medical Corps

International Nepal Fellowship

International Partnership for Human Development

International Rescue Committee

Interplast

Organizations seeking other health professional students *(continued)*

InterServe

Jesuit Refugee Service

Jubilee Volunteer Africa Program of AFRIDEC

Liga International, Inc.

Lighthouse for Christ Mission and Eye Centre

Lumiere Medical Ministries, Inc.

M.E.D.I.C.O.

Magee-Womens Hospital

Maluti Adventist Hospital (Lesotho)

Management Sciences for Health

Maua Methodist Hospital

Medecins Sans Frontieres / Doctors Without Borders USA

Medical Ambassadors International

Medical Care Development International Division

Medical Ministry International

Medical Missionaries of Mary

Mennonite Central Committee

Mexican Medical Ministries

Mima Foundation, Inc.

Minnesota International Health Volunteers

Mission Doctors Association

Moi University Faculty of Health Sciences

Mountain Movers Missions Intl

National Health Service Corps, Recruitment Program

New Missions In Haiti

Nicaraguan Children's Fund

Notre Dame India Mission

Operation Blessing, Medical Division

Operation Rainbow

Operation USA

Our Little Brothers and Sisters

P.C.E.A. Kikuyu Hospital

P.C.E.A. Tumutumu Hospital

P.R.A.Y. (Project Rescue of Amazon Youth)

Pan American Health Organization

Pan American Medical Mission Foundation

Partners of the Americas

PAZAPA

Peacework: Volunteer Medical Projects

Physicians for Peace

Project AmaZon

Project Concern International: OPTIONS

PROMESA

Remote Area Medical

S.E.E. International

Salesian Missions

School Sisters of Saint Francis

Seva Foundation

Simeus Foundation, The

SIM USA

Sister Community Alliances: Ouelessebougou-Utah Alliance

SkillShare International

Special Olympics, Inc.

St. Francis' Hospital

St. John's Medical College

Surgical Medical Assistance Relief Teams

Surgicorps International

Trinity Health International

Tulane University School of Public Health and Tropical Medicine

Unite For Sight

Universidad de Chile, Facultad de Medicina

University of Cincinnati College of Medicine, Dept. of Family Medicine

University of Illinois at Chicago College of Nursing, Global Health Leadership Office

University of Nebraska Medical Center, Office of International Programs and Studies

University of Virginia, Center for Global Health

University of Zimbabwe

Uplift Internationale

UTMB-WHO Collaborating Center for Training in International Health

Vietnam ENT Mission

Virginia Children's Connection, Dept. of Plastic. & Recon. Surgery

Visions in Action

Voluntary Missionary Movement

Volunteer Missionary Movement

Volunteer Optometric Service to Humanity (VOSH) International

Volunteers in Medical Missions

WEC International

World Concern

World Emergency Relief

World Gospel Mission

World Mission Prayer League

World Rehabilitation Fund, Inc.

World Vision International

World Witness - the Associate Reformed Presbyterian Church

Organizations seeking doctors in training

ACCESS

Adventist Development and Relief Agency International

Africa Inland Mission, International

Ak' Tenamit

Aloha Medical Missions (AMM)

Amazon-Africa Aid Organization (3AO)

Organizations seeking doctors in training *(continued)*

American Jewish World Service

American Physicians Fellowship for Medicine in Israel

APUSAN-USA

Associate Reformed Presbyterian Church, World Witness

Bairo Pite Clinic

Baptist General Conference

Baptist Medical and Dental Mission International

Baptist Medical Missions International

Baptist Mid Missions

Beeve Foundation for World Eye and Health, The

Ben Gurion University of the Negev

Board of World Mission of the Moravian Church

Boston International Foundation for Medical Education

Boston University School of Medicine, Section of Preventive Medicine and Epidemiology

Bridges to Community, Inc.

CAM International

Cameroon Baptist Convention Health Board

Cape Cares

CardioStart International, Inc.

Casa Clinica de la Mujer

Catholic Medical Mission Board, Inc.

Catholic Network of Volunteer Service

CB International

CERT International (Christian Emergency Relief Team)

Child Family Health International

Children's Cross Connection, International

Children's Medical Mission

Christian Dental Missions

Christian Dental Society

Christian Medical and Dental Associations-Global Health Outreach

Christian Medical College (Vellore, India) Board

Christian Mission of Pignon Inc.

Church of the Nazarene World Mission Division

Clinica Evangelica Morava Elective

College of Medicine, Malawi

Comitato Collaborazione Medica (Doctors for Developing Countries)

Commonwealth Health Center

Community of Caring

Complete Basic Health 2000

Cross-Cultural Solutions

CrossWorld

Crudem Foundation

Curamericas

DePauw University Winter Term in Service

DoCare International, Inc.

Doctors for Global Health

Duke University Medical Center, Division of Infectious Diseases and Int'l Health

Edmundite Missions Corps

Edward A. Ulzen Memorial Foundation (EAUMF)

Emergency International, Inc.

Evangelical Free Church of America Mission

Evangelical Lutheran Church in America

Father Carr's Place 2B

Fellowship of Associates of Medical Evangelism

Flying Samaritans

Foundation Human Nature (MeHiPro)

General Baptist International

General Board of Global Ministries / The United Methodist Church

Global Operations & Development

Global Outreach International

Global Service Corps/Earth Island Institute

Global Volunteers

Guinea Development Foundation, Inc.

Haitian Health Clinic, Inc.

Hands Together, Inc.

HBS Foundation, Inc. / Hopital Bon Samaritain

Healing the Children Northeast, Inc.

Health Alliance International

Health Teams International

Health Volunteers Overseas

Helen Keller International

Helping Hands Health Education

Helps International

Hillside Healthcare Center

Himalayan Health Exchange

Himalayan HealthCare Inc.

Honduras Outreach, Inc

Hope Alliance

Hope Worldwide

Hospital Albert Schweitzer

Infectious Diseases Society of America, The, and The HIV Medicine Association

Intercultural Nursing, Inc.

Interface UCSD

International Aid, Inc.

International Health Service

International Nepal Fellowship

International Partnership for Human Development

International Relief Teams

International Rescue Committee

Interplast

InterServe

Organizations seeking doctors in training *(continued)*

Johns Hopkins Univ. School of Public Health, Dept. of International Health

Jubilee Volunteer Africa Program of AFRIDEC

Liga International, Inc.

Lighthouse for Christ Mission and Eye Centre

Ludhiana Christian Medical College Board USA

Lumiere Medical Ministries, Inc.

M.E.D.I.C.O.

Magee-Womens Hospital

Maluti Adventist Hospital (Lesotho)

Maryknoll Mission Association of the Faithful

Maua Methodist Hospital

Medical Ministry International

Medical Missionaries of Mary

Medicine for Humanity

Mexican Medical Ministries

Mima Foundation, Inc.

Minnesota International Health Volunteers

Moi University Faculty of Health Sciences

Mountain Movers Missions Intl

National Health Service Corps, Recruitment Program

New Missions In Haiti

Nicaraguan Children's Fund

North American Baptist Conference Missions

Notre Dame India Mission

Omni Med

Operation Blessing, Medical Division

Operation Luz del Sol

Operation Rainbow

Operation Smile International

Our Little Brothers and Sisters

P.C.E.A. Kikuyu Hospital

P.C.E.A. Tumutumu Hospital

P.R.A.Y. (Project Rescue of Amazon Youth)

Palestine Children's Relief Fund

Palms Australia

Pan American Health Organization

Partners of the Americas

PAZAPA

Peacework: Volunteer Medical Projects

Physicians for Peace

Presbyterian Church USA, Mission Service Recruitment

Project AmaZon

Project Concern International: OPTIONS

Project Hope / People to People Health Foundation

PROMESA

Remote Area Medical

Saint Joseph's Medical Center, Family Practice Residency Program, Int'l Health Track

Sanyati Baptist Hospital, Baptist Convention of Zimbabwe

Selian Lutheran Hospital

Seva Foundation

Simeus Foundation, The

SIM USA

Sister Community Alliances: Ouelessebougou-Utah Alliance

Sons of Mary Missionary Society

Special Olympics, Inc.

St. Francis' Hospital

St. John's Medical College

St. Jude Hospital

Surgical Medical Assistance Relief Teams

Surgicorps International

Trans-World Overseas Employment Service

Tulane University School of Public Health and Tropical Medicine

UCSD, Division of International Health

Unite For Sight

Univ. of Wisconsin Med., Office of International Health Affairs

Universidad de Chile, Facultad de Medicina

University of Cincinnati College of Medicine, Dept. of Family Medicine

University of Illinois College of Medicine at Rockford

University of Nebraska Medical Center, Office of International Programs and Studies

University of Virginia, Center for Global Health

University of Zimbabwe

Uplift Internationale

UTMB-WHO Collaborating Center for Training in International Health

Vietnam ENT Mission

Virginia Children's Connection, Dept. of Plastic. & Recon. Surgery

Visions in Action

Voluntary Missionary Movement

Voluntary Service Overseas Canada

Volunteer Missionary Movement

Volunteer Optometric Service to Humanity (VOSH) International

Volunteers in Medical Missions

WEC International

World Concern

World Emergency Relief

World Hearing Network

World Medical Mission

World Mission Prayer League

World Witness - the Associate Reformed Presbyterian Church

Zuma Memorial Hospital

Organizations seeking health personnel who are US citizens

ACCESS

Action Against Hunger

Adventist Development and Relief Agency International

Africa Inland Mission, International

African Inter-Mennonite Mission

Africare

Aid for International Medicine

Ak' Tenamit

Albert Schweitzer Fellowship

Aloha Medical Missions (AMM)

Amazon-Africa Aid and Fundacao Esperanca

Amazon-Africa Aid Organization (3AO)

American Baptist Board of International Ministries

American College of Nurse-Midwives

American Jewish World Service

American Leprosy Missions Inc.

American Physicians Fellowship for Medicine in Israel

American Refugee Committee

Anderson University School of Nursing

Ann Foundation Inc

APUSAN-USA

Armenian Eye Care Project

Armenian Social Transition Program

ASAPROSAR: The Salvadoran Association for Rural Health

Associate Reformed Presbyterian Church, World Witness

Associazione Italiana 'Amici Raoul Follereau'

Bairo Pite Clinic

Baptist General Conference

Baptist Medical and Dental Mission International

Baptist Medical Missions International

Baptist Mid Missions

Beeve Foundation for World Eye and Health, The

Board of World Mission of the Moravian Church

Boston International Foundation for Medical Education

Boston University School of Medicine, Section of Preventive Medicine and Epidemiology

Bridges to Community, Inc.

CAM International

Cameroon Baptist Convention Health Board

Campus Crusade for Christ International

Canvasback Missions, Inc.

Cape Cares

Cape Verde Care Agency, Inc.

CardioStart International, Inc.

Casa Clinica de la Mujer

Catholic Medical Mission Board, Inc.

Catholic Network of Volunteer Service

CB International

CERT International (Christian Emergency Relief Team)

Chanet Community Organization

Child Family Health International

Children's Cross Connection, International

Children's Heartlink

Children's Medical Mission

Christian Dental Missions

Christian Dental Society

Christian Medical and Dental Associations-Global Health Outreach

Christian Medical College (Vellore, India) Board

Christian Mission of Pignon Inc.

Christoffel-Blindenmission EV

Church of the Nazarene World Mission Division

Clinica Evangelica Morava Elective

Clínica Maxena

College of Medicine, Malawi

Commonwealth Health Center

Community of Caring

Complete Basic Health 2000

CONCERN

CONCERN America

Cross-Cultural Solutions

CrossWorld

Crudem Foundation

Curamericas

Dental Health International

DePauw University Winter Term in Service

DoCare International, Inc.

Doctors for Global Health

Doctors of the World

Edmundite Missions Corps

Edward A. Ulzen Memorial Foundation (EAUMF)

Emergency International, Inc.

Esperanca, Inc.

Evangelical Alliance Mission (TEAM World)

Evangelical Covenant Church

Evangelical Free Church of America Mission

Evangelical Lutheran Church in America

Father Carr's Place 2B

Feed the Children

Fellowship of Associates of Medical Evangelism

FIENS Foundation of International Education in Neurological Surgery

Filipino-American Medical Inc.

Florida Association for Volunteer Action in the Caribbean and the Americas (FAVACA)

Flying Doctors of America

Flying Samaritans

FOCUS Inc.

Foundation for International Medical Relief of Children

Organizations seeking health personnel who are US citizens *(continued)*

Foundation Human Nature (MeHiPro)
Foundation of Compassionate American Samaritans
Friends Lugulu Hospital
Fulbright Scholar Award, Council for the International Exchange of Students

General Baptist International
General Board of Global Ministries / The United Methodist Church
General Dept. of World Missions, The Wesleyan Church
Global Operations & Development
Global Outreach International
Global Service Corps/Earth Island Institute
Global Volunteers
Grace Ministries International
Grokha Association of Social Health
Guinea Development Foundation, Inc.

Haitian Health Clinic, Inc.
Hands Together, Inc.
Harlem Hospital, Plastic Surgery Program
HBS Foundation, Inc. / Hopital Bon Samaritain
Healing the Children Northeast, Inc.
Health Alliance International
Health and Child Survival Fellows Program
Health Teams International
Health Volunteers Overseas
Helen Keller International
Helping Hands Health Education
Helps International
Hillside Healthcare Center
Himalayan Health Exchange
Himalayan HealthCare Inc.
Honduras Outreach, Inc
Hope Alliance
Hope Worldwide
Hospital Albert Schweitzer

Indochina Surgical Educational Exchange
Infectious Diseases Society of America, The, and The HIV Medicine Association
Intercultural Nursing, Inc.
Interface UCSD
International Aid, Inc.
International Children's Heart Foundation
International Committee of the Red Cross
International Cooperation for Development (formerly CIIR Overseas Programme)
International Eye Foundation, Inc.
International Federation of Red Cross and Red Crescent Societies
International Health Exchange
International Health Service
International Lifeline
International Medical Corps
International Ministries, American Baptist Churches, USA
International Nepal Fellowship
International Partnership for Human Development
International Relief Teams
International Rescue Committee
Interplast
InterServe

Jesuit Refugee Service
Johns Hopkins Univ. School of Public Health, Dept. of International Health
Jubilee Volunteer Africa Program of AFRIDEC

Lalmba Association
Lay Mission-Helpers Association
Liga International, Inc.
Lighthouse for Christ Mission and Eye Centre
Loma Linda University International Programs
Ludhiana Christian Medical College Board USA
Lumiere Medical Ministries, Inc.

M.E.D.I.C.O.
Magee-Womens Hospital
Maluti Adventist Hospital (Lesotho)
Management Sciences for Health
Maryknoll Mission Association of the Faithful
Maua Methodist Hospital
Medecins Sans Frontieres / Doctors Without Borders USA
Medical Aid for Palestinians
Medical Ambassadors International
Medical Care Development International Division
Medical Ministry International
Medical Missionaries of Mary
Medicine for Humanity
Medicine for Peace
Mennonite Central Committee
Mercy Ships
Mexican Medical Ministries
Michigan State University Institute for International Health
Mima Foundation, Inc.
Minnesota International Health Volunteers
Mission Doctors Association
Moi University Faculty of Health Sciences
Mountain Movers Missions Intl

National Eye Care Project for Armenia
National Health Service Corps, Recruitment Program
New Missions In Haiti
Nicaraguan Children's Fund

Organizations seeking health personnel who are US citizens *(continued)*

North American Baptist Conference Missions

Northwest Medical Teams International, Inc.

Notre Dame India Mission

Omni Med

Operation Blessing, Medical Division

Operation Luz del Sol

Operation Rainbow

Operation Smile International

Operation USA

Our Little Brothers and Sisters

P.C.E.A. Chogoria Hospital

P.C.E.A. Kikuyu Hospital

P.C.E.A. Tumutumu Hospital

P.R.A.Y. (Project Rescue of Amazon Youth)

Palestine Children's Relief Fund

Pan American Health Organization

Partners of the Americas

PAZAPA

Peacework: Volunteer Medical Projects

Physicians for Human Rights

Physicians for Peace

Presbyterian Church USA, Mission Service Recruitment

Project AmaZon

Project Concern International: OPTIONS

Project Hope / People to People Health Foundation

Project Open Hearts

Project ORBIS International, Inc.

Project Skye

PROMESA

Remote Area Medical

Saint Joseph's Medical Center, Family Practice Residency Program, Int'l Health Track

Salesian Missions

Sanyati Baptist Hospital, Baptist Convention of Zimbabwe

School Sisters of Saint Francis

Selian Lutheran Hospital

Seva Foundation

Simeus Foundation, The

SIM USA

Sister Community Alliances: Ouelessebougou-Utah Alliance

Special Olympics, Inc.

St. Francis' Hospital

St. John's Medical College

St. Jude Hospital

St. Mary's Hospital, Vunapope

Surfer's Medical Association

Surgical Eye Expeditions International (S.E.E.), Inc.

Surgical Medical Assistance Relief Teams

Surgicorps International

Trans-World Overseas Employment Service

Trinity Health International

Tulane University School of Public Health and Tropical Medicine

Unite For Sight

Univ. of Wisconsin Med., Office of International Health Affairs

University of Cincinnati College of Medicine, Dept. of Family Medicine

University of Illinois at Chicago College of Nursing, Global Health Leadership Office

University of Illinois College of Medicine at Rockford

University of Nebraska Medical Center, Office of International Programs and Studies

University of Virginia, Center for Global Health

University of Zimbabwe

Uplift Internationale

US Committee for Scientific Cooperation with Vietnam

UTMB-WHO Collaborating Center for Training in International Health

Vietnam ENT Mission

Virginia Children's Connection, Dept. of Plastic. & Recon. Surgery

Visions in Action

Voluntary Service Overseas Canada

Volunteer Missionary Movement

Volunteer Optometric Service to Humanity (VOSH) International

Volunteers in Medical Missions

VSO

WEC International

World Association for Children and Parents

World Concern

World Emergency Relief

World Gospel Mission

World Hearing Network

World Medical Mission

World Mission Prayer League

World Rehabilitation Fund, Inc.

World Vision, Inc.

World Witness - the Associate Reformed Presbyterian Church

Zuma Memorial Hospital

Organizations seeking health personnel who are non-US citizens

ACCESS

Action Against Hunger

Adventist Development and Relief Agency International

Africa Inland Mission, International

African Inter-Mennonite Mission

Africare

Aid for International Medicine

Ak' Tenamit

Albert Schweitzer Fellowship

Organizations seeking health personnel who are non-US citizens *(continued)*

Aloha Medical Missions (AMM)

Amazon-Africa Aid and Fundacao Esperanca

Amazon-Africa Aid Organization (3AO)

American College of Nurse-Midwives

American Jewish World Service

American Leprosy Missions Inc.

American Physicians Fellowship for Medicine in Israel

American Refugee Committee

Anderson University School of Nursing

Ann Foundation Inc

APUSAN-USA

Aremenian Eye Care Project

Armenian Social Transition Program

ASAPROSAR: The Salvadoran Association for Rural Health

Associate Reformed Presbyterian Church, World Witness

Associazione Italiana 'Amici Raoul Follereau'

Bairo Pite Clinic

Baptist General Conference

Baptist Medical and Dental Mission International

Baptist Medical Missions International

Baptist Mid Missions

Beeve Foundation for World Eye and Health, The

Ben Gurion University of the Negev

Board of World Mission of the Moravian Church

Bread for the World (Brot fur die Welt)

Bridges to Community, Inc.

CAM International

Cameroon Baptist Convention Health Board

Campus Crusade for Christ International

Canadian Society for International Health

Canvasback Missions, Inc.

Cape Cares

Cape Verde Care Agency, Inc.

CardioStart International, Inc.

Casa Clinica de la Mujer

Catholic Medical Mission Board, Inc.

Catholic Network of Volunteer Service

CERT International (Christian Emergency Relief Team)

Chanet Community Organization

Child Family Health International

Children's Cross Connection, International

Children's Heartlink

Children's Medical Mission

Children-Surgical Aid International

Christian Dental Missions

Christian Dental Society

Christian Medical and Dental Associations-Global Health Outreach

Christian Medical College (Vellore, India) Board

Christian Mission of Pignon Inc.

Christoffel-Blindenmission EV

Church of the Nazarene World Mission Division

Clinica Evangelica Morava Elective

Clínica Maxena

College of Medicine, Malawi

Comitato Collaborazione Medica (Doctors for Developing Countries)

Commonwealth Health Center

Community of Caring

Complete Basic Health 2000

CONCERN

CONCERN America

Cross-Cultural Solutions

Crudem Foundation

DePauw University Winter Term in Service

Doctors for Global Health

Doctors of the World

Edmundite Missions Corps

Emergency International, Inc.

Esperanca, Inc.

Evangelical Alliance Mission (TEAM World)

Evangelical Free Church of America Mission

Feed the Children

FIENS Foundation of International Education in Neurological Surgery

Filipino-American Medical Inc.

FOCUS Inc.

Foundation for International Medical Relief of Children

Foundation Human Nature (MeHiPro)

Foundation of Compassionate American Samaritans

Friends Lugulu Hospital

General Baptist International

General Board of Global Ministries / The United Methodist Church

Global Operations & Development

Global Service Corps/Earth Island Institute

Global Volunteers

Grace Ministries International

Grokha Association of Social Health

Guinea Development Foundation, Inc.

Haitian Health Clinic, Inc.

Hands Together, Inc.

HBS Foundation, Inc. / Hopital Bon Samaritain

Healing the Children Northeast, Inc.

Health Alliance International

Health Teams International

Health Volunteers Overseas

Helen Keller International

Organizations seeking health personnel who are non-US citizens *(continued)*

Helping Hands Health Education

Helps International

Hillside Healthcare Center

Himalayan Health Exchange

Himalayan HealthCare Inc.

Honduras Outreach, Inc

Hope Alliance

Hope Worldwide

Hospital Albert Schweitzer

Indochina Surgical Educational Exchange

Infectious Diseases Society of America, The, and The HIV Medicine Association

Intercultural Nursing, Inc.

International Aid, Inc.

International Children's Heart Foundation

International Committee of the Red Cross

International Cooperation for Development (formerly CIIR Overseas Programme)

International Federation of Red Cross and Red Crescent Societies

International Health Exchange

International Health Service

International Medical Corps

International Nepal Fellowship

International Partnership for Human Development

International Rescue Committee

Interplast

INTERTEAM

Jesuit Refugee Service

Johns Hopkins Univ. School of Public Health, Dept. of International Health

Jubilee Volunteer Africa Program of AFRIDEC

Lalmba Association

Liga International, Inc.

Lighthouse for Christ Mission and Eye Centre

Loma Linda University International Programs

Lumiere Medical Ministries, Inc.

M.E.D.I.C.O.

Magee-Womens Hospital

Maluti Adventist Hospital (Lesotho)

Management Sciences for Health

Maua Methodist Hospital

Medecins Sans Frontieres / Doctors Without Borders USA

Medical Aid for Palestinians

Medical Ambassadors International

Medical Care Development International Division

Medical Ministry International

Medical Missionaries of Mary

Medicine for Humanity

Memisa Medicus Mundi

Mennonite Central Committee

Mercy Ships

Mexican Medical Ministries

Mima Foundation, Inc.

Minnesota International Health Volunteers

Moi University Faculty of Health Sciences

National Eye Care Project for Armenia

New Missions In Haiti

Nicaraguan Children's Fund

North American Baptist Conference Missions

Notre Dame India Mission

Omni Med

Operation Blessing, Medical Division

Operation Rainbow

Operation Smile International

Operation USA

Our Little Brothers and Sisters

P.C.E.A. Chogoria Hospital

P.C.E.A. Kikuyu Hospital

P.C.E.A. Tumutumu Hospital

P.R.A.Y. (Project Rescue of Amazon Youth)

Palestine Children's Relief Fund

Palms Australia

Pan American Health Organization

Partners of the Americas

PAZAPA

Physicians for Peace

Project Concern International: OPTIONS

Project Hope / People to People Health Foundation

Project Open Hearts

Project ORBIS International, Inc.

PROMESA

Reconstructive Surgery Foundation

Remote Area Medical

Sanyati Baptist Hospital, Baptist Convention of Zimbabwe

Seva Foundation

Simeus Foundation, The

Sister Community Alliances: Ouelessebougou-Utah Alliance

SkillShare International

Special Olympics, Inc.

St. Francis' Hospital

St. John's Medical College

St. Jude Hospital

St. Mary's Hospital, Vunapope

Surfer's Medical Association

Surgical Eye Expeditions International (S.E.E.), Inc.

Surgical Medical Assistance Relief Teams

Trans-World Overseas Employment Service

Trinity Health International

Tulane University School of Public Health and Tropical Medicine

Organizations seeking health personnel who are non-US citizens *(continued)*

Unite For Sight

Univ. of Wisconsin Med., Office of International Health Affairs

University of Cincinnati College of Medicine, Dept. of Family Medicine

University of Illinois at Chicago College of Nursing, Global Health Leadership Office

University of Nebraska Medical Center, Office of International Programs and Studies

University of Virginia, Center for Global Health

University of Zimbabwe

Uplift Internationale

US Committee for Scientific Cooperation with Vietnam

UTMB-WHO Collaborating Center for Training in International Health

Virginia Children's Connection, Dept. of Plastic. & Recon. Surgery

Visions in Action

Voluntary Service Overseas Canada

Volunteer Missionary Movement

Volunteer Optometric Service to Humanity (VOSH) International

Volunteers in Medical Missions

VSO

WEC International

World Association for Children and Parents

World Concern

World Emergency Relief

World Gospel Mission

World Hearing Network

World Medical Mission

World Mission Prayer League

World Rehabilitation Fund, Inc.

World Vision, Inc.

Zuma Memorial Hospital

Organizations seeking health personnel with no prior experience in developing countries

ACCESS

Action Against Hunger

Adventist Development and Relief Agency International

Africa Inland Mission, International

Aid for International Medicine

Ak' Tenamit

Albert Schweitzer Fellowship

Aloha Medical Missions (AMM)

Amazon-Africa Aid and Fundacao Esperanca

Amazon-Africa Aid Organization (3AO)

American Baptist Board of International Ministries

American Jewish World Service

American Leprosy Missions Inc.

American Physicians Fellowship for Medicine in Israel

Anderson University School of Nursing

Ann Foundation Inc

APUSAN-USA

Armenian Eye Care Project

ASAPROSAR: The Salvadoran Association for Rural Health

Associate Reformed Presbyterian Church, World Witness

Associazione Italiana 'Amici Raoul Follereau'

Bairo Pite Clinic

Baptist General Conference

Baptist Medical and Dental Mission International

Baptist Medical Missions International

Baptist Mid Missions

Beeve Foundation for World Eye and Health, The

Board of World Mission of the Moravian Church

Boston International Foundation for Medical Education

Boston University School of Medicine, Section of Preventive Medicine and Epidemiology

Bridges to Community, Inc.

CAM International

Cameroon Baptist Convention Health Board

Campus Crusade for Christ International

Canadian Society for International Health

Canvasback Missions, Inc.

Cape Cares

CardioStart International, Inc.

Casa Clinica de la Mujer

Catholic Medical Mission Board, Inc.

Catholic Network of Volunteer Service

CB International

CERT International (Christian Emergency Relief Team)

Chanet Community Organization

Child Family Health International

Children's Cross Connection, International

Children's Heartlink

Children's Medical Mission

Children-Surgical Aid International

Christian Dental Missions

Christian Dental Society

Christian Medical and Dental Associations-Global Health Outreach

Christian Medical College (Vellore, India) Board

Christian Mission of Pignon Inc.

Church of the Nazarene World Mission Division

Clinica Evangelica Morava Elective

Organizations seeking health personnel with no prior experience in developing countries *(continued)*

Clínica Maxena
College of Medicine, Malawi
Commonwealth Health Center
Community of Caring
Complete Basic Health 2000
CONCERN America
Cross-Cultural Solutions
CrossWorld
Crudem Foundation
Curamericas

Dental Health International
DePauw University Winter Term in Service
DoCare International, Inc.
Doctors for Global Health

Edmundite Missions Corps
Emergency International, Inc.
Esperanca, Inc.
Evangelical Alliance Mission (TEAM World)
Evangelical Free Church of America Mission
Evangelical Lutheran Church in America

Father Carr's Place 2B
Feed the Children
Fellowship of Associates of Medical Evangelism
FIENS Foundation of International Education in Neurological Surgery
Filipino-American Medical Inc.
Flying Doctors of America
Flying Samaritans
FOCUS Inc.
Foundation for International Medical Relief of Children
Foundation Human Nature (MeHiPro)
Friends Lugulu Hospital
Fulbright Scholar Award, Council for the International Exchange of Students

General Board of Global Ministries / The United Methodist Church
Global Operations & Development
Global Outreach International
Global Service Corps/Earth Island Institute
Global Volunteers
Grace Ministries International
Grokha Association of Social Health
Guinea Development Foundation, Inc.

Haitian Health Clinic, Inc.
Hands Together, Inc.
Harlem Hospital, Plastic Surgery Program
HBS Foundation, Inc. / Hopital Bon Samaritain
Healing the Children National Headquarters
Healing the Children Northeast, Inc.
Health and Child Survival Fellows Program
Health Teams International
Health Volunteers Overseas
Helen Keller International
Helping Hands Health Education
Helps International
Hillside Healthcare Center
Himalayan Health Exchange
Himalayan HealthCare Inc.
Honduras Outreach, Inc
Hope Alliance
Hope Worldwide
Hospital Albert Schweitzer
Humanity International, Inc.

Indochina Surgical Educational Exchange
Infectious Diseases Society of America, The, and The HIV Medicine Association
Intercultural Nursing, Inc.
Interface UCSD
International Aid, Inc.
International Children's Heart Foundation
International Committee of the Red Cross
International Cooperation for Development (formerly CIIR Overseas Programme)
International Health Exchange
International Health Service
International Medical Corps
International Ministries, American Baptist Churches, USA
International Nepal Fellowship
International Partnership for Human Development
International Relief Teams
Interplast
InterServe
INTERTEAM

Jubilee Volunteer Africa Program of AFRIDEC

Lalmba Association
Lay Mission-Helpers Association
Liga International, Inc.
Loma Linda University International Programs
Ludhiana Christian Medical College Board USA
Lumiere Medical Ministries, Inc.

M.E.D.I.C.O.
Magee-Womens Hospital
Maluti Adventist Hospital (Lesotho)
Maryknoll Mission Association of the Faithful
Maua Methodist Hospital
Medecins Sans Frontieres / Doctors Without Borders USA
Medical Aid for Palestinians

Organizations seeking health personnel with no prior experience in developing countries *(continued)*

Medical Ambassadors International

Medical Ministry International

Medical Missionaries of Mary

Medicine for Humanity

Medicine for Peace

Mennonite Central Committee

Mercy Ships

Mexican Medical Ministries

Mima Foundation, Inc.

Minnesota International Health Volunteers

Mission Doctors Association

Moi University Faculty of Health Sciences

Mountain Movers Missions Intl

National Eye Care Project for Armenia

New Missions In Haiti

Nicaraguan Children's Fund

North American Baptist Conference Missions

Northwest Medical Teams International, Inc.

Notre Dame India Mission

Omni Med

Operation Blessing, Medical Division

Operation Luz del Sol

Operation Rainbow

Operation Smile International

Our Little Brothers and Sisters

P.C.E.A. Kikuyu Hospital

P.C.E.A. Tumutumu Hospital

P.R.A.Y. (Project Rescue of Amazon Youth)

Palestine Children's Relief Fund

Palms Australia

Partners of the Americas

PAZAPA

Peacework: Volunteer Medical Projects

Physicians for Human Rights

Physicians for Peace

Presbyterian Church USA, Mission Service Recruitment

Project AmaZon

Project Concern International: OPTIONS

Project Hope / People to People Health Foundation

Project Open Hearts

Project ORBIS International, Inc.

Project Skye

Remote Area Medical

Saint Joseph's Medical Center, Family Practice Residency Program, Int'l Health Track

Salesian Missions

Sanyati Baptist Hospital, Baptist Convention of Zimbabwe

School Sisters of Saint Francis

Selian Lutheran Hospital

Simeus Foundation, The

SIM USA

Sister Community Alliances: Ouelessebougou-Utah Alliance

SkillShare International

Sons of Mary Missionary Society

Special Olympics, Inc.

St. Francis' Hospital

St. John's Medical College

St. Jude Hospital

St. Mary's Hospital, Vunapope

Surfer's Medical Association

Surgical Eye Expeditions International (S.E.E.), Inc.

Surgical Medical Assistance Relief Teams

Surgicorps International

Trinity Health International

Tulane University School of Public Health and Tropical Medicine

UCSD, Division of International Health

Unite For Sight

Univ. of Wisconsin Med., Office of International Health Affairs

University of Cincinnati College of Medicine, Dept. of Family Medicine

University of Illinois at Chicago College of Nursing, Global Health Leadership Office

University of Illinois College of Medicine at Rockford

University of Nebraska Medical Center, Office of International Programs and Studies

University of Zimbabwe

Uplift Internationale

US Committee for Scientific Cooperation with Vietnam

UTMB-WHO Collaborating Center for Training in International Health

Vietnam ENT Mission

Virginia Children's Connection, Dept. of Plastic. & Recon. Surgery

Visions in Action

Voluntary Service Overseas Canada

Volunteer Missionary Movement

Volunteer Optometric Service to Humanity (VOSH) International

Volunteers in Medical Missions

VSO

WEC International

World Association for Children and Parents

World Concern

World Emergency Relief

World Gospel Mission

World Hearing Network

World Medical Mission

World Mission Prayer League

World Witness - the Associate Reformed Presbyterian Church

Zuma Memorial Hospital

Organizations seeking health personnel with prior experience in developing countries

African Inter-Mennonite Mission

Africare

American College of Nurse-Midwives

American Refugee Committee

Amigos de las Americas

Bread for the World (Brot fur die Welt)

Cape Verde Care Agency, Inc.

Capiz Emmanuel Hospital

Christoffel-Blindenmission EV

Comitato Collaborazione Medica (Doctors for Developing Countries)

CONCERN

Doctors of the World

Duke University Medical Center, Division of Infectious Diseases and Int'l Health

Florida Association for Volunteer Action in the Caribbean and the Americas (FAVACA)

Foundation of Compassionate American Samaritans

General Baptist International

General Dept. of World Missions, The Wesleyan Church

Health Alliance International

International Eye Foundation, Inc.

International Federation of Red Cross and Red Crescent Societies

International Federation of Social Workers

International Rescue Committee

Jesuit Refugee Service

Johns Hopkins Univ. School of Public Health, Dept. of International Health

Management Sciences for Health

Medical Care Development International Division

Memisa Medicus Mundi

Michigan State University Institute for International Health

National Health Service Corps, Recruitment Program

Operation USA

P.C.E.A. Chogoria Hospital

Pan American Health Organization

PROMESA

Seva Foundation

Universidad de Chile, Facultad de Medicina

University of Virginia, Center for Global Health

Women's Commission for Refugee Women and Children

World Rehabilitation Fund, Inc.

World Vision International

World Vision, Inc.

Organizations seeking health personnel who are not current members of your hospital, university, or organization

ACCESS

Action Against Hunger

Adventist Development and Relief Agency International

Africa Inland Mission, International

Aid for International Medicine

Ak' Tenamit

Albert Schweitzer Fellowship

Aloha Medical Missions (AMM)

Amazon-Africa Aid and Fundacao Esperanca

Amazon-Africa Aid Organization (3AO)

American Baptist Board of International Ministries

American College of Nurse-Midwives

American Jewish World Service

American Leprosy Missions Inc.

American Physicians Fellowship for Medicine in Israel

American Refugee Committee

Ann Foundation Inc

APUSAN-USA

Armenian Eye Care Project

Armenian Social Transition Program

ASAPROSAR: The Salvadoran Association for Rural Health

Associate Reformed Presbyterian Church, World Witness

Associazione Italiana 'Amici Raoul Follereau'

Bairo Pite Clinic

Baptist General Conference

Baptist Medical and Dental Mission International

Baptist Medical Missions International

Baptist Mid Missions

Beeve Foundation for World Eye and Health, The

Ben Gurion University of the Negev

Board of World Mission of the Moravian Church

Boston University School of Medicine, Section of Preventive Medicine and Epidemiology

Bread for the World (Brot fur die Welt)

Bridges to Community, Inc.

CAM International

Cameroon Baptist Convention Health Board

Organizations seeking health personnel who are not current members of your hospital, university, or organization *(continued)*

Campus Crusade for Christ International

Canadian Society for International Health

Canvasback Missions, Inc.

Cape Cares

Cape Verde Care Agency, Inc.

CardioStart International, Inc.

Casa Clinica de la Mujer

Catholic Medical Mission Board, Inc.

Catholic Network of Volunteer Service

CB International

CERT International (Christian Emergency Relief Team)

Chanet Community Organization

Child Family Health International

Childreach PLAN International

Children's Cross Connection, International

Children's Heartlink

Children's Medical Mission

Christian Dental Missions

Christian Dental Society

Christian Medical and Dental Associations-Global Health Outreach

Christian Medical College (Vellore, India) Board

Christian Mission of Pignon Inc.

Christoffel-Blindenmission EV

Church of the Nazarene World Mission Division

Clinica Evangelica Morava Elective

Clínica Maxena

College of Medicine, Malawi

Comitato Collaborazione Medica (Doctors for Developing Countries)

Commonwealth Health Center

Community of Caring

Complete Basic Health 2000

CONCERN

CONCERN America

Cross-Cultural Solutions

CrossWorld

Crudem Foundation

Dental Health International

DePauw University Winter Term in Service

Doctors for Global Health

Doctors of the World

Edmundite Missions Corps

Edward A. Ulzen Memorial Foundation (EAUMF)

Emergency International, Inc.

Esperanca, Inc.

Evangelical Alliance Mission (TEAM World)

Evangelical Lutheran Church in America

Father Carr's Place 2B

Feed the Children

FIENS Foundation of International Education in Neurological Surgery

Filipino-American Medical Inc.

Flying Doctors of America

Flying Samaritans

FOCUS Inc.

Foundation for International Medical Relief of Children

Foundation Human Nature (MeHiPro)

Foundation of Compassionate American Samaritans

Friends Lugulu Hospital

Fulbright Scholar Award, Council for the International Exchange of Students

General Baptist International

General Board of Global Ministries / The United Methodist Church

General Dept. of World Missions, The Wesleyan Church

Global Operations & Development

Global Outreach International

Global Service Corps/Earth Island Institute

Global Volunteers

Grace Ministries International

Grokha Association of Social Health

Guinea Development Foundation, Inc.

Haitian Health Clinic, Inc.

Hands Together, Inc.

Harlem Hospital, Plastic Surgery Program

HBS Foundation, Inc. / Hopital Bon Samaritain

Healing the Children Northeast, Inc.

Health Alliance International

Health and Child Survival Fellows Program

Health Teams International

Health Volunteers Overseas

Helen Keller International

Helping Hands Health Education

Helps International

Hillside Healthcare Center

Himalayan Health Exchange

Himalayan HealthCare Inc.

Honduras Outreach, Inc

Hope Alliance

Hope Worldwide

Hospital Albert Schweitzer

Indochina Surgical Educational Exchange

Intercultural Nursing, Inc.

Interface UCSD

International Aid, Inc.

International Children's Heart Foundation

International Committee of the Red Cross

International Cooperation for Development (formerly CIIR Overseas Programme)

Organizations seeking health personnel who are not current members of your hospital, university, or organization *(continued)*

International Eye Foundation, Inc.

International Federation of Red Cross and Red Crescent Societies

International Health Exchange

International Health Service

International Medical Corps

International Ministries, American Baptist Churches, USA

International Nepal Fellowship

International Partnership for Human Development

International Relief Teams

International Rescue Committee

Interplast

InterServe

INTERTEAM

Jesuit Refugee Service

Jubilee Volunteer Africa Program of AFRIDEC

Lalmba Association

Lay Mission-Helpers Association

Liga International, Inc.

Lighthouse for Christ Mission and Eye Centre

Loma Linda University International Programs

Ludhiana Christian Medical College Board USA

Lumiere Medical Ministries, Inc.

M.E.D.I.C.O.

Maluti Adventist Hospital (Lesotho)

Management Sciences for Health

Maryknoll Mission Association of the Faithful

Maua Methodist Hospital

Medecins Sans Frontieres / Doctors Without Borders USA

Medical Aid for Palestinians

Medical Ambassadors International

Medical Care Development International Division

Medical Ministry International

Medical Missionaries of Mary

Medicine for Humanity

Medicine for Peace

Mennonite Central Committee

Mercy Ships

Mexican Medical Ministries

Mima Foundation, Inc.

Minnesota International Health Volunteers

Mission Doctors Association

Moi University Faculty of Health Sciences

Mountain Movers Missions Intl

National Eye Care Project for Armenia

National Health Service Corps, Recruitment Program

New Missions In Haiti

Nicaraguan Children's Fund

North American Baptist Conference Missions

Northwest Medical Teams International, Inc.

Notre Dame India Mission

Omni Med

Operation Blessing, Medical Division

Operation Luz del Sol

Operation Rainbow

Operation Smile International

Operation USA

Our Little Brothers and Sisters

P.C.E.A. Chogoria Hospital

P.C.E.A. Kikuyu Hospital

P.C.E.A. Tumutumu Hospital

P.R.A.Y. (Project Rescue of Amazon Youth)

Palms Australia

Pan American Health Organization

Partners of the Americas

PAZAPA

Peacework: Volunteer Medical Projects

Physicians for Human Rights

Physicians for Peace

Presbyterian Church USA, Mission Service Recruitment

Project AmaZon

Project Concern International: OPTIONS

Project Hope / People to People Health Foundation

Project Open Hearts

Project ORBIS International, Inc.

Project Skye

PROMESA

Remote Area Medical

Salesian Missions

Sanyati Baptist Hospital, Baptist Convention of Zimbabwe

School Sisters of Saint Francis

Selian Lutheran Hospital

Simeus Foundation, The

SIM USA

Sister Community Alliances: Ouelessebougou-Utah Alliance

SkillShare International

Special Olympics, Inc.

St. Francis' Hospital

St. John's Medical College

St. Jude Hospital

St. Mary's Hospital, Vunapope

Surfer's Medical Association

Surgical Eye Expeditions International (S.E.E.), Inc.

Surgical Medical Assistance Relief Teams

Surgicorps International

Trinity Health International

UCSD, Division of International Health

Organizations seeking health personnel who are not current members of your hospital, university, or organization *(continued)*

Unite For Sight

Univ. of Wisconsin Med., Office of International Health Affairs

University of Cincinnati College of Medicine, Dept. of Family Medicine

University of Illinois at Chicago College of Nursing, Global Health Leadership Office

University of Nebraska Medical Center, Office of International Programs and Studies

University of Zimbabwe

Uplift Internationale

US Committee for Scientific Cooperation with Vietnam

UTMB-WHO Collaborating Center for Training in International Health

Vietnam ENT Mission

Virginia Children's Connection, Dept. of Plastic. & Recon. Surgery

Visions in Action

Voluntary Service Overseas Canada

Volunteer Optometric Service to Humanity (VOSH) International

Volunteers in Medical Missions

VSO

WEC International

World Association for Children and Parents

World Concern

World Emergency Relief

World Gospel Mission

World Hearing Network

World Medical Mission

World Mission Prayer League

World Rehabilitation Fund, Inc.

World Vision, Inc.

World Witness - the Associate Reformed Presbyterian Church

Zuma Memorial Hospital

Organizations with funding available for travel

Action Against Hunger

Africare

Albert Schweitzer Fellowship

American Baptist Board of International Ministries

American College of Nurse-Midwives

American Jewish World Service

American Leprosy Missions Inc.

American Physicians Fellowship for Medicine in Israel

American Refugee Committee

Amigos de las Americas

Anderson University School of Nursing

Armenian Social Transition Program

Associazione Italiana 'Amici Raoul Follereau'

Baptist General Conference

Beeve Foundation for World Eye and Health, The

Boston International Foundation for Medical Education

Bread for the World (Brot fur die Welt)

Canadian Society for International Health

Catholic Medical Mission Board, Inc.

Catholic Network of Volunteer Service

Children's Heartlink

Christoffel-Blindenmission EV

Church of the Nazarene World Mission Division

Comitato Collaborazione Medica (Doctors for Developing Countries)

Commonwealth Health Center

CONCERN

CONCERN America

Covenant House

Doctors of the World

Duke University Medical Center, Division of Infectious Diseases and Int'l Health

Edmundite Missions Corps

FIENS Foundation of International Education in Neurological Surgery

Florida Association for Volunteer Action in the Caribbean and the Americas (FAVACA)

Fulbright Grant Award, Institute of International Education, US Student Programs

Fulbright Scholar Award, Council for the International Exchange of Students

Guinea Development Foundation, Inc.

Harlem Hospital, Plastic Surgery Program

Health Alliance International

Health and Child Survival Fellows Program

Health Teams International

Health Volunteers Overseas

Hope Alliance

Hope Worldwide

Hospital Albert Schweitzer

Infectious Diseases Society of America, The, and The HIV Medicine Association

International Children's Heart Foundation

International Committee of the Red Cross

International Cooperation for Development (formerly CIIR Overseas Programme)

International Eye Foundation, Inc.

International Health Exchange

Organizations with funding available for travel *(continued)*

International Medical Corps
International Ministries, American Baptist Churches, USA
International Partnership for Human Development
International Relief Teams
International Rescue Committee
Interplast
INTERTEAM

Jesuit Refugee Service

Lalmba Association
Lay Mission-Helpers Association

Magee-Womens Hospital
Maryknoll Mission Association of the Faithful
Medecins Sans Frontieres / Doctors Without Borders USA
Medical Aid for Palestinians
Medical Care Development International Division
Medicine for Humanity
Medicine for Peace
Memisa Medicus Mundi
Mennonite Central Committee
Minnesota International Health Volunteers
Mission Doctors Association

Operation Luz del Sol
Operation Rainbow
Operation Smile International

Palestine Children's Relief Fund
Palms Australia
Pan American Health Organization
Partners of the Americas
Physicians for Peace
Presbyterian Church USA, Mission Service Recruitment
Project Hope / People to People Health Foundation
Project ORBIS International, Inc.

Saint Joseph's Medical Center, Family Practice Residency Program, Int'l Health Track
Salesian Missions
SkillShare International
St. Mary's Hospital, Vunapope

Trinity Health International

University of Illinois at Chicago College of Nursing, Global Health Leadership Office
University of Illinois College of Medicine at Rockford
University of Virginia, Center for Global Health

Virginia Children's Connection, Dept. of Plastic. & Recon. Surgery
Voluntary Service Overseas Canada
Volunteer Missionary Movement
VSO

World Association for Children and Parents
World Emergency Relief
World Hearing Network
World Vision International
World Vision, Inc.

Organizations that provide room and board

Action Against Hunger
Adventist Development and Relief Agency International
Africa Inland Mission, International
Africare
Ak' Tenamit
Albert Schweitzer Fellowship
Amazon-Africa Aid and Fundacao Esperanca
Amazon-Africa Aid Organization (3AO)
American Baptist Board of International Ministries
American College of Nurse-Midwives
American Leprosy Missions Inc.
American Physicians Fellowship for Medicine in Israel
American Refugee Committee
Amigos de las Americas
Armenian Eye Care Project
Armenian Social Transition Program
Associazione Italiana 'Amici Raoul Follereau'

Baptist Medical Missions International
Baptist Mid Missions
Beeve Foundation for World Eye and Health, The
Board of World Mission of the Moravian Church
Boston International Foundation for Medical Education
Boston University School of Medicine, Section of Preventive Medicine and Epidemiology
Bread for the World (Brot fur die Welt)
Bridges to Community, Inc.

Cameroon Baptist Convention Health Board
Canadian Society for International Health
Canvasback Missions, Inc.
Cape Cares
Cape Verde Care Agency, Inc.
Capiz Emmanuel Hospital
CardioStart International, Inc.
Catholic Medical Mission Board, Inc.
Catholic Network of Volunteer Service
Child Family Health International
Children's Cross Connection, International
Children's Heartlink

Organizations that provide room and board *(continued)*

Christian Dental Missions

Christoffel-Blindenmission EV

Church of the Nazarene World Mission Division

College of Medicine, Malawi

Comitato Collaborazione Medica (Doctors for Developing Countries)

Commonwealth Health Center

Community of Caring

Complete Basic Health 2000

CONCERN

CONCERN America

Crudem Foundation

DePauw University Winter Term in Service

Doctors of the World

Edmundite Missions Corps

Esperanca, Inc.

Evangelical Free Church of America Mission

Father Carr's Place 2B

FIENS Foundation of International Education in Neurological Surgery

Filipino-American Medical Inc.

Florida Association for Volunteer Action in the Caribbean and the Americas (FAVACA)

FOCUS Inc.

Foreign Ophthalmological Care from the United States, Inc.

Foundation for International Medical Relief of Children

Friends Lugulu Hospital

Friends Without a Border

Fulbright Grant Award, Institute of International Education, US Student Programs

Fulbright Scholar Award, Council for the International Exchange of Students

General Baptist International

Global Operations & Development

Global Service Corps/Earth Island Institute

Grace Ministries International

Guinea Development Foundation, Inc.

Hands Together, Inc.

Harlem Hospital, Plastic Surgery Program

HBS Foundation, Inc. / Hopital Bon Samaritain

Healing the Children Northeast, Inc.

Health Alliance International

Health and Child Survival Fellows Program

Health Volunteers Overseas

Himalayan Health Exchange

Hope Alliance

Hope Worldwide

Hospital Albert Schweitzer

Indochina Surgical Educational Exchange

Infectious Diseases Society of America, The, and The HIV Medicine Association

Intercultural Nursing, Inc.

International Aid, Inc.

International Children's Heart Foundation

International Committee of the Red Cross

International Cooperation for Development (formerly CIIR Overseas Programme)

International Eye Foundation, Inc.

International Federation of Red Cross and Red Crescent Societies

International Health Exchange

International Medical Corps

International Ministries, American Baptist Churches, USA

International Partnership for Human Development

International Relief Teams

International Rescue Committee

Interplast

InterServe

INTERTEAM

Jesuit Refugee Service

Jubilee Volunteer Africa Program of AFRIDEC

Lalmba Association

Lay Mission-Helpers Association

Lighthouse for Christ Mission and Eye Centre

Loma Linda University International Programs

Ludhiana Christian Medical College Board USA

Lumiere Medical Ministries, Inc.

Magee-Womens Hospital

Maluti Adventist Hospital (Lesotho)

Maryknoll Mission Association of the Faithful

Maua Methodist Hospital

Medecins Sans Frontieres / Doctors Without Borders USA

Medical Aid for Palestinians

Medical Care Development International Division

Medical Missionaries of Mary

Medicine for Humanity

Medicine for Peace

Memisa Medicus Mundi

Mennonite Central Committee

Mexican Medical Ministries

Minnesota International Health Volunteers

Mission Doctors Association

National Eye Care Project for Armenia

North American Baptist Conference Missions

Notre Dame India Mission

Omni Med

Operation Blessing, Medical Division

Organizations that provide room and board *(continued)*

Operation Luz del Sol

Operation Rainbow

Operation Smile International

Our Little Brothers and Sisters

P.C.E.A. Chogoria Hospital

P.C.E.A. Kikuyu Hospital

P.C.E.A. Tumutumu Hospital

P.R.A.Y. (Project Rescue of Amazon Youth)

Palestine Children's Relief Fund

Palms Australia

Partners of the Americas

PAZAPA

Peacework: Volunteer Medical Projects

Physicians for Peace

Presbyterian Church USA, Mission Service Recruitment

Project Concern International: OPTIONS

Project Hope / People to People Health Foundation

Project Open Hearts

Project ORBIS International, Inc.

Remote Area Medical

Saint Joseph's Medical Center, Family Practice Residency Program, Int'l Health Track

Salesian Missions

School Sisters of Saint Francis

Selian Lutheran Hospital

Seva Foundation

Simeus Foundation, The

SIM USA

Sister Community Alliances: Ouelessebougou-Utah Alliance

SkillShare International

Sons of Mary Missionary Society

St. Francis' Hospital

St. Jude Hospital

St. Mary's Hospital, Vunapope

Surgical Eye Expeditions International (S.E.E.), Inc.

Surgical Medical Assistance Relief Teams

Trans-World Overseas Employment Service

Trinity Health International

Univ. of Wisconsin Med., Office of International Health Affairs

University of Cincinnati College of Medicine, Dept. of Family Medicine

University of Illinois at Chicago College of Nursing, Global Health Leadership Office

US Committee for Scientific Cooperation with Vietnam

UTMB-WHO Collaborating Center for Training in International Health

Virginia Children's Connection, Dept. of Plastic. & Recon. Surgery

Voluntary Service Overseas Canada

Volunteer Missionary Movement

Volunteer Optometric Service to Humanity (VOSH) International

Volunteers in Medical Missions

VSO

World Association for Children and Parents

World Emergency Relief

World Hearing Network

World Medical Mission

World Mission Prayer League

World Rehabilitation Fund, Inc.

World Vision International

World Vision, Inc.

Organizations that provide other funding

Action Against Hunger

Adventist Development and Relief Agency International

Africare

Albert Schweitzer Fellowship

American College of Nurse-Midwives

American Jewish World Service

American Leprosy Missions Inc.

American Refugee Committee

Armenian Social Transition Program

Associazione Italiana 'Amici Raoul Follereau'

Beeve Foundation for World Eye and Health, The

Boston International Foundation for Medical Education

Bridges to Community, Inc.

Cameroon Baptist Convention Health Board

Canadian Society for International Health

Canvasback Missions, Inc.

Cape Cares

Catholic Network of Volunteer Service

Child Family Health International

Christoffel-Blindenmission EV

Church of the Nazarene World Mission Division

Comitato Collaborazione Medica (Doctors for Developing Countries)

Complete Basic Health 2000

CONCERN

CONCERN America

Doctors of the World

Foundation of Compassionate American Samaritans

Friends Without a Border

Fulbright Grant Award, Institute of International Education, US Student Programs

Fulbright Scholar Award, Council for the International Exchange of Students

Organizations that provide other funding *(continued)*

Global Operations & Development

Grace Ministries International

Guinea Development Foundation, Inc.

Healing the Children Northeast, Inc.

Health Alliance International

Health and Child Survival Fellows Program

Health Volunteers Overseas

Hillside Healthcare Center

Himalayan Health Exchange

Hope Alliance

Hope Worldwide

Infectious Diseases Society of America, The, and The HIV Medicine Association

International Committee of the Red Cross

International Cooperation for Development (formerly CIIR Overseas Programme)

International Federation of Red Cross and Red Crescent Societies

International Health Exchange

International Medical Corps

International Ministries, American Baptist Churches, USA

International Partnership for Human Development

International Relief Teams

International Rescue Committee

INTERTEAM

Jesuit Refugee Service

Lalmba Association

Lay Mission-Helpers Association

M.E.D.I.C.O.

Magee-Womens Hospital

Maryknoll Mission Association of the Faithful

Medecins Sans Frontieres / Doctors Without Borders USA

Medical Aid for Palestinians

Medical Care Development International Division

Memisa Medicus Mundi

Mennonite Central Committee

Minnesota International Health Volunteers

Mission Doctors Association

National Health Service Corps, Recruitment Program

Northwest Medical Teams International, Inc.

Operation Blessing, Medical Division

Our Little Brothers and Sisters

P.C.E.A. Chogoria Hospital

P.C.E.A. Tumutumu Hospital

Palms Australia

Pan American Health Organization

Presbyterian Church USA, Mission Service Recruitment

Project Concern International: OPTIONS

Project ORBIS International, Inc.

Saint Joseph's Medical Center, Family Practice Residency Program, Int'l Health Track

School Sisters of Saint Francis

SkillShare International

St. Mary's Hospital, Vunapope

Trinity Health International

University of Illinois at Chicago College of Nursing, Global Health Leadership Office

University of Zimbabwe

Voluntary Missionary Movement

Volunteers in Medical Missions

VSO

World Association for Children and Parents

World Vision International

World Vision, Inc.

Organizations in which training is provided or available

ACCESS

Action Against Hunger

Africa Inland Mission, International

Albert Schweitzer Fellowship

Amazon-Africa Aid and Fundacao Esperanca

American Leprosy Missions Inc.

American Physicians Fellowship for Medicine in Israel

American Refugee Committee

Amigos de las Americas

Anderson University School of Nursing

Ann Foundation Inc

APUSAN-USA

ASAPROSAR: The Salvadoran Association for Rural Health

Associazione Italiana 'Amici Raoul Follereau'

Baptist General Conference

Baptist Medical and Dental Mission International

Beeve Foundation for World Eye and Health, The

Board of World Mission of the Moravian Church

Boston International Foundation for Medical Education

Cameroon Baptist Convention Health Board

Campus Crusade for Christ International

Canadian Society for International Health

Capiz Emmanuel Hospital

Casa Clinica de la Mujer

Organizations in which training is provided or available *(continued)*

Catholic Network of Volunteer Service

Child Family Health International

Children's Cross Connection, International

Children's Medical Mission

Christian Dental Society

Christoffel-Blindenmission EV

College of Medicine, Malawi

Commonwealth Health Center

Community of Caring

CONCERN

CONCERN America

CrossWorld

Curamericas

Dental Health International

Evangelical Alliance Mission (TEAM World)

Evangelical Lutheran Church in America

Fellowship of Associates of Medical Evangelism

Foundation for International Medical Relief of Children

Foundation of Compassionate American Samaritans

Friends Without a Border

Fulbright Grant Award, Institute of International Education, US Student Programs

General Board of Global Ministries / The United Methodist Church

General Dept. of World Missions, The Wesleyan Church

Global Operations & Development

Global Outreach International

Global Service Corps/Earth Island Institute

Grace Ministries International

Guinea Development Foundation, Inc.

Hands Together, Inc.

Harlem Hospital, Plastic Surgery Program

HBS Foundation, Inc. / Hopital Bon Samaritain

Healing the Children National Headquarters

Healing the Children Northeast, Inc.

Health and Child Survival Fellows Program

Health Teams International

Helping Hands Health Education

Hillside Healthcare Center

Honduras Outreach, Inc

Hope Alliance

Hope Worldwide

Hospital Albert Schweitzer

Infectious Diseases Society of America, The, and The HIV Medicine Association

Intercultural Nursing, Inc.

International Committee of the Red Cross

International Cooperation for Development (formerly CIIR Overseas Programme)

International Federation of Red Cross and Red Crescent Societies

International Health Exchange

International Health Service

International Ministries, American Baptist Churches, USA

International Nepal Fellowship

InterServe

INTERTEAM

Jesuit Refugee Service

Johns Hopkins Univ. School of Public Health, Dept. of International Health

Jubilee Volunteer Africa Program of AFRIDEC

Lalmba Association

Lay Mission-Helpers Association

Liga International, Inc.

Lighthouse for Christ Mission and Eye Centre

Loma Linda University International Programs

Ludhiana Christian Medical College Board USA

Lumiere Medical Ministries, Inc.

Magee-Womens Hospital

Maluti Adventist Hospital (Lesotho)

Maryknoll Mission Association of the Faithful

Maua Methodist Hospital

Medecins Sans Frontieres / Doctors Without Borders USA

Medical Ambassadors International

Medical Care Development International Division

Medicine for Peace

Mennonite Central Committee

Mexican Medical Ministries

Michigan State University Institute for International Health

Minnesota International Health Volunteers

Mission Doctors Association

Moi University Faculty of Health Sciences

Mountain Movers Missions Intl

North American Baptist Conference Missions

Northwest Medical Teams International, Inc.

Notre Dame India Mission

Omni Med

Operation Blessing, Medical Division

Operation Luz del Sol

Operation Smile International

P.C.E.A. Chogoria Hospital

P.C.E.A. Kikuyu Hospital

P.C.E.A. Tumutumu Hospital

Organizations in which training is provided or available *(continued)*

Palms Australia
Pan American Health Organization
Partners of the Americas
Physicians for Human Rights
Presbyterian Church USA, Mission Service Recruitment
Project Concern International: OPTIONS
Project Hope / People to People Health Foundation
Project ORBIS International, Inc.
PROMESA

Remote Area Medical

Saint Joseph's Medical Center, Family Practice Residency Program, Int'l Health Track
Salesian Missions
School Sisters of Saint Francis
Selian Lutheran Hospital
Simeus Foundation, The
SIM USA
Sister Community Alliances: Ouelessebougou-Utah Alliance
SkillShare International
Special Olympics, Inc.
St. Francis' Hospital
St. John's Medical College
St. Jude Hospital
Surgicorps International

Trinity Health International
Tulane University School of Public Health and Tropical Medicine

UCSD, Division of International Health
Unite For Sight
Univ. of Wisconsin Med., Office of International Health Affairs
Universidad de Chile, Facultad de Medicina
University of Arizona College of Medicine
University of Cincinnati College of Medicine, Dept. of Family Medicine
University of Illinois at Chicago College of Nursing, Global Health Leadership Office
University of Illinois College of Medicine at Rockford
University of Virginia, Center for Global Health
University of Zimbabwe
US Committee for Scientific Cooperation with Vietnam

Vietnam ENT Mission
Visions in Action
Voluntary Service Overseas Canada
Volunteer Missionary Movement
Volunteer Optometric Service to Humanity (VOSH) International
VSO

Women's Commission for Refugee Women and Children
World Association for Children and Parents
World Emergency Relief
World Gospel Mission
World Hearing Network
World Medical Mission
World Mission Prayer League
World Relief Corp.
World Witness - the Associate Reformed Presbyterian Church

Zuma Memorial Hospital

Minimum length of stay: ≤ 2 weeks

Aid for International Medicine
Aloha Medical Missions (AMM)
American Baptist Board of International Ministries
American College of Nurse-Midwives
ASAPROSAR: The Salvadoran Association for Rural Health
Associate Reformed Presbyterian Church, World Witness

Baptist Medical and Dental Mission International
Baptist Medical Missions International
Baptist Mid Missions
Beeve Foundation for World Eye and Health, The
CAM International
Campus Crusade for Christ International
Canvasback Missions, Inc.
Cape Cares
Cape Verde Care Agency, Inc.
CardioStart International, Inc.
Casa Clinica de la Mujer
Catholic Medical Mission Board, Inc.
Catholic Network of Volunteer Service
CERT International (Christian Emergency Relief Team)
Children's Heartlink
Children's Medical Mission
Christian Dental Missions
Christian Dental Society
Christian Medical and Dental Associations-Global Health Outreach
Christian Medical College (Vellore, India) Board
Christian Mission of Pignon Inc.
Clinica Evangelica Morava Elective
Commonwealth Health Center
Community of Caring
CrossWorld
Crudem Foundation
Curamericas

DePauw University Winter Term in Service

Minimum length of stay: ≤ 2 weeks *(continued)*

DoCare International, Inc.

Edmundite Missions Corps

Edward A. Ulzen Memorial Foundation (EAUMF)

Emergency International, Inc.

Esperanca, Inc.

Evangelical Alliance Mission (TEAM World)

Fellowship of Associates of Medical Evangelism

Filipino-American Medical Inc.

Florida Association for Volunteer Action in the Caribbean and the Americas (FAVACA)

Flying Samaritans

FOCUS Inc.

Foundation for International Medical Relief of Children

General Baptist International

General Board of Global Ministries / The United Methodist Church

Global Operations & Development

Global Outreach International

Global Service Corps/Earth Island Institute

Global Volunteers

Grace Ministries International

Haitian Health Clinic, Inc.

Hands Together, Inc.

Harlem Hospital, Plastic Surgery Program

Healing the Children Northeast, Inc.

Health Volunteers Overseas

Helping Hands Health Education

Hillside Healthcare Center

Himalayan Health Exchange

Honduras Outreach, Inc

Hope Alliance

Hope Worldwide

Hospital Albert Schweitzer

Indochina Surgical Educational Exchange

Intercultural Nursing, Inc.

International Aid, Inc.

International Children's Heart Foundation

International Eye Foundation, Inc.

International Health Service

International Partnership for Human Development

International Relief Teams

Interplast

Johns Hopkins Univ. School of Public Health, Dept. of International Health

Jubilee Volunteer Africa Program of AFRIDEC

Lighthouse for Christ Mission and Eye Centre

Lumiere Medical Ministries, Inc.

M.E.D.I.C.O.

Magee-Womens Hospital

Maluti Adventist Hospital (Lesotho)

Medical Ambassadors International

Medical Care Development International Division

Medical Ministry International

Medical Teams International, Inc.

Medicine for Humanity

Medicine for Peace

Mercy Ships

Mexican Medical Ministries

Michigan State University Institute for International Health

Mima Foundation, Inc.

Mountain Movers Missions Intl

North American Baptist Conference Missions

Northwest Medical Teams International, Inc.

Omni Med

Operation Blessing, Medical Division

Operation Rainbow

Operation Smile International

Operation USA

P.C.E.A. Kikuyu Hospital

Palestine Children's Relief Fund

Pan American Health Organization

Partners of the Americas

Peacework: Volunteer Medical Projects

Physicians for Peace

Project AmaZon

Project Concern International: OPTIONS

Project Open Hearts

Project Skye

Remote Area Medical

Saint Joseph's Medical Center, Family Practice Residency Program, Int'l Health Track

Sanyati Baptist Hospital, Baptist Convention of Zimbabwe

Seva Foundation

Sister Community Alliances: Ouelessebougou-Utah Alliance

Special Olympics, Inc.

Surfer's Medical Association

Surgical Eye Expeditions International (S.E.E.), Inc.

Surgicorps International

Trinity Health International

Unite For Sight

University of Cincinnati College of Medicine, Dept. of Family Medicine

University of Illinois College of Medicine at Rockford

Uplift Internationale

Vietnam ENT Mission

Virginia Children's Connection, Dept. of Plastic. & Recon. Surgery

Volunteer Optometric Service to Humanity (VOSH) International

Volunteers in Medical Missions

Minimum length of stay: ≤ 2 weeks *(continued)*

WEC International

Women's Commission for Refugee Women and Children

World Emergency Relief

World Hearing Network

World Rehabilitation Fund, Inc.

World Witness - the Associate Reformed Presbyterian Church

Minimum length of stay: 2 weeks–3 months

ACCESS

Africa Inland Mission, International

Ak' Tenamit

Albert Schweitzer Fellowship

Amazon-Africa Aid and Fundacao Esperanca

Amazon-Africa Aid Organization (3AO)

American Academy of Pediatrics, Office of International Health

American Jewish World Service

American Leprosy Missions Inc.

Amigos de las Americas

APUSAN-USA

Armenian Social Transition Program

Associazione Italiana 'Amici Raoul Follereau'

Bairo Pite Clinic

Board of World Mission of the Moravian Church

Boston International Foundation for Medical Education

Boston University School of Medicine, Section of Preventive Medicine and Epidemiology

Cameroon Baptist Convention Health Board

CB International

Chanet Community Organization

Child Family Health International

Church of the Nazarene World Mission Division

Clínica Maxena

College of Medicine, Malawi

Comitato Collaborazione Medica (Doctors for Developing Countries)

Complete Basic Health 2000

Cross-Cultural Solutions

Dental Health International

Doctors for Global Health

Doctors of the World

Duke University Medical Center, Division of Infectious Diseases and Int'l Health

Evangelical Covenant Church

Evangelical Free Church of America Mission

Evangelical Lutheran Church in America

FIENS Foundation of International Education in Neurological Surgery

Foundation Human Nature (MeHiPro)

Friends Lugulu Hospital

Fulbright Scholar Award, Council for the International Exchange of Students

Global Outreach Mission

Grokha Association of Social Health

Health Alliance International

Himalayan HealthCare Inc.

Hospital Clinico Jose J. Aguirre

Humanity International, Inc.

Infectious Diseases Society of America, The, and The HIV Medicine Association

International Committee of the Red Cross

International Federation of Red Cross and Red Crescent Societies

International Health Exchange

International Nepal Fellowship

International Rescue Committee

InterServe

Ludhiana Christian Medical College Board USA

Maua Methodist Hospital

Minnesota International Health Volunteers

Mission Doctors Association

Moi University Faculty of Health Sciences

Notre Dame India Mission

P.C.E.A. Chogoria Hospital

P.C.E.A. Tumutumu Hospital

P.R.A.Y. (Project Rescue of Amazon Youth)

Project ORBIS International, Inc.

PROMESA

Selian Lutheran Hospital

SIM USA

St. Francis' Hospital

St. John's Medical College

St. Jude Hospital

UCSD, Division of International Health

Univ. of Wisconsin Med., Office of International Health Affairs

University of Nebraska Medical Center, Office of International Programs and Studies

University of Virginia, Center for Global Health

UTMB-WHO Collaborating Center for Training in International Health

World Association for Children and Parents

World Gospel Mission

World Medical Mission

World Mission Prayer League

Zuma Memorial Hospital

Minimum length of stay: 3 months–6 months

Baptist General Conference
Canadian Society for International Health
Capiz Emmanuel Hospital
Father Carr's Place 2B
Guinea Development Foundation, Inc.
International Medical Corps
Medecins Sans Frontieres / Doctors Without Borders USA
Medical Aid for Palestinians
St. Mary's Hospital, Vunapope
Visions in Action
VSO
World Concern

Minimum length of stay: < 6 months

Action Against Hunger
Africare
American Refugee Committee
Christoffel-Blindenmission EV
CONCERN
CONCERN America
Fulbright Grant Award, Institute of International Education, US Student Programs
General Dept. of World Missions, The Wesleyan Church
Health and Child Survival Fellows Program
International Cooperation for Development (formerly CIIR Overseas Programme)
International Ministries, American Baptist Churches, USA
INTERTEAM
Jesuit Refugee Service
Lalmba Association
Lay Mission-Helpers Association
Management Sciences for Health
Maryknoll Mission Association of the Faithful
Medical Missionaries of Mary
Memisa Medicus Mundi
Mennonite Central Committee
National Health Service Corps, Recruitment Program
Our Little Brothers and Sisters
Palms Australia
Presbyterian Church USA, Mission Service Recruitment
Salesian Missions
SkillShare International
Sons of Mary Missionary Society
Voluntary Missionary Movement
World Vision International
World Vision, Inc.

Health profession usage:

Administrative health positions

Adventist Development and Relief Agency International
Africare
Aloha Medical Missions (AMM)
American Jewish World Service
American Physicians Fellowship for Medicine in Israel
American Refugee Committee
Ann Foundation Inc
Archdiocesan Health Care Network for Catholic Charities
Bairo Pite Clinic
Baptist Medical Missions International
Beeve Foundation for World Eye and Health, The
Ben Gurion University of the Negev
Cameroon Baptist Convention Health Board
Capiz Emmanuel Hospital
Casa Clinica de la Mujer
CB International
Children's Cross Connection, International
Christian Medical College (Vellore, India) Board
Christian Mission of Pignon Inc.
Church of the Nazarene World Mission Division
Clinica Evangelica Morava Elective
College of Medicine, Malawi
Comitato Collaborazione Medica (Doctors for Developing Countries)
Doctors for Global Health
Doctors of the World
Evangelical Alliance Mission (TEAM World)
Foundation Human Nature (MeHiPro)
Friends Without a Border
General Board of Global Ministries/The United Methodist Church
Global Operations & Development
Global Service Corps/Earth Island Institute
Global Volunteers

Health profession usage: *(continued)*

Administrative health positions *(continued)*

Grace Ministries International
HBS Foundation, Inc./Hopital Bon Samaritain
Healing the Children Northeast, Inc.
Health Alliance International
Health and Child Survival Fellows Program
Health Teams International
Hope Alliance
Hope Worldwide
Hospital Albert Schweitzer
International Committee of the Red Cross
International Cooperation for Development (formerly CIIR Overseas Programme)
International Health Exchange
International Medical Corps
International Nepal Fellowship
InterServe
Johns Hopkins Univ. School of Public Health, Dept. of International Health
Lay Mission-Helpers Association
Ludhiana Christian Medical College Board USA
Lumiere Medical Ministries, Inc.
M.E.D.I.C.O.
Magee-Womens Hospital
Medical Aid for Palestinians
Medical Care Development International Division
Medical Ministry International
Mercy Ships
Mima Foundation, Inc.
Minnesota International Health Volunteers
Mission Doctors Association
Moi University Faculty of Health Sciences
Mountain Movers Missions Intl
Nicaraguan Children's Fund
Northwest Medical Teams International, Inc.
Omni Med
Operation Smile International
P.C.E.A. Kikuyu Hospital
P.C.E.A. Tumutumu Hospital
Pan American Health Organization
Project AmaZon
Project Concern International: OPTIONS
Project Hope/People to People Health Foundation
Project ORBIS International, Inc.
Remote Area Medical
School Sisters of Saint Francis
Simeus Foundation, The
St. John's Medical College
St. Jude Hospital
Surgical Medical Assistance Relief Teams
Trinity Health International
Tulane University School of Public Health and Tropical Medicine
Univ. of Wisconsin Med., Office of International Health Affairs
Universidad de Chile, Facultad de Medicina
University of Cincinnati College of Medicine, Dept. of Family Medicine
University of Zimbabwe
US Committee for Scientific Cooperation with Vietnam
Voluntary Service Overseas Canada
Volunteer Missionary Movement
VSO
WEC International
World Gospel Mission

Anesthesiologists

Adventist Development and Relief Agency International
Africa Inland Mission, International
Aid for International Medicine
Aloha Medical Missions (AMM)
Amazon-Africa Aid Organization (3AO)
American Baptist Board of International Ministries
American Physicians Fellowship for Medicine in Israel
Ann Foundation Inc
Archdiocesan Health Care Network for Catholic Charities
ASAPROSAR: The Salvadoran Association for Rural Health
Associate Reformed Presbyterian Church, World Witness
Bairo Pite Clinic
Baptist Medical Missions International
Beeve Foundation for World Eye and Health, The
Ben Gurion University of the Negev
Cameroon Baptist Convention Health Board
Canvasback Missions, Inc.
Capiz Emmanuel Hospital
CardioStart International, Inc.
Casa Clinica de la Mujer
Catholic Medical Mission Board, Inc.
CB International
Children's Cross Connection, International
Children's Heartlink
Christian Medical College (Vellore, India) Board
Christian Mission of Pignon Inc.
Clinica Evangelica Morava Elective
College of Medicine, Malawi
Commonwealth Health Center
CrossWorld
Crudem Foundation
Curamericas
Esperanca, Inc.
Evangelical Alliance Mission (TEAM World)

Health profession usage: *(continued)*

Anesthesiologists *(continued)*

Filipino-American Medical Inc.

Foundation Human Nature (MeHiPro)

Friends Without a Border

Global Volunteers

Grace Ministries International

Guinea Development Foundation, Inc.

HBS Foundation, Inc./Hopital Bon Samaritain

Healing the Children Northeast, Inc.

Health Teams International

Health Volunteers Overseas

Helps International

Hope Alliance

Hope Worldwide

Hospital Albert Schweitzer

Interface UCSD

International Committee of the Red Cross

International Cooperation for Development (formerly CIIR Overseas Programme)

International Federation of Red Cross and Red Crescent Societies

International Health Exchange

International Health Service

International Medical Corps

International Nepal Fellowship

Interplast

InterServe

Liga International, Inc.

Ludhiana Christian Medical College Board USA

Lumiere Medical Ministries, Inc.

M.E.D.I.C.O.

Magee-Womens Hospital

Medecins Sans Frontieres/ Doctors Without Borders USA

Medical Ministry International

Medicine for Humanity

Mercy Ships

Mexican Medical Ministries

Mima Foundation, Inc.

Mission Doctors Association

Moi University Faculty of Health Sciences

Mountain Movers Missions Intl

Nicaraguan Children's Fund

Northwest Medical Teams International, Inc.

Omni Med

Operation Blessing, Medical Division

Operation Rainbow

Operation Smile International

P.C.E.A. Kikuyu Hospital

P.R.A.Y. (Project Rescue of Amazon Youth)

Palestine Children's Relief Fund

PAZAPA

Project AmaZon

Project Concern International: OPTIONS

Project Hope/People to People Health Foundation

Project Open Hearts

Project ORBIS International, Inc.

Remote Area Medical

Simeus Foundation, The

Sister Community Alliances: Ouelessebougou-Utah Alliance

St. John's Medical College

St. Jude Hospital

Surgical Medical Assistance Relief Teams

Surgicorps International

Univ. of Wisconsin Med., Office of International Health Affairs

Universidad de Chile, Facultad de Medicina

University of Cincinnati College of Medicine, Dept. of Family Medicine

University of Illinois College of Medicine at Rockford

University of Virginia, Center for Global Health

University of Zimbabwe

Uplift Internationale

US Committee for Scientific Cooperation with Vietnam

Virginia Children's Connection, Dept. of Plastic. & Recon. Surgery

Voluntary Service Overseas Canada

Volunteer Missionary Movement

WEC International

World Hearing Network

Cardiologists

Adventist Development and Relief Agency International

Aid for International Medicine

Aloha Medical Missions (AMM)

Amazon-Africa Aid Organization (3AO)

American Baptist Board of International Ministries

American Jewish World Service

American Physicians Fellowship for Medicine in Israel

Ann Foundation Inc

Archdiocesan Health Care Network for Catholic Charities

Bairo Pite Clinic

Baptist Medical Missions International

Ben Gurion University of the Negev

Cameroon Baptist Convention Health Board

Capiz Emmanuel Hospital

CardioStart International, Inc.

Casa Clinica de la Mujer

Children's Cross Connection, International

Children's Heartlink

Christian Medical College (Vellore, India) Board

Christian Mission of Pignon Inc.

Clinica Evangelica Morava Elective

Health profession usage: *(continued)*

Cardiologists *(continued)*

College of Medicine, Malawi

Commonwealth Health Center

Crudem Foundation

DoCare International, Inc.

Evangelical Alliance Mission (TEAM World)

Evangelical Lutheran Church in America

Filipino-American Medical Inc.

Foundation Human Nature (MeHiPro)

Friends Without a Border

General Board of Global Ministries/The United Methodist Church

Global Volunteers

Guinea Development Foundation, Inc.

Healing the Children Northeast, Inc.

Health Teams International

Himalayan HealthCare Inc.

Honduras Outreach, Inc

Hope Alliance

Hope Worldwide

International Children's Heart Foundation

InterServe

Liga International, Inc.

Ludhiana Christian Medical College Board USA

Lumiere Medical Ministries, Inc.

Magee-Womens Hospital

Medical Ministry International

Mercy Ships

Mission Doctors Association

Moi University Faculty of Health Sciences

Mountain Movers Missions Intl

Nicaraguan Children's Fund

Omni Med

Operation Blessing, Medical Division

P.C.E.A. Kikuyu Hospital

P.R.A.Y. (Project Rescue of Amazon Youth)

Palestine Children's Relief Fund

PAZAPA

Physicians for Peace

Project AmaZon

Project Concern International: OPTIONS

Project Hope/People to People Health Foundation

Project Open Hearts

Remote Area Medical

Simeus Foundation, The

St. John's Medical College

St. Jude Hospital

Surgical Medical Assistance Relief Teams

Universidad de Chile, Facultad de Medicina

University of Illinois College of Medicine at Rockford

University of Virginia, Center for Global Health

University of Zimbabwe

Volunteer Missionary Movement

WEC International

World Hearing Network

Dental hygienists

Adventist Development and Relief Agency International

Ak' Tenamit

American Physicians Fellowship for Medicine in Israel

Ann Foundation Inc

Archdiocesan Health Care Network for Catholic Charities

Bairo Pite Clinic

Baptist Medical Missions International

Beeve Foundation for World Eye and Health, The

Cameroon Baptist Convention Health Board

Canvasback Missions, Inc.

Cape Cares

Casa Clinica de la Mujer

Catholic Medical Mission Board, Inc.

CERT International (Christian Emergency Relief Team)

Chanet Community Organization

Children's Cross Connection, International

Christian Dental Missions

Christian Dental Society

Christian Medical College (Vellore, India) Board

Christian Mission of Pignon Inc.

Clinica Evangelica Morava Elective

DePauw University Winter Term in Service

Doctors for Global Health

Edward A. Ulzen Memorial Foundation (EAUMF)

Evangelical Alliance Mission (TEAM World)

Flying Samaritans

Foundation Human Nature (MeHiPro)

Foundation of Compassionate American Samaritans

Friends Without a Border

General Board of Global Ministries/The United Methodist Church

Global Volunteers

Grokha Association of Social Health

Guinea Development Foundation, Inc.

Haitian Health Clinic, Inc.

Healing the Children Northeast, Inc.

Health Teams International

Helps International

Honduras Outreach, Inc

Hope Alliance

Hope Worldwide

Health profession usage: *(continued)*
Dental hygienists *(continued)*

International Health Service
Lumiere Medical Ministries, Inc.
M.E.D.I.C.O.
Maua Methodist Hospital
Medical Ministry International
Mercy Ships
Mima Foundation, Inc.
Moi University Faculty of Health Sciences
Mountain Movers Missions Intl
National Health Service Corps, Recruitment Program
Nicaraguan Children's Fund
Northwest Medical Teams International, Inc.
Operation Blessing, Medical Division
P.C.E.A. Tumutumu Hospital
P.R.A.Y. (Project Rescue of Amazon Youth)
Project AmaZon
Project Concern International: OPTIONS
Project Hope/People to People Health Foundation
Remote Area Medical
School Sisters of Saint Francis
Simeus Foundation, The
Sister Community Alliances: Ouelessebougou-Utah Alliance
Special Olympics, Inc.
St. Jude Hospital
St. Mary's Hospital, Vunapope
Surgical Medical Assistance Relief Teams
University of Zimbabwe
Uplift Internationale
Volunteer Missionary Movement
WEC International

Dentists

Adventist Development and Relief Agency International
Africa Inland Mission, International
Ak' Tenamit
Aloha Medical Missions (AMM)
Amazon-Africa Aid and Fundacao Esperanca
Amazon-Africa Aid Organization (3AO)
American Physicians Fellowship for Medicine in Israel
Ann Foundation Inc
Archdiocesan Health Care Network for Catholic Charities
Bairo Pite Clinic
Baptist Medical and Dental Mission International
Baptist Medical Missions International
Baptist Mid Missions
Beeve Foundation for World Eye and Health, The
Board of World Mission of the Moravian Church
CAM International
Cameroon Baptist Convention Health Board
Campus Crusade for Christ International
Canvasback Missions, Inc.
Cape Cares
Capiz Emmanuel Hospital
Casa Clinica de la Mujer
Catholic Medical Mission Board, Inc.
CERT International (Christian Emergency Relief Team)
Chanet Community Organization
Children's Cross Connection, International
Christian Dental Missions
Christian Dental Society
Christian Medical College (Vellore, India) Board
Christian Mission of Pignon Inc.
Clinica Evangelica Morava Elective
Clínica Maxena
College of Medicine, Malawi
Commonwealth Health Center
CrossWorld
Curamericas
Dental Health International
DePauw University Winter Term in Service
DoCare International, Inc.
Doctors for Global Health
Edward A. Ulzen Memorial Foundation (EAUMF)
Evangelical Alliance Mission (TEAM World)
Evangelical Lutheran Church in America
Father Carr's Place 2B
Feed the Children
Flying Doctors of America
Flying Samaritans
Foundation Human Nature (MeHiPro)
Foundation of Compassionate American Samaritans
Friends Without a Border
General Board of Global Ministries/The United Methodist Church
Global Outreach International
Global Volunteers
Grace Ministries International
Grokha Association of Social Health
Guinea Development Foundation, Inc.
Haitian Health Clinic, Inc.
Hands Together, Inc.
Healing the Children Northeast, Inc.
Health Teams International
Health Volunteers Overseas
Helping Hands Health Education
Helps International
Hillside Healthcare Center
Himalayan Health Exchange
Himalayan HealthCare Inc.
Honduras Outreach, Inc

Health profession usage: *(continued)*

Dentists *(continued)*

Hope Alliance

Hope Worldwide

Hospital Albert Schweitzer

Intercultural Nursing, Inc.

International Aid, Inc.

International Cooperation for Development (formerly CIIR Overseas Programme)

International Health Exchange

International Health Service

International Nepal Fellowship

International Partnership for Human Development

InterServe

Liga International, Inc.

Ludhiana Christian Medical College Board USA

Lumiere Medical Ministries, Inc.

M.E.D.I.C.O.

Maluti Adventist Hospital (Lesotho)

Maua Methodist Hospital

Medical Ambassadors International

Medical Ministry International

Mercy Ships

Mexican Medical Ministries

Mima Foundation, Inc.

Moi University Faculty of Health Sciences

Mountain Movers Missions Intl

National Health Service Corps, Recruitment Program

Nicaraguan Children's Fund

North American Baptist Conference Missions

Northwest Medical Teams International, Inc.

Operation Blessing, Medical Division

Operation Rainbow

Operation Smile International

Our Little Brothers and Sisters

P.C.E.A. Chogoria Hospital

P.R.A.Y. (Project Rescue of Amazon Youth)

Pan American Health Organization

PAZAPA

Physicians for Human Rights

Physicians for Peace

Project AmaZon

Project Concern International: OPTIONS

Project Hope/People to People Health Foundation

PROMESA

Remote Area Medical

Sanyati Baptist Hospital, Baptist Convention of Zimbabwe

School Sisters of Saint Francis

Simeus Foundation, The

Special Olympics, Inc.

St. Francis' Hospital

St. John's Medical College

St. Jude Hospital

St. Mary's Hospital, Vunapope

Surgical Medical Assistance Relief Teams

University of Cincinnati College of Medicine, Dept. of Family Medicine

University of Zimbabwe

Uplift Internationale

Virginia Children's Connection, Dept. of Plastic. & Recon. Surgery

Voluntary Service Overseas Canada

Volunteer Missionary Movement

Volunteer Optometric Service to Humanity (VOSH) International

VSO

WEC International

World Concern

World Medical Mission

Dermatologists

Adventist Development and Relief Agency International

Aloha Medical Missions (AMM)

Amazon-Africa Aid and Fundacao Esperanca

Amazon-Africa Aid Organization (3AO)

American Leprosy Missions Inc.

American Physicians Fellowship for Medicine in Israel

Ann Foundation Inc

Archdiocesan Health Care Network for Catholic Charities

Associazione Italiana 'Amici Raoul Follereau'

Bairo Pite Clinic

Baptist Medical Missions International

Beeve Foundation for World Eye and Health, The

Ben Gurion University of the Negev

Board of World Mission of the Moravian Church

Cameroon Baptist Convention Health Board

Canvasback Missions, Inc.

Capiz Emmanuel Hospital

Casa Clinica de la Mujer

Catholic Medical Mission Board, Inc.

Children's Cross Connection, International

Christian Medical College (Vellore, India) Board

Clinica Evangelica Morava Elective

Clínica Maxena

College of Medicine, Malawi

Commonwealth Health Center

Curamericas

DePauw University Winter Term in Service

DoCare International, Inc.

Evangelical Alliance Mission (TEAM World)

Foundation Human Nature (MeHiPro)

Friends Without a Border

Health profession usage: *(continued)*
<u>Dermatologists</u> *(continued)*

General Board of Global Ministries/The United Methodist Church
Global Volunteers
Guinea Development Foundation, Inc.
Haitian Health Clinic, Inc.
HBS Foundation, Inc./Hopital Bon Samaritain
Health Teams International
Health Volunteers Overseas
Helps International
Hillside Healthcare Center
Himalayan HealthCare Inc.
Honduras Outreach, Inc
Hope Alliance
Intercultural Nursing, Inc.
Liga International, Inc.
Ludhiana Christian Medical College Board USA
Lumiere Medical Ministries, Inc.
M.E.D.I.C.O.
Medical Ministry International
Mercy Ships
Mission Doctors Association
Moi University Faculty of Health Sciences
Mountain Movers Missions Intl
Nicaraguan Children's Fund
Omni Med
Operation Blessing, Medical Division
P.C.E.A. Kikuyu Hospital
P.R.A.Y. (Project Rescue of Amazon Youth)
PAZAPA
Project AmaZon
Project Concern International: OPTIONS
Project Hope/People to People Health Foundation
Remote Area Medical
Simeus Foundation, The
St. John's Medical College
St. Jude Hospital
Surgical Medical Assistance Relief Teams
Universidad de Chile, Facultad de Medicina
University of Illinois College of Medicine at Rockford
University of Zimbabwe
UTMB-WHO Collaborating Center for Training in International Health
Volunteer Missionary Movement
WEC International
World Hearing Network

<u>Emergency medicine physicians</u>

Adventist Development and Relief Agency International
Aid for International Medicine
Ak' Tenamit
Aloha Medical Missions (AMM)
American Baptist Board of International Ministries
American Jewish World Service
American Physicians Fellowship for Medicine in Israel
American Refugee Committee
Ann Foundation Inc
Archdiocesan Health Care Network for Catholic Charities
Armenian Social Transition Program
Bairo Pite Clinic
Baptist Medical Missions International
Beeve Foundation for World Eye and Health, The
Ben Gurion University of the Negev
Board of World Mission of the Moravian Church
Cameroon Baptist Convention Health Board
Canvasback Missions, Inc.
Cape Cares
Casa Clinica de la Mujer
Catholic Medical Mission Board, Inc.
CERT International (Christian Emergency Relief Team)
Children's Cross Connection, International
Christian Medical College (Vellore, India) Board
Clinica Evangelica Morava Elective
Clínica Maxena
College of Medicine, Malawi
Commonwealth Health Center
Complete Basic Health 2000
Curamericas
DePauw University Winter Term in Service
DoCare International, Inc.
Doctors for Global Health
Doctors of the World
Emergency International Inc.
Fellowship of Associates of Medical Evangelism
Flying Samaritans
Foundation Human Nature (MeHiPro)
Friends Without a Border
General Board of Global Ministries/The United Methodist Church
Global Volunteers
Guinea Development Foundation, Inc.
Healing the Children Northeast, Inc.
Health Teams International
Helps International
Honduras Outreach, Inc
Hope Alliance
Hope Worldwide
Hospital Albert Schweitzer
Intercultural Nursing, Inc.
International Cooperation for Development (formerly CIIR Overseas Programme)

Health profession usage: *(continued)*
<u>**Emergency medicine physicians**</u> *(continued)*

International Federation of Red Cross and Red Crescent Societies
International Health Exchange
International Health Service
International Medical Corps
International Nepal Fellowship
International Relief Teams
International Rescue Committee
Liga International, Inc.
Ludhiana Christian Medical College Board USA
Lumiere Medical Ministries, Inc.
M.E.D.I.C.O.
Magee-Womens Hospital
Medecins Sans Frontieres/ Doctors Without Borders USA
Medical Care Development International Division
Medical Ministry International
Medicine for Peace
Memisa Medicus Mundi
Mercy Ships
Mexican Medical Ministries
Michigan State University Institute for International Health
Mission Doctors Association
Moi University Faculty of Health Sciences
Mountain Movers Missions Intl
Nicaraguan Children's Fund
Northwest Medical Teams International, Inc.
Omni Med
Operation Blessing, Medical Division
Operation Smile International
P.C.E.A. Kikuyu Hospital
P.R.A.Y. (Project Rescue of Amazon Youth)
Palestine Children's Relief Fund
Pan American Health Organization
PAZAPA
Physicians for Human Rights
Project AmaZon
Project Hope/People to People Health Foundation
PROMESA
Remote Area Medical
Sanyati Baptist Hospital, Baptist Convention of Zimbabwe
School Sisters of Saint Francis
Simeus Foundation, The
Sister Community Alliances: Ouelessebougou-Utah Alliance
Special Olympics, Inc.
St. Jude Hospital
Surgical Medical Assistance Relief Teams
Tulane University School of Public Health and Tropical Medicine
Univ. of Wisconsin Med., Office of International Health Affairs
Universidad de Chile, Facultad de Medicina
University of Illinois College of Medicine at Rockford
University of Nebraska Medical Center, Office of International Programs and Studies
University of Zimbabwe
US Committee for Scientific Cooperation with Vietnam
Volunteer Missionary Movement
WEC International
World Emergency Relief
World Gospel Mission
World Hearing Network

<u>**Endocrinologists**</u>

Adventist Development and Relief Agency International
Aloha Medical Missions (AMM)
American Physicians Fellowship for Medicine in Israel
Ann Foundation Inc
Archdiocesan Health Care Network for Catholic Charities
Bairo Pite Clinic
Baptist Medical Missions International
Beeve Foundation for World Eye and Health, The
Ben Gurion University of the Negev
Cameroon Baptist Convention Health Board
Capiz Emmanuel Hospital
Casa Clinica de la Mujer
Children's Cross Connection, International
Christian Medical College (Vellore, India) Board
Clinica Evangelica Morava Elective
Clínica Maxena
College of Medicine, Malawi
Doctors for Global Health
Foundation Human Nature (MeHiPro)
Friends Without a Border
Global Volunteers
Guinea Development Foundation, Inc.
Healing the Children Northeast, Inc.
Health Teams International
Honduras Outreach, Inc
Hope Alliance
Hope Worldwide
Liga International, Inc.
Ludhiana Christian Medical College Board USA
Lumiere Medical Ministries, Inc.
Magee-Womens Hospital
Mercy Ships
Michigan State University Institute for International Health
Mission Doctors Association
Moi University Faculty of Health Sciences
Mountain Movers Missions Intl
Nicaraguan Children's Fund

Health profession usage: *(continued)*

Endocrinologists *(continued)*

Omni Med

Operation Blessing, Medical Division

P.C.E.A. Kikuyu Hospital

P.R.A.Y. (Project Rescue of Amazon Youth)

Palestine Children's Relief Fund

Project AmaZon

Project Hope/People to People Health Foundation

Remote Area Medical

Simeus Foundation, The

Special Olympics, Inc.

St. John's Medical College

St. Jude Hospital

Surgical Medical Assistance Relief Teams

Univ. of Wisconsin Med., Office of International Health Affairs

Universidad de Chile, Facultad de Medicina

University of Illinois College of Medicine at Rockford

University of Zimbabwe

US Committee for Scientific Cooperation with Vietnam

Volunteer Missionary Movement

WEC International

World Hearing Network

Epidemiologists and health educators

ACCESS

Action Against Hunger

Adventist Development and Relief Agency International

Africare

American College of Nurse-Midwives

American Jewish World Service

American Leprosy Missions Inc.

American Physicians Fellowship for Medicine in Israel

American Refugee Committee

Ann Foundation Inc

Bairo Pite Clinic

Baptist Medical Missions International

Beeve Foundation for World Eye and Health, The

Ben Gurion University of the Negev

Cameroon Baptist Convention Health Board

Campus Crusade for Christ International

Casa Clinica de la Mujer

CB International

Chanet Community Organization

Child Family Health International

Children's Cross Connection, International

Christian Medical College (Vellore, India) Board

Christian Mission of Pignon Inc.

Clinica Evangelica Morava Elective

Clínica Maxena

College of Medicine, Malawi

CONCERN

CONCERN America

Crudem Foundation

Curamericas

DePauw University Winter Term in Service

DoCare International, Inc.

Doctors for Global Health

Doctors of the World

Evangelical Alliance Mission (TEAM World)

Flying Samaritans

Foundation Human Nature (MeHiPro)

Foundation of Compassionate American Samaritans

Friends Without a Border

Global Operations & Development

Global Service Corps/Earth Island Institute

Global Volunteers

Grokha Association of Social Health

Guinea Development Foundation, Inc.

Haitian Health Clinic, Inc.

Hands Together, Inc.

HBS Foundation, Inc./Hopital Bon Samaritain

Health Alliance International

Health and Child Survival Fellows Program

Health Teams International

Himalayan HealthCare Inc.

Honduras Outreach, Inc

Hope Alliance

Hope Worldwide

Hospital Albert Schweitzer

International Committee of the Red Cross

International Cooperation for Development (formerly CIIR Overseas Programme)

International Eye Foundation, Inc.

International Federation of Red Cross and Red Crescent Societies

International Health Exchange

International Medical Corps

International Nepal Fellowship

International Rescue Committee

InterServe

INTERTEAM

Jesuit Refugee Service

Johns Hopkins Univ. School of Public Health, Dept. of International Health

Lalmba Association

Ludhiana Christian Medical College Board USA

Lumiere Medical Ministries, Inc.

Magee-Womens Hospital

Management Sciences for Health

Medical Aid for Palestinians

Medical Care Development International Division

Health profession usage: *(continued)*
Epidemiologists and health educators *(continued)*

Medical Ministry International
Medicine for Peace
Memisa Medicus Mundi
Mennonite Central Committee
Mercy Ships
Michigan State University Institute for International Health
Mima Foundation, Inc.
Minnesota International Health Volunteers
Mission Doctors Association
Moi University Faculty of Health Sciences
Mountain Movers Missions Intl
Nicaraguan Children's Fund
Northwest Medical Teams International, Inc.
Operation Blessing, Medical Division
P.C.E.A. Kikuyu Hospital
P.C.E.A. Tumutumu Hospital
P.R.A.Y. (Project Rescue of Amazon Youth)
Presbyterian Church USA, Mission Service Recruitment
Project AmaZon
Project Hope/People to People Health Foundation
Remote Area Medical
Seva Foundation
Simeus Foundation, The
Sister Community Alliances: Ouelessebougou-Utah Alliance
SkillShare International
Sons of Mary Missionary Society
Special Olympics, Inc.
St. John's Medical College
Surgical Medical Assistance Relief Teams
Trinity Health International
Tulane University School of Public Health and Tropical Medicine
UCSD, Division of International Health
Univ. of Wisconsin Med., Office of International Health Affairs
Universidad de Chile, Facultad de Medicina
University of Cincinnati College of Medicine, Dept. of Family Medicine
University of Illinois College of Medicine at Rockford
University of Zimbabwe
US Committee for Scientific Cooperation with Vietnam
UTMB-WHO Collaborating Center for Training in International Health
Visions in Action
Voluntary Service Overseas Canada
Volunteer Missionary Movement
VSO
WEC International
Women's Commission for Refugee Women and Children
World Concern
World Emergency Relief
World Gospel Mission
World Mission Prayer League
World Rehabilitation Fund, Inc.
World Vision International
World Vision, Inc.

Family practitioners

Adventist Development and Relief Agency International
Africa Inland Mission, International
Aid for International Medicine
Ak' Tenamit
Aloha Medical Missions (AMM)
Amazon-Africa Aid and Fundacao Esperanca
Amazon-Africa Aid Organization (3AO)
American Jewish World Service
American Physicians Fellowship for Medicine in Israel
American Refugee Committee
Ann Foundation Inc
Archdiocesan Health Care Network for Catholic Charities
Armenian Social Transition Program
Bairo Pite Clinic
Baptist Medical Missions International
Baptist Mid Missions
Beeve Foundation for World Eye and Health, The
Ben Gurion University of the Negev
Board of World Mission of the Moravian Church
Cameroon Baptist Convention Health Board
Campus Crusade for Christ International
Canvasback Missions, Inc.
Casa Clinica de la Mujer
Catholic Medical Mission Board, Inc.
CB International
CERT International (Christian Emergency Relief Team)
Chanet Community Organization
Child Family Health International
Children's Cross Connection, International
Children's Medical Mission
Christian Medical College (Vellore, India) Board
Christian Mission of Pignon Inc.
Clinica Evangelica Morava Elective
Clínica Maxena
College of Medicine, Malawi
Community of Caring
CONCERN America
CrossWorld
Crudem Foundation
Curamericas
DePauw University Winter Term in Service
DoCare International, Inc.

Health profession usage: *(continued)*
Family practitioners *(continued)*

Doctors for Global Health
Doctors of the World
Edward A. Ulzen Memorial Foundation (EAUMF)
Evangelical Alliance Mission (TEAM World)
Evangelical Free Church of America Mission
Evangelical Lutheran Church in America
Father Carr's Place 2B
Fellowship of Associates of Medical Evangelism
Filipino-American Medical Inc.
Flying Samaritans
Foundation Human Nature (MeHiPro)
Friends Without a Border
General Board of Global Ministries/The United Methodist Church
Global Operations & Development
Global Outreach International
Global Volunteers
Grace Ministries International
Grokha Association of Social Health
Guinea Development Foundation, Inc.
Haitian Health Clinic, Inc.
Hands Together, Inc.
HBS Foundation, Inc./Hopital Bon Samaritain
Healing the Children Northeast, Inc.
Health Teams International
Helps International
Himalayan Health Exchange
Himalayan HealthCare Inc.
Honduras Outreach, Inc
Hope Alliance
Hope Worldwide
Hospital Albert Schweitzer
Intercultural Nursing, Inc.
International Aid, Inc.
International Cooperation for Development (formerly CIIR Overseas Programme)
International Federation of Red Cross and Red Crescent Societies
International Health Service
International Medical Corps
International Ministries, American Baptist Churches, USA
International Nepal Fellowship
International Partnership for Human Development
InterServe
Lalmba Association
Liga International, Inc.
Lumiere Medical Ministries, Inc.
M.E.D.I.C.O.
Magee-Womens Hospital
Maua Methodist Hospital
Medecins Sans Frontieres/ Doctors Without Borders USA
Medical Aid for Palestinians
Medical Ambassadors International
Medical Care Development International Division
Medical Ministry International
Medicine for Peace
Mennonite Central Committee
Mercy Ships
Mexican Medical Ministries
Mima Foundation, Inc.
Mission Doctors Association
Moi University Faculty of Health Sciences
Mountain Movers Missions Intl
National Health Service Corps, Recruitment Program
Nicaraguan Children's Fund
Northwest Medical Teams International, Inc.
Omni Med
Operation Blessing, Medical Division
Our Little Brothers and Sisters
P.C.E.A. Kikuyu Hospital
P.C.E.A. Tumutumu Hospital
P.R.A.Y. (Project Rescue of Amazon Youth)
PAZAPA
Presbyterian Church USA, Mission Service Recruitment
Project AmaZon
Project Hope/People to People Health Foundation
Remote Area Medical
Saint Joseph's Medical Center, Family Practice Residency Program, Int'l Health Track
Salesian Missions
Sanyati Baptist Hospital, Baptist Convention of Zimbabwe
School Sisters of Saint Francis
Simeus Foundation, The
SkillShare International
Special Olympics, Inc.
St. Francis' Hospital
St. John's Medical College
St. Jude Hospital
St. Mary's Hospital, Vunapope
Surgical Medical Assistance Relief Teams
Trinity Health International
UCSD, Division of International Health
Universidad de Chile, Facultad de Medicina
University of Illinois College of Medicine at Rockford
University of Nebraska Medical Center, Office of International Programs and Studies
University of Zimbabwe
Uplift Internationale
Volunteer Missionary Movement
Volunteer Optometric Service to Humanity (VOSH) International
VSO
WEC International
World Gospel Mission
World Hearing Network
World Mission Prayer League

Health profession usage: *(continued)*

Gastroenterologists

Adventist Development and Relief Agency International
Ak' Tenamit
Aloha Medical Missions (AMM)
Amazon-Africa Aid Organization (3AO)
American Physicians Fellowship for Medicine in Israel
Ann Foundation Inc
Archdiocesan Health Care Network for Catholic Charities
Bairo Pite Clinic
Baptist Medical Missions International
Ben Gurion University of the Negev
Cameroon Baptist Convention Health Board
Capiz Emmanuel Hospital
Casa Clinica de la Mujer
Children's Cross Connection, International
Christian Medical College (Vellore, India) Board
Clinica Evangelica Morava Elective
College of Medicine, Malawi
Commonwealth Health Center
Complete Basic Health 2000
Curamericas
DoCare International, Inc.
Foundation Human Nature (MeHiPro)
Friends Without a Border
Global Volunteers
Guinea Development Foundation, Inc.
Haitian Health Clinic, Inc.
Healing the Children Northeast, Inc.
Health Teams International
Himalayan HealthCare Inc.
Hope Alliance
Lumiere Medical Ministries, Inc.
Magee-Womens Hospital
Medical Ministry International
Mercy Ships
Mission Doctors Association
Moi University Faculty of Health Sciences
Mountain Movers Missions Intl
Nicaraguan Children's Fund
Omni Med
Operation Blessing, Medical Division
P.C.E.A. Kikuyu Hospital
P.R.A.Y. (Project Rescue of Amazon Youth)
Project AmaZon
Project Hope/People to People Health Foundation
Remote Area Medical
Simeus Foundation, The
Special Olympics, Inc.
St. John's Medical College
Surgical Medical Assistance Relief Teams
Universidad de Chile, Facultad de Medicina
University of Illinois College of Medicine at Rockford
University of Zimbabwe
Volunteer Missionary Movement
WEC International
World Hearing Network

General surgeons

Adventist Development and Relief Agency International
Africa Inland Mission, International
Aid for International Medicine
Aloha Medical Missions (AMM)
Amazon-Africa Aid and Fundacao Esperanca
Amazon-Africa Aid Organization (3AO)
American Leprosy Missions Inc.
American Physicians Fellowship for Medicine in Israel
Ann Foundation Inc
Archdiocesan Health Care Network for Catholic Charities
Associate Reformed Presbyterian Church, World Witness
Bairo Pite Clinic
Baptist Medical Missions International
Baptist Mid Missions
Ben Gurion University of the Negev
Cameroon Baptist Convention Health Board
Canvasback Missions, Inc.
Capiz Emmanuel Hospital
CardioStart International, Inc.
Casa Clinica de la Mujer
Catholic Medical Mission Board, Inc.
CB International
CERT International (Christian Emergency Relief Team)
Child Family Health International
Children's Cross Connection, International
Children's Heartlink
Christian Medical College (Vellore, India) Board
Christian Mission of Pignon Inc.
Clinica Evangelica Morava Elective
College of Medicine, Malawi
Comitato Collaborazione Medica (Doctors for Developing Countries)
Commonwealth Health Center
Complete Basic Health 2000
CrossWorld
Crudem Foundation
Curamericas
DoCare International, Inc.
Esperanca, Inc.
Evangelical Alliance Mission (TEAM World)

Health profession usage: *(continued)*

General surgeons *(continued)*

Evangelical Free Church of America Mission
Evangelical Lutheran Church in America
Fellowship of Associates of Medical Evangelism
Filipino-American Medical Inc.
Flying Samaritans
Foundation Human Nature (MeHiPro)
Friends Without a Border
General Board of Global Ministries/The United Methodist Church
Global Volunteers
Grace Ministries International
Guinea Development Foundation, Inc.
Hands Together, Inc.
HBS Foundation, Inc./Hopital Bon Samaritain
Healing the Children Northeast, Inc.
Health Teams International
Health Volunteers Overseas
Helping Hands Health Education
Helps International
Hillside Healthcare Center
Honduras Outreach, Inc
Hope Alliance
Hope Worldwide
Hospital Albert Schweitzer
International Children's Heart Foundation
International Committee of the Red Cross
International Cooperation for Development (formerly CIIR Overseas Programme)
International Federation of Red Cross and Red Crescent Societies
International Health Exchange
International Health Service
International Medical Corps
International Ministries, American Baptist Churches, USA
International Nepal Fellowship
InterServe
Jesuit Refugee Service
Liga International, Inc.
Loma Linda University International Programs
Ludhiana Christian Medical College Board USA
Lumiere Medical Ministries, Inc.
M.E.D.I.C.O.
Magee-Womens Hospital
Maluti Adventist Hospital (Lesotho)
Maua Methodist Hospital
Medecins Sans Frontieres/ Doctors Without Borders USA
Medical Care Development International Division
Medical Ministry International
Medicine for Peace
Mennonite Central Committee
Mercy Ships
Mexican Medical Ministries
Mima Foundation, Inc.
Mission Doctors Association
Moi University Faculty of Health Sciences
Mountain Movers Missions Intl
Nicaraguan Children's Fund
Northwest Medical Teams International, Inc.
Omni Med
Operation Blessing, Medical Division
Operation Rainbow
P.C.E.A. Chogoria Hospital
P.C.E.A. Kikuyu Hospital
P.C.E.A. Tumutumu Hospital
P.R.A.Y. (Project Rescue of Amazon Youth)
PAZAPA
Presbyterian Church USA, Mission Service Recruitment
Project AmaZon
Project Hope/People to People Health Foundation
Project Open Hearts
Remote Area Medical
Sanyati Baptist Hospital, Baptist Convention of Zimbabwe
School Sisters of Saint Francis
Simeus Foundation, The
SIM USA
Sister Community Alliances: Ouelessebougou-Utah Alliance
Special Olympics, Inc.
St. Francis' Hospital
St. John's Medical College
St. Jude Hospital
St. Mary's Hospital, Vunapope
Surgical Medical Assistance Relief Teams
Surgicorps International
Univ. of Wisconsin Med., Office of International Health Affairs
Universidad de Chile, Facultad de Medicina
University of Illinois College of Medicine at Rockford
University of Virginia, Center for Global Health
University of Zimbabwe
US Committee for Scientific Cooperation with Vietnam
Voluntary Service Overseas Canada
Volunteer Missionary Movement
WEC International
World Gospel Mission
World Hearing Network
World Mission Prayer League
Zuma Memorial Hospital

Hematologists and oncologists

Adventist Development and Relief Agency International
Aloha Medical Missions (AMM)
Amazon-Africa Aid Organization (3AO)

Health profession usage: *(continued)*
Hematologists and oncologists *(continued)*

American Physicians Fellowship for Medicine in Israel
Ann Foundation Inc
Archdiocesan Health Care Network for Catholic Charities
Bairo Pite Clinic
Baptist Medical Missions International
Ben Gurion University of the Negev
Cameroon Baptist Convention Health Board
Capiz Emmanuel Hospital
Casa Clinica de la Mujer
Children's Cross Connection, International
Christian Medical College (Vellore, India) Board
Christian Mission of Pignon Inc.
Clinica Evangelica Morava Elective
College of Medicine, Malawi
Crudem Foundation
Foundation Human Nature (MeHiPro)
Friends Without a Border
Global Volunteers
Grace Ministries International
Guinea Development Foundation, Inc.
Health Teams International
Himalayan HealthCare Inc.
Hope Alliance
Hope Worldwide
International Health Exchange
Ludhiana Christian Medical College Board USA
Lumiere Medical Ministries, Inc.
Magee-Womens Hospital
Medicine for Peace
Mercy Ships
Mission Doctors Association
Moi University Faculty of Health Sciences
Mountain Movers Missions Intl
Nicaraguan Children's Fund
Omni Med
Operation Blessing, Medical Division
Operation USA
P.C.E.A. Kikuyu Hospital
P.R.A.Y. (Project Rescue of Amazon Youth)
Palestine Children's Relief Fund
Project AmaZon
Project Hope/People to People Health Foundation
Remote Area Medical
School Sisters of Saint Francis
Simeus Foundation, The
St. John's Medical College
Surgical Medical Assistance Relief Teams
Univ. of Wisconsin Med., Office of International Health Affairs
Universidad de Chile, Facultad de Medicina
University of Illinois College of Medicine at Rockford
University of Zimbabwe
US Committee for Scientific Cooperation with Vietnam
Volunteer Missionary Movement
WEC International
World Hearing Network

Infectious disease specialists

Adventist Development and Relief Agency International
Aid for International Medicine
Ak' Tenamit
Aloha Medical Missions (AMM)
Amazon-Africa Aid Organization (3AO)
American Jewish World Service
American Physicians Fellowship for Medicine in Israel
American Refugee Committee
Ann Foundation Inc
Archdiocesan Health Care Network for Catholic Charities
Armenian Social Transition Program
Associazione Italiana 'Amici Raoul Follereau'
Bairo Pite Clinic
Baptist Medical Missions International
Beeve Foundation for World Eye and Health, The
Ben Gurion University of the Negev
Board of World Mission of the Moravian Church
Cameroon Baptist Convention Health Board
Canvasback Missions, Inc.
Cape Cares
Capiz Emmanuel Hospital
Casa Clinica de la Mujer
Child Family Health International
Children's Cross Connection, International
Children's Heartlink
Christian Medical College (Vellore, India) Board
Christian Mission of Pignon Inc.
Clinica Evangelica Morava Elective
Clínica Maxena
College of Medicine, Malawi
Commonwealth Health Center
Crudem Foundation
DePauw University Winter Term in Service
DoCare International, Inc.
Doctors for Global Health
Doctors of the World
Evangelical Alliance Mission (TEAM World)
Evangelical Lutheran Church in America
Foundation Human Nature (MeHiPro)
Friends Without a Border
Global Volunteers
Grace Ministries International

Health profession usage: *(continued)*

Infectious disease specialists *(continued)*

Grokha Association of Social Health

Guinea Development Foundation, Inc.

Haitian Health Clinic, Inc.

Hands Together, Inc.

HBS Foundation, Inc./Hopital Bon Samaritain

Health and Child Survival Fellows Program

Health Teams International

Helps International

Himalayan HealthCare Inc.

Honduras Outreach, Inc

Hope Alliance

Hope Worldwide

Infectious Diseases Society of America, The, and The HIV Medicine Association

Intercultural Nursing, Inc.

International Cooperation for Development (formerly CIIR Overseas Programme)

International Federation of Red Cross and Red Crescent Societies

International Health Exchange

International Medical Corps

International Nepal Fellowship

International Partnership for Human Development

International Rescue Committee

InterServe

Ludhiana Christian Medical College Board USA

Lumiere Medical Ministries, Inc.

Magee-Womens Hospital

Maua Methodist Hospital

Medical Care Development International Division

Medical Ministry International

Medicine for Peace

Mercy Ships

Michigan State University Institute for International Health

Mima Foundation, Inc.

Mission Doctors Association

Moi University Faculty of Health Sciences

Mountain Movers Missions Intl

Nicaraguan Children's Fund

Omni Med

P.C.E.A. Kikuyu Hospital

P.R.A.Y. (Project Rescue of Amazon Youth)

Pan American Health Organization

PAZAPA

Physicians for Peace

Presbyterian Church USA, Mission Service Recruitment

Project AmaZon

Project Concern International: OPTIONS

Project Hope/People to People Health Foundation

Remote Area Medical

Sanyati Baptist Hospital, Baptist Convention of Zimbabwe

School Sisters of Saint Francis

Seva Foundation

Simeus Foundation, The

Sister Community Alliances: Ouelessebougou-Utah Alliance

Special Olympics, Inc.

St. John's Medical College

Surgical Medical Assistance Relief Teams

Tulane University School of Public Health and Tropical Medicine

Univ. of Wisconsin Med., Office of International Health Affairs

Universidad de Chile, Facultad de Medicina

University of Illinois College of Medicine at Rockford

University of Nebraska Medical Center, Office of International Programs and Studies

University of Virginia, Center for Global Health

University of Zimbabwe

US Committee for Scientific Cooperation with Vietnam

Visions in Action

Voluntary Service Overseas Canada

Volunteer Missionary Movement

WEC International

World Hearing Network

Internal medicine, general practitioners, and primary care providers

ACCESS

Action Against Hunger

Adventist Development and Relief Agency International

Africa Inland Mission, International

Aid for International Medicine

Ak' Tenamit

Aloha Medical Missions (AMM)

Amazon-Africa Aid and Fundacao Esperanca

Amazon-Africa Aid Organization (3AO)

American Jewish World Service

American Physicians Fellowship for Medicine in Israel

American Refugee Committee

Ann Foundation Inc

APUSAN-USA

Archdiocesan Health Care Network for Catholic Charities

Armenian Social Transition Program

Bairo Pite Clinic

Baptist Medical Missions International

Beeve Foundation for World Eye and Health, The

Ben Gurion University of the Negev

Board of World Mission of the Moravian Church

Cameroon Baptist Convention Health Board

Campus Crusade for Christ International

Health profession usage: *(continued)*

Internal medicine, general practitioners, and primary care providers *(continued)*

Canvasback Missions, Inc.
Cape Cares
Capiz Emmanuel Hospital
Casa Clinica de la Mujer
Catholic Medical Mission Board, Inc.
CB International
CERT International (Christian Emergency Relief Team)
Chanet Community Organization
Child Family Health International
Children's Cross Connection, International
Christian Medical College (Vellore, India) Board
Christian Mission of Pignon Inc.
Clinica Evangelica Morava Elective
Clínica Maxena
College of Medicine, Malawi
Comitato Collaborazione Medica (Doctors for Developing Countries)
Commonwealth Health Center
Complete Basic Health 2000
CONCERN
CONCERN America
CrossWorld
Crudem Foundation
Curamericas
DePauw University Winter Term in Service
Doctors for Global Health
Doctors of the World
Edward A. Ulzen Memorial Foundation (EAUMF)
Evangelical Lutheran Church in America
Filipino-American Medical Inc.
Foundation Human Nature (MeHiPro)
Foundation of Compassionate American Samaritans
Friends Without a Border
General Board of Global Ministries/The United Methodist Church
Global Operations & Development
Global Volunteers
Grokha Association of Social Health
Guinea Development Foundation, Inc.
Haitian Health Clinic, Inc.
Hands Together, Inc.
Healing the Children Northeast, Inc.
Health and Child Survival Fellows Program
Health Teams International
Health Volunteers Overseas
Helping Hands Health Education
Helps International
Himalayan Health Exchange
Himalayan HealthCare Inc.
Honduras Outreach, Inc
Hope Alliance
Hope Worldwide
Hospital Albert Schweitzer
Intercultural Nursing, Inc.
International Aid, Inc.
International Committee of the Red Cross
International Federation of Red Cross and Red Crescent Societies
International Health Exchange
International Health Service
International Medical Corps
International Ministries, American Baptist Churches, USA
International Rescue Committee
InterServe
Lalmba Association
Liga International, Inc.
Lumiere Medical Ministries, Inc.
M.E.D.I.C.O.
Magee-Womens Hospital
Maluti Adventist Hospital (Lesotho)
Maua Methodist Hospital
Medical Aid for Palestinians
Medical Ambassadors International
Medical Care Development International Division
Medical Ministry International
Medical Missionaries of Mary
Medicine for Peace
Mercy Ships
Mexican Medical Ministries
Mima Foundation, Inc.
Mission Doctors Association
Moi University Faculty of Health Sciences
Mountain Movers Missions Intl
National Health Service Corps, Recruitment Program
Nicaraguan Children's Fund
Northwest Medical Teams International, Inc.
Omni Med
Operation Blessing, Medical Division
Our Little Brothers and Sisters
P.C.E.A. Kikuyu Hospital
P.C.E.A. Tumutumu Hospital
P.R.A.Y. (Project Rescue of Amazon Youth)
Palms Australia
PAZAPA
Physicians for Human Rights
Project AmaZon
Project Concern International: OPTIONS
Project Hope/People to People Health Foundation
PROMESA
Remote Area Medical
Salesian Missions
Sanyati Baptist Hospital, Baptist Convention of Zimbabwe
School Sisters of Saint Francis
Simeus Foundation, The

Health profession usage: *(continued)*

Internal medicine, general practitioners, and primary care providers *(continued)*

SkillShare International

Special Olympics, Inc.

St. Francis' Hospital

St. John's Medical College

St. Jude Hospital

Surgical Medical Assistance Relief Teams

Tulane University School of Public Health and Tropical Medicine

Univ. of Wisconsin Med., Office of International Health Affairs

Universidad de Chile, Facultad de Medicina

University of Cincinnati College of Medicine, Dept. of Family Medicine

University of Illinois College of Medicine at Rockford

University of Nebraska Medical Center, Office of International Programs and Studies

University of Zimbabwe

Uplift Internationale

US Committee for Scientific Cooperation with Vietnam

Visions in Action

Voluntary Service Overseas Canada

Volunteer Missionary Movement

WEC International

World Emergency Relief

World Gospel Mission

World Hearing Network

World Mission Prayer League

World Vision International

World Vision, Inc.

Medical technicians

Adventist Development and Relief Agency International

Africa Inland Mission, International

American Physicians Fellowship for Medicine in Israel

American Refugee Committee

Ann Foundation Inc

Bairo Pite Clinic

Baptist Medical Missions International

Baptist Mid Missions

Beeve Foundation for World Eye and Health, The

Ben Gurion University of the Negev

Board of World Mission of the Moravian Church

Cameroon Baptist Convention Health Board

Canvasback Missions, Inc.

Capiz Emmanuel Hospital

Casa Clinica de la Mujer

Catholic Medical Mission Board, Inc.

Chanet Community Organization

Children's Cross Connection, International

Christian Medical College (Vellore, India) Board

Christian Mission of Pignon Inc.

Clinica Evangelica Morava Elective

Clínica Maxena

College of Medicine, Malawi

Commonwealth Health Center

Complete Basic Health 2000

Crudem Foundation

Curamericas

Evangelical Alliance Mission (TEAM World)

Evangelical Free Church of America Mission

Evangelical Lutheran Church in America

Foundation Human Nature (MeHiPro)

Friends Without a Border

Global Volunteers

Grokha Association of Social Health

Guinea Development Foundation, Inc.

Haitian Health Clinic, Inc.

HBS Foundation, Inc./Hopital Bon Samaritain

Health Teams International

Honduras Outreach, Inc

Hope Alliance

Hope Worldwide

Hospital Albert Schweitzer

International Aid, Inc.

International Committee of the Red Cross

International Cooperation for Development (formerly CIIR Overseas Programme)

International Health Exchange

International Health Service

International Nepal Fellowship

InterServe

INTERTEAM

Liga International, Inc.

Lumiere Medical Ministries, Inc.

Magee-Womens Hospital

Maluti Adventist Hospital (Lesotho)

Maua Methodist Hospital

Medical Aid for Palestinians

Medical Ministry International

Mercy Ships

Mexican Medical Ministries

Moi University Faculty of Health Sciences

Mountain Movers Missions Intl

Nicaraguan Children's Fund

North American Baptist Conference Missions

Northwest Medical Teams International, Inc.

Operation Blessing, Medical Division

P.C.E.A. Kikuyu Hospital

P.C.E.A. Tumutumu Hospital

P.R.A.Y. (Project Rescue of Amazon Youth)

PAZAPA

Physicians for Peace

Project AmaZon

Health profession usage: *(continued)*

Medical technicians *(continued)*

Nephrologists

Neurologists

Health profession usage: *(continued)*

Neurologists *(continued)*

Guinea Development Foundation, Inc.

Healing the Children Northeast, Inc.

Health Teams International

Honduras Outreach, Inc

Hope Alliance

Hope Worldwide

Ludhiana Christian Medical College Board USA

Lumiere Medical Ministries, Inc.

M.E.D.I.C.O.

Medecins Sans Frontieres/ Doctors Without Borders USA

Medical Ministry International

Mission Doctors Association

Moi University Faculty of Health Sciences

Mountain Movers Missions Intl

Nicaraguan Children's Fund

Omni Med

P.C.E.A. Kikuyu Hospital

P.R.A.Y. (Project Rescue of Amazon Youth)

Project AmaZon

Project Hope/People to People Health Foundation

Simeus Foundation, The

Special Olympics, Inc.

St. John's Medical College

Surgical Medical Assistance Relief Teams

Univ. of Wisconsin Med., Office of International Health Affairs

US Committee for Scientific Cooperation with Vietnam

Universidad de Chile, Facultad de Medicina

University of Illinois College of Medicine at Rockford

University of Zimbabwe

Volunteer Missionary Movement

WEC International

World Hearing Network

Neurosurgeons

Adventist Development and Relief Agency International

American Physicians Fellowship for Medicine in Israel

Ann Foundation Inc

Archdiocesan Health Care Network for Catholic Charities

Associate Reformed Presbyterian Church, World Witness

Bairo Pite Clinic

Ben Gurion University of the Negev

Cameroon Baptist Convention Health Board

Casa Clinica de la Mujer

Catholic Medical Mission Board, Inc.

Children's Cross Connection, International

Christian Medical College (Vellore, India) Board

Clinica Evangelica Morava Elective

College of Medicine, Malawi

FIENS Foundation of International Education in Neurological Surgery

Foundation Human Nature (MeHiPro)

Friends Without a Border

Global Volunteers

Guinea Development Foundation, Inc.

Healing the Children Northeast, Inc.

Health Teams International

Hope Alliance

Ludhiana Christian Medical College Board USA

Lumiere Medical Ministries, Inc.

Medical Ministry International

Mission Doctors Association

Moi University Faculty of Health Sciences

Mountain Movers Missions Intl

Nicaraguan Children's Fund

Northwest Medical Teams International, Inc.

Omni Med

Operation Blessing, Medical Division

P.C.E.A. Kikuyu Hospital

P.R.A.Y. (Project Rescue of Amazon Youth)

Palestine Children's Relief Fund

Project AmaZon

Project Hope/People to People Health Foundation

Simeus Foundation, The

St. John's Medical College

Surgical Medical Assistance Relief Teams

Universidad de Chile, Facultad de Medicina

University of Illinois College of Medicine at Rockford

University of Zimbabwe

Volunteer Missionary Movement

WEC International

World Hearing Network

Nurse midwives

Adventist Development and Relief Agency International

Africa Inland Mission, International

Ak' Tenamit

American College of Nurse-Midwives

American Jewish World Service

American Physicians Fellowship for Medicine in Israel

American Refugee Committee

Ann Foundation Inc

Bairo Pite Clinic

Baptist Medical Missions International

Baptist Mid Missions

Health profession usage: *(continued)*
Nurse midwives *(continued)*

Beeve Foundation for World Eye and Health, The
Ben Gurion University of the Negev
Cameroon Baptist Convention Health Board
Canvasback Missions, Inc.
Casa Clinica de la Mujer
Chanet Community Organization
Children's Cross Connection, International
Christian Medical College (Vellore, India) Board
Clinica Evangelica Morava Elective
Comitato Collaborazione Medica (Doctors for Developing Countries)
Commonwealth Health Center
Community of Caring
CONCERN
CONCERN America
CrossWorld
Curamericas
DePauw University Winter Term in Service
DoCare International, Inc.
Doctors for Global Health
Doctors of the World
Evangelical Alliance Mission (TEAM World)
Evangelical Lutheran Church in America
Foundation Human Nature (MeHiPro)
Foundation of Compassionate American Samaritans
Friends Without a Border
Global Outreach International
Global Volunteers
Grokha Association of Social Health
Guinea Development Foundation, Inc.
Hands Together, Inc.
HBS Foundation, Inc./Hopital Bon Samaritain
Health and Child Survival Fellows Program
Health Teams International
Himalayan HealthCare Inc.
Honduras Outreach, Inc
Hope Alliance
Intercultural Nursing, Inc.
International Cooperation for Development (formerly CIIR Overseas Programme)
International Health Exchange
International Medical Corps
International Nepal Fellowship
International Relief Teams
International Rescue Committee
INTERTEAM
Jesuit Refugee Service
Johns Hopkins Univ. School of Public Health, Dept. of International Health
Lalmba Association
Liga International, Inc.
Lumiere Medical Ministries, Inc.
Magee-Womens Hospital
Maluti Adventist Hospital (Lesotho)
Maua Methodist Hospital
Medical Aid for Palestinians
Medical Care Development International Division
Medical Ministry International
Medical Missionaries of Mary
Medicine for Peace
Mercy Ships
Moi University Faculty of Health Sciences
Mountain Movers Missions Intl
Nicaraguan Children's Fund
Northwest Medical Teams International, Inc.
P.C.E.A. Kikuyu Hospital
P.C.E.A. Tumutumu Hospital
P.R.A.Y. (Project Rescue of Amazon Youth)
Pan American Health Organization
Project AmaZon
Project Concern International: OPTIONS
Project Hope/People to People Health Foundation
PROMESA
School Sisters of Saint Francis
Selian Lutheran Hospital
Simeus Foundation, The
SkillShare International
St. Francis' Hospital
St. John's Medical College
St. Jude Hospital
Surgical Medical Assistance Relief Teams
Tulane University School of Public Health and Tropical
UCSD, Division of International Health
Univ. of Wisconsin Med., Office of International Health Affairs
Universidad de Chile, Facultad de Medicina
University of Illinois at Chicago College of Nursing, Global Health Leadership Office
University of Zimbabwe
US Committee for Scientific Cooperation with Vietnam
UTMB-WHO Collaborating Center for Training in International Health
Visions in Action
Voluntary Service Overseas Canada
Volunteer Missionary Movement
VSO
WEC International
World Emergency Relief
World Gospel Mission
World Mission Prayer League
World Vision International
World Vision, Inc.

Health profession usage: *(continued)*

Nurse practitioners

Action Against Hunger

Adventist Development and Relief Agency International

Aid for International Medicine

Ak' Tenamit

Aloha Medical Missions (AMM)

American College of Nurse-Midwives

American Jewish World Service

American Physicians Fellowship for Medicine in Israel

American Refugee Committee

Anderson University School of Nursing

Ann Foundation Inc

Bairo Pite Clinic

Baptist Medical Missions International

Beeve Foundation for World Eye and Health, The

Ben Gurion University of the Negev

Board of World Mission of the Moravian Church

CAM International

Cameroon Baptist Convention Health Board

Canvasback Missions, Inc.

Cape Cares

CardioStart International, Inc.

Casa Clinica de la Mujer

CERT International (Christian Emergency Relief Team)

Chanet Community Organization

Children's Cross Connection, International

Christian Medical College (Vellore, India) Board

Christian Mission of Pignon Inc.

Clinica Evangelica Morava Elective

Clínica Maxena

Commonwealth Health Center

CONCERN America

Curamericas

DePauw University Winter Term in Service

DoCare International, Inc.

Doctors for Global Health

Doctors of the World

Esperanca, Inc.

Evangelical Alliance Mission (TEAM World)

Feed the Children

Fellowship of Associates of Medical Evangelism

Filipino-American Medical Inc.

Flying Samaritans

Foundation Human Nature (MeHiPro)

Friends Without a Border

General Board of Global Ministries/The United Methodist Church

Global Outreach International

Global Volunteers

Grokha Association of Social Health

Guinea Development Foundation, Inc.

Haitian Health Clinic, Inc.

Hands Together, Inc.

HBS Foundation, Inc./Hopital Bon Samaritain

Healing the Children Northeast, Inc.

Health and Child Survival Fellows Program

Health Teams International

Helps International

Hillside Healthcare Center

Himalayan HealthCare Inc.

Honduras Outreach, Inc

Hope Alliance

Hope Worldwide

Intercultural Nursing, Inc.

International Children's Heart Foundation

International Cooperation for Development (formerly CIIR Overseas Programme)

International Health Exchange

International Health Service

International Medical Corps

International Nepal Fellowship

International Partnership for Human Development

International Relief Teams

International Rescue Committee

InterServe

Johns Hopkins Univ. School of Public Health, Dept. of International Health

Lalmba Association

Liga International, Inc.

Lumiere Medical Ministries, Inc.

M.E.D.I.C.O.

Magee-Womens Hospital

Maluti Adventist Hospital (Lesotho)

Maua Methodist Hospital

Medical Aid for Palestinians

Medical Care Development International Division

Medical Ministry International

Medical Missionaries of Mary

Medicine for Peace

Mennonite Central Committee

Mercy Ships

Mima Foundation, Inc.

Moi University Faculty of Health Sciences

Mountain Movers Missions Intl

National Health Service Corps, Recruitment Program

Nicaraguan Children's Fund

North American Baptist Conference Missions

Northwest Medical Teams International, Inc.

Omni Med

Operation Blessing, Medical Division

Our Little Brothers and Sisters

P.C.E.A. Kikuyu Hospital

Health profession usage: *(continued)*

Nurse practitioners *(continued)*

P.C.E.A. Tumutumu Hospital

P.R.A.Y. (Project Rescue of Amazon Youth)

Palms Australia

Pan American Health Organization

PAZAPA

Project AmaZon

Project Concern International: OPTIONS

Project Hope/People to People Health Foundation

Project Open Hearts

Remote Area Medical

School Sisters of Saint Francis

Selian Lutheran Hospital

Simeus Foundation, The

Sister Community Alliances: Ouelessebougou-Utah Alliance

Special Olympics, Inc.

St. Francis' Hospital

St. Jude Hospital

Surgery

Surgical Medical Assistance Relief Teams

Tulane University School of Public Health and Tropical Medicine

UCSD, Division of International Health

Univ. of Wisconsin Med., Office of International Health Affairs

Universidad de Chile, Facultad de Medicina

University of Cincinnati College of Medicine, Dept. of Family Medicine

University of Illinois at Chicago College of Nursing, Global Health Leadership Office

University of Illinois College of Medicine at Rockford

University of Nebraska Medical Center, Office of International Programs and Studies

University of Zimbabwe

US Committee for Scientific Cooperation with Vietnam

Virginia Children's Connection, Dept. of Plastic. & Recon. Surgery

Visions in Action

Voluntary Service Overseas Canada

Volunteer Missionary Movement

Volunteer Optometric Service to Humanity (VOSH) International

WEC International

World Emergency Relief

World Mission Prayer League

Nurses

Action Against Hunger

Adventist Development and Relief Agency International

Africa Inland Mission, International

African Inter-Mennonite Mission

Aid for International Medicine

Ak' Tenamit

Aloha Medical Missions (AMM)

American Baptist Board of International Ministries

American College of Nurse-Midwives

American Jewish World Service

American Leprosy Missions Inc.

American Physicians Fellowship for Medicine in Israel

American Refugee Committee

Anderson University School of Nursing

Ann Foundation Inc

APUSAN-USA

Archdiocesan Health Care Network for Catholic Charities

ASAPROSAR: The Salvadoran Association for Rural Health

Bairo Pite Clinic

Baptist General Conference

Baptist Medical Missions International

Baptist Mid Missions

Beeve Foundation for World Eye and Health, The

Ben Gurion University of the Negev

Board of World Mission of the Moravian Church

CAM International

Cameroon Baptist Convention Health Board

Canvasback Missions, Inc.

Cape Cares

CardioStart International, Inc.

Casa Clinica de la Mujer

Catholic Medical Mission Board, Inc.

CB International

CERT International (Christian Emergency Relief Team)

Chanet Community Organization

Children's Cross Connection, International

Children's Heartlink

Children's Medical Mission

Christian Medical College (Vellore, India) Board

Christian Mission of Pignon Inc.

Christoffel-Blindenmission EV

Church of the Nazarene World Mission Division

Clinica Evangelica Morava Elective

Clínica Maxena

CONCERN America

Crudem Foundation

Curamericas

DePauw University Winter Term in Service

DoCare International, Inc.

Doctors for Global Health

Doctors of the World

Edward A. Ulzen Memorial Foundation (EAUMF)

Esperanca, Inc.

Evangelical Alliance Mission (TEAM World)

Health profession usage: *(continued)*

Nurses *(continued)*

Evangelical Free Church of America Mission

Evangelical Lutheran Church in America

Father Carr's Place 2B

Feed the Children

Fellowship of Associates of Medical Evangelism

Filipino-American Medical Inc.

Flying Doctors of America

Flying Samaritans

Foundation Human Nature (MeHiPro)

Foundation of Compassionate American Samaritans

Friends Without a Border

General Board of Global Ministries/The United Methodist Church

General Dept. of World Missions, The Wesleyan Church

Global Operations & Development

Global Outreach International

Global Volunteers

Grokha Association of Social Health

Guinea Development Foundation, Inc.

Haitian Health Clinic, Inc.

Hands Together, Inc.

HBS Foundation, Inc./Hopital Bon Samaritain

Healing the Children Northeast, Inc.

Health Alliance International

Health and Child Survival Fellows Program

Health Teams International

Health Volunteers Overseas

Helping Hands Health Education

Helps International

Hillside Healthcare Center

Himalayan Health Exchange

Himalayan HealthCare Inc.

Honduras Outreach, Inc

Hope Alliance

Hope Worldwide

Intercultural Nursing, Inc.

Interface UCSD

International Children's Heart Foundation

International Committee of the Red Cross

International Cooperation for Development (formerly CIIR Overseas Programme)

International Health Exchange

International Health Service

International Medical Corps

International Ministries, American Baptist Churches, USA

International Nepal Fellowship

International Partnership for Human Development

International Relief Teams

Interplast

InterServe

INTERTEAM

Jesuit Refugee Service

Johns Hopkins Univ. School of Public Health, Dept. of International Health

Jubilee Volunteer Africa Program of AFRIDEC

Lalmba Association

Lay Mission-Helpers Association

Liga International, Inc.

Lighthouse for Christ Mission and Eye Centre

Loma Linda University International Programs

Ludhiana Christian Medical College Board USA

Lumiere Medical Ministries, Inc.

M.E.D.I.C.O.

Magee-Womens Hospital

Maluti Adventist Hospital (Lesotho)

Maua Methodist Hospital

Medecins Sans Frontieres/ Doctors Without Borders USA

Medical Aid for Palestinians

Medical Ambassadors International

Medical Care Development International Division

Medical Ministry International

Medicine for Peace

Mennonite Central Committee

Mercy Ships

Mexican Medical Ministries

Mima Foundation, Inc.

Moi University Faculty of Health Sciences

Mountain Movers Missions Intl

National Health Service Corps, Recruitment Program

Nicaraguan Children's Fund

North American Baptist Conference Missions

Northwest Medical Teams International, Inc.

Notre Dame India Mission

Omni Med

Operation Blessing, Medical Division

Operation Luz del Sol

Operation Rainbow

Operation Smile International

Our Little Brothers and Sisters

P.C.E.A. Kikuyu Hospital

P.C.E.A. Tumutumu Hospital

P.R.A.Y. (Project Rescue of Amazon Youth)

Palestine Children's Relief Fund

Pan American Health Organization

PAZAPA

Physicians for Peace

Project AmaZon

Project Concern International: OPTIONS

Project Hope/People to People Health Foundation

Project Open Hearts

Project ORBIS International, Inc.

PROMESA

Health profession usage: *(continued)*

Nurses *(continued)*

Remote Area Medical

Salesian Missions

School Sisters of Saint Francis

Simeus Foundation, The

SIM USA

Sister Community Alliances: Ouelessebougou-Utah Alliance

SkillShare International

Sons of Mary Missionary Society

Special Olympics, Inc.

St. Francis' Hospital

St. John's Medical College

St. Jude Hospital

Surgical Medical Assistance Relief Teams

Surgicorps International

Tulane University School of Public Health and Tropical Medicine

UCSD, Division of International Health

Universidad de Chile, Facultad de Medicina

University of Cincinnati College of Medicine, Dept. of Family Medicine

University of Illinois at Chicago College of Nursing, Global Health Leadership Office

University of Virginia, Center for Global Health

University of Zimbabwe

Uplift Internationale

Virginia Children's Connection, Dept. of Plastic. & Recon. Surgery

Visions in Action

Voluntary Service Overseas Canada

Volunteer Missionary Movement

VSO

WEC International

World Concern

World Emergency Relief

World Gospel Mission

World Hearing Network

World Mission Prayer League

World Vision International

World Vision, Inc.

World Witness - the Associate Reformed Presbyterian Church

Nutritionists and dieticians

ACCESS

Action Against Hunger

Adventist Development and Relief Agency International

Africare

Aloha Medical Missions (AMM)

American Jewish World Service

American Physicians Fellowship for Medicine in Israel

Ann Foundation Inc

Archdiocesan Health Care Network for Catholic Charities

Bairo Pite Clinic

Baptist Medical and Dental Mission International

Baptist Medical Missions International

Beeve Foundation for World Eye and Health, The

Cameroon Baptist Convention Health Board

Capiz Emmanuel Hospital

Casa Clinica de la Mujer

Chanet Community Organization

Children's Cross Connection, International

Christian Medical College (Vellore, India) Board

Clinica Evangelica Morava Elective

Clínica Maxena

College of Medicine, Malawi

Commonwealth Health Center

CONCERN

CONCERN America

Crudem Foundation

DePauw University Winter Term in Service

Evangelical Alliance Mission (TEAM World)

Foundation Human Nature (MeHiPro)

Foundation of Compassionate American Samaritans

Friends Without a Border

General Board of Global Ministries/The United Methodist Church

Global Volunteers

Guinea Development Foundation, Inc.

Haitian Health Clinic, Inc.

HBS Foundation, Inc./Hopital Bon Samaritain

Health and Child Survival Fellows Program

Health Teams International

Honduras Outreach, Inc

Hope Alliance

Hope Worldwide

Intercultural Nursing, Inc.

International Committee of the Red Cross

International Cooperation for Development (formerly CIIR Overseas Programme)

International Federation of Red Cross and Red Crescent Societies

International Health Exchange

International Medical Corps

International Partnership for Human Development

International Rescue Committee

INTERTEAM

Johns Hopkins Univ. School of Public Health, Dept. of International Health

Lumiere Medical Ministries, Inc.

Magee-Womens Hospital

Maluti Adventist Hospital (Lesotho)

Medical Ambassadors International

Medical Ministry International

Health profession usage: *(continued)*
Nutritionists and dieticians *(continued)*

Medicine for Peace
Mennonite Central Committee
Mercy Ships
Moi University Faculty of Health Sciences
Mountain Movers Missions Intl
Nicaraguan Children's Fund
Operation Blessing, Medical Division
Operation Smile International
P.C.E.A. Kikuyu Hospital
P.C.E.A. Tumutumu Hospital
P.R.A.Y. (Project Rescue of Amazon Youth)
Project AmaZon
Project Concern International: OPTIONS
Project Hope/People to People Health Foundation
Remote Area Medical
Seva Foundation
Simeus Foundation, The
Special Olympics, Inc.
St. John's Medical College
Surgical Medical Assistance Relief Teams
Tulane University School of Public Health and Tropical Medicine
Universidad de Chile, Facultad de Medicina
University of Zimbabwe
Visions in Action
Volunteer Missionary Movement
VSO
WEC International
World Vision International
World Vision, Inc.

Obstetricians and gynecologists

Adventist Development and Relief Agency International
Africa Inland Mission, International
Aid for International Medicine
Ak' Tenamit
Aloha Medical Missions (AMM)
Amazon-Africa Aid and Fundacao Esperanca
Amazon-Africa Aid Organization (3AO)
American College of Nurse-Midwives
American Jewish World Service
American Physicians Fellowship for Medicine in Israel
American Refugee Committee
Ann Foundation Inc
APUSAN-USA
Archdiocesan Health Care Network for Catholic Charities
Armenian Social Transition Program
Bairo Pite Clinic
Baptist Medical Missions International
Baptist Mid Missions
Beeve Foundation for World Eye and Health, The
Ben Gurion University of the Negev
Cameroon Baptist Convention Health Board
Canvasback Missions, Inc.
Capiz Emmanuel Hospital
CardioStart International, Inc.
Casa Clinica de la Mujer
Catholic Medical Mission Board, Inc.
CB International
Child Family Health International
Children's Cross Connection, International
Children's Medical Mission
Christian Medical College (Vellore, India) Board
Christian Mission of Pignon Inc.
Clinica Evangelica Morava Elective
Clínica Maxena
College of Medicine, Malawi
Commonwealth Health Center
Complete Basic Health 2000
CONCERN America
CrossWorld
Crudem Foundation
Curamericas
DePauw University Winter Term in Service
DoCare International, Inc.
Doctors for Global Health
Doctors of the World
Evangelical Lutheran Church in America
Fellowship of Associates of Medical Evangelism
Foundation Human Nature (MeHiPro)
Foundation of Compassionate American Samaritans
Friends Without a Border
General Board of Global Ministries/The United Methodist Church
Global Volunteers
Grace Ministries International
Guinea Development Foundation, Inc.
Haitian Health Clinic, Inc.
Hands Together, Inc.
HBS Foundation, Inc./Hopital Bon Samaritain
Healing the Children Northeast, Inc.
Health and Child Survival Fellows Program
Health Teams International
Helping Hands Health Education
Helps International
Hillside Healthcare Center
Himalayan Health Exchange
Himalayan HealthCare Inc.
Honduras Outreach, Inc
Hope Alliance

Health profession usage: *(continued)*
Obstetricians and gynecologists *(continued)*

Hope Worldwide
Hospital Albert Schweitzer
Intercultural Nursing, Inc.
International Health Exchange
International Medical Corps
International Nepal Fellowship
International Relief Teams
International Rescue Committee
InterServe
Liga International, Inc.
Ludhiana Christian Medical College Board USA
Lumiere Medical Ministries, Inc.
M.E.D.I.C.O.
Magee-Womens Hospital
Maua Methodist Hospital
Medical Aid for Palestinians
Medical Care Development International Division
Medical Ministry International
Medical Missionaries of Mary
Medicine for Humanity
Medicine for Peace
Mercy Ships
Mexican Medical Ministries
Mima Foundation, Inc.
Mission Doctors Association
Moi University Faculty of Health Sciences
Mountain Movers Missions Intl
National Health Service Corps, Recruitment Program
Nicaraguan Children's Fund
Northwest Medical Teams International, Inc.
Omni Med
Operation Blessing, Medical Division
P.C.E.A. Chogoria Hospital
P.C.E.A. Kikuyu Hospital
P.C.E.A. Tumutumu Hospital
P.R.A.Y. (Project Rescue of Amazon Youth)
Palestine Children's Relief Fund
Physicians for Human Rights
Physicians for Peace
Project AmaZon
Project Hope/People to People Health Foundation
Project Open Hearts
Remote Area Medical
Sanyati Baptist Hospital, Baptist Convention of Zimbabwe
School Sisters of Saint Francis
Simeus Foundation, The
SIM USA
Sister Community Alliances: Ouelessebougou-Utah Alliance
St. Francis' Hospital
St. John's Medical College
St. Jude Hospital
St. Mary's Hospital, Vunapope
Surgical Medical Assistance Relief Teams
Tulane University School of Public Health and Tropical Medicine
Universidad de Chile, Facultad de Medicina
University of Illinois College of Medicine at Rockford
University of Zimbabwe
UTMB-WHO Collaborating Center for Training in International Health
Voluntary Service Overseas Canada
Volunteer Missionary Movement
WEC International
World Emergency Relief
World Hearing Network
World Mission Prayer League
Zuma Memorial Hospital

Ophthalmologists

Adventist Development and Relief Agency International
Aloha Medical Missions (AMM)
Amazon-Africa Aid and Fundacao Esperanca
Amazon-Africa Aid Organization (3AO)
American Jewish World Service
American Leprosy Missions Inc.
American Physicians Fellowship for Medicine in Israel
Ann Foundation Inc
Archdiocesan Health Care Network for Catholic Charities
Aremenian EyeCare Project
ASAPROSAR: The Salvadoran Association for Rural Health
Bairo Pite Clinic
Baptist Medical Missions International
Baptist Mid Missions
Beeve Foundation for World Eye and Health, The
Ben Gurion University of the Negev
Cameroon Baptist Convention Health Board
Canvasback Missions, Inc.
Cape Cares
Capiz Emmanuel Hospital
Casa Clinica de la Mujer
Catholic Medical Mission Board, Inc.
Children's Cross Connection, International
Christian Medical College (Vellore, India) Board
Christian Mission of Pignon Inc.
Christoffel-Blindenmission EV
Clinica Evangelica Morava Elective
Clínica Maxena
College of Medicine, Malawi
Crudem Foundation
Curamericas
DoCare International, Inc.
Doctors of the World
Evangelical Alliance Mission (TEAM World)

Health profession usage: *(continued)*

<u>**Ophthalmologists**</u> *(continued)*

Evangelical Lutheran Church in America

FOCUS Inc.

Foundation Human Nature (MeHiPro)

Friends Without a Border

General Board of Global Ministries/The United Methodist Church

Global Volunteers

Grace Ministries International

Guinea Development Foundation, Inc.

Haitian Health Clinic, Inc.

Healing the Children Northeast, Inc.

Health Teams International

Helen Keller International

Helping Hands Health Education

Helps International

Hillside Healthcare Center

Honduras Outreach, Inc

Hope Alliance

Hope Worldwide

Hospital Albert Schweitzer

International Aid, Inc.

International Eye Foundation, Inc.

International Health Exchange

International Health Service

International Ministries, American Baptist Churches, USA

International Partnership for Human Development

International Relief Teams

InterServe

Liga International, Inc.

Lighthouse for Christ Mission and Eye Centre

Ludhiana Christian Medical College Board USA

Lumiere Medical Ministries, Inc.

Maluti Adventist Hospital (Lesotho)

Maua Methodist Hospital

Medical Ministry International

Mercy Ships

Mexican Medical Ministries

Mima Foundation, Inc.

Mission Doctors Association

Moi University Faculty of Health Sciences

Mountain Movers Missions Intl

National Eye Care Project for Armenia

Nicaraguan Children's Fund

Northwest Medical Teams International, Inc.

Omni Med

Operation Blessing, Medical Division

Operation USA

P.R.A.Y. (Project Rescue of Amazon Youth)

Palestine Children's Relief Fund

Pan American Health Organization

PAZAPA

Physicians for Peace

Project AmaZon

Project Concern International: OPTIONS

Project Hope/People to People Health Foundation

Project ORBIS International, Inc.

Remote Area Medical

Sanyati Baptist Hospital, Baptist Convention of Zimbabwe

School Sisters of Saint Francis

Seva Foundation

Simeus Foundation, The

SIM USA

Sister Community Alliances: Ouelessebougou-Utah Alliance

Special Olympics, Inc.

St. Francis' Hospital

St. John's Medical College

St. Jude Hospital

Surgical Eye Expeditions International (S.E.E.), Inc.

Surgical Medical Assistance Relief Teams

Unite For Sight

Univ. of Wisconsin Med., Office of International Health Affairs

Universidad de Chile, Facultad de Medicina

University of Illinois College of Medicine at Rockford

University of Zimbabwe

US Committee for Scientific Cooperation with Vietnam

Virginia Children's Connection, Dept. of Plastic. & Recon. Surgery

Volunteer Missionary Movement

Volunteer Optometric Service to Humanity (VOSH) International

WEC International

World Hearing Network

Zuma Memorial Hospital

<u>**Optometrists**</u>

Adventist Development and Relief Agency International

American Physicians Fellowship for Medicine in Israel

Ann Foundation Inc

Archdiocesan Health Care Network for Catholic Charities

ASAPROSAR: The Salvadoran Association for Rural Health

Bairo Pite Clinic

Baptist Medical Missions International

Beeve Foundation for World Eye and Health, The

Cameroon Baptist Convention Health Board

Casa Clinica de la Mujer

Children's Cross Connection, International

Christian Medical College (Vellore, India) Board

Christian Mission of Pignon Inc.

Health profession usage: *(continued)*

Optometrists *(continued)*

Christoffel-Blindenmission EV

Clinica Evangelica Morava Elective

Crudem Foundation

Curamericas

DePauw University Winter Term in Service

DoCare International, Inc.

Feed the Children

Flying Samaritans

Foundation Human Nature (MeHiPro)

Friends Without a Border

General Board of Global Ministries/The United Methodist Church

Global Volunteers

Grace Ministries International

Guinea Development Foundation, Inc.

Haitian Health Clinic, Inc.

Healing the Children Northeast, Inc.

Health Teams International

Helen Keller International

Hillside Healthcare Center

Himalayan Health Exchange

Hope Alliance

Hope Worldwide

International Aid, Inc.

International Cooperation for Development (formerly CIIR Overseas Programme)

International Nepal Fellowship

InterServe

Liga International, Inc.

Lighthouse for Christ Mission and Eye Centre

Lumiere Medical Ministries, Inc.

M.E.D.I.C.O.

Maluti Adventist Hospital (Lesotho)

Medical Ministry International

Mercy Ships

Mexican Medical Ministries

Mima Foundation, Inc.

Moi University Faculty of Health Sciences

Mountain Movers Missions Intl

Nicaraguan Children's Fund

Northwest Medical Teams International, Inc.

Operation Blessing, Medical Division

P.R.A.Y. (Project Rescue of Amazon Youth)

Project AmaZon

Project Concern International: OPTIONS

Project Hope/People to People Health Foundation

Remote Area Medical

School Sisters of Saint Francis

Simeus Foundation, The

Sister Community Alliances: Ouelessebougou-Utah Alliance

Special Olympics, Inc.

St. Jude Hospital

Surgical Medical Assistance Relief Teams

Unite For Sight

University of Zimbabwe

Volunteer Missionary Movement

Volunteer Optometric Service to Humanity (VOSH) International

WEC International

Oral surgeons

Adventist Development and Relief Agency International

Ak' Tenamit

Aloha Medical Missions (AMM)

Amazon-Africa Aid Organization (3AO)

American Physicians Fellowship for Medicine in Israel

Ann Foundation Inc

Archdiocesan Health Care Network for Catholic Charities

Bairo Pite Clinic

Baptist Medical Missions International

Beeve Foundation for World Eye and Health, The

Ben Gurion University of the Negev

Cameroon Baptist Convention Health Board

Cape Cares

Casa Clinica de la Mujer

Chanet Community Organization

Children's Cross Connection, International

Christian Dental Society

Christian Medical College (Vellore, India) Board

Christian Mission of Pignon Inc.

Clinica Evangelica Morava Elective

Clínica Maxena

College of Medicine, Malawi

Dental Health International

DoCare International, Inc.

Evangelical Lutheran Church in America

Foundation Human Nature (MeHiPro)

Friends Without a Border

General Board of Global Ministries/The United Methodist Church

Global Volunteers

Guinea Development Foundation, Inc.

Haitian Health Clinic, Inc.

Hands Together, Inc.

Healing the Children Northeast, Inc.

Health Teams International

Health Volunteers Overseas

Helps International

Hillside Healthcare Center

Himalayan HealthCare Inc.

Honduras Outreach, Inc

Hope Alliance

International Health Exchange

Health profession usage: *(continued)*

<u>Oral surgeons</u> *(continued)*

International Nepal Fellowship
Lumiere Medical Ministries, Inc.
Maua Methodist Hospital
Medical Ministry International
Mercy Ships
Mima Foundation, Inc.
Mission Doctors Association
Moi University Faculty of Health Sciences
Mountain Movers Missions Intl
Nicaraguan Children's Fund
Northwest Medical Teams International, Inc.
Omni Med
Operation Blessing, Medical Division
Operation Luz del Sol
Operation Rainbow
P.C.E.A. Kikuyu Hospital
P.R.A.Y. (Project Rescue of Amazon Youth)
Palestine Children's Relief Fund
Pan American Health Organization
PAZAPA
Project AmaZon
Project Hope/People to People Health Foundation
Remote Area Medical
Sanyati Baptist Hospital, Baptist Convention of Zimbabwe
Simeus Foundation, The
Sister Community Alliances: Ouelessebougou-Utah Alliance
Special Olympics, Inc.
St. John's Medical College
St. Jude Hospital
Surgical Medical Assistance Relief Teams
Surgicorps International
Universidad de Chile, Facultad de Medicina
University of Cincinnati College of Medicine, Dept. of Family Medicine
University of Illinois College of Medicine at Rockford
University of Zimbabwe
Uplift Internationale
Volunteer Missionary Movement
WEC International
World Hearing Network

<u>Orthopedic surgeons</u>

Adventist Development and Relief Agency International
Africa Inland Mission, International
Aid for International Medicine
Aloha Medical Missions (AMM)
Amazon-Africa Aid Organization (3AO)
American Physicians Fellowship for Medicine in Israel
Ann Foundation Inc
APUSAN-USA
Archdiocesan Health Care Network for Catholic Charities
Associate Reformed Presbyterian Church, World Witness
Bairo Pite Clinic
Baptist Medical Missions International
Ben Gurion University of the Negev
Cameroon Baptist Convention Health Board
Canvasback Missions, Inc.
Capiz Emmanuel Hospital
Casa Clinica de la Mujer
Catholic Medical Mission Board, Inc.
Children's Cross Connection, International
Christian Medical College (Vellore, India) Board
Christian Mission of Pignon Inc.
Christoffel-Blindenmission EV
Clinica Evangelica Morava Elective
Clínica Maxena
College of Medicine, Malawi
Commonwealth Health Center
Complete Basic Health 2000
Crudem Foundation
Curamericas
DoCare International, Inc.
Esperanca, Inc.
Evangelical Lutheran Church in America
Foundation Human Nature (MeHiPro)
Friends Without a Border
General Board of Global Ministries/The United Methodist Church
Global Volunteers
Grace Ministries International
Guinea Development Foundation, Inc.
HBS Foundation, Inc./Hopital Bon Samaritain
Healing the Children Northeast, Inc.
Health Teams International
Health Volunteers Overseas
Honduras Outreach, Inc
Hope Alliance
Hope Worldwide
Hospital Albert Schweitzer
International Committee of the Red Cross
International Cooperation for Development (formerly CIIR Overseas Programme)
International Health Service
International Medical Corps
Liga International, Inc.
Loma Linda University International Programs
Ludhiana Christian Medical College Board USA
Lumiere Medical Ministries, Inc.
M.E.D.I.C.O.
Maua Methodist Hospital

Health profession usage: *(continued)*

Orthopedic surgeons *(continued)*

Medical Ministry International
Mercy Ships
Mima Foundation, Inc.
Moi University Faculty of Health Sciences
Mountain Movers Missions Intl
Nicaraguan Children's Fund
Northwest Medical Teams International, Inc.
Omni Med
Operation Blessing, Medical Division
Operation Luz del Sol
Operation Rainbow
Operation USA
P.C.E.A. Kikuyu Hospital
P.R.A.Y. (Project Rescue of Amazon Youth)
Palestine Children's Relief Fund
PAZAPA
Physicians for Peace
Project AmaZon
Project Concern International: OPTIONS
Project Hope/People to People Health Foundation
Remote Area Medical
Sanyati Baptist Hospital, Baptist Convention of Zimbabwe
Simeus Foundation, The
Special Olympics, Inc.
St. John's Medical College
St. Jude Hospital
Surgical Medical Assistance Relief Teams
Univ. of Wisconsin Med., Office of International Health Affairs
Universidad de Chile, Facultad de Medicina
University of Illinois College of Medicine at Rockford
University of Virginia, Center for Global Health
University of Zimbabwe
US Committee for Scientific Cooperation with Vietnam
Volunteer Missionary Movement
WEC International
World Hearing Network
World Witness - the Associate Reformed Presbyterian Church

Otolaryngologists

Adventist Development and Relief Agency International
Aloha Medical Missions (AMM)
American Physicians Fellowship for Medicine in Israel
Ann Foundation Inc
Archdiocesan Health Care Network for Catholic Charities
Bairo Pite Clinic
Baptist Medical Missions International
Baptist Mid Missions
Ben Gurion University of the Negev
Cameroon Baptist Convention Health Board
Casa Clinica de la Mujer
Children's Cross Connection, International
Christian Medical College (Vellore, India) Board
Clinica Evangelica Morava Elective
College of Medicine, Malawi
Commonwealth Health Center
Crudem Foundation
DoCare International, Inc.
Foundation Human Nature (MeHiPro)
Friends Without a Border
Global Volunteers
Guinea Development Foundation, Inc.
Haitian Health Clinic, Inc.
Healing the Children Northeast, Inc.
Health Teams International
Hope Alliance
International Nepal Fellowship
Lumiere Medical Ministries, Inc.
Maua Methodist Hospital
Medical Ministry International
Mercy Ships
Mima Foundation, Inc.
Mission Doctors Association
Moi University Faculty of Health Sciences
Mountain Movers Missions Intl
Nicaraguan Children's Fund
Omni Med
Operation Blessing, Medical Division
Operation Luz del Sol
Operation Smile International
P.C.E.A. Kikuyu Hospital
P.R.A.Y. (Project Rescue of Amazon Youth)
Palestine Children's Relief Fund
Physicians for Peace
Project AmaZon
Project Hope/People to People Health Foundation
Remote Area Medical
Sanyati Baptist Hospital, Baptist Convention of Zimbabwe
Simeus Foundation, The
Special Olympics, Inc.
St. John's Medical College
Surgical Medical Assistance Relief Teams
Universidad de Chile, Facultad de Medicina
University of Illinois College of Medicine at Rockford
University of Zimbabwe
Uplift Internationale
Vietnam ENT Mission
Volunteer Missionary Movement
WEC International
World Hearing Network

Health profession usage: *(continued)*

Paramedics

Adventist Development and Relief Agency International
Africare
Ak' Tenamit
Aloha Medical Missions (AMM)
American Physicians Fellowship for Medicine in Israel
Ann Foundation Inc
Bairo Pite Clinic
Baptist Medical Missions International
Beeve Foundation for World Eye and Health, The
Ben Gurion University of the Negev
CAM International
Cameroon Baptist Convention Health Board
Casa Clinica de la Mujer
Chanet Community Organization
Children's Cross Connection, International
Christian Medical College (Vellore, India) Board
Clinica Evangelica Morava Elective
College of Medicine, Malawi
DePauw University Winter Term in Service
DoCare International, Inc.
Fellowship of Associates of Medical Evangelism
Foundation Human Nature (MeHiPro)
Friends Without a Border
Global Outreach International
Global Volunteers
Grokha Association of Social Health
Guinea Development Foundation, Inc.
Health Teams International
Hope Alliance
Hope Worldwide
International Health Exchange
International Health Service
International Medical Corps
International Nepal Fellowship
INTERTEAM
Liga International, Inc.
Lumiere Medical Ministries, Inc.
M.E.D.I.C.O.
Maua Methodist Hospital
Medical Aid for Palestinians
Medical Care Development International Division
Medical Ministry International
Mercy Ships
Moi University Faculty of Health Sciences
Mountain Movers Missions Intl
Nicaraguan Children's Fund
Northwest Medical Teams International, Inc.
Operation Blessing, Medical Division
Operation Smile International
P.C.E.A. Tumutumu Hospital
P.R.A.Y. (Project Rescue of Amazon Youth)
Project AmaZon
Project Concern International: OPTIONS
Project Hope/People to People Health Foundation
Remote Area Medical
Seva Foundation
Simeus Foundation, The
Special Olympics, Inc.
St. John's Medical College
St. Jude Hospital
Surgical Medical Assistance Relief Teams
UCSD, Division of International Health
University of Zimbabwe
Volunteer Missionary Movement
WEC International

Pathologists

Adventist Development and Relief Agency International
Aloha Medical Missions (AMM)
American Physicians Fellowship for Medicine in Israel
Ann Foundation Inc
Archdiocesan Health Care Network for Catholic Charities
Bairo Pite Clinic
Ben Gurion University of the Negev
Cameroon Baptist Convention Health Board
Capiz Emmanuel Hospital
Casa Clinica de la Mujer
Children's Cross Connection, International
Christian Medical College (Vellore, India) Board
Clinica Evangelica Morava Elective
College of Medicine, Malawi
Commonwealth Health Center
DePauw University Winter Term in Service
Evangelical Alliance Mission (TEAM World)
Evangelical Lutheran Church in America
Foundation Human Nature (MeHiPro)
Friends Without a Border
Global Volunteers
Haitian Health Clinic, Inc.
Health Teams International
Hope Alliance
Hope Worldwide
Lumiere Medical Ministries, Inc.
Magee-Womens Hospital
Maua Methodist Hospital
Medical Ministry International
Medicine for Humanity
Mercy Ships
Mission Doctors Association

Health profession usage: *(continued)*
Pathologists *(continued)*

Moi University Faculty of Health Sciences
Mountain Movers Missions Intl
Nicaraguan Children's Fund
Omni Med
P.C.E.A. Kikuyu Hospital
Project AmaZon
Project Hope/People to People Health Foundation
Simeus Foundation, The
St. John's Medical College
St. Jude Hospital
Surgical Medical Assistance Relief Teams
Univ. of Wisconsin Med., Office of International Health Affairs
Universidad de Chile, Facultad de Medicina
University of Illinois College of Medicine at Rockford
University of Zimbabwe
US Committee for Scientific Cooperation with Vietnam
Volunteer Missionary Movement
WEC International
World Hearing Network

Pediatricians

ACCESS
Adventist Development and Relief Agency International
Africa Inland Mission, International
Ak' Tenamit
Aloha Medical Missions (AMM)
Amazon-Africa Aid and Fundacao Esperanca
Amazon-Africa Aid Organization (3AO)
American Baptist Board of International Ministries
American Jewish World Service
American Physicians Fellowship for Medicine in Israel
American Refugee Committee
Ann Foundation Inc
APUSAN-USA
Archdiocesan Health Care Network for Catholic Charities
Armenian Social Transition Program
Bairo Pite Clinic
Baptist Medical Missions International
Beeve Foundation for World Eye and Health, The
Ben Gurion University of the Negev
Board of World Mission of the Moravian Church
Cameroon Baptist Convention Health Board
Canvasback Missions, Inc.
Cape Cares
Capiz Emmanuel Hospital
Casa Clinica de la Mujer
Catholic Medical Mission Board, Inc.
CB International
CERT International (Christian Emergency Relief Team)
Chanet Community Organization
Child Family Health International
Children's Cross Connection, International
Children's Medical Mission
Christian Medical College (Vellore, India) Board
Christian Mission of Pignon Inc.
Clinica Evangelica Morava Elective
Clínica Maxena
College of Medicine, Malawi
Commonwealth Health Center
CONCERN America
CrossWorld
Crudem Foundation
Curamericas
DePauw University Winter Term in Service
DoCare International, Inc.
Doctors for Global Health
Doctors of the World
Evangelical Alliance Mission (TEAM World)
Evangelical Free Church of America Mission
Evangelical Lutheran Church in America
Filipino-American Medical Inc.
Foundation Human Nature (MeHiPro)
Foundation of Compassionate American Samaritans
Friends Lugulu Hospital
Friends Without a Border
General Board of Global Ministries/The United Methodist Church
Global Volunteers
Grace Ministries International
Grokha Association of Social Health
Guinea Development Foundation, Inc.
Haitian Health Clinic, Inc.
Hands Together, Inc.
Healing the Children Northeast, Inc.
Health and Child Survival Fellows Program
Health Teams International
Health Volunteers Overseas
Helping Hands Health Education
Helps International
Hillside Healthcare Center
Himalayan Health Exchange
Himalayan HealthCare Inc.
Honduras Outreach, Inc
Hope Alliance
Hope Worldwide
Hospital Albert Schweitzer
Intercultural Nursing, Inc.
International Aid, Inc.

Health profession usage: *(continued)*

Pediatricians *(continued)*

International Cooperation for Development (formerly CIIR Overseas Programme)
International Federation of Red Cross and Red Crescent Societies
International Health Exchange
International Medical Corps
International Relief Teams
International Rescue Committee
Interplast
InterServe
Lalmba Association
Liga International, Inc.
Lumiere Medical Ministries, Inc.
M.E.D.I.C.O.
Magee-Womens Hospital
Maua Methodist Hospital
Medecins Sans Frontieres/ Doctors Without Borders USA
Medical Aid for Palestinians
Medical Care Development International Division
Medical Ministry International
Medicine for Peace
Memisa Medicus Mundi
Mercy Ships
Mima Foundation, Inc.
Minnesota International Health Volunteers
Mission Doctors Association
Moi University Faculty of Health Sciences
Mountain Movers Missions Intl
National Health Service Corps, Recruitment Program
Nicaraguan Children's Fund
Northwest Medical Teams International, Inc.
Omni Med
Operation Blessing, Medical Division
Operation USA
Our Little Brothers and Sisters
P.C.E.A. Chogoria Hospital
P.C.E.A. Kikuyu Hospital
P.C.E.A. Tumutumu Hospital
P.R.A.Y. (Project Rescue of Amazon Youth)
P.R.A.Y. (Project Rescue of Amazon Youth)
Palestine Children's Relief Fund
Pan American Health Organization
PAZAPA
Physicians for Peace
Presbyterian Church USA, Mission Service Recruitment
Project AmaZon
Project Hope/People to People Health Foundation
PROMESA
Remote Area Medical
Salesian Missions
Sanyati Baptist Hospital, Baptist Convention of Zimbabwe
School Sisters of Saint Francis
Seva Foundation
Simeus Foundation, The
Special Olympics, Inc.
St. Francis' Hospital
St. John's Medical College
St. Jude Hospital
Surgical Medical Assistance Relief Teams
Tulane University School of Public Health and Tropical Medicine
Universidad de Chile, Facultad de Medicina
University of Cincinnati College of Medicine, Dept. of Family Medicine
University of Illinois College of Medicine at Rockford
University of Zimbabwe
Uplift Internationale
Virginia Children's Connection, Dept. of Plastic. & Recon. Surgery
Visions in Action
Voluntary Service Overseas Canada
Volunteer Missionary Movement
WEC International
World Emergency Relief
World Gospel Mission
World Hearing Network
World Mission Prayer League

Pharmacists

Adventist Development and Relief Agency International
Aloha Medical Missions (AMM)
American Physicians Fellowship for Medicine in Israel
Ann Foundation Inc
Bairo Pite Clinic
Baptist General Conference
Baptist Medical Missions International
Beeve Foundation for World Eye and Health, The
Ben Gurion University of the Negev
Board of World Mission of the Moravian Church
Cameroon Baptist Convention Health Board
Cape Cares
Capiz Emmanuel Hospital
Casa Clinica de la Mujer
CB International
Chanet Community Organization
Children's Cross Connection, International
Christian Medical College (Vellore, India) Board
Christian Mission of Pignon Inc.
Clinica Evangelica Morava Elective
Commonwealth Health Center
CrossWorld
Crudem Foundation
Curamericas

Health profession usage: *(continued)*

<u>**Pharmacists**</u> *(continued)*

DePauw University Winter Term in Service

DoCare International, Inc.

Feed the Children

Fellowship of Associates of Medical Evangelism

Filipino-American Medical Inc.

Flying Samaritans

Foundation Human Nature (MeHiPro)

Friends Without a Border

Global Volunteers

Grokha Association of Social Health

Guinea Development Foundation, Inc.

Haitian Health Clinic, Inc.

Health and Child Survival Fellows Program

Health Teams International

Hillside Healthcare Center

Honduras Outreach, Inc

Hope Alliance

Hope Worldwide

International Committee of the Red Cross

International Cooperation for Development (formerly CIIR Overseas Programme)

International Health Exchange

International Health Service

International Medical Corps

International Nepal Fellowship

International Relief Teams

International Rescue Committee

InterServe

Liga International, Inc.

Lumiere Medical Ministries, Inc.

M.E.D.I.C.O.

Magee-Womens Hospital

Maluti Adventist Hospital (Lesotho)

Maua Methodist Hospital

Medical Ministry International

Memisa Medicus Mundi

Mercy Ships

Moi University Faculty of Health Sciences

Mountain Movers Missions Intl

Nicaraguan Children's Fund

Operation Blessing, Medical Division

Our Little Brothers and Sisters

P.C.E.A. Chogoria Hospital

P.C.E.A. Kikuyu Hospital

P.C.E.A. Tumutumu Hospital

P.R.A.Y. (Project Rescue of Amazon Youth)

PAZAPA

Project AmaZon

Project Concern International: OPTIONS

Project Hope/People to People Health Foundation

Remote Area Medical

School Sisters of Saint Francis

Simeus Foundation, The

SIM USA

Sister Community Alliances: Ouelessebougou-Utah Alliance

St. Francis' Hospital

St. John's Medical College

St. Jude Hospital

Surgical Medical Assistance Relief Teams

Universidad de Chile, Facultad de Medicina

University of Cincinnati College of Medicine, Dept. of Family Medicine

University of Zimbabwe

Voluntary Service Overseas Canada

Volunteer Missionary Movement

WEC International

<u>**Physical and occupational therapists**</u>

Adventist Development and Relief Agency International

Africa Inland Mission, International

Aloha Medical Missions (AMM)

Amazon-Africa Aid Organization (3AO)

American Leprosy Missions Inc.

American Physicians Fellowship for Medicine in Israel

Ann Foundation Inc

Archdiocesan Health Care Network for Catholic Charities

Associazione Italiana 'Amici Raoul Follereau'

Bairo Pite Clinic

Baptist Medical and Dental Mission International

Baptist Medical Missions International

Cameroon Baptist Convention Health Board

Canvasback Missions, Inc.

Capiz Emmanuel Hospital

Casa Clinica de la Mujer

Catholic Medical Mission Board, Inc.

CB International

Chanet Community Organization

Children's Cross Connection, International

Christian Medical College (Vellore, India) Board

Christian Mission of Pignon Inc.

Christoffel-Blindenmission EV

Clinica Evangelica Morava Elective

Commonwealth Health Center

Complete Basic Health 2000

Crudem Foundation

Curamericas

DePauw University Winter Term in Service

DoCare International, Inc.

Evangelical Alliance Mission (TEAM World)

Evangelical Lutheran Church in America

Health profession usage: *(continued)*
<u>Physical and occupational therapists</u> *(continued)*

Foundation Human Nature (MeHiPro)

Friends Without a Border

Global Volunteers

Grokha Association of Social Health

Guinea Development Foundation, Inc.

Haitian Health Clinic, Inc.

HBS Foundation, Inc./Hopital Bon Samaritain

Healing the Children Northeast, Inc.

Health Teams International

Health Volunteers Overseas

Hillside Healthcare Center

Honduras Outreach, Inc

Hope Alliance

Hospital Albert Schweitzer

Intercultural Nursing, Inc.

International Committee of the Red Cross

International Cooperation for Development (formerly CIIR Overseas Programme)

International Health Exchange

InterServe

Liga International, Inc.

Lumiere Medical Ministries, Inc.

M.E.D.I.C.O.

Maluti Adventist Hospital (Lesotho)

Maua Methodist Hospital

Medical Aid for Palestinians

Medical Ministry International

Medicine for Peace

Mercy Ships

Moi University Faculty of Health Sciences

Mountain Movers Missions Intl

Nicaraguan Children's Fund

Northwest Medical Teams International, Inc.

Operation Blessing, Medical Division

Operation Smile International

P.C.E.A. Kikuyu Hospital

P.C.E.A. Tumutumu Hospital

P.R.A.Y. (Project Rescue of Amazon Youth)

Palestine Children's Relief Fund

PAZAPA

Physicians for Peace

Project AmaZon

Project Hope/People to People Health Foundation

School Sisters of Saint Francis

Simeus Foundation, The

SIM USA

SkillShare International

Special Olympics, Inc.

St. Francis' Hospital

St. John's Medical College

St. Jude Hospital

Surgical Medical Assistance Relief Teams

Surgicorps International

Universidad de Chile, Facultad de Medicina

University of Zimbabwe

Visions in Action

Voluntary Service Overseas Canada

Volunteer Missionary Movement

VSO

WEC International

World Association for Children and Parents

World Rehabilitation Fund, Inc.

<u>Physician assistants</u>

Adventist Development and Relief Agency International

Aid for International Medicine

Aloha Medical Missions (AMM)

American Baptist Board of International Ministries

American Jewish World Service

American Physicians Fellowship for Medicine in Israel

American Refugee Committee

Ann Foundation Inc

Bairo Pite Clinic

Baptist Medical Missions International

Beeve Foundation for World Eye and Health, The

Ben Gurion University of the Negev

Board of World Mission of the Moravian Church

CAM International

Cameroon Baptist Convention Health Board

Canvasback Missions, Inc.

Cape Cares

CardioStart International, Inc.

Casa Clinica de la Mujer

Catholic Medical Mission Board, Inc.

CERT International (Christian Emergency Relief Team)

Chanet Community Organization

Children's Cross Connection, International

Christian Medical College (Vellore, India) Board

Clinica Evangelica Morava Elective

Clínica Maxena

Commonwealth Health Center

Community of Caring

CONCERN America

Crudem Foundation

Curamericas

DePauw University Winter Term in Service

DoCare International, Inc.

Doctors for Global Health

Doctors of the World

Edward A. Ulzen Memorial Foundation (EAUMF)

Feed the Children

Fellowship of Associates of Medical Evangelism

Health profession usage: *(continued)*

Physician assistants *(continued)*

Filipino-American Medical Inc.
Flying Samaritans
Foundation Human Nature (MeHiPro)
Friends Without a Border
General Dept. of World Missions, The Wesleyan Church
Global Volunteers
Grace Ministries International
Grokha Association of Social Health
Guinea Development Foundation, Inc.
Haitian Health Clinic, Inc.
HBS Foundation, Inc./Hopital Bon Samaritain
Healing the Children Northeast, Inc.
Health Teams International
Helps International
Hillside Healthcare Center
Honduras Outreach, Inc
Hope Alliance
International Cooperation for Development (formerly CIIR Overseas Programme)
International Medical Corps
InterServe
Jubilee Volunteer Africa Program of AFRIDEC
Lalmba Association
Lay Mission-Helpers Association
Liga International, Inc.
Lumiere Medical Ministries, Inc.
M.E.D.I.C.O.
Maua Methodist Hospital
Medical Ambassadors International
Medical Ministry International
Mercy Ships
Mima Foundation, Inc.
Moi University Faculty of Health Sciences
Mountain Movers Missions Intl
National Health Service Corps, Recruitment Program
Nicaraguan Children's Fund
North American Baptist Conference Missions
Northwest Medical Teams International, Inc.
Omni Med
Operation Blessing, Medical Division
Operation Luz del Sol
Our Little Brothers and Sisters
P.C.E.A. Kikuyu Hospital
P.C.E.A. Tumutumu Hospital
P.R.A.Y. (Project Rescue of Amazon Youth)
PAZAPA
Physicians for Peace
Project AmaZon
Project Concern International: OPTIONS
Project Hope/People to People Health Foundation
Remote Area Medical
School Sisters of Saint Francis
Simeus Foundation, The
Sister Community Alliances: Ouelessebougou-Utah Alliance
Special Olympics, Inc.
St. Francis' Hospital
St. Jude Hospital
Surgical Medical Assistance Relief Teams
Surgicorps International
University of Cincinnati College of Medicine, Dept. of Family Medicine
University of Zimbabwe
Uplift Internationale
Voluntary Service Overseas Canada
Volunteer Missionary Movement
WEC International
World Gospel Mission

Physicians

Adventist Development and Relief Agency International
Africa Inland Mission, International
African Inter-Mennonite Mission
Aid for International Medicine
Ak' Tenamit
Aloha Medical Missions (AMM)
Amazon-Africa Aid and Fundacao Esperanca
Amazon-Africa Aid Organization (3AO)
American Baptist Board of International Ministries
American Jewish World Service
American Leprosy Missions Inc.
American Physicians Fellowship for Medicine in Israel
American Refugee Committee
Ann Foundation Inc
Archdiocesan Health Care Network for Catholic Charities
Armenian Social Transition Program
ASAPROSAR: The Salvadoran Association for Rural Health
Associate Reformed Presbyterian Church, World Witness
Bairo Pite Clinic
Baptist General Conference
Baptist Medical and Dental Mission International
Baptist Medical Missions International
Baptist Mid Missions
Beeve Foundation for World Eye and Health, The
Ben Gurion University of the Negev
Board of World Mission of the Moravian Church
Boston International Foundation for Medical Education
CAM International
Cameroon Baptist Convention Health Board

Health profession usage: *(continued)*
Physicians *(continued)*

Campus Crusade for Christ International

Canvasback Missions, Inc.

Cape Cares

Capiz Emmanuel Hospital

Casa Clinica de la Mujer

Catholic Medical Mission Board, Inc.

CB International

Chanet Community Organization

Child Family Health International

Children's Cross Connection, International

Children's Heartlink

Christian Medical College (Vellore, India) Board

Christian Mission of Pignon Inc.

Clinica Evangelica Morava Elective

Clínica Maxena

College of Medicine, Malawi

Commonwealth Health Center

Community of Caring

Complete Basic Health 2000

CONCERN America

CrossWorld

Crudem Foundation

Curamericas

DePauw University Winter Term in Service

DoCare International, Inc.

Doctors for Global Health

Doctors of the World

Edward A. Ulzen Memorial Foundation (EAUMF)

Esperanca, Inc.

Evangelical Alliance Mission (TEAM World)

Evangelical Free Church of America Mission

Evangelical Lutheran Church in America

Feed the Children

Filipino-American Medical Inc.

Flying Doctors of America

Flying Samaritans

Foundation Human Nature (MeHiPro)

Foundation of Compassionate American Samaritans

Friends Without a Border

General Baptist International

General Board of Global Ministries/The United Methodist Church

General Dept. of World Missions, The Wesleyan Church

Global Service Corps/Earth Island Institute

Global Volunteers

Grace Ministries International

Grokha Association of Social Health

Guinea Development Foundation, Inc.

Haitian Health Clinic, Inc.

Hands Together, Inc.

Harlem Hospital, Plastic Surgery Program

HBS Foundation, Inc./Hopital Bon Samaritain

Healing the Children Northeast, Inc.

Health Teams International

Helping Hands Health Education

Helps International

Hillside Healthcare Center

Honduras Outreach, Inc

Hope Alliance

Hope Worldwide

Hospital Albert Schweitzer

International Aid, Inc.

International Children's Heart Foundation

International Committee of the Red Cross

International Cooperation for Development (formerly CIIR Overseas Programme)

International Federation of Red Cross and Red Crescent Societies

International Health Exchange

International Health Service

International Medical Corps

International Nepal Fellowship

International Rescue Committee

Interplast

InterServe

Jubilee Volunteer Africa Program of AFRIDEC

Liga International, Inc.

Ludhiana Christian Medical College Board USA

Lumiere Medical Ministries, Inc.

M.E.D.I.C.O.

Magee-Womens Hospital

Maua Methodist Hospital

Medecins Sans Frontieres/ Doctors Without Borders USA

Medical Care Development International Division

Medical Ministry International

Medicine

Medicine for Humanity

Medicine for Peace

Mercy Ships

Mexican Medical Ministries

Mima Foundation, Inc.

Mission Doctors Association

Moi University Faculty of Health Sciences

Mountain Movers Missions Intl

National Health Service Corps, Recruitment Program

Nicaraguan Children's Fund

North American Baptist Conference Missions

Northwest Medical Teams International, Inc.

Notre Dame India Mission

Omni Med

Operation Blessing, Medical Division

Operation Rainbow

Operation Smile International

Operation USA

Health profession usage: *(continued)*

Physicians *(continued)*

Our Little Brothers and Sisters
P.R.A.Y. (Project Rescue of Amazon Youth)
Palestine Children's Relief Fund
PAZAPA
Physicians for Human Rights
Project AmaZon
Project Concern International: OPTIONS
Project Hope/People to People Health Foundation
Project ORBIS International, Inc.
Remote Area Medical
School Sisters of Saint Francis
Selian Lutheran Hospital
Simeus Foundation, The
Sister Community Alliances: Ouelessebougou-Utah Alliance
Sons of Mary Missionary Society
St. Francis' Hospital
St. John's Medical College
St. Jude Hospital
Surgical Medical Assistance Relief Teams
Surgicorps International
Univ. of Wisconsin Med., Office of International Health Affairs
Universidad de Chile, Facultad de Medicina
University of Cincinnati College of Medicine, Dept. of Family
University of Illinois College of Medicine at Rockford
University of Nebraska Medical Center, Office of International Programs and Studies
University of Virginia, Center for Global Health
University of Zimbabwe
Uplift Internationale
US Committee for Scientific Cooperation with Vietnam
Vietnam ENT Mission
Virginia Children's Connection, Dept. of Plastic. & Recon. Surgery
Volunteer Missionary Movement
Volunteer Optometric Service to Humanity (VOSH) International
Volunteers in Medical Missions
WEC International
World Hearing Network
World Mission Prayer League
Zuma Memorial Hospital

Plastic, hand, and reconstructive surgeons

Adventist Development and Relief Agency International
Aid for International Medicine
Aloha Medical Missions (AMM)
Amazon-Africa Aid Organization (3AO)
American Physicians Fellowship for Medicine in Israel
Ann Foundation Inc
Archdiocesan Health Care Network for Catholic Charities
Associate Reformed Presbyterian Church, World Witness
Bairo Pite Clinic
Baptist Medical Missions International
Beeve Foundation for World Eye and Health, The
Ben Gurion University of the Negev
Cameroon Baptist Convention Health Board
Casa Clinica de la Mujer
Catholic Medical Mission Board, Inc.
CB International
Child Family Health International
Children's Cross Connection, International
Christian Medical College (Vellore, India) Board
Christian Mission of Pignon Inc.
Clinica Evangelica Morava Elective
College of Medicine, Malawi
Crudem Foundation
Esperanca, Inc.
Evangelical Lutheran Church in America
Filipino-American Medical Inc.
Foundation Human Nature (MeHiPro)
Friends Lugulu Hospital
Friends Without a Border
Global Volunteers
Guinea Development Foundation, Inc.
Hands Together, Inc.
Harlem Hospital, Plastic Surgery Program
Healing the Children Northeast, Inc.
Health Teams International
Health Volunteers Overseas
Helps International
Honduras Outreach, Inc
Hope Alliance
Hope Worldwide
Hospital Albert Schweitzer
Indochina Surgical Educational Exchange
Interface UCSD
International Cooperation for Development (formerly CIIR Overseas Programme)
International Health Service
International Nepal Fellowship
International Relief Teams
Interplast
Liga International, Inc.
Lumiere Medical Ministries, Inc.
Magee-Womens Hospital
Maua Methodist Hospital
Medical Ministry International
Medicine for Peace
Mercy Ships
Mexican Medical Ministries
Mima Foundation, Inc.

Health profession usage: *(continued)*

Plastic, hand, and reconstructive surgeons *(continued)*

Moi University Faculty of Health Sciences

Mountain Movers Missions Intl

Nicaraguan Children's Fund

Northwest Medical Teams International, Inc.

Omni Med

Operation Blessing, Medical Division

Operation Luz del Sol

Operation Rainbow

Operation Smile International

Operation USA

P.C.E.A. Kikuyu Hospital

P.R.A.Y. (Project Rescue of Amazon Youth)

Palestine Children's Relief Fund

PAZAPA

Physicians for Peace

Project AmaZon

Project Hope/People to People Health Foundation

Remote Area Medical

Simeus Foundation, The

SIM USA

Sister Community Alliances: Ouelessebougou-Utah Alliance

St. John's Medical College

Surgical Medical Assistance Relief Teams

Surgicorps International

Univ. of Wisconsin Med., Office of International Health Affairs

Universidad de Chile, Facultad de Medicina

University of Illinois College of Medicine at Rockford

University of Virginia, Center for Global Health

University of Zimbabwe

Uplift Internationale

US Committee for Scientific Cooperation with Vietnam

Virginia Children's Connection, Dept. of Plastic. & Recon. Surgery

Volunteer Missionary Movement

WEC International

World Emergency Relief

World Hearing Network

World Witness - the Associate Reformed Presbyterian Church

Podiatrists

Adventist Development and Relief Agency International

Aloha Medical Missions (AMM)

American Leprosy Missions Inc.

American Physicians Fellowship for Medicine in Israel

Ann Foundation Inc

Archdiocesan Health Care Network for Catholic Charities

Bairo Pite Clinic

Baptist Medical Missions International

Beeve Foundation for World Eye and Health, The

Cameroon Baptist Convention Health Board

Canvasback Missions, Inc.

Casa Clinica de la Mujer

Children's Cross Connection, International

Christian Medical College (Vellore, India) Board

Clinica Evangelica Morava Elective

DoCare International, Inc.

Foundation Human Nature (MeHiPro)

Friends Without a Border

Global Volunteers

Guinea Development Foundation, Inc.

Health Teams International

Hillside Healthcare Center

Hope Alliance

Hope Worldwide

Liga International, Inc.

Lumiere Medical Ministries, Inc.

M.E.D.I.C.O.

Mercy Ships

Mima Foundation, Inc.

Moi University Faculty of Health Sciences

Mountain Movers Missions Intl

Nicaraguan Children's Fund

P.R.A.Y. (Project Rescue of Amazon Youth)

Project AmaZon

Project Hope/People to People Health Foundation

School Sisters of Saint Francis

Simeus Foundation, The

Special Olympics, Inc.

Surgical Medical Assistance Relief Teams

University of Zimbabwe

Volunteer Missionary Movement

WEC International

Prosthetists

Adventist Development and Relief Agency International

American Physicians Fellowship for Medicine in Israel

Ann Foundation Inc

Archdiocesan Health Care Network for Catholic Charities

Associazione Italiana 'Amici Raoul Follereau'

Bairo Pite Clinic

Baptist Medical Missions International

Beeve Foundation for World Eye and Health, The

Ben Gurion University of the Negev

Cameroon Baptist Convention Health Board

Casa Clinica de la Mujer

Children's Cross Connection, International

Health profession usage: *(continued)*

Prosthetists *(continued)*

Christian Medical College (Vellore, India) Board
Clinica Evangelica Morava Elective
Community of Caring
Curamericas
Foundation Human Nature (MeHiPro)
Friends Without a Border
Global Volunteers
Guinea Development Foundation, Inc.
Health Teams International
Hope Alliance
Hope Worldwide
International Committee of the Red Cross
International Health Exchange
International Medical Corps
International Nepal Fellowship
InterServe
Liga International, Inc.
Lumiere Medical Ministries, Inc.
Maua Methodist Hospital
Medical Ministry International
Mercy Ships
Mexican Medical Ministries
Moi University Faculty of Health Sciences
Mountain Movers Missions Intl
Nicaraguan Children's Fund
Northwest Medical Teams International, Inc.
Operation USA
P.C.E.A. Kikuyu Hospital
P.R.A.Y. (Project Rescue of Amazon Youth)
Palestine Children's Relief Fund
Project AmaZon
Project Hope/People to People Health Foundation
Simeus Foundation, The
St. Jude Hospital
Surgical Medical Assistance Relief Teams
Universidad de Chile, Facultad de Medicina
University of Zimbabwe
Volunteer Missionary Movement
WEC International
World Emergency Relief
World Rehabilitation Fund, Inc.

Psychiatrists

Adventist Development and Relief Agency International
Africa Inland Mission, International
Aloha Medical Missions (AMM)
American Jewish World Service
American Physicians Fellowship for Medicine in Israel
American Refugee Committee
Ann Foundation Inc
Archdiocesan Health Care Network for Catholic Charities
Bairo Pite Clinic
Baptist Medical Missions International
Ben Gurion University of the Negev
Cameroon Baptist Convention Health Board
Casa Clinica de la Mujer
Catholic Medical Mission Board, Inc.
Children's Cross Connection, International
Christian Medical College (Vellore, India) Board
Clinica Evangelica Morava Elective
College of Medicine, Malawi
Commonwealth Health Center
Curamericas
DePauw University Winter Term in Service
DoCare International, Inc.
Doctors of the World
Evangelical Alliance Mission (TEAM World)
Foundation Human Nature (MeHiPro)
Friends Without a Border
Global Volunteers
Health Teams International
Himalayan HealthCare Inc.
Hope Alliance
Hope Worldwide
International Health Exchange
Lumiere Medical Ministries, Inc.
Magee-Womens Hospital
Maua Methodist Hospital
Medecins Sans Frontieres/ Doctors Without Borders USA
Medical Ministry International
Medicine for Peace
Mercy Ships
Mission Doctors Association
Moi University Faculty of Health Sciences
Mountain Movers Missions Intl
National Health Service Corps, Recruitment Program
Nicaraguan Children's Fund
Northwest Medical Teams International, Inc.
Omni Med
Operation Blessing, Medical Division
Operation USA
P.R.A.Y. (Project Rescue of Amazon Youth)
Pan American Health Organization
Physicians for Human Rights
Presbyterian Church USA, Mission Service Recruitment
Project AmaZon
Project Hope/People to People Health Foundation
Simeus Foundation, The
St. John's Medical College
St. Jude Hospital
Surgical Medical Assistance Relief Teams

Health profession usage: *(continued)*

Psychiatrists *(continued)*

Tulane University School of Public Health and Tropical Medicine
Universidad de Chile, Facultad de Medicina
University of Illinois College of Medicine at Rockford
University of Zimbabwe
Voluntary Service Overseas Canada
Volunteer Missionary Movement
WEC International

Psychologists

Adventist Development and Relief Agency International
Africa Inland Mission, International
American Physicians Fellowship for Medicine in Israel
Ann Foundation Inc
Archdiocesan Health Care Network for Catholic Charities
Bairo Pite Clinic
Ben Gurion University of the Negev
Cameroon Baptist Convention Health Board
Casa Clinica de la Mujer
CB International
Children's Cross Connection, International
Christian Medical College (Vellore, India) Board
Clinica Evangelica Morava Elective
College of Medicine, Malawi
Community of Caring
Curamericas
DePauw University Winter Term in Service
Doctors for Global Health
Foundation Human Nature (MeHiPro)
Friends Without a Border
Global Volunteers
Guinea Development Foundation, Inc.
Health Teams International
Hope Alliance
International Health Exchange
International Medical Corps
International Nepal Fellowship
Lumiere Medical Ministries, Inc.
Mercy Ships
Moi University Faculty of Health Sciences
Mountain Movers Missions Intl
Nicaraguan Children's Fund
Northwest Medical Teams International, Inc.
Operation Blessing, Medical Division
Operation Smile International
Operation USA
P.R.A.Y. (Project Rescue of Amazon Youth)
Pan American Health Organization
Physicians for Human Rights
Presbyterian Church USA, Mission Service Recruitment
Project AmaZon
Project Hope/People to People Health Foundation
Simeus Foundation, The
St. John's Medical College
St. Jude Hospital
Surgical Medical Assistance Relief Teams
Tulane University School of Public Health and Tropical Medicine
Universidad de Chile, Facultad de Medicina
University of Illinois College of Medicine at Rockford
University of Zimbabwe
Visions in Action
Voluntary Service Overseas Canada
Volunteer Missionary Movement
WEC International
World Rehabilitation Fund, Inc.

Pulmonary specialists

Adventist Development and Relief Agency International
Aloha Medical Missions (AMM)
American Physicians Fellowship for Medicine in Israel
Ann Foundation Inc
Archdiocesan Health Care Network for Catholic Charities
Bairo Pite Clinic
Ben Gurion University of the Negev
Cameroon Baptist Convention Health Board
Capiz Emmanuel Hospital
Casa Clinica de la Mujer
Children's Cross Connection, International
Christian Medical College (Vellore, India) Board
Christian Mission of Pignon Inc.
Clinica Evangelica Morava Elective
Clínica Maxena
College of Medicine, Malawi
Curamericas
DePauw University Winter Term in Service
Doctors of the World
Foundation Human Nature (MeHiPro)
Friends Without a Border
Global Volunteers
Guinea Development Foundation, Inc.
Healing the Children Northeast, Inc.
Health Teams International
Himalayan HealthCare Inc.

Health profession usage: *(continued)*

Pulmonary specialists *(continued)*

Hope Alliance
Hope Worldwide
Hospital Albert Schweitzer
International Health Exchange
Lumiere Medical Ministries, Inc.
Maua Methodist Hospital
Medical Ministry International
Mission Doctors Association
Moi University Faculty of Health Sciences
Mountain Movers Missions Intl
Nicaraguan Children's Fund
Omni Med
P.C.E.A. Kikuyu Hospital
P.R.A.Y. (Project Rescue of Amazon Youth)
Physicians for Peace
Project AmaZon
Project Hope/People to People Health Foundation
Simeus Foundation, The
St. John's Medical College
Surgical Medical Assistance Relief Teams
Universidad de Chile, Facultad de Medicina
University of Illinois College of Medicine at Rockford
University of Zimbabwe
Volunteer Missionary Movement
WEC International
World Hearing Network

Radiologists

Adventist Development and Relief Agency International
American Baptist Board of International Ministries
American Physicians Fellowship for Medicine in Israel
Ann Foundation Inc
Archdiocesan Health Care Network for Catholic Charities
Bairo Pite Clinic
Ben Gurion University of the Negev
Cameroon Baptist Convention Health Board
Campus Crusade for Christ International
Capiz Emmanuel Hospital
Casa Clinica de la Mujer
Children's Cross Connection, International
Christian Medical College (Vellore, India) Board
Clinica Evangelica Morava Elective
Clínica Maxena
College of Medicine, Malawi
Commonwealth Health Center
DePauw University Winter Term in Service
Evangelical Alliance Mission (TEAM World)
Foundation Human Nature (MeHiPro)
Friends Without a Border
Global Volunteers
Guinea Development Foundation, Inc.
Haitian Health Clinic, Inc.
Healing the Children Northeast, Inc.
Health Teams International
Helps International
Honduras Outreach, Inc
Hope Alliance
Hope Worldwide
Hospital Albert Schweitzer
International Health Exchange
InterServe
Ludhiana Christian Medical College Board USA
Lumiere Medical Ministries, Inc.
M.E.D.I.C.O.
Magee-Womens Hospital
Maua Methodist Hospital
Medical Ministry International
Mercy Ships
Mission Doctors Association
Moi University Faculty of Health Sciences
Mountain Movers Missions Intl
Nicaraguan Children's Fund
Omni Med
Operation Blessing, Medical Division
P.C.E.A. Kikuyu Hospital
P.R.A.Y. (Project Rescue of Amazon Youth)
Palestine Children's Relief Fund
Project AmaZon
Project Hope/People to People Health Foundation
Remote Area Medical
School Sisters of Saint Francis
Simeus Foundation, The
St. John's Medical College
St. Jude Hospital
Surgical Medical Assistance Relief Teams
Universidad de Chile, Facultad de Medicina
University of Illinois College of Medicine at Rockford
University of Zimbabwe
Voluntary Service Overseas Canada
Volunteer Missionary Movement
VSO
WEC International
World Hearing Network

Respiratory therapists

Adventist Development and Relief Agency International
Aloha Medical Missions (AMM)
American Physicians Fellowship for Medicine in Israel
Ann Foundation Inc
Bairo Pite Clinic
Baptist Medical Missions International

Health profession usage: *(continued)*
Respiratory therapists *(continued)*

Ben Gurion University of the Negev
Cameroon Baptist Convention Health Board
Capiz Emmanuel Hospital
Casa Clinica de la Mujer
Chanet Community Organization
Children's Cross Connection, International
Christian Medical College (Vellore, India) Board
Christian Mission of Pignon Inc.
Clinica Evangelica Morava Elective
Commonwealth Health Center
Curamericas
DePauw University Winter Term in Service
Foundation Human Nature (MeHiPro)
Foundation of Compassionate American Samaritans
Friends Without a Border
Global Volunteers
Guinea Development Foundation, Inc.
Healing the Children Northeast, Inc.
Health Teams International
Hope Alliance
Hope Worldwide
International Relief Teams
Lumiere Medical Ministries, Inc.
M.E.D.I.C.O.
Medical Ministry International
Mercy Ships
Moi University Faculty of Health Sciences
Mountain Movers Missions Intl
Nicaraguan Children's Fund
Operation Smile International
P.C.E.A. Kikuyu Hospital
P.R.A.Y. (Project Rescue of Amazon Youth)
Project AmaZon
Project Hope/People to People Health Foundation
Remote Area Medical
Simeus Foundation, The
Special Olympics, Inc.
Surgical Medical Assistance Relief Teams
Tulane University School of Public Health and Tropical Medicine
Universidad de Chile, Facultad de Medicina
University of Zimbabwe
Volunteer Missionary Movement
WEC International

Social workers

ACCESS
Adventist Development and Relief Agency International
Africare
American Physicians Fellowship for Medicine in Israel
Ann Foundation Inc
APUSAN-USA
Bairo Pite Clinic
Baptist Medical Missions International
Beeve Foundation for World Eye and Health
Ben Gurion University of the Negev
Board of World Mission of the Moravian Church
Bread for the World (Brot fur die Welt)
Cameroon Baptist Convention Health Board
Canvasback Missions, Inc.
Casa Clinica de la Mujer
CB International
Chanet Community Organization
Children's Cross Connection, International
Christian Medical College (Vellore, India) Board
Clinica Evangelica Morava Elective
Clínica Maxena
CONCERN
DePauw University Winter Term in Service
Doctors for Global Health
Evangelical Alliance Mission (TEAM World)
Foundation Human Nature (MeHiPro)
Foundation of Compassionate American Samaritans
Friends Without a Border
General Board of Global Ministries/The United Methodist
Global Volunteers
Guinea Development Foundation, Inc.
HBS Foundation, Inc./Hopital Bon Samaritain
Healing the Children Northeast, Inc.
Health Teams International
Honduras Outreach, Inc
Hope Alliance
Hope Worldwide
International Cooperation for Development (formerly CIIR Overseas Programme)
International Federation of Social Workers
International Health Exchange
International Partnership for Human Development
International Rescue Committee
InterServe
INTERTEAM
Jesuit Refugee Service
Lay Mission-Helpers Association
Liga International, Inc.
Lumiere Medical Ministries, Inc.
M.E.D.I.C.O.

Health profession usage: *(continued)*
Social workers *(continued)*

Medical Care Development International Division
Medicine for Peace
Mennonite Central Committee
Mercy Ships
Moi University Faculty of Health Sciences
Mountain Movers Missions Intl
National Health Service Corps, Recruitment Program
Nicaraguan Children's Fund
Operation Rainbow
P.C.E.A. Kikuyu Hospital
P.R.A.Y. (Project Rescue of Amazon Youth)
Physicians for Human Rights
Presbyterian Church USA, Mission Service Recruitment
Project AmaZon
Project Hope/People to People Health Foundation
Remote Area Medical
Salesian Missions
School Sisters of Saint Francis
Seva Foundation
Simeus Foundation, The
Sons of Mary Missionary Society
Special Olympics, Inc.
St. John's Medical College
Surgical Medical Assistance Relief Teams
Tulane University School of Public Health and Tropical
Universidad de Chile, Facultad de Medicina
University of Illinois College of Medicine at Rockford
Visions in Action
Voluntary Service Overseas Canada
Volunteer Missionary Movement
VSO
WEC International
World Association for Children and Parents
World Rehabilitation Fund, Inc.

Urologists

Adventist Development and Relief Agency International
Aloha Medical Missions (AMM)
Amazon-Africa Aid Organization (3AO)
American Physicians Fellowship for Medicine in Israel
Ann Foundation Inc
Archdiocesan Health Care Network for Catholic Charities
Associate Reformed Presbyterian Church, World Witness
Bairo Pite Clinic
Baptist Medical Missions International
Ben Gurion University of the Negev
Cameroon Baptist Convention Health Board
Canvasback Missions, Inc.
Capiz Emmanuel Hospital
Casa Clinica de la Mujer
Catholic Medical Mission Board, Inc.
Children's Cross Connection, International
Christian Medical College (Vellore, India) Board
Clinica Evangelica Morava Elective
College of Medicine, Malawi
Complete Basic Health 2000
Crudem Foundation
DePauw University Winter Term in Service
DoCare International, Inc.
Evangelical Alliance Mission (TEAM World)
Foundation Human Nature (MeHiPro)
Friends Without a Border
Global Volunteers
Grace Ministries International
Grokha Association of Social Health
Guinea Development Foundation, Inc.
Healing the Children Northeast, Inc.
Health Teams International
Helps International
Hope Alliance
Hope Worldwide
Hospital Albert Schweitzer
Lumiere Medical Ministries, Inc.
M.E.D.I.C.O.
Medical Ministry International
Mercy Ships
Mexican Medical Ministries
Mima Foundation, Inc.
Mission Doctors Association
Moi University Faculty of Health Sciences
Mountain Movers Missions Intl
Nicaraguan Children's Fund
Omni Med
Operation Blessing, Medical Division
Operation Luz del Sol
P.C.E.A. Kikuyu Hospital
P.R.A.Y. (Project Rescue of Amazon Youth)
Palestine Children's Relief Fund
Physicians for Peace
Project AmaZon
Project Hope/People to People Health Foundation
Sanyati Baptist Hospital, Baptist Convention of Zimbabwe
Simeus Foundation, The
St. John's Medical College
St. Jude Hospital
Surgical Medical Assistance Relief Teams
Universidad de Chile, Facultad de Medicina
University of Illinois College of Medicine at Rockford
University of Zimbabwe

Health profession usage: *(continued)*

Urologists *(continued)*

Volunteer Missionary Movement
WEC International
World Hearing Network

Water and sanitation specialists

Action Against Hunger
Adventist Development and Relief Agency International
Africare
American Jewish World Service
American Physicians Fellowship for Medicine in Israel
American Refugee Committee
Ann Foundation Inc
Bairo Pite Clinic
Baptist Medical Missions International
Beeve Foundation for World Eye and Health, The
Cameroon Baptist Convention Health Board
Canvasback Missions, Inc.
Casa Clinica de la Mujer
CB International
CERT International (Christian Emergency Relief Team)
Chanet Community Organization
Children's Cross Connection, International
Christian Medical College (Vellore, India) Board
Christian Mission of Pignon Inc.
Clinica Evangelica Morava Elective
Clínica Maxena
Community of Caring
CrossWorld
DePauw University Winter Term in Service
Doctors for Global Health
Evangelical Alliance Mission (TEAM World)
Foundation Human Nature (MeHiPro)
Foundation of Compassionate American Samaritans
Friends Without a Border
Global Outreach International
Global Volunteers
Grokha Association of Social Health
Guinea Development Foundation, Inc.
Hands Together, Inc.
HBS Foundation, Inc./Hopital Bon Samaritain
Health and Child Survival Fellows Program
Health Teams International
Helping Hands Health Education
Honduras Outreach, Inc
Hope Alliance
Hospital Albert Schweitzer
International Committee of the Red Cross
International Cooperation for Development (formerly CIIR Overseas Programme)
International Federation of Red Cross and Red Crescent Societies
International Health Exchange
International Medical Corps
International Nepal Fellowship
International Partnership for Human Development
International Rescue Committee
InterServe
INTERTEAM
Lumiere Medical Ministries, Inc.
Maua Methodist Hospital
Medecins Sans Frontieres/ Doctors Without Borders USA
Medical Care Development International Division
Medical Ministry International
Medicine for Peace
Mennonite Central Committee
Mercy Ships
Michigan State University Institute for International Health
Moi University Faculty of Health Sciences
Mountain Movers Missions Intl
Nicaraguan Children's Fund
P.C.E.A. Kikuyu Hospital
P.C.E.A. Tumutumu Hospital
Pan American Health Organization
Project AmaZon
Project Hope/People to People Health Foundation
PROMESA
Remote Area Medical
School Sisters of Saint Francis
Simeus Foundation, The
Sister Community Alliances: Ouelessebougou-Utah Alliance
St. John's Medical College
Surgical Medical Assistance Relief Teams
University of Cincinnati College of Medicine, Dept. of Family Medicine
Voluntary Service Overseas Canada
Volunteer Missionary Movement
WEC International
World Concern
World Vision International
World Vision, Inc.

Specific continent: Africa

Action Against Hunger
Africa Inland Mission, Int'l
African Inter-Mennonite Mission
Africare
Aid for International Medicine
Albert Schweitzer Fellowship

Specific continent: Africa *(continued)*

American Baptist Board of International Ministries

American College of Nurse-Midwives

American Jewish World Service

American Leprosy Missions Inc.

American Refugee Committee

American Society of Plastic Surgeons - Reconstructive Surgeons Volunteer Program

Ann Foundation Inc

Associazione Italiana 'Amici Raoul Follereau'

Baptist General Conference

Baptist Medical Missions International

Baptist Mid Missions

Ben Gurion University of the Negev

Boston University School of Medicine, Section of Preventive Medicine and Epidemiology

Bread for the World (Brot fur die Welt)

Bridges to Community, Inc.

Campus Crusade for Christ International

Cape Verde Care Agency, Inc.

Catholic Medical Mission Board, Inc.

Catholic Network of Volunteer Service

CB International

CERT International (Christian Emergency Relief Team)

Child Family Health International

Children's Cross Connection, International

Children's Heartlink

Christian Dental Missions

Christian Dental Society

Christian Medical and Dental Associations-Global Health Outreach

Christoffel-Blindenmission EV

Church of the Nazarene World Mission Division

College of Medicine, Malawi

Comitato Collaborazione Medica (Doctors for Developing Countries)

Community of Caring

Complete Basic Health 2000

CONCERN

CONCERN America

Cross-Cultural Solutions

CrossWorld

Dental Health International

DePauw University Winter Term in Service

Doctors for Global Health

Doctors of the World

Duke University Medical Center, Division of Infectious Diseases and Int'l Health

Edward A. Ulzen Memorial Foundation (EAUMF)

Esperanca, Inc.

Evangelical Alliance Mission (TEAM World)

Evangelical Covenant Church

Evangelical Free Church of America Mission

Evangelical Lutheran Church in America

Fellowship of Associates of Medical Evangelism

FIENS Foundation of International Education in Neurological Surgery

FOCUS Inc.

Foreign Ophthalmological Care from the United States, Inc.

Foundation for International Medical Relief of Children

Foundation Human Nature (MeHiPro)

Friends Lugulu Hospital

General Board of Global Ministries / The United Methodist Church

General Dept. of World Missions, The Wesleyan Church

Global Operations & Development

Global Outreach International

Global Service Corps/Earth Island Institute

Global Volunteers

Grace Ministries International

Guinea Development Foundation, Inc.

Harlem Hospital, Plastic Surgery Program

Healing the Children Northeast, Inc.

Health Alliance International

Health and Child Survival Fellows Program

Health Teams International

Health Volunteers Overseas

Helen Keller International

Hope Alliance

Hope Worldwide

Infectious Diseases Society of America, The, and The HIV Medicine Association

International Aid, Inc.

International Children's Heart Foundation

International Committee of the Red Cross

International Cooperation for Development (formerly CIIR Overseas Programme)

International Eye Foundation, Inc.

International Federation of Red Cross and Red Crescent Societies

International Federation of Social Workers

International Health Exchange

International Medical Corps

International Ministries, American Baptist Churches, USA

International Partnership for Human Development

International Rescue Committee

InterServe

Specific continent: Africa *(continued)*

INTERTEAM

Jesuit Refugee Service

Johns Hopkins Univ. School of Public Health, Dept. of International Health

Jubilee Volunteer Africa Program of AFRIDEC

Lalmba Association

Lay Mission-Helpers Association

Lighthouse for Christ Mission and Eye Centre

Maluti Adventist Hospital (Lesotho)

Management Sciences for Health

Maryknoll Mission Association of the Faithful

Maua Methodist Hospital

Medical Ambassadors International

Medical Care Development International Division

Medical Ministry International

Medical Missionaries of Mary

Medical Teams International, Inc.

Medicine for Humanity

Memisa Medicus Mundi

Mennonite Central Committee

Mercy Ships

Michigan State University Institute for International Health

Minnesota International Health Volunteers

Mission Doctors Association

Moi University Faculty of Health Sciences

North American Baptist Conference Missions

Northwest Medical Teams International, Inc.

Omni Med

Operation Blessing, Medical Division

Operation Smile International

Operation USA

P.C.E.A. Chogoria Hospital

P.C.E.A. Kikuyu Hospital

P.C.E.A. Tumutumu Hospital

Palms Australia

Partners for Development

Physicians for Human Rights

Physicians for Peace

Presbyterian Church USA, Mission Service Recruitment

Project Concern International: OPTIONS

Project Open Hearts

Project ORBIS International, Inc.

Saint Joseph's Medical Center, Family Practice Residency Program, Int'l Health Track

Sanyati Baptist Hospital, Baptist Convention of Zimbabwe

Selian Lutheran Hospital

Seva Foundation

SIM USA

Sister Community Alliances: Ouelessebougou-Utah Alliance

SkillShare International

Special Olympics, Inc.

St. Francis' Hospital

Surgical Eye Expeditions International (S.E.E.), Inc.

Surgicorps International

Trinity Health International

Tulane University School of Public Health and Tropical Medicine

UCSD, Division of International Health

Unite For Sight

University of Illinois at Chicago College of Nursing, Global Health Leadership Office

University of Virginia, Center for Global Health

University of Zimbabwe

Visions in Action

Voluntary Missionary Movement

Volunteer Missionary Movement

Volunteer Optometric Service to Humanity (VOSH) Int'l

Volunteers in Medical Missions

VSO

WEC International

Women's Commission for Refugee Women and Children

World Concern

World Emergency Relief

World Gospel Mission

World Medical Mission

World Mission Prayer League

World Rehabilitation Fund, Inc.

World Relief Corp.

World Vision, Inc.

Zuma Memorial Hospital

Specific continent: Asia

ACCESS

Action Against Hunger

Aid for International Medicine

Aloha Medical Missions (AMM)

American Baptist Board of International Ministries

American College of Nurse-Midwives

American Jewish Joint Distribution Committee

American Jewish World Service

American Leprosy Missions Inc.

American Physicians Fellowship for Medicine in Israel

American Refugee Committee

Anderson University School of Nursing

Ann Foundation Inc

Specific continent: Asia *(continued)*

Associate Reformed Presbyterian Church, World Witness

Associazione Italiana 'Amici Raoul Follereau'

Bairo Pite Clinic

Baptist Medical Missions International

Baptist Mid Missions

Beeve Foundation for World Eye and Health, The

Ben Gurion University of the Negev

Bridges to Community, Inc.

Campus Crusade for Christ International

Canadian Society for International Health

Canvasback Missions, Inc.

Capiz Emmanuel Hospital

CardioStart International, Inc.

Catholic Medical Mission Board, Inc.

Catholic Network of Volunteer Service

CB International

CERT International (Christian Emergency Relief Team)

Child Family Health International

Children's Heartlink

Children's Medical Mission

Christian Dental Missions

Christian Dental Society

Christian Medical and Dental Associations-Global Health Outreach

Christian Medical College (Vellore, India) Board

Christoffel-Blindenmission EV

Church of the Nazarene World Mission Division

Clínica Maxena

Commonwealth Health Center

CONCERN

Cross-Cultural Solutions

CrossWorld

Dental Health International

DePauw University Winter Term in Service

Doctors of the World

Duke University Medical Center, Division of Infectious Diseases and Int'l Health

Emergency International, Inc.

Evangelical Alliance Mission (TEAM World)

Evangelical Covenant Church

Evangelical Free Church of America Mission

Evangelical Lutheran Church in America

Feed the Children

Fellowship of Associates of Medical Evangelism

FIENS Foundation of International Education in Neurological Surgery

Filipino-American Medical Inc.

Flying Doctors of America

Foundation for International Medical Relief of Children

Foundation for International Scientific Cooperation

General Baptist International

General Board of Global Ministries / The United Methodist Church

Global Operations & Development

Global Outreach International

Global Service Corps/Earth Island Institute

Global Volunteers

Grokha Association of Social Health

Healing the Children Northeast, Inc.

Health Alliance International

Health Teams International

Health Volunteers Overseas

Helen Keller International

Helping Hands Health Education

Himalayan Health Exchange

Himalayan HealthCare Inc.

Hope Alliance

Hope Worldwide

Indochina Surgical Educational Exchange

International Aid, Inc.

International Children's Heart Foundation

International Committee of the Red Cross

International Cooperation for Development (formerly CIIR Overseas Programme)

International Federation of Red Cross and Red Crescent Societies

International Federation of Social Workers

International Health Exchange

International Health Medical Education Consortium

International Medical Corps

International Ministries, American Baptist Churches, USA

International Nepal Fellowship

International Relief Teams

International Rescue Committee

Interplast

InterServe

INTERTEAM

Jesuit Refugee Service

Johns Hopkins Univ. School of Public Health, Dept. of International Health

Lay Mission-Helpers Association

Liga International, Inc.

Ludhiana Christian Medical College Board USA

Management Sciences for Health

Maryknoll Mission Association of the Faithful

Medical Aid for Palestinians

Medical Ambassadors International

Specific continent: Asia *(continued)*

Medical Care Development International Division

Medical Ministry International

Medicine for Humanity

Medicine for Peace

Memisa Medicus Mundi

Mennonite Central Committee

Mercy Ships

Michigan State University Institute for International Health

Minnesota International Health Volunteers

Mission Doctors Association

Northwest Medical Teams International, Inc.

Notre Dame India Mission

Omni Med

Operation Blessing, Medical Division

Operation Rainbow

Operation Smile International

Operation USA

Palestine Children's Relief Fund

Palms Australia

Physicians for Human Rights

Physicians for Peace

Presbyterian Church USA, Mission Service Recruitment

Project Concern International: OPTIONS

Project Open Hearts

Project ORBIS International, Inc.

Remote Area Medical

Saint Joseph's Medical Center, Family Practice Residency Program, Int'l Health Track

School Sisters of Saint Francis

Seva Foundation

SIM USA

SkillShare International

Sons of Mary Missionary Society

Special Olympics, Inc.

St. John's Medical College

St. Mary's Hospital, Vunapope

Surfer's Medical Association

Surgical Eye Expeditions International (S.E.E.), Inc.

Surgicorps International

Trinity Health International

Tulane University School of Public Health and Tropical Medicine

UCSD, Division of International Health

Unite For Sight

University of Illinois at Chicago College of Nursing, Global Health Leadership Office

University of Illinois College of Medicine at Rockford

University of Virginia, Center for Global Health

Uplift Internationale

Vietnam ENT Mission

Virginia Children's Connection, Dept. of Plastic. & Recon. Surgery

Volunteer Optometric Service to Humanity (VOSH) International

Volunteers in Medical Missions

VSO

WEC International

Women's Commission for Refugee Women and Children

World Association for Children and Parents

World Concern

World Emergency Relief

World Gospel Mission

World Hearing Network

World Medical Mission

World Mission Prayer League

World Rehabilitation Fund, Inc.

World Relief Corp.

World Vision International

World Vision, Inc.

World Witness - the Associate Reformed Presbyterian Church

Specific continent: Europe

Action Against Hunger

American College of Nurse-Midwives

American Jewish World Service

American Refugee Committee

Anderson University School of Nursing

Armenian Eye Care Project

Armenian Social Transition Program

Baptist Medical Missions International

Baptist Mid Missions

Ben Gurion University of the Negev

Bread for the World (Brot fur die Welt)

CAM International

Campus Crusade for Christ International

Canadian Society for International Health

CardioStart International, Inc.

Catholic Network of Volunteer Service

CB International

CERT International (Christian Emergency Relief Team)

Children's Heartlink

Christian Dental Society

Christian Medical and Dental Associations-Global Health Outreach

Christoffel-Blindenmission EV

Clínica Maxena

Specific continent: Europe *(continued)*

Cross-Cultural Solutions

Doctors of the World

Feed the Children

Fellowship of Associates of Medical Evangelism

General Board of Global Ministries / The United Methodist Church

General Dept. of World Missions, The Wesleyan Church

Global Operations & Development

Global Outreach International

Global Volunteers

Healing the Children Northeast, Inc.

Health and Child Survival Fellows Program

Health Teams International

Helen Keller International

Hope Worldwide

International Aid, Inc.

International Children's Heart Foundation

International Committee of the Red Cross

International Eye Foundation, Inc.

International Federation of Red Cross and Red Crescent Societies

International Federation of Social Workers

International Health Exchange

International Medical Corps

International Partnership for Human Development

International Relief Teams

International Rescue Committee

Interplast

Jesuit Refugee Service

Magee-Womens Hospital

Management Sciences for Health

Medical Ambassadors International

Medical Ministry International

Medical Teams International, Inc.

Medicine for Humanity

Medicine for Peace

Mennonite Central Committee

Mercy Ships

Michigan State University Institute for International Health

National Eye Care Project for Armenia

Northwest Medical Teams International, Inc.

Operation Blessing, Medical Division

Operation Rainbow

Operation Smile International

Operation USA

Pan American Health Organization

Physicians for Human Rights

Presbyterian Church USA, Mission Service Recruitment

Project Concern International: OPTIONS

Project Open Hearts

Project ORBIS International, Inc.

School Sisters of Saint Francis

Special Olympics, Inc.

Surgical Eye Expeditions International (S.E.E.), Inc.

Trinity Health International

UCSD, Division of International Health

Unite For Sight

University of Illinois at Chicago College of Nursing, Global Health Leadership Office

University of Illinois College of Medicine at Rockford

Volunteer Optometric Service to Humanity (VOSH) International

Volunteers in Medical Missions

VSO

WEC International

World Association for Children and Parents

World Emergency Relief

World Gospel Mission

World Medical Mission

World Mission Prayer League

World Vision International

World Vision, Inc.

World Witness - the Associate Reformed Presbyterian Church

Specific continent: Oceania

Baptist Mid Missions

General Baptist International

Trinity Health International

Specific continent: The Americas

Action Against Hunger

Aid for International Medicine

Ak' Tenamit

Aloha Medical Missions (AMM)

Amazon-Africa Aid and Fundacao Esperanca

Amazon-Africa Aid Organization (3AO)

American Baptist Board of International Ministries

American College of Nurse-Midwives

Specific continent: The Americas *(continued)*

American Jewish Joint Distribution Committee

American Jewish World Service

Amigos de las Americas

Anderson University School of Nursing

Ann Foundation Inc

APUSAN-USA

Archdiocesan Health Care Network for Catholic Charities

ASAPROSAR: The Salvadoran Association for Rural Health

Associazione Italiana 'Amici Raoul Follereau'

Baptist Medical and Dental Mission International

Baptist Medical Missions International

Baptist Mid Missions

Ben Gurion University of the Negev

Board of World Mission of the Moravian Church

Bridges to Community, Inc.

CAM International

Canadian Society for International Health

Cape Cares

Capiz Emmanuel Hospital

CardioStart International, Inc.

Casa Clinica de la Mujer

Catholic Medical Mission Board, Inc.

Catholic Network of Volunteer Service

CB International

CERT International (Christian Emergency Relief Team)

Child Family Health International

Children's Cross Connection, International

Children's Heartlink

Christian Dental Missions

Christian Dental Society

Christian Medical and Dental Associations-Global Health Outreach

Christian Mission of Pignon Inc.

Christoffel-Blindenmission EV

Church of the Nazarene World Mission Division

Clinica Evangelica Morava Elective

Clínica Maxena

Comitato Collaborazione Medica (Doctors for Developing Countries)

Community of Caring

CONCERN

CONCERN America

Cross-Cultural Solutions

CrossWorld

Crudem Foundation

Curamericas

DePauw University Winter Term in Service

DoCare International, Inc.

Doctors for Global Health

Doctors of the World

Duke University Medical Center, Division of Infectious Diseases and Int'l Health

Edmundite Missions Corps

Emergency International, Inc.

Esperanca, Inc.

Father Carr's Place 2B

Feed the Children

Fellowship of Associates of Medical Evangelism

FIENS Foundation of International Education in Neurological Surgery

Florida Association for Volunteer Action in the Caribbean and the Americas (FAVACA)

Flying Doctors of America

Foundation for International Medical Relief of Children

Foundation Human Nature (MeHiPro)

Foundation of Compassionate American Samaritans

General Baptist International

General Board of Global Ministries / The United Methodist Church

General Dept. of World Missions, The Wesleyan Church

Global Operations & Development

Global Outreach International

Global Volunteers

Haitian Health Clinic, Inc.

Hands Together, Inc.

Harlem Hospital, Plastic Surgery Program

HBS Foundation, Inc. / Hopital Bon Samaritain

Healing the Children Northeast, Inc.

Health and Child Survival Fellows Program

Health Teams International

Health Volunteers Overseas

Helps International

Hillside Healthcare Center

Honduras Outreach, Inc

Hope Alliance

Hope Worldwide

Hospital Albert Schweitzer

Intercultural Nursing, Inc.

Interface UCSD

International Aid, Inc.

International Children's Heart Foundation

International Committee of the Red Cross

International Cooperation for Development (formerly CIIR Overseas Programme)

International Eye Foundation, Inc.

International Federation of Red Cross and Red Crescent Societies

International Federation of Social Workers

International Health Exchange

International Health Service

International Medical Corps

Specific continent: The Americas *(continued)*

International Ministries, American Baptist Churches, USA
International Relief Teams
International Rescue Committee
Interplast
INTERTEAM

Jesuit Refugee Service
Johns Hopkins Univ. School of Public Health, Dept. of International Health

Lay Mission-Helpers Association
Liga International, Inc.
Lumiere Medical Ministries, Inc.

M.E.D.I.C.O.
Management Sciences for Health
Maryknoll Mission Association of the Faithful
Medical Ambassadors International
Medical Ministry International
Medical Missionaries of Mary
Medicine for Humanity
Medicine for Peace
Memisa Medicus Mundi
Mennonite Central Committee
Mercy Ships
Mexican Medical Ministries
Michigan State University Institute for International Health
Mima Foundation, Inc.
Minnesota International Health Volunteers
Mission Doctors Association
Mountain Movers Missions Intl

National Health Service Corps, Recruitment Program
New Missions In Haiti
Northwest Medical Teams International, Inc.

Omni Med
Operation Blessing, Medical Division
Operation Luz del Sol
Operation Rainbow
Operation Smile International
Operation USA
Our Little Brothers and Sisters

P.R.A.Y. (Project Rescue of Amazon Youth)
Pan American Health Organization
Pan American Medical Mission Foundation
Partners of the Americas
PAZAPA
Peacework: Volunteer Medical Projects
Physicians for Human Rights
Physicians for Peace
Presbyterian Church USA, Mission Service Recruitment
Project AmaZon
Project Concern International: OPTIONS
Project ORBIS International, Inc.
Project Skye
PROMESA

Remote Area Medical

Saint Joseph's Medical Center, Family Practice Residency Program, Int'l Health Track
School Sisters of Saint Francis
Simeus Foundation, The
SIM USA
Sons of Mary Missionary Society
Special Olympics, Inc.
St. Jude Hospital
Surgical Eye Expeditions International (S.E.E.), Inc.
Surgical Medical Assistance Relief Teams
Surgicorps International

Trinity Health International
Tulane University School of Public Health and Tropical Medicine

UCSD, Division of International Health
Unite For Sight
Universidad de Chile, Facultad de Medicina
University of Arizona College of Medicine
University of Cincinnati College of Medicine, Dept. of Family Medicine
University of Illinois at Chicago College of Nursing, Global Health Leadership Office
University of Illinois College of Medicine at Rockford
University of Nebraska Medical Center, Office of International Programs and Studies
University of Virginia, Center for Global Health

Vietnam ENT Mission
Visions in Action
Volunteer Missionary Movement
Volunteer Optometric Service to Humanity (VOSH) International
Volunteers in Medical Missions

WEC International
Women's Commission for Refugee Women and Children
World Concern
World Emergency Relief
World Gospel Mission
World Hearing Network
World Medical Mission
World Mission Prayer League
World Rehabilitation Fund, Inc.
World Vision International
World Vision, Inc.
World Witness - the Associate Reformed Presbyterian Church

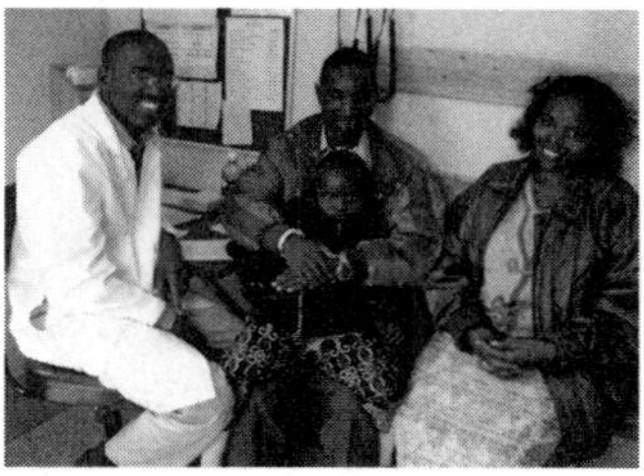

Chapter 5

Other Relevant Organizations

And it's true we are immune
When fact is fiction and TV reality
And today the millions cry
We eat and drink while tomorrow they die

—U2

Let the future say of our generation that we sent forth mighty currents of hope, and that we worked together to heal the world.

—Jeffrey Sachs

I cannot help but feel the suffering all around me, not only of humanity, but of the whole of creation. . . . I have never tried to withdraw myself from this community of suffering. It seemed to me a matter of course that we should all take our share of the burden of pain that lies upon the world. . . . But however concerned I was with the suffering in the world, I never let myself become lost in brooding over it. I always held firmly to the thought that each one of us can do a little to bring some portion of it to an end. . . . If people can be found who revolt against the spirit of thoughtlessness and are sincere and profound enough to spread the ideals of ethical progress, we will witness the emergence of a new spiritual force strong enough to evoke a new spirit in mankind.

—Albert Schweitzer

The organizations that follow in this chapter comprise a diverse and useful list. Few of them send health personnel abroad, but all offer something of value to those engaged in the struggle to bring quality health to those in poor countries. Some organizations like MAP International provide low-cost medical supply packages for transport abroad that any health provider can purchase—at a considerable discount. Other organizations like GW Associates provide informational packages on how to share one's international health experiences with the media. Still others like MedShare International ship medical supplies all over the world. Anyone considering working abroad should peruse the organizations that follow. You are sure to find a few that can help you in your work.

Not all of the organizations listed in this chapter offer benefits specifically to those traveling abroad. In the prequel to this book, *Awakening Hippocrates: A Primer on Health, Poverty, and Global Service,* I made the point that many of the efforts to improve health in the developing world have come from non-health providers. In fact, those who work in the fields of human rights, conflict resolution, public policy, and grassroots advocacy may have contributed more through the years than those who go overseas and serve directly. Influencing the levers of power in the United States may offer the most direct and effective means of improving the health of the global poor. Organizations like Jubilee 2000, which presses for debt cancellation in the least developed countries, have saved tens of thousands of lives through their work. Similarly, ACT UP, Partners In Health, the Institute for Policy Studies, and Fifty Years is Enough have greatly influenced the leaders in the United States and in the multilateral organizations that control the way the world responds to poverty and health inequality.

Other storied organizations like CARE, Oxfam, IPPNW, Lions International, Rotary International, Save the Children, and the United Nations Development Program offer educational and advocacy programs, outreach, informational materials, or grant support. The Foundation Center should be familiar to anyone involved in running a non-profit organization. Some reading this might just be ideal candidates for a Fulbright Scholar Award, though may never consider it otherwise.

I recognize that not everyone can go overseas due to constraints posed by young children, practice obligations, mortgages, and the like. Yet for those who can't travel abroad now, there is still much they can do to affect the larger structural changes that perpetuate poverty. Many of the organizations in this chapter allow you that opportunity right here at home.

A Glimmer of Hope

Address: **4407 Bee Caves Road, Suite 301, Austin, TX 78746 U.S.A.**

Phone: **(512) 328-9944** Fax: **(512) 328-8872**

E-Mail: **inquiries@aglimmerofhope.org** Web: **www.aglimmerofhope.org/index.htm**

Description: A Glimmer of Hope is a family foundation. Founded in 2000, it serves to ease some of the pain and suffering on the planet. It currently operates a national aid program in Ethiopia, one of the oldest yet poorest nations in the world. With their people left destitute by years of war, clinics and health posts depleted, and a government health budget of only US$4 per person per year, the need is dire. In 2004, A Glimmer of Hope funded over 30 health projects throughout Ethiopia at a total cost of more than $580,000. They include the construction and upkeep of health posts and the Dembi Dollo Hospital Restoration Project. The projects will benefit around 200,000. By the end of 2003, the foundation had completed 45 health related projects worth more than $1.35 million.

ACCION International

Address: **56 Roland St., Suite 300, Boston, MA 02129 U.S.A.**

Phone: **(617) 625-7080** Fax: **(617) 625-7020**

E-Mail: **info@accion.org** Web: **www.accion.org**

Description: Founded in 1961 by an idealistic law student named Joseph Blatchford, ACCION today is one of the premier microfinance organizations in the world, with a network of lending partners that spans Latin America, the United States and Africa. Over the last four decades, ACCION has built a tradition of developing innovative solutions to poverty. By providing "micro" loans and business training to poor women and men who start their own businesses, ACCION's partner lending organizations help people work their own way up the economic ladder, with dignity and pride. With capital, people can grow their own businesses. They can earn enough to afford basics like running water, better food and schooling for their children. A small loan can cut the cost of raw goods or buy a sewing machine. Sales grow, and so do profits. With a growing income, people can work their way out of poverty. A focus on financial sustainability has helped ACCION's partner programs increase the number of people served from 13,000 in 1988 to 740,000 in 2002.

ACT UP

Address: **332 Bleecker St., Suite G5, New York, NY 10014 U.S.A.**

Phone: **(212) 966-4873** Fax:

E-Mail: **actupny@panix.com** Web: **www.actupny.org**

Description: ACT UP stands for AIDS Coalition to Unleash Power. "ACT UP is a diverse, non-partisan group of individuals united in anger and committed to direct action to end the AIDS crisis." This coalition does pro-active demonstrations to support AIDS; advises and supports AIDS victims and their families; and informs the public about the reality of the AIDS epidemic.

Adhoc Committee to Defend Health Care, The

Address: **37 Temple Place, 4th Floor, Boston, MA 02111 U.S.A.**

Phone: **(617) 542-3305** Fax: **(617) 303-2198**

E-Mail: **contact@massdefendhealthcare.org** Web: **www.MassDefendHealthCare.org**

Description: The Ad Hoc Committee to Defend Health Care is a group of health care professionals and others who believe that health care is a fundamental human right, and that the delivery of health care should be guided by science and compassion, not by corporate self-interest. The committee collaborates with others to foster public dialogue and health policy reforms that will help achieve universal access to high quality affordable health care for all.

American Academy of Family Physicians-International Health Care Opportunities, The

Address: **11400 Tomahawk Creek Parkway, Leawood, KS 66211-2672 U.S.A.**

Phone: **(800) 274-2237 or (913) 906-6000** Fax:

E-Mail: **fp@aafp.org** Web: **www.aafp.org/x30617.xml**

Description: The American Academy of Family Physicians is one of the largest national medical organizations, representing more than 94,000 family physicians, family medicine residents, and medical students nationwide. AAFP keeps a listing of International Health Care Opportunities for physicians. One such program is "Physicians With Heart" (www.aafp.org/x14203.xml) – a partnership between the American Academy of Family Physicians (AAFP Foundation) and Heart to Heart International – to mobilize resources to improve health, provide medical education and to foster the development of Family Medicine worldwide.

American Academy of Pediatrics CHILDisaster NETWORK

Address: **141 Northwest Point Boulevard, Elk Grove Village, IL 60007-1098 U.S.A.**

Phone: **(847) 434-4000** Fax: **(847) 434-8000**

E-Mail: **kidsdocs@aap.org** Web: **www.aap.org/disaster/index.htm**

Description: The American Academy of Pediatrics is providing assistance to governmental and non-governmental organizations responding to disasters. AAP recognizes the importance of meeting the needs of children in disaster situations and is developing a network of pediatric professionals who will be available to accompany organizations responding to disasters on short-term notice. Should an organization need child health experts on a project, the AAP will provide a list of practitioners who have completed a comprehensive application process. These disaster relief organizations may require additional information regarding the expert's credentials.

American Academy of Pediatrics, Office of International Health

Address: **141 North West Point Blvd, Elk Grove Village, IL 60007-1098 U.S.A.**

Phone: **(847) 434-4000** Fax: **(847) 434-8000**

E-Mail: **kidsdoc@aap.org** Web: **www.aap.org**

Description: The American Academy of Pediatrics (AAP) and its member pediatricians dedicate their efforts and resources to the health, safety and well-being of infants, children, adolescents and young adults. The AAP has approximately 55,000 members in the United States, Canada and Latin America. Members include pediatricians, pediatric medical subspecialists and pediatric surgical specialists. The mission of the American Academy of Pediatrics is to attain optimal physical, mental and social health and well-being for all infants, children, adolescents and young adults. The AAP sends physicians overseas for 4 week terms. Room and board is provided and there are no language or religious requirements.

American Dental Association

Address: **211 East Chicago Ave., Chicago, IL 60611-2678 U.S.A.**

Phone: **(312) 440-2726** Fax: **(312) 440-2707**

E-Mail: Web: **www.ada.org**

Description: The ADA is the professional association of dentists committed to the public's oral health, ethics, science and professional advancement; leading a unified profession through initiatives in advocacy, education, research and the development of standards. Volunteers can travel to various countries around the world for as short as 2 weeks to provide dental care to those in need. The ADA will help connect volunteer dentists with organizations (such as Health Volunteer Overseas) which run the international programs.

American Medical Association

Address: **515 North State Street, Chicago, IL 60610 U.S.A.**

Phone: **(312) 464-4386 or (800) 621-8335** Fax: **(312) 464-5973**

E-Mail: **robin_menes@ama-assn.org** Web: **www.ama-assn.org**

Description: The American Medical Association takes and voices positions on medical issues important to the nation. The AMA seeks to remain an essential part of the professional life of every physician and an essential force for progress in improving the nation's health. The AMA keeps listings of some volunteer opportunities and the organizations which run them.

American Medical Student Association's International Health Residency Program

Address: **1902 Association Dr., Reston, VA 20191 U.S.A.**

Phone: **(703) 620-6600 x453 or (800) 227-5728** Fax: **(703) 620-5873**

E-Mail: **amsa@www.amsa.org** Web: **www.amsa.org/global/ih/**

Description: AMSA keeps a catalog of international programs on their website for medical student's and residents. Students can search for opportunities to work overseas through internships, fellowships, electives, course work, volunteer/educational and Medical Spanish. International residency programs are offered in family medicine, emergency medicine, internal medicine, and pediatrics.

American Society of Plastic Surgeons - Reconstructive Surgeons Volunteer Program

Address: **444 East Algonquin Rd, Arlington Heights, IL 60005 U.S.A.**

Phone: **(847) 228-9900** Fax: **(847) 228-0628 or (847) 228-9131**

E-Mail: **po@plasticsurgery.org** Web: **www.plasticsurgery.org/**

Description: Formed in 1988 to raise funds and act as a clearing house of information, Reconstructive Surgeons Volunteer Program (RSVP) is an umbrella organization of the Plastic Surgery Educational Foundation. RSVP is comprised of 16 agencies that actively participate in overseas volunteer service, whose mission is to see that the greatest number of people are helped in the most efficient way possible.

American Society of Tropical Medicine and Hygiene

Address: **60 Revere Drive, Suite 500, Northbrook, IL 60062 U.S.A.**

Phone: **(847) 480-9592** Fax: **(847) 480-9282**

E-Mail: **astmh@astmh.org** Web: **www.astmh.org**

Description: The American Society of Tropical Medicine and Hygiene (ASTMH) is an organization representing a network of researchers, clinicians and others with interests in the prevention and control of tropical diseases. The ASTMH is focused on improving and promoting world health by fighting tropical diseases through research and education. The society holds meetings, certification programs, funding opportunities and also maintains a travel clinic directory.

Amerispan

Address: **PO Box 58129, Philadelphia, PA 19102-8129 U.S.A.**

Phone: **(800) 879-6640 or (215) 751-1100** Fax: **(215) 751-1986**

E-Mail: **info@amerispan.com** Web: **www.amerispan.com**

Description: AmeriSpan was created in 1993 and has grown to be one of the leaders in educational travel with over 20,000 past clients. We started out as specialists in Latin America and have since applied our expertise to many other languages and regions. Collectively, our staff has traveled to more than 65 countries - every continent except Antarctica - and speaks 10 languages. We offer a variety of educational travel programs including language programs, volunteer/Internship placements, Academic Study Abroad and Specialized Programs such as SALUD, an AMSA-inspired medical Spanish program.

Amizade

Address: **PO Box 110107, Pittsburgh, PA 15232 U.S.A.**

Phone: **(888) 973-4443** Fax: **(412) 441-6655**

E-Mail: **Volunteer@amizade.org** Web: **amizade.org/**

Description: Amizade encourages intercultural exploration and understanding through community-driven volunteer programs and service-learning courses. Amizade Volunteer Programs offer a rewarding combination of exploration, service and understanding in communities around the world. From Hervey Bay, Australia, to Santarem, Brazil, Amizade volunteers have cooperated with community members to meet shared goals. While programs vary considerably, they often involve construction and manual labor. Individuals are able to join programs on their own, while Amizade customizes programs for groups of six or more. Group rates are available for volunteer programs in several countries. Contact Amizade with your site and dates of interest to arrange a customized volunteer program.

Asian Pacific American Medical Student Association

Address: **1200 East University Ave., Old Main Building, Room 104, Tucson, AZ 85721-0001 U.S.A.**

Phone: Fax:

E-Mail: **mvp_apamsa@hotmail.com** Web: **www.apamsa.org/**

Description: APAMSA a national organization that aims to address those issues important to Asian-American medical students. One part of our mission is to bring together Asians and others interested in the health issues that affect Asians so that we may have a strong, collective, public and political voice. We are interested in both directly promoting the health and well-being of the Asian community as well as in helping all health care workers who work with these communities understand how to care for the Asian patient in a culturally sensitive manner. Finally, APAMSA provides an important forum for APA medical students to meet, exchange information and experiences, and develop personally and professionally. The APAMSA website contains links to other AAPI health organizations and international volunteer opportunities.

Baby Milk Action

Address: **34 Trumpington Street, Cambridge CB2 1QY U.K.**

Phone: **44 1223 46 4420** Fax: **44 1223 46 1417**

E-Mail: **info@babymilkaction.org** Web: **www.babymilkaction.org**

Description: Baby Milk Action works with a network of over 200 citizens groups in more than 100 countries to promote breastfeeding and to raise awareness of the dangers of artifical feeding. Hundreds of thousands of babies die worldwide each year (WHO) because they are not breastfed. Baby Milk Actions aims to enable mothers to make well-informed decisions regarding breastfeeding, while not being pressured by commercial sources. Baby Milk Action also fights for improved maternity rights worldwide.

Blessings International

Address: **5881 South Garnett Rd., Tulsa, OK 74146-6812 U.S.A.**

Phone: **(918) 250-8101** Fax: **(918) 250-1281**

E-Mail: **info@blessing.org** Web: **www.blessing.org**

Description: Blessings International seeks to give hope to destitute children and adults by providing pharmaceuticals and medical supplies for patients in clinics and hospitals in developing nations. Partnering with local Christian churches and humanitarian groups, Blessings primarily assists short term medical teams that carry medicines from Blessings to the designated site of ministry. Blessings does not place physicians or any medical people, but instead serves as a resource for pharmaceuticals for medical teams involved in international medicine.

Bread for the World

Address: **50 F Street, NW, Suite 500, Washington, DC 20001 U.S.A.**

Phone: **(202) 639-9400 or (800) 82-BREAD** Fax: **(202) 639-9401**

E-Mail: **bread@bread.org** Web: **www.bread.org**

Description: Bread for the World is a Christian citizen's movement that consists of 46,000 citizens who contact their senators and representatives about legislation that affects hungry people in the United States and worldwide. While they do not provide direct relief or development assistance, they focus on using the power of citizens in a democracy to support policies that address the causes of hunger and poverty. Local churches and community groups support Bread for the World's efforts by writing letters to Congress and making financial gifts to the organization. Bread for the World groups across the country meet locally to pray, study and take action; members meet with their representatives in Congress, organize telephone trees, win media coverage and reach out to new churches. Bread for the World also publishes an annual report on the state of world hunger.

Casa De Espanol Xelaju

Address: **4701 Zenith Ave. S., Minneapolis, MN 55410 U.S.A.**

Phone: **1-888-796-CASA or (612) 281-5705** Fax:

E-Mail: **jbatres@casaxelaju.com** Web: **members.aol.com/cexspanish/**

Description: Casa Xelajú (shay-la-Hoo') is a socially responsible educational institute in Quetzaltenango, Guatemala, promoting cross-cultural understanding through its Spanish, Quiche languages and cultural programs, social projects, internship program, volunteer work and travel services. Opportunities include teaching, statistical legal work, medical and dental clinic positions. Also offer a Spanish for Healthcare program for those that wish to develop and improve their linguistics ability and Spanish understanding to maintain better communication with Hispanic patients that require attention and medical care in their own language.

Center for Global Education

Address: **Augsburg College, 221 Riverside Avenue, Minneapolis, MN 55454 U.S.A.**

Phone: **(612) 330-1159 or (800) 299-8889** Fax: **(612) 330-1695**

E-Mail: **globaled@augsburg.edu** Web: **www.augsburg.edu/global**

Description: The Center for Global Education provides cross-cultural educational opportunities in Central America, Southern Africa and other global sites. Programs include a semester abroad, short term travel seminary, and customized travel programs.

Christian Connections for International Health

Address: **1817 Rupert Street** **McLean, VA 22101 U.S.A.**

Phone: **(703) 556-0123** Fax: **(703) 917-4251**

E-Mail: **CCIHdirector@aol.com** Web: **www.ccih.org**

Description: The mission of Christian Connections for International Health (CCIH) is to promote international health from a Christian perspective. CCIH has an online listing of organizations which recruit volunteers for work overseas as well as links to organizations with information about additional overseas opportunities. The website also hosts a forum for discussion and networking with Christian organizations and individuals working in international health.

Christian Foundation for Children and Aging

Address: **1 Elmwood Ave., Kansas City, KS 66103-3798 U.S.A.**

Phone: **(800) 875-6564 or (913) 384-6500** Fax: **(913) 384-2211**

E-Mail: **mail@cfcausa.org** Web: **www.cfcausa.org**

Description: CFCA is a lay Catholic organization creating relationships between sponsors in the United States and children and elderly people in 25 developing nations around the world. Funding for travel and room and board is not provided. There are no religious requirements for volunteers, but Spanish is required for some placements. Terms of service range from 6 months to 2 years.

Cooperative for American Relief Everywhere, Inc.

Address: **151 Ellis Street, Atlanta, GA 30303 U.S.A.**

Phone: **(404) 681-2552** Fax: **(404) 589-2651**

E-Mail: **info@care.org** Web: **www.care.org**

Description: CARE International is a secular international relief and development organization that serves individuals and families in the poorest communities in the world. In regards to health, CARE is not a direct service provider and does not place volunteers in underserved areas. Instead, CARE partners with the ministry of health or other organizations to build their capacity for better care. Drawing strength from its global diversity, resources, and experience, CARE promotes innovative solutions and is an advocate for global responsibility. We facilitate lasting change by strengthening capacity for self-help, providing economic opportunity, delivering relief in emergencies, influencing policy decisions at all levels, and addressing discrimination in all its forms. CARE International seeks employees who are health care or public health personnel. There are no opportunities for students.

Corporate Accountability International (formerly INFACT)

Address: **46 Plympton Street, Boston, MA 02118 U.S.A.**

Phone: **(617) 695-2525 or 800 688-8797** Fax: **(617) 695-2626**

E-Mail: **info@stopcorporateabuse.org** Web: **www.infact.org**

Description: Corporate Accountability International (formerly INFACT) works to lead the grassroots challenge to unwarranted corporate influence for years to come. The organization wants to bring an end to all life-threatening abuses committed by transnational organizations. CAI has accomplished much since its founding in 1977, from the Nestle Boycott of the 1970s and 80s over infant formula marketing, to the GE Boycott of the 1980s and 90s to curb nuclear weapons production and promotion, to the Boycott of Kraft Macaroni & Cheese—a product of tobacco giant Philip Morris. CAI also tries to shed light on the overwhelming influence that corporations have on U.S. legislators and the entire electoral process.

Council on International and Public Affairs

Address: **777 United Nations Press, Suite 3C, New York, NY 10017 U.S.A.**

Phone: **(800) 316-2739** Fax: **(800) 316-2739**

E-Mail: Web: **www.cipa-apex.org**

Description: The Council on International and Public Affairs was founded in 1954 and is a non-profit research, education, and publishing group. It seeks to further the study and public understanding of problems and affairs of the peoples of the United States and other nations of the world through conferences, research, seminars and workshops, publications, and other means. The organization operates several programs that analyze public policy issues, particularly issues pertaining to the health and well-being of poor people. Examples of the organizations efforts include the Apex Press; the Program on Economic Democracy; the Corporate Accountability Project; the International Toxics Project; and much more.

Doctors on Call for Service (DOCS)

Address: **PO Box 24597, St. Simon Island, GA 31522 U.S.A.**

Phone: **(912) 634-0065** Fax: **(912) 638-2014**

E-Mail: **docs@docs.org** Web: **docs.org**

Description: Doctors on Call for Service, Inc. (DOCS), is a charitable organization established to assist medical professionals in volunteering their services to other medical professionals in needy countries around the world. DOCS gives volunteers the opportunity to mentor and encourage foreign physicians as they share insight and practical experience.

Family Health International

Address: **P.O. Box 13950, Research Triangle Park, NC 27709 U.S.A.**

Phone: **(919) 544-7040** Fax: **(919) 544-7261**

E-Mail: **services@fhi.org** Web: **www.fhi.org/en/index.htm**

Description: Formed in 1971, Family Health International (FHI) is among the largest and most established nonprofit organizations active in international public health with a mission to improve lives worldwide through research, education, and services in family health. We manage research and field activities in more than 70 countries to meet the public health needs of some of the world's most vulnerable people. We work with a wide variety of partners including governmental and nongovernmental organizations, research institutions, community groups, and the private sector.

Fifty Years is Enough

Address: **3628 12th St NE, Washington, DC 20017 U.S.A.**

Phone: **(202) 463-2265** Fax: **(202) 636-4238**

E-Mail: **info@50years.org** Web: **www.50years.org**

Description: Fifty Years is Enough was founded on the 50th Anniversary of the World Bank and the International Monetary Fund (IMF) with the objective of changing the policies and practices of the two institutions. With a network of more than 200 organizations, the organization is committed to increasing people's ability to shape global economic policies. "We call for the immediate suspension of the policies and practices of the International Monetary Fund (IMF) and World Bank Group which have caused widespread poverty, inequality, and suffering among the world's peoples and damage to the world's environment. Substantial responsibility for the unjust world economic system lies with those institutions and the World Trade Organization (WTO). We note that these institutions are anti-democratic, controlled by the G-7 governments, and that their policies have benefited international private sector financiers, transnational corporations, and corrupt officials and politicians."

Flying Physicians Association

Address: **PO Box 677427, Orlando, FL 32867 U.S.A.**

Phone: **(407) 359-1423** Fax: **(407) 359-1167**

E-Mail: **FPAHQ@aol.com** Web: **FPADRS.org**

Description: As physicians, with knowledge in the effects of Flying (physical, mental and emotional), we strive to increase safety and to preserve health by providing basic information through example and teaching to the medical profession, to aircrews and to the public at large, influencing members of the medical profession to fly and to develop expertise in the effects of flying, which will result in better utilization of aircraft for emergency services, better cooperation with state and federal aviation agencies, better qualified aviation medical examiners and more significant research.

Foundation Center, The

Address: **79 Fifth Avenue, New York, NY 10003-3076 U.S.A.**

Phone: **(212) 620-4230 or (800) 424-9836** Fax: **(212) 807-3677**

E-Mail: **see Web site** Web: **fdncenter.org/**

Description: The Foundation Center's mission is to support and improve philanthropy by promoting public understanding of the field and helping grantseekers succeed. Services provided by the center include compiled information and research on trends in the U.S. philanthropy field; education and training for grantseekers; and provided access to important tools through the worldwide web and five grant library locations. The Foundation Center is a powerful tool that serves grantseekers, grantmakers, researchers, policymakers, the media, and the general public.

Francois-Xavier Bagnoud Center for Health and Human Rights, The

Address: **Harvard School of Public Health, 651 Huntington Ave, 7th Floor, Boston, MA 02115 U.S.A.**

Phone: **(617) 432-0656** Fax: **(617) 432-4310**

E-Mail: **fxbcenter@igc.org** Web: **www.hsph.harvard.edu/fxbcenter/**

Description: The François-Xavier Bagnoud Center for Health and Human Rights was the first academic center to focus exclusively on health and human rights, combining the academic strengths of research and teaching with a strong commitment to service and policy development. Its faculty work at international and national levels through collaboration and partnerships with health and human rights practitioners, governmental and nongovernmental organizations, academic institutions, and international agencies. They strive to expand knowledge through scholarship, professional training, and public education; develop domestic and international policy focusing on the relationship between health and human rights in a global perspective; and engage scholars, public health and human rights practitioners, public officials, donors, and activists in the health and human rights movement.

Freedom from Debt Coalition (FDC)

Address: **34 Matiaga St, Central District, Quezon City 1100 Philippines**

Phone: **(632) 921-1985** Fax: **(632) 924-6399**

E-Mail: **mail@freedomfromdebtcoaliton.org** Web: **www.freedomfromdebtcoalition.org**

Description: The Freedom from Debt Coalition brings individuals, organizations and chapters from throughout the Philippines together to call for debt relief within the country. The members are united in a mission to help the Philippines recover from debt and structural adjustment programs. The FDC believes in economic development as a means towards providing the material requisites to ensure that people can live with integrity and dignity. Since 1988, the Freedom from Debt Coalition has challenged anti-poor and anti-development World Bank/IMF policies in the Philippines. The Coalition does research, provides forums for discussing debt reform and sustainable development, and participates in global campaigns to undo World Bank/IMF-induced damage.

Fresh Start Surgical Gifts, Inc.

Address: **2011 Palomar Airport Rd, Suite 206, Carlsbad, CA 92009 U.S.A.**

Phone: **(760) 944-7774 or (800) 551-1003** Fax: **(760) 944-1729**

E-Mail: **freshstart@freshstart.org** Web: **www.freshstart.org/**

Description: Fresh Start's goal is to answer the hopes of children and their families by providing reconstructive surgery primarily to children who suffer from physical deformities caused by birth defects, accidents, abuse, or disease. Fresh Start treats patients at sites in the United States and India, with the clinical staff volunteering their time and expertise. Patients are referred in from the U.S., Mexico and India and all medical procedures are provided by Fresh Start. They will evaluate any reasonable referrals from anywhere in the world. There are three criteria for acceptance: (1) the condition is fixable or improvable; (2) the condition results from a birth defect, an accident, abuse or disease; and (3) that all other resources have been exhausted and correction will enhance the patient's life. Volunteers can serve for 1 week and a second language is preferred, but not required.

Fulbright Scholar Award, Council for the International Exchange of Students

Address: **3007 Tilden St., NW, Suite 5L, Washington, DC 20008-3009 U.S.A.**

Phone: **(202) 686-4000** Fax: **(202) 362-3442**

E-Mail: **scholars@cies.iie.org** Web: **www.cies.org**

Description: The Fulbright Program, recognized as the U.S. government's flagship program in international educational exchange, was proposed to the U.S. Congress in 1945 for promoting "mutual understanding between the people of the United States and the people of other countries of the world." The program would provide grantees and their hosts the opportunity to better comprehend the institutions, cultures and societies of other parts of the world. Fulbright grants are made to U.S. citizens and nationals of other countries for a variety of educational activities, primarily university lecturing, advanced research, graduate study and teaching in elementary and secondary schools.

Global Exchange

Address: **2017 Mission Street, #303, San Francisco, CA 94110 U.S.A.**

Phone: **(415) 255-7296** Fax: **(415) 255-7498**

E-Mail: **info@globalexchange.org** Web: **www.globalexchange.org**

Description: Global Exchange is an international human rights organization dedicated to promoting environmental, political and social justice. Since being founded in 1988, the exchange has strived to educate people on the status of political, economic and human rights issues in developing coutnries. The Exchange develops newsletters, arranges speakers and does media appearances. In addition, it operates two craft stores to support fair trade and provide income for thousands of craftspeople in developing countries. The Exchange also sends volunteers to conflict zones to influence human rights outcomes.

Global Health Council

Address: **1701 K Street NW, Suite 600, Washington, DC 20006 U.S.A.**

Phone: **(202) 833-5900** Fax: **(202) 833-0075**

E-Mail: **ghc@globalhealth.org** Web: **www.globalhealth.org**

Description: The Global Health Council is the world's largest membership alliance dedicated to saving lives by improving health throughout the world. The Council works to ensure that all who strive for improvement and equity in global health have the information and resources they need to succeed. To achieve this goal, the Council serves as the voice for action on global health issues and the voice for progress in the global health field. The Council informs and educates opinion leaders, policy-makers, the media and concerned citizens about crucial global health issues. The Council mobilizes hundreds of thousands through grassroots efforts; advocates for increased resources and sound policy; generates newspaper, television and radio coverage on key issues;and hold conferences to bring people together on such issues.

Global Health Education Consortium (GHEC)

Address: **305 W. Broadway #332, New York, NY 10013 U.S.A.**

Phone: **(646) 831-3220** Fax: **(646) 839-2707**

E-Mail: **info@globalhealth-ec.org** Web: **www.globalhealth-ec.org**

Description: GHEC is a consortium of faculty and health care educators dedicated to international health education in U.S. and Canadian medical schools and residency programs. Formed in 1991, its mission is to foster international health medical education in four program areas: curriculum, clinical training, career development, and international education policy. GHEC is working to facilitate international educational experiences and exchanges for medical students and residents, encourage the development of courses and curricula related to international health, promote the sharing of resources and information about international health among the members, facilitate the development of international health career tracks and short term work/service/learning opportunities for students, residents, and faculty, develop appropriate positions on international medical education policy, including appropriate implementation strategies, and develop and maintain an active collaborative liaison with other organizations interested in international medical education. Members participate in medical education policy, international health education electives and curriculum, and international heath institutional partnerships. Lengths of term vary from 2 weeks to 2 years, and there may be some funding available.

Global Lawyers and Physicians

Address: **Department of Health Law, Bioethics and Human Rights/B.U. 715 Albany St., Boston, MA 02118 U.S.A.**

Phone: **(617) 638-4626** Fax: **(617) 414-1464**

E-Mail: **glp@bu.edu** Web: **www.glphr.org**

Description: Global Lawyers and Physicians is a non-profit non-governmental organization that focuses on health and human rights issues. GLP was formed to reinvigorate the collaboration of the legal and medical/public health professions to protect the human rights and dignity of all persons. Our mission is to work at the local, national, and international levels through collaboration and partnerships with individuals, NGOs, IGOs, and governments on issues such as the global implementation of the health-related provisions of the Universal Declaration of Human Rights and the Covenants on Civil and Political Rights and Economic, Social, and Cultural Rights, with a focus on health and human rights, patient rights, and human experimentation. Global Lawyers and Physicians: provides information and resources about human rights; serves as a network and referral source for professionals working on health-related human rights issues; and provides support and assistance in developing, implementing, and advocating public policies and legal remedies that protect and enhance human rights in health.

GW Associates

Address: **702 South Beech, Syracuse, NY 13210 U.S.A.**

Phone: **(315) 476-3396** Fax: **(603) 590-8273**

E-Mail: **pwirth@ican.net** Web: **www.peterwirth.net**

Description: GW Associates advises non-profit organizations on how to use mass media and publicity as a resource and how to affect public opinion on important issues. Through a media training workshop that includes how to write news releases, establish relations with reporters and arrange editorial board meetings, among other things, GW Associates makes the non-profit organization more media savvy.

Harvard University School of Public Health, Department of Population and Int'l Health

Address: **665 Huntington Ave., Boston, MA 02115 U.S.A.**

Phone: **(617) 432-0686** Fax: **(617) 432-1251**

E-Mail: **takemi@hsph.harvard.edu** Web: **www.hsph.harvard.edu/takemi**

Description: To create better methods for mobilizing and using health resources in both rich and poor countries. To promote cooperative research and comparative analysis of health policies and programs in different countries. To contribute to individual and institutional development by bringing together leading health professionals and scholars from many nations for research and training.

Healing the Children National Headquarters

Address: **2624 W Beacon Avenue, Spokane, WA 99208 U.S.A.**

Phone: **(509) 327-4281** Fax: **(509) 327-4284**

E-Mail: **national-htc@worldnet.att.net** Web: **www.healingthechildren.org**

Description: Healing the Children provides volunteer medical treatment for foreign children in need in both Africa and South Amercia, as well as the United States. The National Headquarters coordinates placements and refers placements for the 12 regional Healing the Children chapters.

Health Action International (HAI)

Address: **1053 NJ Amsterdam, Amsterdam, The Netherlands**

Phone: **31 (020) 683-3684** Fax: **31 (020) 685-5002**

E-Mail: **info@haiweb.org** Web: **www.haiweb.org**

Description: HAI is a non-profit, global network of health, development, consumer and other public interest groups in more than 70 countries working for a more rational use of medicinal drugs. HAI represents the interests of consumers in drug policy and believes that all drugs marketed should be acceptably safe, effective, affordable and meet real medical needs. HAI campaigns for better controls on drug promotion and the provision of balanced, independent information for prescribers and consumers. The HAI provides public access to a Medicine Prices database on its website (www.haiweb.org).

Health Rights Connection

Address: **c/o Physicians for Human Rights, 100 Boylston Street, Suite 702, Boston, MA 02116 U.S.A.**

Phone: **(617) 695-0041** Fax: **(617) 695-0307**

E-Mail: **phrusa@phrusa.org** Web: **www.phrusa.org/healthrights/index.html**

Description: The Health Rights Connection is a service of Physicians for Human Rights - USA that provides information and reports from colleagues of PHR-USA. The purpose the HealthRights Connection is to provide web space for organizations that lack web sites of their own, as well as to serve as a resource for all manner of health and human rights information. Organizations with their own web sites are encouraged to send links to PHR so that they may be displayed here and receive increased exposure. Medical associations working on health and human rights related projects are also invited to submit materials for display on this site.

Institute for Policy Studies (IPS)

Address: **733 15th St NW, Suite 1020, Washington, DC 20005 U.S.A.**

Phone: **(202) 234-9382** Fax: **(202) 387-7915**

E-Mail: **scott@ips-dc.org** Web: **www.ips-dc.org**

Description: The Institute for Policy Studies is the nation's oldest multi-issue progressive think tank. Since 1963, the Institute has worked with social movements to forge viable and sustainable policies to promote democracy, justice, human rights, and diversity. IPS played key roles in the Civil Rights and anti-war movements in the 1960s, the women's and environmental movements in the 1970s, the anti-apartheid and anti-intervention movements in the 1980s, and the fair trade and environmental justice movements today. Based in Washington, DC, IPS has links to activists and scholars across the nation and around the world, and it serves as a bridge between progressive forces in government and grass-roots activists, and between movements in the U.S. and those in the developing world. IPS provides an alternative voice, helping the least powerful to be heard in the government and in the press.

Interaction

Address: **1717 Massachusetts Ave., N.W., Suite 701, Washington, DC 20036 U.S.A.**

Phone: **(202) 667-8227** Fax: **(202) 667-8236**

E-Mail: **ia@interaction.org** Web: **www.interaction.org/**

Description: InterAction is the largest alliance of U.S.-based international development and humanitarian nongovernmental organizations. With more than 160 members operating in every developing country, we work to overcome poverty, exclusion and suffering by advancing social justice and basic dignity for all. InterAction convenes and coordinates its members can collectively influence policy and debate on issues affecting tens of millions of people worldwide. InterAction's "Global Work" publication highlights volunteer, internship, and fellowship opportunities in international development. Providing information on opportunities from nearly 100 member organizations working in 120 countries, including the U.S., this is the perfect guide for students, mid-career adventures, retired goodwill seekers and persons of any age wishing to donate their time and skills while creating effective change in a developing world.

Interchurch Medical Assistance

Address: **P.O. Box 429, New Windsor, MD 21776 U.S.A.**

Phone: **(410) 635-8720 or (877) 241-7952** Fax: **(410) 635-8726**

E-Mail: **pattypickett@interchurch.org** Web: **www.interchurch.org/medical/index.php**

Description: I.M.A. supplies medicines and medical supplies to health professionals and medical mission teams for short-term, volunteer overseas medical service trips. I.M.A. does not sponsor volunteer medical service teams. I.M.A.'s Member agencies offer many volunteer service opportunities. I.M.A. offers donated medicines and medical supplies to medical service teams through its General Inventory program. Products offered are based on availability. Administrative, packing and shipping fees are calculated based on the order.

International Federation of Medical Students' Association

Address: **IFMSA General Secretariat, c/o WMA, BP 63, Ferney-Voltaire CEDEX 01212 France**

Phone: Fax: **+33-450-405937**

E-Mail: **gs@ifmsa.org** Web: **www.ifmsa.org**

Description: An independent non-political association of medical student associations worldwide, IFMSA catalogs information and helps organize student clinical and research exchanges, and through six standing committees, is involved in medical, public health, professional exchange and other projects. IFMSA also has information on grants and other financial aid opportunities for students wishing to work on overseas projects.

International Foundation for Education and Self-Help

Address: **5040 East Shea Boulevard, Suite 260, Phoenix, AZ 85254-4610 U.S.A.**

Phone: **(480) 443-1800** Fax: **(480) 443-1824**

E-Mail: **ifesh@ifesh.org or info@ifesh.org** Web: **www.ifesh.org**

Description: IFESH focuses on empowering individuals of developing nations through community-based programs in the areas of literacy, education, vocational training, agriculture, nutrition and health care. The organization seeks to help people develop and use technical skills, regardless of their race, color, creed, or sex. The primary area of concern is sub-Saharan Africa. Through its International Fellows Program (IFP) the Foundation has provided nine-month overseas internships for Americans who are graduate students or recent college and university graduates. Fellows assist international nongovernmental organizations working in community development settings.

International Medical Equipment Collaborative

Address: **PO Box 394, Portsmouth, NH 03801 U.S.A.**

Phone: **(978) 388-5522** Fax: **(978) 388-5312**

E-Mail: **imec@imecamerica.org** Web: **www.imecamerica.org/**

Description: The International Medical Equipment Collaborative (IMEC) is a non-profit group in New Hampshire that began in 1995. They ask American hospitals and healthcare companies to donate their surplus equipment, linens, supplies and educational materials to doctors and nurses in developing countries. IMEC works with a global network of established NGOs, in-country health systems, and church groups to identify the neediest health facilities in the world's poorest countries. They deliver medical equipment and supplies to help local providers provide better care.

International Medical Volunteers Association (IMVA)

Address: **P.O. Box 205, Woodville, MA 01784 U.S.A.**

Phone: **(508) 435-7377** Fax: **(508) 497-9568**

E-Mail: **info@imva.org** Web: **www.imva.org/index.html**

Description: The International Medical Volunteers Association (IMVA) is a non-profit organization that promotes, facilitates, and supports voluntary medical activity through education and information exchange. Our interests are primarily in developing countries. While we do not send or sponsor volunteers ourselves, we act as a clearinghouse of detailed information, profiling over 100 organizations that seek healthcare volunteers. We also maintain a Volunteer Registry, where organizations can find people with skills they need. We facilitate volunteering by providing educational materials about health problems in various parts of the world and advice on how to function effectively while working abroad. Most importantly, we attempt to motivate healthcare workers to assist those most in need. In addition to assisting volunteer seeking groups, principally non-governmental organizations (NGOs), in locating volunteers, the IMVA provides a forum for project cooperation, information, equipment, and supply exchange. All services are free.

International Physicians for the Prevention of Nuclear War (IPPNW)

Address: **727 Massachusetts Ave., Cambridge, MA 02139 U.S.A.**

Phone: **(617) 868-5050** Fax: **(617) 868-2560**

E-Mail: **ippnwbos@ippnw.org** Web: **www.ippnw.org**

Description: IPPNW is a non-partisan global federation of medical organizations dedicated to research, education, and advocacy relevant to the prevention of nuclear war. IPPNW seeks to prevent all wars, to promote non-violent conflict resolution, and to minimize the effects of war and preparations for war on health, development, and the environment. Winner of the 1985

Nobel Peace Prize, IPPNW warns all of humanity that nuclear war would cause an epidemic that could not be taken back, with no solutions or cures. Today, IPPNW has extended its resources and efforts to the promotion of alternatives to violence and armed conflict.

International Volunteer Registry - Foundation of the American Academy of Ophthalmology

Address: **655 Beach St., San Francisco, CA 94109-1336 U.S.A.**

Phone: **(415) 561-8500 or (415) 447-0281** Fax: **(415) 561-8567**

E-Mail: **wovaitt@aao.org** Web: **www.aao.org**

Description: The International Volunteer Registry is a computer program that was designed to assist with the enhancement of eye care services in developing nations. The registry connects ophthalmologists and other eye care professionals who are interested in volunteering their skills and expertise to provide eye care services in developing nations with organizations that coordinate medical misisons, and educational institutions in developing nations that need professional eye care personnel. The computer matches your particular skills and interests to the needs of organizations, based on geographic preference, length of service, type of personnel, type of service, specialized training, and financial assistance.

Jubilee 2000/USA

Address: **222 East Capitol Street, NE, Washington, DC 20003-1036 U.S.A.**

Phone: **(202) 783-3566** Fax: **(202) 546-4468**

E-Mail: **coord@j2000usa.org** Web: **www.jubileeusa.org**

Description: Jubilee USA Network began as Jubilee 2000/USA in 1997 when a diverse gathering of people and organizations came together in response to the international call for Jubilee debt cancellation. Now over 60 organizations including labor, churches, religious communities and institutions, AIDS activists, trade campaigners and over 9,000 individuals are active members of the Jubilee USA Network. Together, these members create a strong, diverse and growing network dedicated to working for a world free of debt for billions of people. Jubilee USA continues to protest international governance and lending agencies by coordinating grassroots organizations and media campaigns, as well as creating protest petitions directed at the governments of the world's wealthiest and most influential countries.

Lingua Service Worldwide, Ltd.

Address: **75 Prospect Street, Suite 4, Huntington, NY 11743 U.S.A.**

Phone: **(800) 394-5327 or (631) 424-0777** Fax: **(631) 271-3441**

E-Mail: **itctravel@worldnet.att.net** Web: **www.linguaserviceworldwide.com/**

Description: Lingua Service Worldwide, Ltd., an independent foreign language program agency, represents private foreign language schools all over the world that specialize in offering "full immersion" language program opportunities. These foreign language study abroad programs have been developed with the purpose of teaching a new language within its own setting in a short period of time. Language immersion is available in French, Portuguese, Japanese, Chinese, Spanish, Russian, Italian, and Greek.

Lions Club International Foundation

Address: **300 22nd Street, Oak Brook, IL 60523-8842 U.S.A.**

Phone: **(630) 571-5466 x383** Fax: **(630) 571-8890**

E-Mail: **lcif@lionsclubs.org** Web: **www.lionsclubs.org**

Description: LCIF funds Lion-sponsored medical missions. The projects are initiated at the grass-roots level by our 43,000 clubs. LCIF does not have an active role in developing/organizing individual missions—we only consider grant requests to support these missions. In addition, each mission team must include at least one Lion member plus the active involvement of a Lions Club in the host country.

LCIF's mission is to support the efforts of Lions clubs around the world in serving their local comunities and the world community through humanitarian service, major disaster relief and vocational assistance programs.

MAP International

Address: **2200 Glynco Parkway, P.O. Box 215000, Brunswick, GA 31521-5000 U.S.A.**

Phone: **(800) 225-8550 ext. 6671 or (912) 265-6010** Fax: **(912) 265-6170**

E-Mail: **lcrosby@map.org or map@map.org** Web: **www.map.org**

Description: MAP International is a non-profit, Christian global health organization whose mission is to provide enabling services which promote total health care for needy people in the developing world. Today MAP International provides nearly 300 Church-related hospitals and clinics, 70 agencies, and some 600 U.S. health care workers and physicians every year with donated medicines and medical supplies from approximately 90 pharmaceutical and medical supply companies to provide health for the world's poor.

MedShare International

Address: **5053 Chatooga Drive, Lithonia, GA 30038-2301 U.S.A.**

Phone: **(770) 323-5858** Fax: **(770) 323-4301**

E-Mail: **abshort@medshare.org or info@medshare.org** Web: **www.medshare.org**

Description: MedShare International is a non-profit organization based in metro Atlanta, Georgia that collects surplus medical supplies and transports them to developing countries around the world. MedShare sorts, evaluates, classifies, labels and redistributes these supplies to healthcare institutions and medical teams. Organizations or teams traveling abroad should contact MedShare for assistance. MedShare has its own biomedical technicians who evaluate and repair equipment; only appropriate equipment is sent. It also has a strong track record of sending only locally appropriate supplies abroad. Since its founding in late 1998, the organization has shipped many millions of dollars worth of unused medical supplies to developing countries.

Mission Aviation Fellowship

Address: **1849 N. Wabash Avenue, Redlands, CA 92374 U.S.A.**

Phone: **(909) 794-1151 or (800) 359-7623** Fax: **(909) 794-3016**

E-Mail: **maf-us@maf.org** Web: **www.maf.org/**

Description: With a fleet of 56 aircraft taking off from 41 bases worldwide, our pilots can travel across rough, hostile terrain that could take days or even weeks to travel. MAF also provides telecommunications services in many countries — like electronic mail, satellite phones, HF data radio and other wireless systems. Imagine a missionary doctor struggling to save a person in a jungle with a rare disease. Empowered by the internet he can access the latest treatment data, save a life and demonstrate the compassion of Christ. MAF also provides warehousing, shipping, and demographic mapping services for many Christian agencies.

Mission Finders

Address: **P.O. Box 356, Sunol, CA 94586 U.S.A.**

Phone: **(208) 723-4657** Fax: **(815) 371-1660**

E-Mail: Web: **www.missionfinder.org/medstudents.htm**

Description: We are evangelical Christians. We are not affiliated with any church or mission organization, and unless noted otherwise, the organizations we list aren't either, to the best of our knowledge. Contained on the site are a database of volunteer service opportunities for Medical, Pre-med, Dental, Nursing, and EMT students. The organizations listed specifically invite medical students on their projects. There are also some ideas of where to get funds, rotation assignments, and specialty training.

Missionary Expediters, Inc.

Address: **225 Arabella St, New Orleans, LA 70115 U.S.A.**

Phone: **(800) 299-6363** Fax: **(800) 643-6363**

E-Mail: **mx@solvenet.com** Web: **www.solvenet.com/**

Description: Missionary Expediters, Inc., specializes in customized international transportation services "to the strange places of the world." They will deliver Relief Aid Cargoes; Personal Effects & Household Goods; and Non-routine Commercial Cargoes via ocean, air, motor and rail. They also have an invaluable booklet that answers most questions about getting supplies to developing countries. An on-line budget calculator will give an estimate of the approximate cost of shipping anything anywhere. They also have step-by-step instructions for how to collect, box, and ship supplies.

Operation Crossroads Africa, Inc.

Address: **PO Box 5570, New York, NY 10027 U.S.A.**

Phone: **(212) 289-1949** Fax: **(212) 289-2526**

E-Mail: **oca@igc.org** Web: **operationcrossroadsafrica.org**

Description: Operations Crossroads sends volunteers to Africa to live and work on community-based rural initiatives for six weeks. Operations Crossroads has sent over 11,000 people to work in Africa over 45 years and was hailed as the "progenitor of the Peace Corps" by President John F. Kennedy. Programs are in english and french speaking countries and some projects are health-related.

Outreach International

Address: **PO Box 210, Independence, MO 64051-0210 U.S.A.**

Phone: **(888) 833-1235 or (816) 833-0883** Fax: **(816) 833-0103**

E-Mail: **info@outreachmail.org** Web: **outreach-international.org/**

Description: Outreach International (OUTREACH) was organized to receive and disburse funds and other resources for community development projects focusing on enabling the poor to become self-reliant. The development emphasis was on releasing dormant human potential through projects of livelihood, health, education and sustainable community development. Although in the past they have funded a program which trained local health care workers in Zambia and Zaire, it is not anticipated that this will be expanded, and OI remains primarily a funding organization.

OXFAM America

Address: **26 West St., Boston, MA 02111 U.S.A.**

Phone: **(617) 482-1211 or (800) 776-9326** Fax: **(617) 728-2594**

E-Mail: **info@oxfamamerica.org** Web: **www.oxfamamerica.org/**

Description: Oxfam seeks to find lasting solutions to poverty, hunger, and social justice around the world. Its philosophy is that partnerships between external support and local community groups are essential and need to be sustained over time. International health care service opportunities are related to Oxfam's disaster relief efforts in various parts of the world, in which Oxfam's work includes health workshops on disease prevention and preparation of communities for future crises. Oxfam does not appoint health care personnel to communities in need, but instead seeks volunteers interested in providing services for disaster relief.

Oxfam Great Britain

Address: **274 Banbury Road, Oxford OX27DZ U.K.**

Phone: **44 1865 311 311 or 44 1865 312289**
Fax: **44 1865 312 600 or 44 1865 312 580**

E-Mail: **oxfam@oxfam.org.uk**
Web: **www.oxfam.org.uk/**

Description: Oxfam International, founded in 1995, is an international confederation of 11 autonomous non-government organizations. Member organizations are of diverse cultures, history, and language, but share the commitment to working for an end to the waste and injustice of poverty - both in longer-term development work and in times of urgent humanitarian need. The individual Oxfams work in different ways but have a common purpose: addressing the structural causes of poverty and related injustice. The Oxfams work primarily through local organizations in more than 100 countries.

Partners for Development

Address: **1320 Fenwick Lane, Suite 406, Silver Spring, MD 20910 U.S.A.**

Phone: **(301) 608-0426**
Fax: **(301) 608-0822**

E-Mail: **pfdinfo@pfd.org**
Web: **www.partnersfordevelopment.org/**

Description: PFD's mission is to work with underserved populations in developing countries and improve their quality of life. Partners for Development gives the greatest importance to the role of partners in every aspect of our work. This includes a deep commitment to involving local counterparts in needs assessment, program design, and implementation. PFD's partner-oriented approach also includes working with and harnessing the resources of the international community in meeting the needs of vulnerable populations. With programs currently in Cambodia, Nigeria, and Bosnia and Herzegovina, PFD is addressing local needs in the areas of health, agriculture, water and sanitation, veterinary health, and credit.

Partners In Health

Address: **641 Huntington Ave, 1st Floor, Boston, MA 02115 U.S.A.**

Phone: **(617) 432-5256**
Fax: **(617) 432-5300**

E-Mail: **info@pih.org**
Web: **www.pih.org**

Description: Partners In Health operates on the belief that health is a basic human right. "By establishing long-term relationships with sister organizations based in settings of poverty, Partners In Health strives to achieve two overarching goals: to bring the benefits of modern medical science to those most in need of them and to serve as an antidote to despair." With projects in Latin America, the Caribbean, Russia, Africa, and the United States, Partners In Health works with community-based organizations to address issues such as AIDS, tuberculosis and women's health issues. The organization is also active in the health policy realm, trying to support initiatives on a global level.

Partners in Restoring Vision and Improving Lives

Address: **222 Ridgewood Drive, San Rafael, CA 94901 U.S.A.**

Phone: **(415) 453-9123**
Fax: **(415) 454-3178**

E-Mail: **info@restoringvision.org**
Web: **www.restoringvision.org**

Description: Partners in Restoring Vision and Improving Lives supplies reading and sunglasses to groups helping in less developed countries and low income seniors in the US. Since our beginning in late 2003, we have supplied over 50,000 glasses to people around the world. Many different organizations conduct "missions" to under-developed countries. These missions include eye exams and the distribution of (usually) recycled glasses. We collect and distribute glasses to organizations who can give them to the less fortunate.

Peace Corps, Corp Headquarters

Address: **1111 20th Street, NW, Washington, DC 20526 U.S.A.**

Phone: **(800) 424-8580 or (202) 692-1430** Fax: **(202) 692-1431**

E-Mail: **dcinfo@peacecorps.gov or hotline@peacecorps.gov** Web: **www.peacecorps.gov**

Description: The Peace Corps is the United States government program founded by President John F. Kennedy in 1961. It sends volunteers of all ages to serve in 72 developing countries for mostly two-year terms. Few health providers serve through the Peace Corps; most volunteers are college aged and teach in the areas of education, youth outreach and community development, the environment, and information technology. Some volunteers work in HIV/AIDS awareness, or other health-related projects. Returning Peace Corps volunteers receive preferential job placement through the US government. Non-Competitive Eligibility (NCE) is a special mechanism through which returning Peace Corps volunteers can be appointed to federal positions without competing with the general public in order to be hired. Many work in USAID or elsewhere in the Department of State. The Peace Corps has an excellent website that addresses most concerns.

Public Health Foundation

Address: **1300 L St. NW, Suite 300, Washington, DC 20005 U.S.A.**

Phone: **(202) 218-4400** Fax: **(202) 218-4409**

E-Mail: **info@phf.org** Web: **www.phf.org**

Description: The Public Health Foundation operates a distance learning clearinghouse that may be of interest to those who want to serve internationally. The website is at www.trainingfinder.org and lists courses of all types, particularly focused on public health. It is sponsored by a group of non-profit organizations and the US government.

Rotary Foundation of Rotary International

Address: **One Rotary Center, 1560 Sherman Ave., Evanston, IL 60201 U.S.A.**

Phone: **(847) 866-3000** Fax: **(847) 328-8554 or (847) 328-8281**

E-Mail: **feedback@rotaryintl.org or futae@rotaryintl.org** Web: **www.rotary.org**

Description: Rotary International (RI) is a worldwide organization offering a multitude of humanitarian, intercultural, and educational programs which seek to improve human conditions and advance the ultimate goal of world peace and understanding. RI currently has 1.2 million members (Rotarians) worldwide who represent 31,000 Rotary Foundation clubs and 167 different countries. Rotary has long funded the initiative to eliminate polio. RI runs nine structured programs with international service opportunities, including health care, where they strive to provide essential care to millions in need. Rotarians volunteer through one of the nine programs while also acting as ambassadors of fellowship and goodwill. Rotarians are well established in most developing countries, with clear service objectives for each club, at the discretion of the club and that year's president. Rotarians serve as invaluable partners in many international development projects, particularly in health. "Service above self" is the Rotary motto.

Samaritan's Purse International Relief

Address: **P.O. Box 3000, Boone, NC 28607 U.S.A.**

Phone: **(828) 262-1980** Fax: **(828) 266-1053**

E-Mail: **info@samaritan.org** Web: **www.samaritanspurse.org**

Description: Samaritan's Purse is a nondenominational evangelical Christian organization providing spiritual and physical aid to hurting people around the world. Since 1970, Samaritan's Purse has helped meet needs of people who are victims of war, poverty, natural disasters, disease, and famine with the purpose of sharing God's love through His Son, Jesus Christ. It runs hundreds of projects in more than 100 countries around the world. In addition to organizing conferences, the Prescription for Hope program of Samaritan's Purse supports frontline grassroots HIV/AIDS ministries around the world. The direct service arm of Samaritan's Purse is the World Medical Missions, included elsewhere, that sends doctors, dentists, and residents to serve in poor communities worldwide. A separate program sends college students to its project sites. Samaritan's Purse has a large fund-raising arm and has considerable political impact through Franklin Graham, Jesse Helms, and Bill Frist. The organization serves the Church worldwide to promote the Gospel of the Lord Jesus Christ.

Save the Children Federation

Address: **54 Wilton Rd., PO Box 950, Westport, CT 06880 U.S.A.**

Phone: **(203) 221-4000 or (800) 728-3843** Fax: **(203) 227-5667**

E-Mail: **cmaccorm@savechildren.org** Web: **www.savethechildren.org/**

Description: Save the Children Federation is a secular organization that provides services to families and children in need, primarily by relying on local professionals within the country where the services are provided. Occasionally, however, the organization sends ex-patriate health care personnel for relatively short-term (1-6 month) stays. The federation works to improve health care in various countries in Africa, Asia, Europe, and the Americas.

Spanish Language Schools in Latin America (sponsored by Nicaragua Spanish Schools)

Address: **De la Rotonda Bello Horizonte, Apartado SL-145, Managua, Nicaragua**

Phone: **011 505-244-1699 or 011 805-687-9941** Fax: **011 505-244-1699**

E-Mail: **nssmga@ibw.com.ni** Web: **www.ibw.com.ni/~nssmga/guide.htm#mex**

Description: A directory of Spanish immersion programs, SLSLA is the most comprehensive directory of its kind on the web. The schools included represent the majority of Spanish language schools in each country listed. Each school listing has a brief summary of the school's included features and price of its basic four-week program. Schools searchable by country.

Thomas S. Durant, MD, Fellowship for Refugee Medicine, The

Address: **Massachusetts General Hospital, 55 Fruit St., Bartlett 9, Boston, MA 02114 U.S.A.**

Phone: **(617) 724-3874** Fax: **(617) 726-7491**

E-Mail: **see Web site** Web: **www.durantfellowship.org**

Description: The Thomas S. Durant Fellowship in Refugee Medicine is open to health care professionals and staff at the Massachusetts General Hospital. It seeks to honor and celebrate the life, spirit, humor, passion, joy and legacy of an incredible humanitarian by following Durant's example of aiding victims of war, famine and disaster. Durant fellows seek to make a difference in some of the world's bleakest places and under the most challenging circumstances.

UN Volunteers for Peace and Development

Address: **One United Nations Plaza (UN#7), New York, NY 10017 U.S.A.**

Phone: **(212) 906 3639** Fax: **(212) 906 3659**

E-Mail: **rona@unvolunteers.org** Web: **www.unv.org/**

Description: The United Nations Volunteers programme (UNV) is the volunteer arm of the United Nations. Created by the UN General Assembly in 1970 to serve as an operational partner in development cooperation, it mobilizes qualified UN volunteers and promotes people to volunteer in their own countries. The UNV is administered by the United Nations Development Programme (UNDP) and works through UNDP's country offices worldwide. The UN Volunteers programme has arrangements with cooperating organizations, volunteer sending organizations or national focal points in about 40 countries. They help assess volunteer candidates, interview and brief those selected.

United for a Fair Economy (UFE)

Address: **37 Temple Place, 2nd Floor, Boston, MA 02111 U.S.A.**

Phone: **(617) 423-2148** Fax: **(617) 423-0191**

E-Mail: **info@faireconomy.org** Web: **www.stw.org**

Description: UFE is dedicated to raising awareness that concentrated wealth and power undermine the economy, corrupt democracy, deepen the racial divide, and tear communities apart. They initiatie and support social movements to ensure more equality and to end economic injustices. "United for a Fair Economy is the single most effective group in the country when it comes to publicizing issues of economic injustice, income disparity, the racial underpinnings of the gap between rich and poor, and . . . the yawning chasm between the salaries of corporate CEOs and those of working Americans." — John Nichols, journalist, *The Nation*

United Methodists Volunteers in Mission

Address: **159 Ralph McGill Boulevard Northeast, Suite 305, Atlanta, GA 30308 U.S.A.**

Phone: **(404) 659-5060** Fax: **(404) 659-2977**

E-Mail: **sejinfo@umvim.org** Web: **www.gbgm-umc.org/volunteers**

Description: United Methodist Volunteers in Mission assists volunteer health care organizations and helps develop new ones by maintaining a network of health care volunteers throughout the United Methodist connectional system. UMVIM strives to match potential team members with selected organizations around the world who need medical volunteers. UMVIM also organizes a Medical Fellowship to facilitate and encourage its members to witness to their faith in Jesus Christ while providing volunteer health care services around the world. Training is provided through a variety of workshops to equip the faithful for medical mission work.

United Nations Development Program

Address: **1 United Nations Plaza, New York, NY 10017 U.S.A.**

Phone: **(212) 906-5000** Fax: **(212) 906-5364**

E-Mail: **hq@undp.org** Web: **www.undp.org**

Description: The UNDP helps the UN system and its partners to raise awareness and track progress, while it connects countries to the knowledge and resources needed to achieve these goals. The main focus is helping countries build and share solutions to the challenges of: Democratic Governance; Poverty Reduction; Crisis Prevention and Recovery; Energy and Environment; Information and Communications Technology; and HIV/AIDS. One of the UNDP's most valuable resources is the Human Development Report, which is an independent publication commissioned by UNDP. The annual reports contain realistic analyses of major issues, updated Human Development Indicators that compare the relative levels of human development of over 175 countries, and agendas to help transform development priorities.

University of the Witwatersrand Elective program

Address: **Elective Office, Faculty of H.S., Univ. of the Witwatersrand, 7 York Road, Parktown 2193 South Africa**

Phone: **+27 11 717- 2000** Fax: **+27 11 643- 4318**

E-Mail: **elective@health.wits.ac.za** Web: **www.wits.ac.za/fac/med/elective/index.html**

Description: The University of Witwatersrand is located in the largest metropolitan area and the commercial heart of South Africa. It is recognized nationally and internationally for excellence in teaching, research and service to society. Students from Europe, North America and Australia apply to the Faculty of Health Sciences to complete a wide variety of clinical electives in Johannesburg. Over 500 inquiries are received annually and approximately 200 students are placed in elective clerkships. Basic studies and 1 year of hospital experience required.

West Virginia Department of Health

Address: **State Capitol Complex, Building 3, Room 206, Charleston, WV 25305 U.S.A.**

Phone: **(304) 558-0684** Fax: **(304) 558-1130**

E-Mail: **wvdhhrsecretary@wvdhhr.org** Web: **www.wvdhhr.org**

Description: Our mission is to assist in the development, recruitment, and retention of comptetent primary care providers to serve the people of rural underserved communities in West Virginia and to alleviate and ultimately overcome the State's problem of a substantial maldistribution and shortage of primary care providers in rural communities in West Virginia. Since our office operates a clearing house for both primary care providers and facilities it is impossible to give an accurate accounting of the amount of time each provider is recruited for at a given facility. It is the hope of the West Virginia Division of Recruitment that providers placed will remain at the facility they have been recruited to.

West Virginia University, Byrd Health Sciences Center International Health Program

Address: **PO Box 9164, Morgantown, WV 26506 U.S.A.**

Phone: **(304) 293-5916** Fax: **(304) 293-8677**

E-Mail: **mfisher2@wvu.edu** Web: **www.hsc.wvu.edu/som/tropmed**

Description: Byrd Health Sciences Center facilitates international travel for medical students and faculty at the Robert C. Byrd Health Sciences Center, Morgantown, West Virginia. It also offers a fully accredited 8-week course for Health Care Professionals in Clinical Tropical Medicine and Parasitology every summer.

World Harvest Mission

Address: **100 West Ave. W960, Jenkintown, PA 19046-2697 U.S.A.**

Phone: **(215) 885-1811** Fax: **(215) 885-4762**

E-Mail: **info@whm.org** Web: **www.whm.org**

Description: World Harvest Mission is a mission sending agency that was begun in 1983 and today has over 130 missionaries in 13 countries. Our vision is to see people and communities everywhere being made new by the gospel. To that end, we serve the church by sending people who are being changed by the gospel to begin new churches and strengthen existing churches. We are excited if you are considering career service with WHM. We are always happy to talk and pray with individuals considering serving overseas. We regularly are looking for individuals willing to serve in these areas: doctors, health care workers, and nurses.

WorldScopes (part of AMA Caring for Humanity)

Address: **515 North State Street, Chicago, IL 60610 U.S.A.**

Phone: **(888) 881-6744** Fax: **(312) 464-4799**

E-Mail: **caring@ama-assn.org** Web: **www.caring4humanity.org**

Description: WorldScopes is an AMA Caring for Humanity project that is organizing an effort to equip doctors around the world with stethoscopes. The organization hopes to collect 100,000 stethoscopes from physicians in the United States and then distribute them in concert with humanitarian organizations to needy communities worldwide where medical supplies are scarce.

Appendix A

Useful Web Sites

AEGIS History and Timeline of HIV/AIDS
www.aegis.com/topics/timeline/default.asp
Documents the major events of HIV/AIDS beginning with the first recognized outbreaks in 1978.

American Family Physician
www.aafp.org/afp/980800ap/dick.html
Useful articles on travel medicine.

American Medical Association, Medical Student Section, International Health Database
www.ama-assn.org/ama/pub/category/12675.html
A page with details on international health care opportunities including funding, travel, and organizational information.

Americans and the World
www.americans-world.org/index.cfm
Features results and analysis of Americans polled on international topics.

American Society of Tropical Medicine and Hygiene
www.astmh.org
A comprehensive site devoted to tropical disease medicine, including a directory of travel clinics, funding opportunities, and certification programs.

Amnesty International
www.amnesty.org
An organization devoted to protecting human rights.

AMSA Electives and International Opportunities page
www.amsa.org/global/ih/ihopps.cfm

AMSA International Health Links
www.amsa.org/global/ih/ihres.cfm
American Medical Student Association's page for international health.

The Atlantic
www.theatlantic.com/index/foreign
A great source of fresh information and ideas about "literature, politics, science, and the arts."

Bread for the World-Hunger Basics
www.bread.org/hungerbasics/domestic.html
Facts about poverty and hunger in the United States.

British Medical Journal
www.bmj.com/cgi/collection/travel_medicine
Maintains a constantly updated list of most recent articles related to travel medicine.

Catholic Campaign for Human Development
www.usccb.org/cchd/povertyusa/povfacts.htm
Provides information on the state of poverty in the United States and ways to help.

Center for Disease Control-Media Relations-Public Health Achievements
www.cdc.gov/od/oc/media/tengpha.htm
Links to the CDC's list of the 10 great public health achievements from the 20th century.

Center for Disease Control National Center for Infectious Diseases and Traveler's Health
www.cdc.gov/travel
A great resource for travel information and disease precautions, with a database searchable by region.

Central Intelligence Agency World Factbook
www.cia.gov/cia/publications/factbook/geos/us.html
A great resource for familiarization on a foreign country.

Council on Foreign Relations—Foreign Affairs
www.foreignaffairs.org/current/
A news source from CFR devoted to providing balanced, non-partisan ideas about the world and foreign policy.

The Economist
www.economist.com
An objective source for domestic and world news.

European Court of Human Rights
www.echr.coe.int
Features legal rulings and pending cases from the ECHR and other human rights information.

Foreign Policy in Focus Data Page
www.fpif.org/papers/win_body.html
Index of data corresponding to documents from FPIF.

Foreign Policy in Focus Investments Page
www.fpif.org/indices/topics/financial.html
A page of reports and briefs on global investments and other financial flows.

The François-Xavier Bagnoud Center for Health and Human Rights
www.hsph.harvard.edu/fxbcenter/
An academic center focused exclusively on the interface between health and human rights.

GIDEON
http://gideononline.com
Maintains updated information on global infectious diseases for diagnostic or reference purposes.

Global Health Education Consortium
www.globalhealth-ec.org
Holds conferences designed to train and prepare health care providers for overseas trips.

Global Lawyers and Physicians for Human Rights
www.glphr.org
A group committed to sustaining and improving human rights and global health.

Global Programme for Vaccines and Immunization
www.who.int/vaccines-documents/DocsPDF/www9724.pdf
Suggested guidelines for safe and effective vaccine donations.

Harvard School of Medicine, Department of Social Medicine
www.hms.harvard.edu/dsm/WorkFiles/html/academics/clinical/DSMHI.html#top
Describes the new Division of Social Medicine and Health Inequalities designed to employ medically relevant social science information to improve medical care.

Health Affairs
www.healthaffairs.org/index.php
A public policy journal devoted to health and human welfare.

Healthcare Traveler
www.healthcaretraveler.com/healthcaretraveler
A magazine devoted to traveling health care providers.

Human Rights Internet
www.hri.ca/index.aspx
Contains a catalogue of nongovernmental organizations, human rights databases, and other information.

Human Rights Watch
www.hrw.org
Organization committed to defending human rights, HRW provides information on human rights searchable by country or global issue.

Idealist.org/Action Without Borders
www.idealist.org
A large, interactive database of service organizations and opportunities.

International Campaign to End Genocide
www.genocidewatch.org/Links.htm
Lists member organizations which monitor and aim to prevent genocide.

International Healthcare Opportunities Clearinghouse
http://library.umassmed.edu/ihoc
Contains worldwide listings of international volunteer opportunities and associated programs.

International Medical Corps
www.imcworldwide.org/index.shtml
An international organization dedicated to providing health care training and development programs to needy populations.

International Committee of the Red Cross
www.icrc.org
A humanitarian organization committed to protecting the lives and rights of victims of international war and internal violence.

International Society of Travel Medicine
www.istm.org
Publishes an online directory of travel medicine clinics, as well as the abstracts of the *Journal of Travel Medicine.*

International Travel Healthline
www.travelhealthline.com
Great information on how to safely prepare for you trip abroad including vaccine information, travel advisories, disease risks, and more.

Institute of Medicine and the National Academies Reports
www.iom.edu/reports.asp
A listing of IOM reports, many of which may be ordered and read online.

Jubilee
www.jubileeplus.org/index.htm
An organization devoted to worldwide economic justice, Jubilee also provides news and information on global economic conditions.

Library of Economics and Liberty
www.econlib.org/library/Enc/SavingsandLoanCrisis.html
Contains information on the savings and loan industry in the United States.

Maps.com
www.maps.com
A site providing a huge assortment of domestic and world maps.

Medical College of Wisconsin Healthlink
http://healthlink.mcw.edu/travel-medicine
A good site for new articles related to travel medicine.

Medical Missions
www.medmissions.org
Contains links to current medical missions, mostly through religiously affiliated organizations.

National Academies Press—Article Page
http://books.nap.edu/books/030908265X/html/29.html#pagetop
Feature on the effect of race and ethnicity on health care.

National Center for Health Statistics
www.cdc.gov/nchs/
A great data source about the health of the American public.

National Center for Infectious Diseases Traveler's Health
www.cdc.gov/travel
Provides information about local infectious agents, and recommended vaccines are itemized.

The Nobel Peace Prize
http://nobelprize.org/peace/index.html
Information about the Nobel Peace Prize.

Office of the High Commissioner for Human Rights
www.unhchr.ch/hredu.nsf
Contains information and organizational links on human rights education and advocacy.

Opportunities in Int'l Health (Handbook Published by UNC-CH SOM)
www.med.unc.edu/wrkunits/orgs/ihf/handbook00
Contains information on academic credit, funding, and other resources connected to international health care opportunities.

Organisation for Economic Co-operation and Development
www.oecd.org/home
Provides economic information and statistics on 30 OECD member countries.

Pan American Health Organization
www.paho.org
A regional office of the World Health Organization that provides updated information on health care conditions in the Americas.

Pew Charitable Trusts
www.pewtrusts.org
A non-partisan source for information on public issues and policy decisions.

Practical Nomad
www.practicalnomad.com
A great guide for domestic and international travel.

Program on International Policy Attitudes-Hunger Basics Page
www.pipa.org/OnlineReports/BFW/toc.html
Article exploring the views of Americans on foreign aid and worldwide hunger.

Reality of Aid
www.devinit.org/realityofaid/
Provides an alternative picture of foreign aid.

Rethinking Schools Archive page
www.rethinkingschools.org/archive/17_04/fact174.shtml
A fact sheet about land mines.

Rotary International
www.rotary.org/index.html
A worldwide organization devoted to humanitarian service.

State Department Travel Tips
http://travel.state.gov
A good site for helping to safely plan a trip overseas.

Student National Medical Association
www.snma.org/ihealth/ihealth/index.html
Contains information on how to prepare for an international health mission as well as feedback from health care workers who participated on previous missions, and other resources.

Teaching Human Rights Online
http://homepages.uc.edu/thro/
Offers an online library of human rights case studies.

Thomson Travel Medicine Advisor
www.ahcpub.com/ahc_root_html/products/newsletters/tma.html
Contains updated information on preventing, diagnosing, and treating travel-related diseases.

Travel Clinics Australia
www.travelclinic.com.au
Contains medical advice for international travel such as country-specific immunizations, clinic locations, and more.

Travel Doctor
www.tmvc.com.au
Contains vaccine information, travel advice, and a directory of overseas travel clinics, searchable by city and country.

Travel Health Online
www.tripprep.com
Posts proprietary information for travel medicine clinics; includes detailed information about almost every country, with data about specific health risks and precautions. Fact sheets for each disease and immunization.

Travel Medicine
www.travmed.com
Contains information on what precautions and products travelers need for their overseas trips and a comprehensive product catalog to equip them.

Tufts University Health Sciences Library
www.library.tufts.edu/hsl
A great resource for medical information.

UNAIDS
www.unaids.org/en/default.asp
The major organization concerned with combating HIV and AIDS; site has information about the disease and the global efforts to fight it.

UNESCO
www.unesco.org
The United Nations Educational, Scientific and Cultural Organization strives to disseminate information on each topic and find agreement on emerging ethical issues.

UNICEF—Monitoring the Situation of Children and Women
http://childinfo.org/index2.htm
A statistical database with country-specific information on women and children.

United for a Fair Economy
www.faireconomy.org/
Provides information about how concentrated wealth and power may affect health and social structures.

United Nations
www.un.org/english
The main site for the UN with links to its various organizations.

United Nations Directory of NGOs
www.un.org/dpi/ngosection/asp/form.asp
Good site for checking nongovernmental organization addresses, phone numbers, etc; no descriptions of the organizations.

United Nations High Commissioner for Human Rights
www.ohchr.org/english
Good site on human rights issues.

United Nations Treaty Collection
http://untreaty.un.org
A compilation of UN and international treaties.

United Nations University—World Institute for Development Economics Research
www.wider.unu.edu/publications/dps/dps2002/dp2002-42.pdf
A discussion paper on the effects of international bank lending.

United Press International
www.upi.com/view.cfm?StoryID=05022002-051747-9149r
An article highlighting Omni Med and the author's work in third world nations.

United States National Library of Medicine
www.nlm.nih.gov/
A great resource for medical information.

University of Pittsburgh Supercourse
www.pitt.edu/~super1/index.htm
A great network of over 20,000 faculty members from 151 countries who offer a library of health care and training lectures.

University of Minnesota Human Rights Library
www.1.umn.edu/humanrts/instree/ainstls1.htm
Links to declarations, treaties, and other international human rights instruments.

University of Wisconsin-Milwaukee—Center for International Education
www.uwm.edu/Dept/CIE/Resources/globalization/globalecon.html
A collection of sites containing useful information on the global economy.

US Department of Health and Human Services Indian Health Service
www.ihs.gov/index.asp
An agency devoted to improving the health of American Indians and Alaskan natives, they offer nationwide health care programs and initiatives.

US State Department Human Rights Country Reports
www.state.gov/g/drl/hr/c1470.htm
Searchable reports on human rights for most countries of the world.

World Bank Debt Department
www.worldbank.org/debt
The World Bank's site for information about its current international loan programs and their effects on indebted nations.

World Health Organization
www.who.org
The site to the United Nations' specialized agency for worldwide health.

World Health Organization-Outbreaks
www.who.int/disease-outbreak-news/index.html
Contains up-to-date news on infectious disease outbreaks around the world. Articles contain links to clinically useful fact sheets.

World Health Organization Macroeconomics and Health
www.3.who.int/whosis/menu.cfm?path=whosis,cmh&language=english
A commission that assesses and reports on the relationship between health and the global economy.

World Health Organization's Civil Society Initiative
www.who.int/ina-ngo
Directory of nongovernmental organizations in official relations with the World Health Organization.

Appendix B

About Omni Med

At Omni Med, we believe that *all* people have a right to health and quality health care and that all health professionals, by their very involvement in the profession, share an ethical imperative to make quality health care broadly accessible to all people, regardless of their nationality or income. We work to improve health globally, with a focus on the poor, by following two parallel and synergistic goals: to develop programs cooperatively with host nationals that *they* deem important to improving health for their people and to expand the pool of internationally experienced and engaged US health providers. Specifically, we do the following:

> **Health volunteerism:** Omni Med has programs in several developing countries (Belize, Guyana, and Kenya) that bring health providers with some or no prior international experience to short-term, effective teaching trips, rendering maximal impact for both volunteers and learners. We also publish books on international health service that explore root causes of poverty, review pragmatic steps of health volunteerism, and encourage direct service through our large database of service opportunities.
>
> **Program development:** We encourage our volunteers to develop sustainable, cooperative programs that improve health for the poor. Examples include: a national cervical cancer screening initiative in Guyana; continuing medical education programs in Belize, Guyana, and Kenya; and an eye screening and treatment program in Thailand. Our work is oriented toward social justice, not charity.
>
> **Ethical leadership:** The US medical profession must engage global health disparities far more than it has. Omni Med provides an opportunity for health providers to develop their own leadership skills as part of an overarching, moral vision to improve health for the poor in the countries we serve. Through the transforming experience of direct service in poor countries, many more US health providers will engage the problem directly in an ongoing fashion and, ultimately, exert their influence in the corridors of power in the United States.

For those interested in serving through an Omni Med program, for those who know of an nongovernmental organization or hospital that should become a part of our database, or for those interested in booking Dr O'Neil for a speaking engagement, please visit our Web site (www.omnimed.org) or contact Omni Med directly:

Edward O'Neil, Jr, MD
President, Omni Med
81 Wyman Street, #1
Waban, MA 02468

Phone: 617 332-9614
Fax: 617 332-6623
E-mail: ejoneil@omnimed.org or ejoneil@comcast.net
Web site: www.omnimed.org

Omni Med is a registered 501 (c)(3) under the IRS code and gladly accepts donations to support our work. In 2005, Omni Med was accepted by the Ayuda Federation (www.ayudafederation.org) as a part of the combined federal campaign. Of our funding, 97.9% goes toward programs; 2004 and 2005 audits available upon request.

Glossary

Acute Mountain Sickness (AMS): An illness affecting persons such as mountain climbers, hikers, or other travelers who rapidly ascend to high altitudes. The symptoms are often mild, but severe cases can include pulmonary edema (fluid collection in the lungs causing shortness of breath) or cerebral edema (brain swelling causing disorientation, coma, or even death if untreated). The severity often corresponds to the total altitude, rate of ascent, and level of exertion put forth to reach that altitude.

American Medical Student Association (AMSA): A student-governed independent national association of physicians-in-training in the United States. AMSA strives to represent the interests of current medical students and pre-medical student members.

American Society of Tropical Medicine and Traveler's Health (ASTMH): An American organization embodying scientists, physicians, and others interested in the prevention and control of tropical diseases. ASTMH seeks to promote world health by combating current and emerging tropical diseases through research and education.

ASAPROSAR: *See* Salvadoran Rural Health Association.

Cable News Network (CNN): A cable television network founded in 1980 and widely credited for the birth of 24-hour news coverage.

Centers for Disease Control (CDC): An agency of the Department of Health and Human Services and is designed to safeguard the American people's public health and safety. The CDC works toward providing credible information about current and emerging diseases in order to enhance health decisions. The CDC works with federal agencies, state health departments, and other organizations to prevent and control diseases and educate the public about infectious diseases, environmental health, and general health promotion. The CDC is headquartered in Atlanta, Georgia.

Deep Venous Thrombosis (DVT): A clot that obstructs blood flow in the veins and usually takes place in the lower extremities (legs). The clots can occasionally migrate to the lungs, causing a PE (pulmonary embolism). DVT most often afflicts certain high-risk groups, like those immediately after surgery, on birth control pills, obese, with a recent history of cancer, or with clotting disorders. DVTs and PEs have occurred on long-distance flights, mostly in high-risk people.

DEET: *See* N-diethyl-3-methyl-benzamide (N,N-dimethyl-m-toluamide).

European Union (EU): A union of 25 independent states drawn from the European Community, founded to enhance political, economic, and social co-operation between members. The 1993 treaty establishing the European Union expanded the political scope of foreign and security policy, and created a central European bank, which adopted the euro as a common currency at the end of the 20th century.

Food and Drug Administration (FDA): A federal agency responsible for regulating the production, use, and safety of food, dietary supplements, drugs, cosmetics, medical devices, and related products. The FDA is a branch agency of the Department of Health and Human Services.

High Altitude Cerebral Edema (HACE): A life-threatening form of altitude sickness resulting in swelling brain tissue from fluid leakage. HACE can occur after extended periods of time at high altitudes with severe effects. Symptoms include headaches, seizures, reduced motor functions, disorientation, hallucinations, and even coma. Persons suffering from HACE must quickly descend and receive treatment to avoid death.

High Altitude Pulmonary Edema (HAPE): A life-threatening condition afflicting a small percentage of people suffering from Acute Mountain Sickness. HAPE causes pulmonary blood vessels to leak fluid into the lung tissue. The victim experiences increasing shortness of breath as the fluid builds up in the lungs (pulmonary edema). Almost anyone can experience HAPE regardless of their individual fitness level.

Hospital Albert Schweitzer (HAS): An integrated rural health system providing health care and community development programs for impoverished people in central Haiti. HAS teams visiting health care professionals with a permanent Haitian staff of almost 900 people to serve the poor. Partnering organizations and private donors worldwide combine to support the work of HAS.

Human Immunodeficiency Virus (HIV): A retrovirus that attacks the human immune system and compromises the ability to fight off infections such as pneumonia, diarrhea, tumors, and other illnesses. HIV is the virus which eventually causes AIDS.

International Health Medical Education Consortium (IHMEC): An association of faculty and educators dedicated to promoting international health education in US and Canadian medical schools and residency programs. IHMEC focuses its efforts on curriculum, clinical training, career development, and international education policy.

Low Molecular Weight Heparin (LMWH): A class of the heparin anticoagulants used therapeutically to prevent or reduce blood from clotting. LMWH has a lower mean molecular weight than standard heparin and is used to treat diseases featuring thrombosis, or as a prophylactic measure for situations with a high risk of thrombosis.

Multidrug-Resistant Tuberculosis (MDR-TB): A form of tuberculosis with resistance to two or more of the primary drugs used to treatment TB. Resistance can occur after the bacteria are exposed to an antibiotic and develop an ability to withstand the drug (often as a result of inadequate treatment or improper use of the drugs). Resistance to several first-line drugs is now widespread.

N-diethyl-3-methyl-benzamide (N,N-dimethyl-m-toluamide) (DEET): A powerful insect repellent intended for application to the skin and clothing. DEET has caused neurologic and allergic complications in a small number of users, mostly children, but has been declared one of the safest and most effective insect repellents available. DEET is particularly effective against malaria and lyme disease transmission from mosquitoes and ticks.

Non-Governmental Organization (NGO): A civic organization maintaining its own funding and independence from any central, local, or municipal government. The term “NGO” is generally restricted to social and cultural groups with non-commercial goals.

Oral Rehydration Solution (ORS): A solution containing salt and a form of sugar (preferably glucose) made to prevent dehydration in children suffering from diarrhea. ORS has become widely available and is hailed as one of the most important medical discoveries of the twentieth century. The UN claimed in 1997 that ORS saves 1 million lives annually.

Peace Corps Volunteer (PCV): A volunteer from the Peace Corps, a federal government agency that trains and sends American volunteers to developing countries to work on projects of technological, agricultural, and educational improvement, usually for two-year terms. The Peace Corps was initiated by President Kennedy’s executive order in 1961, and has been an independent agency since 1981. Peace Corps volunteers are preferentially hired by some federal agencies, like US AID.

Pulmonary Embolism (PE): A blood clot in the pulmonary artery of the lungs resulting in sudden shortness of breath, chest pains, and rapid heart and respiratory rates. The clots normally form from a deep vein thrombosis (clot in a vein in the legs) that has broken free and traveled in the bloodstream to the lungs. The condition can be fatal.

Salvadoran Rural Health Association (ASAPROSAR): An organization committed to empowering the poor sector of El Salvador. ASAPROSAR trains community leaders in the areas of health, nutrition, family planning, the environment, and sustainable agriculture. ASAPROSAR also offers small loans to local female entrepreneurs and helps provide eye care to the poor.

Severe Acute Respiratory Syndrome (SARS): A respiratory disease caused by a previously unknown type of coronavirus and first documented in mainland China in 2003 and characterized by fever, coughing, and difficulty breathing. SARS is transmitted by close contact with infected persons and can be life-threatening.

Traveler's Diarrhea (TD): An illness common to travelers in which ingestion of bacteria like *E coli, Campylobactyer, Salmonella, Shigella,* or certain viruses or parasites causes diarrhea, often self-limited over a few days. More severe cases involve fever, abdominal pain, vomiting, or bloody diarrhea (dysentery). Most cases are self-limited but may respond to antibiotics like Cipro. Prevention of TD is best accomplished by drinking only water that is bottled, boiled, or first passed through a purifier, and by steering clear of peeled fruits, or any food washed in non-purified water.

United Nations (UN): An international organization founded in 1945 that includes most of the sovereign nations of the world. The UN coordinates international cooperation in promoting global peace, security, and economic development and acts through its members to respond to social, political, or humanitarian crises.

United Nations Children's Fund (*formerly United Nations International Children's Emergency Fund*) (UNICEF): A United Nations organization that provides long-term humanitarian and developmental assistance to needy children and mothers worldwide. Established in 1946, UNICEF delivers food, clothing, shelter, and other assistance to wherever extreme hardships exist.

World Health Organization (WHO): An organization run by the United Nations and committed to improving worldwide public health. The WHO helps countries strengthen their health services, provides technical aid in health emergencies, promotes disease control, and helps establish food and medical safety standards. The WHO has over 190 member countries.

Bibliography

Abelson, R. 1999. Report Outlines Problems with Donated Drugs Sent Overseas. *The New York Times.* August 16.

Adachi, J.A. et al. 2000. Empirical Antimicrobial Therapy for Traveler's Diarrhea. *Clinical Infectious Diseases.* 31(4):1079–1083.

"A Great Time to Work." 1999. *The Economist.* July 22.

American College of Physicians. 1995. Single-Dose Ciprofloxacin Stemmed Traveler's Diarrhea. *ACP Journal Club.* 122(1):43–44.

American Medical Student Association. 2004. Creative Funding for International Health Electives. Available online at www.amsa.org/resource/amsarc/creative/creative.cfm.

Ansell, J.E. 2001. Air travel and Venous Thromboembolism—Is the Evidence in? *New England Journal of Medicine.* 345(11):828–829.

Arendt, J. 2000. Melatonin, Circadian Rhythms, and Sleep. *New England Journal of Medicine.* 343(15):1114–1116.

ASAPROSAR. 2005. The ASAPROSAR Development Fund. Available online at www.thegreenresource.com/asaprosar.

Baker, T. and Quinley, J. 1987. A U.S. International Health Service Corps, Options, and Constraints. *JAMA.* 257(19):2622–2625.

Baker, T. et al. 1984. US Physicians in International Health: Report of a Current Survey. *JAMA.* 251(4):502–504.

Becker, E. 2003. Western Farmers Fear Third-World Challenge to Subsidies. *The New York Times.* September 9.

Behrens, R.H. et al. 1994. Travel Medicine: Before Departure. *Medical Journal of Australia.* 160:143–147.

Behrman, G. 2004. *Invisible People.* New York, NY: Free Press.

Belcaro, G. et al. 2003. Prevention of Venous Thrombosis with Elastic Stockings During Long-Haul Flights: The LONFLIT 5 JAP Study. *Clinical and Applied Thrombosis/Hemostasis.* 9(3):197–201.

———. 2002. Prevention of Edema, Flight Microangiopathy, and Venous Thrombosis in Long Flights with Elastic Stockings, a Randomized Trial: The LONFLIT4 Concorde-SSL Study. *Angiology.* 53(6):635–645.

———. 2001. Venous Thromboembolism from Air Travel: the LONFLIT Study. *Angiology.* 52(6):369–374.

Bellingham, C. 2001. News Feature: Giving Advice on Traveler's Thrombosis. *The Pharmaceutical Journal.* 266(7132):116–117.

Bent, S. et al. 1999. Antibiotics in Acute Bronchitis: A Meta-Analysis. *American Journal of Medicine.* 107(1):62–67.

Bernard, K.W. et al. 1989. Epidemiological Surveillance in Peace Corps Volunteers: A Model for Monitoring Health in Temporary Residents in Developing Countries. *International Journal of Epidemiology.* 18(1):220–226.

Bloor, M. et al. 1998. Differences in Sexual Risk Behavior Between Young Men and Women Traveling Abroad from the UK. *Lancet.* 353(9141):1664–1668.

Brown, R. 1990. *Gustavo Gutierrez: An Introduction to Liberation Theology.* Maryknoll, NY: Orbis Books.

Budd, W. 1931. *Typhoid Fever, Its Nature, Mode of Spreading, and Prevention.* New York, NY: Arno Press.

Busch, M. et al. 1995. Time course Detection of Viral and Serologic Markers Preceding Human Immunodeficiency Virus Type I Seroconversion: Implications for Screening of Blood and Tissue Donors. *Transfusion.* 35(2):91–97.

Cardo, D.M. et al. 1997. A Case-control Study of HIV Seroconversion in Health Care Workers After Percutaneous Exposure. *New England Journal of Medicine.* 337(21):1485–1490.

Carnethon, M.R. et al. 2003. Cardiorespiratory Fitness in Young Adulthood and the Development of Cardiovascular Disease Risk Factors. *Journal of the American Medical Association.* 290(23):3092–3100.

Center for Defense Information (CDI). 2002. *2002 CDI Military Almanac.* Washington, DC: Center for Defense Information.

Centers for Disease Control and Prevention (CDC). 2002. Life Expectancy. Available online at www.cdc.gov/nchs/fastats/lifexpec.htm.

———. 2001a. Exposure to Patients with Meningococcal Disease on Aircrafts—United States, 1999–2001. *Morbidity and Mortality Weekly Report.* 50(23):485–489.

———. 2001b. Malaria Deaths Following Inappropriate Malaria Chemoprophylaxis—United States, 2001. *Morbidity and Mortality Weekly Report.* 50(28):597–599.

———. 1999. Achievements in Public Health: Decline in Deaths from Heart Disease and Stroke—United States, 1900–1999. *Morbidity and Mortality Weekly Report.* 48(30):649–656.

———. 1993. Schistosomiasis in US Peace Corps Volunteers: Malawi, 1992. *Morbidity and Mortality Weekly Report.* 42(29):565–570.

Cesarone, M.R. et al. 2002. Venous Thrombosis from Air Travel: Prevention with Aspirin vs Low-Molecular-Weight Heparin (LMWH) in High-Risk Subjects. *Angiology.* 53(1):1–6.

Cloud, S. 1996. The Opportunities and Challenges of a More Diverse American Society as We Enter a New Century. Speech presented at the Lahey Clinic North Shore; Peabody, Mass.

Cohen, J. 2000. *The Traveler's Pocket Medical Guide and International Certificate of Vaccination.* Self-published.

Congressional Research Service. 2004. Foreign Aid: An Introductory Overview of US Programs and Policy. April 15. Available online at www.crs.gov.

Corbin, M. and Pemberton, M. 2004. A Unified Security Budget for the United States. Foreign Policy in Focus and Center for Defense Information, March. Available online at www.cdi.org.

Covey, S.R. et al. 1994. *First Things First: To Live, to Love, to Learn, to Leave a Legacy.* New York, NY: Simon and Schuster.

Dalen, J.E. 2003. Economy Class Syndrome, Too Much Flying or Too Much Sitting? *Archives of Internal Medicine.* 163(22):2674–2676.

Daniel, D. 2002. Packing with a Light Touch. *The Boston Globe.* April 28.

De Bruyn, G. et al. 2002. Antibiotic Treatment for Travelers' Diarrhea. *The Cochrane Database of Systematic Reviews.* Oxford, England.

Diamond, J. 1999. *Guns, Germs, and Steel.* New York, NY: W.W. Norton & Co.

Dominguez, J. and Robin, V. 1992. *Your Money or Your Life.* New York, NY: Penguin Books.
Driver, C.R. et al. 1994. Transmission of Mycobacterium tuberculosis Associated with Air Travel. *Journal of the American Medical Association.* 272(13):1031–1035.
"Drugs for Parasitic Infections." 2002. *The Medical Letter.* Available online at www.medletter.com.
Eaton, J. and Etue, K. 2002. *The aWAKE Project, Uniting Against the African AIDS Crisis.* Nashville, Tenn: W. Publishing Group.
Epstein, D. 1999. Malaria: Failure, Puzzle, and Challenge. *Perspectives in Health: Magazine of the Pan American Health Organization.* 4(1):2–7.
Fahey, T. et al. 1998. Quantitative Systematic Review of Randomized Controlled Trials Comparing Antibiotic With Placebo for Acute Cough in Adults. *British Medical Journal.* 316(7135):906–910.
Farmer, P. 2001. The Major Infectious Diseases in the World—To Treat of Not to Treat? *New England Journal of Medicine.* 345(3):208–210.
———. 1999. *Infections and Inequalities: The Modern Plagues.* Berkeley, Calif: University of California Press.
———. 1994. *The Uses of Haiti.* Monroe, Maine: Common Courage Press.
Ferrari, E. et al. 1999. Travel as a Risk Factor for Venous Thrombosis Disease: A Case Study. *Chest.* 115(2):440–444.
Fisher, J.T. 1997. *Dr. America the Lives of Thomas A. Dooley, 1927–1961.* Amherst, Mass: University of Massachusetts Press.
Fradin, M.S. 1998. Mosquitoes and Mosquito Repellents: A Clinician's Guide. *Annals of Internal Medicine.* 128(11):931–940.
Fradin, M.S. and Day, J.F. 2002. Comparative Efficacy of Insect Repellents Against Mosquito Bites. *New England Journal of Medicine.* 347(1):1–18.
Freire, P. 1970. *A Pedagogy of the Oppressed.* New York, NY: Continuum Publishing.
Garrett, L. 2003. Local Transmission of Plasmodium Vivax Malaria—Palm Beach County, Florida. *Journal of the American Medical Association.* 290(22): 2931–2934.
———. 1994. *The Coming Plague.* New York, NY: Penguin Books.
Gawande, A. 2002. Dispatch from India. *New England Journal of Medicine.* 349(25):2383–2386.
Gendreau, M.A. and DeJohn, C. 2002. Responding to Medical Events During Commercial Airline Flights. *New England Journal of Medicine.* 346(14):1067–1073.
Gerberding, J.L. 2003. Occupational Exposure to HIV in Health Care Settings. *New England Journal of Medicine.* 348(9):826–833.
Gilbert, S. 2004. Long Flights and Thrombosis. *The New York Times.* February 29.
Glendon, M.A. 2001. *A World Made New: Eleanor Roosevelt and the Universal Declaration of Human Rights.* New York, NY: Random House.
Gonzales, R., and Sande, M.A. 2000. Uncomplicated Acute Bronchitis. *Annals of Internal Medicine.* 133(12):981–991.
Goodwin, D.K. 1994. *No Ordinary Time.* New York, NY: Simon and Schuster.
Green, H. 2003. Doctors Abroad. *Harvard Magazine.* January–February.
Guerrant, R.L. et al. 2001. Practice Guidelines for the Management of Infectious Diarrhea, Infectious Disease Society of America (IDSA) Guidelines. *Clinical Infectious Diseases.* 32(3):331–350.
Hackett, P.H. and Roach, R.C. 2001. High-Altitude Illness. *New England Journal of Medicine.* 345(2):107–114.
Hancock, G. 1989. *Lords of Poverty.* New York, NY: Atlantic Monthly Press.
Hargarten, S.W. 1991. Epidemiology of Travel-Related Deaths. In: Jong E.D. (ed). *Travel Medicine Advisor.* Atlanta, Ga.: American Health Consultants.

Hargarten, S.W. and Baker, S.P. 1991. Overseas Fatalities of United States Citizen Travelers: An Analysis of Deaths Related to International Travel. *Annals of Emergency Medicine.* 20(6):622–626.

———. 1985. Fatalities in the Peace Corps. A Retrospective Study: 1962 Through 1983. *Journal of the American Medical Association.* 254(10):1326–1329.

Hasbrouck, E. 2000. *The Practical Nomad: How to Travel Around the World.* 2nd ed. Emeryville, Calif: Avalon Travel Publishing.

Hitchens, C. 1997. *The Missionary Position.* New York, NY: Verso Press.

Hogerzeil, H.V. et al. 1997. Guidelines for Drug Donations. *British Medical Journal.* 314(7082):737–740.

"How to Make Aid Work." 1999. *The Economist.* June 24.

Isayev, Y. et al. 2002. Economy Class' Syndrome? *Neurology.* 58(6):960–961.

Jehil, D. 1997. Cairo Reports 6 Militants Died in Fighting. *The New York Times.* November 18.

Johnson, P.W. 2005. RFK: What We Lost. *The Boston Globe.* November 20.

Johnston, R. 2000. Clinical Aviation Medicine: Safe Travel by Air. *Clinical Medicine.* 1(5):385–388.

Kain, K.C. and Keystone, J.S. 1998. Malaria in Travelers, Epidemiology, Disease, and Prevention. *Infectious Disease Clinics of North America.* 12(2):267–283.

Kenyon, T.A. et al. 1996. Transmission of Multidrug-Resistant Mycobacterium Tuberculosis During a Long Airplane Flight. *New England Journal of Medicine.* 334(15):933–938.

Keystone, J.S. 2003. Malaria Prevention. *ASTMH Intensive Update Course in Clinical Tropical Medicine and Traveler's Health.* San Diego, Calif: October 7–8.

Kidder, T. 2002. *Mountains Beyond Mountains: The Quest of Dr. Paul Farmer, a Man Who Would Cure the World.* New York, NY: Random House.

Kim, J.Y. et al. 2000. *Dying for Growth.* Monroe, Maine: Common Courage Press.

Kindig, D.A. et al. 1984. Share Our Doctors Abroad. *The New Physician.* September.

King, C.H. 2002. Book Reviews: *Traveler's Malaria* (Schlagenhauf-Lawlor, P., ed). *New England Journal of Medicine.* 346(16):1256–1257.

Kohls, R. 1996. *Survival Kit for Overseas Living: For Americans Planning to Live and Work Abroad.* 3rd ed. Yarmouth, Maine: Intercultural Press.

Kozarsky, P.E. 1998. Prevention of Common Travel Ailments. *Infectious Disease Clinics of North America.* 12(2):305–323.

Kristoff, N.D. 2004. 117 Deaths Each Day. *The New York Times.* March 13.

Lapostolle, F. et al. 2001. Severe Pulmonary Embolism Associated with Air Travel. *New England Journal of Medicine.* 345(11):779–783.

Leggat, P.A. 2001. Book Reviews: *The Traveler's Pocket Guide and International Certificate of Vaccination* (Cohen, J.). *New England Journal of Medicine.* 285(12):1642–1643.

Mahon, F. 1998. The Legacy of a Legend. *Notre Dame Magazine.* Spring 27(1).

Magill, A.J. 1998. Fever in the Returned Traveler. *Infectious Disease Clinics of North America.* 12(2):445–469.

Martinson F.E. et al. 1996. Seroepidemiological Survey of Hepatitis B and C Virus Infections in Ghanian Children. *Journal of Medical Virology.* 8(3):278–283.

McNeil, D.G. 1999. The Dicey Game of Travel Risk. *The New York Times.* March 7.

Merriam-Webster. 1991. *Webster's New World Dictionary, Third College Edition.* New York, NY: Prentice Hall.

Metlay, J.P. et al. 1997. Does This Patient Have Community-Acquired Pneumonia? Diagnosing Pneumonia by History and Physical Examination. *JAMA.* 278:1440–1445.

Moore, J. et al. 1995. HIV Risk Behavior Among Peace Corps Volunteers. *AIDS.* 9(7):795–799.

Mungai, M. et al. 2000. Transfusion-Transmitted Malaria in the United States from 1963 Through 1999. *New England Journal of Medicine.* 344(26):1973–1978.
Newman, R.D. et al. 1999. Malaria Surveillance—United States, 1999. *Morbidity and Mortality Weekly Report.* 51(SS-1):15–28.
National Transportation Safety Board (NTSB). 1998. We are all Safer, NTSB-Inspired Improvements in Transportation Safety. Available online at www.ntsb.gov/publictn/1998/SR9801.pdf.
Nickerson, C. 1997. Relief Workers Shoulder a World of Conflict: Aid Agencies Encounter Growing Dangers as Nations Withhold Peacekeeping Troops. *The Boston Globe.* July 27.
Olsen, S.J. et al. 2003. Transmission of the Severe Acute Respiratory Syndrome on Aircraft. *New England Journal of Medicine.* 349(25):2416–2422.
Organization for Economic Co-operation and Development (OECD). 2004. *The Development Assistance Committee Journal of Development Co-Operation 2003 Report (Volume 5, No.1).* Development Assistance Committee of the Organization for Economic Co-operation and Development. Paris, France: OECD Publications.
Overbosch, D. et al. 2001. Atovaquone-Proguanil versus Mefloquine for Malaria Prophylaxis in Nonimmune Travelers: Results from a Randomized, Double-Blind Study. *Clinical Infectious Diseases.* 33(7):1015–1021.
Oxfam. 2002. Rigged Rules and Double Standards: Trade, Globalization and the Fight Against Poverty. *Oxfam/Make Trade Fair.* Available online at www.oxfamamerica.org/pdfs/rigged_rules_report_summary.pdf.
Pérez-Rodriguez, E. et al. 2003. Incidence of Air Travel-Related Pulmonary Embolism at the Madrid-Barajas Airport. *Archives of Internal Medicine.* 163(22):2766–2770.
Perry, K. 2000. Blood Clot Kills Woman after Flight. *The Guardian.* October 23.
Ramzan, N.N. 2001. Traveler's Diarrhea. *Gastroenterology Clinics of North America.* 30(3):665–678.
Ryan E.T. and Kain, K.C. 2000. Health Advice and Immunizations for Travelers. *New England Journal of Medicine.* 342(23):1716–1725.
Sachs, J. 2005. *The End of Poverty: Economic Possibilities For Our Time.* New York, NY: The Penguin Press.
———. 2002. Realizing the Vision: The Global Fund to Fight AIDS, Tuberculosis, and Malaria. A one-day conference held by the United Nations Association of Greater Boston at the American Academy of Arts and Sciences in Cambridge, Mass; May 2.
———. 2001a. The Strategic Significance of Global Inequality. *Washington Quarterly.* Summer.
———. 2001b. *Macroeconomics and Health: Investing in Health for Economic Development, Report of the Commission on Macroeconomics and Health.* Geneva, Switzerland: World Health Organization.
Sagoe-Moses, C. et al. 2001. Risks to Health Care Workers in Developing Countries. *New England Journal of Medicine.* 345(7):538–541.
Schweitzer, A. 1949. *Out of My Life and Thought: An Autobiography.* New York, NY: Henry Holt and Co.
———. 1933. *Out of My Life and Thought: An Autobiography.* Baltimore, Md: Johns Hopkins University Press.
Scurr, J.H. et al. 2001. Frequency and Prevention of Symptomless Deep-Vein Thrombosis in Long-Haul Flights: A Randomized Trial. *The Lancet.* 357(9267):1485–1489.
Sen, A. 1999. *Development as Freedom.* New York, NY: Random House.
———. 1993. The Economics of Life and Death. *Scientific American.* March:40–47.
Sennott, C.M. 1997. Egypt Tourist Attack Leaves 71 Dead. *The Boston Globe.* November 18.
Stinson, K. 1940. Shelter Deaths from Pulmonary Embolism. *The Lancet.* 11:744.

Steffen, R. et al. 1999. Epidemiology, Etiology, and Impact of Traveler's Diarrhea in Jamaica. *Journal of the American Medical Association.* 281(9):811–817.

Strickland, G.T. 2000. Treatment and Control of Malaria. In: Strickland G.T. (ed). *Hunter's Tropical Medicine.* 8th ed. Philadelphia, Pa: W.B. Saunders.

Sutton, M. 1994. *Bear in Mind These Dead: An Index of Deaths from the Conflict in Ireland 1969–1993.* Belfast, Ireland: Beyond the Pale Publications.

Symington, I.S. and Stack, B.H.R. 1977. Pulmonary Thromboembolism After Travel. *British Journal of Diseases of the Chest.* 71(2):138–140.

"The Cost of AIDS: An Imprecise Catastrophe." 2004. *The Economist.* May 20.

UNAIDS. 2004. UNAIDS web site. Available online at www.unaids.org/EN/Resources/Epidemiology/EPI_Search.asp.

United Nations Development Program (UNDP). 2005. *Human Development Report, 2005.* New York, NY: Oxford University Press.

———. 2002. *Human Development Report, 2002.* New York, NY: Oxford University Press.

———. 1997. *Human Development Report, 1997.* New York, NY: Oxford University Press.

———. 1995. *Human Development Report, 1995.* New York, NY: Oxford University Press.

US Agency for International Development (USAID). 2002. *Foreign Aid in the National Interest, Promoting Freedom, Security and Opportunity.* Washington, DC: USAID.

US Congress. 1987. House of Representatives. H.R. 3669, A Bill to Amend the Public Health Service Act to Establish an International Health Corps. 100th Congress, 1st session.

US Department of Justice. 2002. Summary of Forum Held on March 1, 2002: Police-Probation Teams Address Juvenile Violence in Boston Through Operation Night Light. Available online at www.ojp.usdoj.gov/eows/forumcj3.htm.

US Peace Corps. 2002. The 2002 Annual Report of Volunteer Safety. Available online at www.peacecorps.gov/policies/pdf/volsafety2002.pdf.

Verespej, M. 1999. Work vs Life vs The World. *Industryweek.com.* April 19. Available online at www.industryweek.com/CurrentArticles/asp/articles.asp?ArticleID=521.

Vidal, J. 2004. Tuberculosis. Available online at www.who.int/tb/en.

———. 2003. Farmer Commits Suicide at Protests. *The Guardian.* September 11.

Virk, A. 2001. Medical advice for international travelers. *Mayo Clinic Proceedings.* 76(8):831–840.

Weiss, E. 2003. Altitude, Diving, and Fish. American Society of Tropical Medicine and Hygiene's "Intensive Update Course in Clinical Tropical Medicine and Traveler's Health," San Diego, Calif: October 7–8.

Wenzel, R.P. 1996. Airline travel and infection. *New England Journal of Medicine.* 334(15):981–982.

Werner, D. and Sanders, D. 1997. *Questioning the Solution: The Politics of Primary Health Care and Child Survival, With an In-Depth Critique of Oral Rehydration Therapy.* Palo Alto, Calif: Healthrights Press.

Wong, E. 2003. Lawsuits Cast Attention on Passenger Blood Clots on Long Flights. *The New York Times.* December 2.

World Health Organization (WHO). 2002. *World Report on Violence and Health.* Geneva, Switzerland: WHO Press. Also available online at www.who.int/violence_injury_prevention/violence/world_report/en/full_en.pdf.

———. 2001. WRIGHT Project: DVT and air travel. Available online at www.who.int/cardiovascular_diseases/wright_project/en.

———. 1999. Guidelines for Drug Donations, Revised 1999. Available online at www.who.int/en.

Zitter, J.N. et al. 2002. Aircraft Cabin Air Recirculation and Symptoms of the Common Cold. *Journal of the American Medical Association.* 288(4):483–486.

About the Author

Edward O'Neil Jr, MD, is a practicing emergency physician at Caritas St Elizabeth's Medical Center in Boston and an assistant professor of emergency medicine at Tufts University School of Medicine. Dr O'Neil is an alumnus of the W.K. Kellogg National Leadership Program and is the founder and president of Omni Med (www.omnimed.org), a nongovernmental organization founded in 1998 that runs innovative, cooperatively designed programs emphasizing health volunteerism and ethical leadership in Belize, Kenya, Thailand, and Guyana. Since its inception, volunteer health providers have made over 100 trips abroad—mostly educational—through its various programs. Omni Med was founded on the philosophy that *all* people have a right to health and quality health care, and that all health professionals, by their very involvement in the profession, share an ethical imperative to make quality health care broadly accessible to all people, regardless of their nationality or income. For a number of years prior to and during medical training, Dr O'Neil played piano professionally in Washington, DC, and Boston, as well as during travels through the United States, Europe, Asia, and Africa. He and his wife, Judy, live in Newton, Mass, with their three children, James, Michaela, and Sean.